Aging, Heart Disease, and Its Management

CONTEMPORARY CARDIOLOGY

CHRISTOPHER P. CANNON, MD
SERIES EDITOR

AGING, HEART DISEASE, AND ITS MANAGEMENT

Facts and Controversies

Edited by

NILOO M. EDWARDS, MD
Columbia University, New York, NY

MATHEW S. MAURER, MD
Columbia University, New York, NY

RACHEL B. WELLNER, MPH
University of Connecticut School of Medicine, Farmington, CT

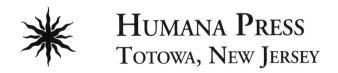

HUMANA PRESS
TOTOWA, NEW JERSEY

© 2003 Humana Press Inc.
999 Riverview Drive, Suite 208
Totowa, New Jersey 07512

www.humanapress.com

Production Editor: Jessica Jannicelli.
Cover design by Patricia F. Cleary.

For additional copies, pricing for bulk purchases, and/or information about other Humana titles, contact Humana at the above address or at any of the following numbers: Tel.: 973-256-1699; Fax: 973-256-8341, E-mail: humana@humanapr.com; or visit our Website: http://humanapr.com

This publication is printed on acid-free paper. ∞
ANSI Z39.48-1984 (American National Standards Institute) Permanence of Paper for Printed Library Materials.

Printed in the United States of America.   10 9 8 7 6 5 4 3 2 1

Library of Congress Cataloging-in-Publication Data

Aging, heart disease, and its management : facts and controversies / edited by Niloo M.
Edwards, Mathew S. Maurer, Rachel B. Wellner.
    p. ; cm. -- (Contemporary cardiology)
  Includes bibliographical references and index.
  ISBN 1-58829-056-5 (alk. paper)
   1. Cardiovascular diseases in old age. I. Edwards, Niloo M. II. Maurer, Mathew S. III.
  Wellner, Rachel B. IV. Contemporary cardiology (Totowa, N.J. : unnumbered)
   [DNLM: 1. Aging--physiology. 2. Heart Diseases--therapy--Aged. WG 210 A267 2003]
   RC669.7 .A36 2003
   618.97'61--dc21
                                                                              2002027387

Preface

The past century heralded a significant shift in the age composition of the world's population. Both as a nation and a world community, we are aging. Currently, older Americans (age 65 years and over) constitute approximately 13% of the population and this group is its fastest growing segment. As the "Baby Boom" generation ages, the role of the gerontologist and other practitioners caring for the elderly will become increasingly important. The demand for clinicians to become proficient in elder care is great. Issues unique to the elderly span the gamut, from the medical challenges they must meet to the vast life experience they contribute to society, their loved ones, and their caregivers. Older adults, often having "weathered many storms," merit the highest level of deference and care in the clinical setting. The challenge for caregivers is to consistently show respect and caring for their elderly patients while dealing with complex clinical, technical, economic, social, and ethical issues. Perhaps what is most alarming is that despite the vast number of older individuals with cardiovascular disease and the complexity involved in providing their care, providers often do so in the absence of any data to guide their treatment strategies. Indeed, a review of all clinical research articles in four premier medical journals determined that less than 50% had enough elderly participants to enable any conclusions to be drawn from these studies concerning older patients themselves (1). With this in mind, we have collaborated with experts in various clinical fields to bring you this textbook. The primary purpose of *Aging, Heart Disease, and Its Management: Facts and Controversies* is to highlight what is presently known and not known in the arena of cardiovascular medicine and cardiac surgery as it pertains to the elderly patient.

The text is organized into four sections, which are described in greater detail below. Section I delineates the epidemiologic and demographic imperative that we face in caring for the rising tide of elderly individuals with cardiovascular disease and specifically highlights health care policy issues that arise. Section II provides the practitioner with several chapters covering fundamental concerns outside of the cardiovascular domain that are essential in providing care for the elderly subject, including nutritional, neurological, pharmacologic, psychiatric, ethical, and rehabilitative issues. Section III, after delineating age-related changes in cardiovascular structure and function as well as the role for risk factor modification, goes on to highlight cardiovascular syndromes that disproportionately afflict the older individual including arrhythmias (particularly atrial fibrillation), syncope, heart failure (particularly diastolic heart failure), and ischemic heart disease. Finally, in Section IV, the surgical management of the elderly cardiac patient is delineated including postoperative management and complications as well as specific surgical procedures such as coronary artery bypass grafting, valve surgery, pacemaker, and defibrillators as well as surgical management of heart failure.

PRINCIPLES OF AGING

Aging is an inevitable process common to all species. The physiologic changes that accompany aging form a natural part of the maturation process. As the numbers of elderly individuals continue to rise at staggering rates, continued study of biological, clinical, sociological, ethical, and economic factors is essential to accommodate our elders and improve our systems of care for them and the ensuing generations.

Several important principles of geriatrics have been delineated and are an essential backdrop for this text. First, as individuals age they become more dissimilar. Thus, attributing age-related changes to a particular patient's clinical syndrome should be accompanied by a healthy amount of skepticism. Second, an abrupt decline in any system or function is always caused by disease and not by "normal aging." Though many providers and even patients will attribute their symptoms or conditions to "getting old," a practitioner well versed in the principles of geriatric medicine will often find a precipitating pathophysiologic condition. Third, "normal" aging can be attenuated by modification of risk factors. Thus, many of the proposals for a healthy lifestyle, such as exercise, a well-balanced diet, and avoidance of tobacco products, are equally important in attenuating the ill effects of aging. Finally, "healthy old age" is not an oxymoron. It is quite possible for people to live healthy, active, productive lives well into their eighties and nineties.

BASIC TENETS OF GERIATRIC MEDICINE

The basic tenets of geriatric medicine that have been described to reflect the fundamentals of geriatric care offer the clinician both a set of "cardinal" rules and a practical guideline for the management of elderly patients. In the reading of various chapters, we encourage the reader to keep these principles in mind.

Tenets of Geriatric Medicine

• The onset of new disease in the elderly generally affects an organ system made vulnerable by physiologic and pathologic changes.

• Because of an impaired physiologic reserve, older patients often present at an earlier stage of their disease.

• Since many homeostatic mechanisms may be compromised concurrently, there are usually multiple abnormalities amenable to treatment, and small improvements in each may yield dramatic benefits overall.

• Many findings that are abnormal in younger patients are relatively common in older patients. They may not be responsible for a particular symptom but only be incidental findings that result in misdiagnosis or misdirected therapy.

• Since symptoms in older people are often due to multiple causes, the diagnostic "law of parsimony" often does not apply.

• Because the older patient is more likely to suffer the adverse consequences of disease, treatment (and even prevention) may be equally or more effective than in younger patients.

REVIEW OF HUMAN AGING

From a physiologic standpoint, aging can be described as the progressive decline in homeostatic reserve (homeostenosis) of every organ system. As humans age a number of physiologic changes occur that are related to senescence and many of the aging theories. Essentially, each and every organ system becomes modified to some degree, though the aging process is selective. Generally speaking, these modifications occur in the negative direction, reflecting loss of organ reserve capacity. Notably, there is considerable overlap between physiologic changes and pathophysiologic processes. Often, one or more organ systems will fail secondary to some pathophysiologic mechanism, and the remaining healthy yet senescent components of the body may respond inadequately to other insults. In this sense the organs' interdependence upon one another is truly illustrative.

The aging human organism undergoes a series of general and organ-specific changes. The overall body composition changes, manifest by a loss of lean body mass and a decrease in total body water. Body fat is subsequently redistributed. Various organs are also affected. The cardiovascular system experiences vascular calcification and increased stiffness, as well as reduced vessel compliance. Pulmonary changes include a decrease in vital capacity, chest wall strength, and forced expiratory volume per one second (FEV1), resulting clinically in an increased work of breathing, diminished pulmonary reserve, decreased effective cough needed to clear secretions and microbes, and overall chronic obstruction. In the aged kidney, total nephron mass is decreased, renal blood flow is slowed, creatinine clearance is diminished, and the ability to concentrate urine is decreased. Clinically, elderly individuals are prone to dehydration and experience reduced clearance rates of drugs and drug metabolites. This latter feature is partially responsible for the sensitivity of this subpopulation to drug therapy. There are high rates of drug interaction and increased likelihood of toxicity and organ damage secondary to drug intake and the potential side effects from drug interactions. The elderly immune system demonstrates decreased T-cell function and decreased antibody production, leaving individuals more susceptible to infectious illness. As humans age, progressive bone loss, particularly in postmenopausal females, ensues. This leads to brittleness of bones and an increased risk of hip fracture and its associated morbidity. The gastrointestinal tracts of aged individuals also experience changes, including gastric atrophy as well as decreased gastrin activity and parietal cell secretion of hydrochloric acid. There is a high incidence of dysphagia among the elderly as well, a clinical syndrome leading to morbidity secondary to aspiration of gastric contents. Integumentary changes include thinning of the skin with a reduction of subcutaneous fat. Thinning of the skin often puts older adults at risk for developing decubitus ulcers, or bed sores, resulting in marked discomfort and associated morbidity. Additionally, these people become intolerant to colder temperatures, manifesting increased susceptibility to experiencing hypothermia, particularly when undergoing cardiopulmonary bypass. Individuals commonly experience neuropsychiatric and neurocognitive changes as they age. Cortical atrophy is prominent. Nerve conduction velocity declines. The incidence of Alzheimer's disease in the elderly is notably high. Figure 1 demonstrates declining organ function with age.

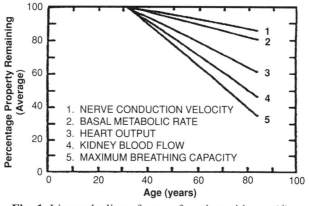

Fig. 1. Linear decline of organ function with age (*1*).

IMPACT OF AGE ON CARDIAC SURGERY AND CARDIAC DISEASE

In the setting of an intensive care unit or under perioperative circumstances, advanced age often translates into high risk. Elderly individuals have altered drug excretion caused by their 25% decrease in renal mass and decline in renal blood flow. Often surgery increases the risk of renal failure. For example, cross-clamping and cardiopulmonary bypass cause a reduction in blood flow, further compromising renal perfusion pressure. Accumulation of certain drug products, particularly anesthetic agents and opioids, results in prolonged intubation time. Weaning an elderly patient off of a ventilator becomes increasingly difficult with multisystem decompensation (2). Patients undergoing cardiac surgery are typically instrumented with a transesophogeal echocardiogram (TEE) probe. Advanced age and TEE instrumentation increase an elderly person's risk for developing dysphagia. In turn, the risk of aspiration pneumonia increases, creating a complex picture of co-morbidity. Since human organ systems are intrinsically connected, damage to one system invariably affects other systems, particularly in an elderly individual whose organ reserve capacity is diminished.

These various alterations in cardiac function in the older individual often create the need for polypharmacy and potentially multiple interventions. For example, a person with hypertension, atherosclerosis, and an arrhythmia will require treatment with a series of pharmaceutical agents. Often, employing one medication to treat a single disease creates the need to use another medication to counterbalance the effect of the first drug. For example, a hypertensive elderly patient placed on beta-blockers who has intrinsic conduction defects may experience symptomatic bradycardia, necessitating the placement of a pacemaker. Dealing with older individuals often creates complex scenarios. Our hope is that after reading this text, providers will be better able to tackle the multitude of issues they and their patients face.

EPIDEMIOLOGY, DEMOGRAPHICS, AND HEALTH CARE POLICY

Americans are living longer, healthier, more active lives than ever before. Longevity has increased by 28 years since 1900, and recent studies indicate that many older citizens have fewer disabilities today than people the same age had just 15 years ago. Nevertheless, older Americans who do require medical attention tend to have multiple and complicated problems. The ever-increasing population of older patients who have cardiovascular disease parallels the demographic imperative that is changing the face of the world's population. Last year, 6,145,000 patients discharged with cardiovascular disease were over the age of 65 years. This same age group contributed to eighty-five percent of all myocardial infarction deaths. Fifty-six percent of coronary artery bypass graft (CABG) patients and 51% of the percutaneous transluminal coronary angioplasty (PTCA) procedures were performed in individuals over 65. The numbers of elderly patients comprising the cardiac patient population are staggering.

Section I of the text provides the backdrop for the rest of the text. In Chapter 1, the demography and epidemiologic data are described drawing attention to the crisis looming in health care. Subsequently, Drs. Ridge and Cassell describe the history of health care policy specifically as it pertains to the elderly in the United States in Chapter 2.

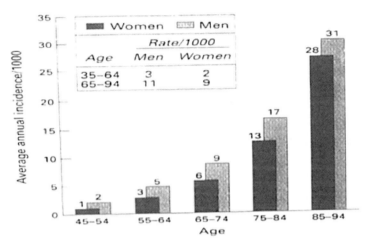

Fig. 2. Increasing incidence of heart failure in the aging population (*3*).

FUNDAMENTALS OF CARE FOR THE ELDERLY

Caring for the elderly patient with cardiovascular disease requires a multidisciplinary approach. Therefore, in this section of the text, we have asked our contributing authors to delineate age-related changes in organ systems outside of the cardiovascular system and how they impact on the manifestations and management of the cardiovascular disease in the elderly. Drs. Elkind, Kenny, Muskin, and Shapiro as well as Dr. Chong and colleagues provide valuable information regarding neurologic, psychiatric, and nutritional issues, respectively. Subsequently, Dr. King provides insights into the process of rehabilitation, an essential step in improving the quality of life in the elderly subject with cardiovascular disease who has undergone cardiac surgery. As our pharmacopoeia enlarges and the benefits of various agents are realized, concerns regarding the appropriate use of pharmacologic agents are of paramount importance in the elderly as described by Drs. Odeh-Ramadan and Remington. Finally, with all of the ethical issues that surround the care of our older patients, we would be remiss without considering carefully the concerns presented by Dr. Prager in his chapter on ethical issues.

CARDIOVASCULAR CARE FOR THE ELDERLY

Changes in cardiovascular structure and function are selective, with some portions of the cardiovascular system affected dramatically even as others are well maintained during normal human aging. In this section of the text, Drs. Maurer and Weisfeldt delineate these normative age-related changes and place them in clinical context. Subsequently, Dr. Wenger emphasizes the role of preventive strategies that can attenuate many of the disorders that disproportionately afflict the elderly. Finally, Drs. Reiffel, Bloomfield, Kitzman, Zieman, Schulman, and Fleg provide a comprehensive evaluation of the current facts and controversies that surround the management of dominant geriatric cardiovascular syndromes: atrial fibrillation, syncope, heart failure, and ischemic heart disease, respectively.

CARDIAC SURGICAL CARE FOR THE ELDERLY

A crucial aspect of surgical management of the elderly is the ability to make the right decision when one is faced with a multitude of imperfect options. The decision to operate should not be based on age alone, but reflect an assessment of the risk–benefit ratio of individual cases. Though it has been demonstrated that cardiovascular reserve capacity decreases with aging, chronological age alone should not be relied upon as a predictor of outcome. Instead, more emphasis should be placed on the functional status of the patient. In the earlier days of cardiac surgery, advanced age was considered a relative contra-indication for revascularization procedures. However, as surgical techniques and peri-operative management have improved, more elderly patients are now accepted for surgical intervention.

With an increasingly aging population, surgeons can expect a greater proportion of their workload to include patients aged over 75 years. During the 1990s we performed cardiac surgical procedures on 1448 subjects 75 years of age and older at our institution. This represented more than 10% of all cardiac surgical procedures. The number of patients over 75 years old presenting to a cardiac surgeon in our institution has in-creased over the past five years resulting in the initiation of the AGE (American Geriatric Experience) Program. This program is designed to foster clinical care, research, and education in the arena of cardiovascular disease in the elderly.

Our contributing authors in this section define the issues essential to providing cutting-edge surgical management of the elderly cardiac patient. Drs. Garrido, Argenziano, and Rose describe the surgical management of ischemic heart disease, while Drs. Oz and Smith cover the surgical management of heart failure and valvular disorders, respec-tively. Inasmuch as indications for pacemakers and defibrillators have expanded, Dr. Spotnitz provides a practical guide regarding the application of these technologies to the older individual. Finally, Dr. Edwards delineates the outcomes, both positive and nega-tive, that accompany the expansion of cardiac surgical procedures for the elderly, and Dr. Playford provides instructions regarding postoperative management.

CLOSING THOUGHTS

You will find throughout your reading of the various chapters of *Aging, Heart Dis-ease, and Its Management: Facts and Controversies* that there are perhaps far more "controversies" than "facts." This leads us to our second purpose, namely, to delineate the present issues that require immediate attention by the clinical and research commu-nity in order to improve the quality of care that we provide to our older patients with cardiovascular disease. To that end, we hope our book will serve as a simple step in the right direction.

Niloo M. Edwards, MD
Mathew S. Maurer, MD
Rachel B. Wellner, MPH

REFERENCES

1. Clarfield AM, Friedman R. A survey of the eye structure of "age-relevant" articles in four medical journals. J Am Geriatr Soc 1985;33:773–778.

2.Cope S, Hawley R, et. al. Needs of the older patient in the intensive care unit following heart surgery. Prog Cardiovasc Nurs 2001;16(2):44–48.

3. Kannel WB, Ho K, Thorn T. Changing epidemiological features of cardiac failure. (Framingham). Br Heart J 1994;72(Supp.2): 53.

CONTENTS

CONTRIBUTORS

PATRICK ARCHDEACON, MD • *Department of Medicine, Milstein Hospital, Columbia University College of Physicians and Surgeons, New York, NY*

MICHAEL ARGENZIANO, MD • *Division of Cardiothoracic Surgery, New York Presbyterian Hospital, Columbia University College of Physicians and Surgeons, New York, NY*

DANIEL M. BLOOMFIELD, MD, FACC • *Division of Cardiology, Department of Medicine, Columbia University College of Physicians and Surgeons, and Syncope Center, New York Presbyterian Hospital, Columbia Presbyterian Medical Center, New York, NY*

CHRISTINE CASSEL, MD • *Oregon Health and Science University School of Medicine, Portland, OR; and Henry L. Schwartz Department of Geriatrics and Adult Development, Mount Sinai School of Medicine, New York, NY*

DAVID H. CHONG, MD • *Department of Medicine, Columbia Presbyterian Medical Center, New York, NY*

NILOO M. EDWARDS, MD • *Division of Cardiothoracic Surgery, Columbia University College of Physicians and Surgeons, New York, NY*

MITCHELL S. V. ELKIND, MD, MS • *Department of Neurology, Neurological Institute, New York, NY*

JEROME L. FLEG, MD • *Gerontology Research Center, National Institute of Aging/NIH, Baltimore, MD*

MAURICIO J. GARRIDO, MD • *Cardiothoracic Research Fellow, Columbia University College of Physicians and Surgeons, New York Presbyterian Hospital, New York, NY*

ASHLEY S. IM, MS, MPH • *Joseph L. Mailman School of Public Health at Columbia University, New York, NY*

EDWARD T. KENNY, MD • *Consultation Liaison, Department of Psychiatry, Columbia University Medical Center, New York, NY*

AFTAB R. KHERANI, MD • *Duke University Medical Center, Durham, NC; and Division of Cardiothoracic Surgery, Columbia University College of Physicians and Surgeons, New York, NY*

MARJORIE L. KING, MD, FACC, FAACVPR • *Cardiac Services, Columbia University, New York; and Department of Internal Medicine, Helen Hayes Hospital, West Haverstraw, NY*

DALANE W. KITZMAN, MD • *Department of Internal Medicine/Cardiology, Wake Forest University School of Medicine, Winston-Salem, NC*

EUGENE KUKUY, MD • *Cardiothoracic Research Fellow, Columbia University College of Physicians and Surgeons, New York, NY*

CHANDRA KUNAVARAPU, MD • *Division of Cardiology, Department of Medicine, Columbia University College of Physicians and Surgeons, New York, NY*

MATHEW S. MAURER, MD • *Division of Circulatory Physiology/Department of Medicine, Columbia University College of Physicians and Surgeons, New York, NY*

PHILIP R. MUSKIN, MD • *Consultation Liaison, Department of Psychiatry, Columbia University Medical Center, New York, NY*

RUDINA M. ODEH-RAMADAN, PHARMD • *Department of Pharmacy, Center for Liver Disease and Transplantation, New York-Presbyterian Hospital, Columbia Presbyterian Medical Center, New York, NY*

MEHMET C. OZ, MD • *Division of Cardiothoracic Surgery, Columbia University College of Physicians and Surgeons, New York, NY*

HUGH R. PLAYFORD, MB, BS, FANZCA, FFICANZCA • *Department of Anesthesiology, Columbia University College of Physicians and Surgeons, New York, NY*

KENNETH M. PRAGER, MD • *Department of Medicine, Columbia University College of Physicians and Surgeons, New York, NY*

JAMES A. REIFFEL, MD • *Division of Cardiology, Department of Medicine, Columbia University College of Physicians and Surgeons, New York, NY*

TAMI L. REMINGTON, PHARMD • *Department of Pharmacy Services and College of Pharmacy, University of Michigan Health System, Ann Arbor, MI*

S. BRENT RIDGE, MD • *Department of Internal Medicine, Columbia University, New York, NY*

ERIC A. ROSE, MD • *Division of Cardiothoracic Surgery, Columbia University College of Physicians and Surgeons, New York Presbyterian Hospital, New York, NY*

STEVEN P. SCHULMAN, MD • *Division of Cardiology, Johns Hopkins Medical Institutions, Johns Hopkins Hospital, Baltimore, MD*

PETER A. SHAPIRO, MD • *Consultation Liaison, Department of Psychiatry, Columbia University Medical Center, New York, NY*

CRAIG R. SMITH, MD • *Division of Cardiothoracic Surgery, Columbia University College of Physicians and Surgeons, New York, NY*

HENRY M. SPOTNITZ, MD • *Columbia University College of Physicians and Surgeons, New York, NY*

WINDSOR TING, MD • *Division of Cardiothoracic Surgery, Columbia University College of Physicians and Surgeons, New York, NY*

MYRON L. WEISFELDT, MD • *Department of Medicine, The Johns Hopkins Medical Institutions, The John Hopkins Hospital, Baltimore, MD*

RACHEL B. WELLNER, BA, MPH • *University of Connecticut School of Medicine, Farmington, CT*

NANETTE K. WENGER, MD • *Division of Cardiology, Department of Medicine, Emory University School of Medicine, Grady Memorial Hospital, Atlanta, GA*

SUSAN J. ZIEMAN, MD • *Division of Cardiology, Johns Hopkins Medical Institutions, Johns Hopkins Hospital; and Gerontology Research Center, National Institute of Aging/NIH, Baltimore, MD*

I   Epidemiology, Demographics, and Health Care Policy

1

Demography and Epidemiology
An Examination of Cardiovascular Disease in the Elderly

Rachel B. Wellner, BA, MPH

CONTENTS

INTRODUCTION
DEFINING AGING AS A BIOLOGICAL CONSTRUCT
THEORIES OF AGING
THE CULTURAL CONTEXT OF AGING
DEMOGRAPHY OF THE ELDERLY POPULATION:
  YESTERDAY, TODAY, AND TOMORROW
QUALITY-OF-LIFE ISSUES
REFERENCES

The challenge of global aging, like a massive iceberg, looms ahead in the future of the largest and most affluent economies of the world. Visible above the waterline are the unprecedented growth in the number of elderly and the unprecedented decline in the number of youth over the next several decades.

From Peter G. Peterson, *Gray Dawn*

INTRODUCTION

As the 21st century commences, the aged constitutes a growing proportion of the world's population. This growth is occurring in America at unprecedented rates. The "graying" of America is a popular expression describing the phenomenon of a uniformly aging population. The upward trend in the growth of America's elders promises to have a significant impact socially, economically, and culturally, particularly by 2030, when the country's cohort of baby boomers will reach the age of 85 and over.

According to the United States Bureau of the Census, from the beginning of the 20th century to its close, the percentage of the US population comprised by seniors over the age of 65 has increased from 3.1 million people to 34.1 million (*1*). The oldest old, those above the age of 80, have also experienced an astounding population explosion, increasing from 4% of the population in 1900 to 10% in 1990. This proportion is expected to exceed 13% by the year 2050 (*2*). This burgeoning of elderly individuals has and will continue to increase the demand for more assisted-living facilities, improved long-term-

From: *Aging, Heart Disease, and Its Management: Facts and Controversies*
Edited by: N. Edwards, M. Maurer, and R. Wellner © Humana Press Inc., Totowa, NJ

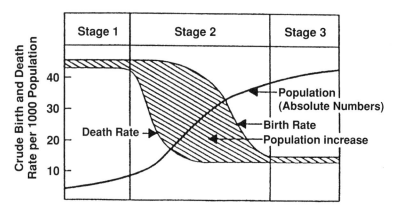

Fig. 1. Stages in demographic transition. Stage 1 (common to developing countries) is marked by a high death rate compensating for a high birth rate, effectively controlling population. Stage 2: As the death rate declines rapidly and the birth rate declines at a slower rate, population growth is inevitable. Stage 3: Birth rate declines sufficiently to lower the population.

care program options, broader health maintenance organization (HMO) coverage, and more stringent Social Security safeguarding.

The graying of the industrialized world results from an interplay of two independent trends. The first of these trends is a sharp decline in overall mortality. The decrease in mortality represents the outcome that many years of intense public health measures to reduce all-cause mortality, particularly the incidence of infectious disease and associated mortality. Second, in many industrialized countries, the birth rate has also declined dramatically. Having multiple children is a trend that has lost popularity in developed nations for various socioeconomic and cultural reasons. The developing world, in contrast, continues to boast a very high birth rate, as children are often considered an economic resource and source of livelihood for many families. Additionally, infant and child mortality rates are exceedingly high in developing nations, increasing the rationale for birthing multiple children.

In less industrialized countries the demographic picture historically has exhibited a high proportion of national populations under the age of 15 and a paucity of seniors over the age of 65. High case-fatality rates from diseases of infectious and other etiologies persist in the developing world but are beginning to decline as industrialization, improved medical technology, and delivery systems permeate these societies. As a result, developing populations are expected to undergo demographic transition, a trend marked by declining death rate and birth rate that will ultimately lead to a decrease in population size (*see* Fig. 1). A cross-national comparison of proportional elderly populations is presented in Table 1.

DEFINING AGING AS A BIOLOGICAL CONSTRUCT

Aging, in its broadest sense, can be seen as a loss of adaptability and an increase in vulnerability over time *(3)*. Crews introduced a more comprehensive definition of the aging process: "all time-dependent structural and functional changes both maturational and senescent, that normally occur in the postpubertal period among males and females of a species" *(4)*. The concept of senescence is integral to the aging process. According to Albert and Cattell, senescence "includes the progressive and cumulative functional deter-

Table 1
Cross-Comparison of Population Types Ranging from Aged to Youthful in Various Nations

	Aged populations (≥100%)[a]
18[b]	Sweden
16	Norway
15	Austria, Germany–Federal Republic, United Kingdom
14	Belgium, France, Italy
12	United States, Uruguay, Bulgaria
11	Barbados, Canada, Japan, Czechoslovakia, Ireland, Australia, New Zealand
10	Cyprus, Poland
	Maturing populations ($7 \leq N \leq 9\%$)
9	Puerto Rico, Argentina, Israel, USSR
7	Dominica
	Youthful populations ($4 \leq N \leq 6\%$)
6	Antigua–Barbuda, Jamaica, Chile, China, Singapore, Taiwan
5	Costa Rica, Haiti, Panama, Republic of Korea, Lebanon
4	South Africa, Mexico, Nicaragua, Bolivia, Brazil, Colombia, Ecuador, Sri Lanka, Syria, Thailand, Turkey, Vietnam, Belize
	Young populations (<4%)
3	India, Indonesia, Iran, Iraq, Ghana, Honduras, Nepal, Oman, Philippines, Saudi Arabia, Zimbabwe, Sudan, Somalia, Yemen Arab Republic, Dominican Republic, Central African Republic, Congo, Mozambique
2	United Arab Emirates, Rwanda, Jordan, Kenya, Ivory Coast, Zambia, Uganda
1	Qatar, Kuwait

[a]The percentages refer to the relative number of elderly individuals within each population, e.g., the top group demonstrates that the elderly comprise about 10% of their populations.

[b]The numbers on the left order the countries in terms of having the most elderly to having the least.

Source: Modified from Population Reference Bureau 1991: World Data Disk (World Game Institute).

Note: Data missing for 21 countries or territories.

ioration associated with longer lifespan" *(5)*. Senescence does not encompass definitions of disease, which refers to specific pathological processes resulting in damage to one or more target organs. Aging is a natural biological process that allows all organisms to grow and develop; it is also responsible for the progressive functional decline that occurs at some critical point in maturation. Because of this complex process of senescence and maturation, to declare biological age and chronological age as synonymous would be incorrect. After all, each individual ages at his or her own pace. An unhealthy 65-yr-old may be biologically much older than a spry 85-yr-old, despite the reverse chronological relationship.

THEORIES OF AGING

The process of aging is multidimensional and complex. As one ages, there are significant declines in some physiological parameters, whereas other changes appear to have minimal impact on overall function. Scientists have tried to understand and describe the aging process for decades. Presently, no one theory has been proposed to explain aging in its entirety. Conversely, the individual explanatory mechanisms that have been described most likely interact to cause aging. Selected theories of aging include Autoimmune Theory, Wear and Tear Theory, Crosslinkage Theory, Free-Radical Theory, and Cellular Age Theory

Table 2
Theories of Aging

Theory	Explanation
Autoimmune Theory (Walford, 1969)	• Aging is function of body's immune system—becomes defective and attacks not only foreign proteins, bacteria, and virus but also producing antibodies against self. • Theory is consistent with diseases associated with increase age such as cancer, diabetes, and rheumatoid arthritis.
Wear and Tear Theory (Wilson, 1974)	• Organism wears out as time progresses. • Aging is a preprogrammed process. • Each species has a biological clock that determines maximum life-span. • External factors stresses the organism so eventually cells in the organisms wear out and cannot repair itself.
Crosslinkage Theory (Bjorksten, 1974)	• With increasing age, collagen changes—elasticity in connective tissue are lost.
Free Radical Theory (Harman, 1956, 1981)	• Free radicals in the body cause damage to cells, tissues, and organs. • Antioxidants such as vitamin C and E can reduce the free-radical damage.
Cellular Aging Theory (Hayflick and Moorehead, 1961)	• Aging occurs as cells slow their number of replications. • Cells are programmed to follow their biological clock and stop replicating after a given number of times.

(*see* Table 2). The process we appreciate as aging is most likely the result of a complex interplay between each theory presented and perhaps other unexplained mechanisms.

THE CULTURAL CONTEXT OF AGING

The definition of aging varies across cultures. It is essential to account for distinctions in classification systems, however subtle they may seem. Doing so successfully requires minimizing ethnocentricity and bias. The various stages in life can carry great significance in a culture. In some societies elders are appointed as community leaders and are assigned specific privileges that juniors to which are not entitled. Albert and Cattell *(5)* write:

> Aging is linked to social distinction, as societies use age to categorize individuals. The distinction between the relatively junior and senior is central for allocating resources, knowing to whom to defer, and indexing cultural expertise.

Among populations with low average life expectancies, the concept of "old age" bears a different significance than it does to societies that experience high average life expectancies. The truncated life cycle characteristic of the former population type must provide for the acceleration of social markers and rites of passage (e.g., puberty, marriage, reproduction, menopause). Examples of these populations include the foraging peoples of the !Kung tribe of the Kalahari Desert (mean age of onset of menopause is 40, vs 51 for American women) and the preindustrial Yanomama Indians of South America *(5)*.

Elders residing in industrialized nations certainly command societal respect for their longevity, years, and cumulative wisdom. However, older individuals are sometimes viewed as burdensome to families and the greater society. The advancement of technology and

Table 3
Average Life Expectancies in Different Nations over Time

	Life expectancy at birth (in yr)	Infant mortality rate (per 1000 live births)
Prehistoric	20–35	200–300
Sweden, 1750s	37	210
India, 1880s	25	230
United States, 1900	48	133
France, 1950	66	52
Japan, 1996	80	4

industry has frequently signified the dissolution of the nuclear family, creating a rift between elders and their natural caregivers. Part of this perceived strain results from the sheer increase in numbers of older individuals:

> These demographic trends ultimately will place unprecedented demands on the nation's caregivers. As families become older and more linear, there will be fewer sons, daughters, cousins, aunts and uncles to care for their longer-lived elders *(6)*.

DEMOGRAPHY OF THE ELDERLY POPULATION: *YESTERDAY, TODAY, AND TOMORROW*

From centuries of historical record, scientists and historians have ascertained with a high degree of accuracy how prehistoric human and modern-day human average life expectancies and life-spans have evolved over time. First, the two measures must be distinguished. The average life expectancy refers to the average age to which an individual is likely to live. The human life-span represents a maximal number of years the human organism can live. The early hominids probably demonstrated a maximal life-span of approx 50 yr *(5)*. Conversely, *Australopithecines* had an average life expectancy of about 15 yr *(5)*. Often, the two definitions are thought of as interchangeable, but, as demonstrated by the respective life-span and average life expectancy of our distant ancestors, the distinction is self-evident. The maximum life-span for humans doubled between approx 3 million and 100,000 yr ago *(5)*. On the other hand, average human life expectancy, highly sensitive to infant and child mortality, ranges across different cultures and societies. Table 3 compares average life expectancies in different nations over time.

Over the next four decades, the composition of the elderly population will undergo a metamorphosis resulting from the significant increase in the absolute number of seniors. The oldest old (≥80 yr) currently constitute 14% of the world's elderly population. As a result of sharply declining mortality rates, particularly cardiovascular mortality, individuals above the age of 85 are predicted to be the fastest growing constituent of the elderly population over the next century *(2)*. Additionally, by 2050, the average life expectancy is projected to be 81.8 yr for males and 88.2 yr for females *(2)*. Presently, the life expectancy for females is higher than that for males, and similar trends will continue. Consequential to this gender disparity is the creation of a vulnerable population: the widowed female, who is often left with little social support in her last years. The ramifications of this increasing social and financial burden will likely increase the incidence of depression, neurocognitive changes, overall morbidity, and mortality in this subset of people, as well as hospital costs.

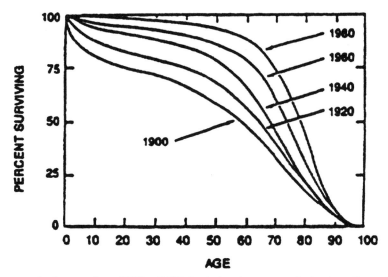

Fig. 2. Human survival curves from 1900 to 1980, depicting the rectangularization of overall survival. From ref. *1*.

Shifts in the racial makeup of the elderly population will inevitably occur at increasing rates as a result of the overall graying trend. Approximately one-third of the nation's elderly are projected to be other than non-Hispanic white by 2050. Social and cultural norms for many minority groups must also help shape policy and access issues regarding elder care.

The industrialized world has, as a whole, experienced a rectangularization of overall survival for entire populations. This phenomenon is depicted graphically in Fig. 2. Fries *(7)* describes the trend:

> In 1900 mortality occurred at a relatively steady rate throughout the life span. In successive decades, the curves have begun to bend upward and to the right, each considerably different from the last. The form of the curve is increasingly rectangular, having an increasingly flat top and an increasingly sharp downslope.

The rectangularization of survival reflects epidemiologic transitions over time, as societies have adapted from primarily foragers to a technology-based culture *(5)*. With the transition from a hunter–gatherer society to an agrarian society, primary cause of mortality shifted from external injuries to infectious diseases. That trend was followed by the change to an industrial society, at which point chronic conditions such as cardiovascular disease overtook infection as the major cause of mortality. Following industrialization, cancer rates exceeded those of most chronic diseases. This epidemiologic transition has resulted from the gradual reduction of multiple causes of death with advancing technology. Clearly, this reduction produces the survival-rate rectangularization.

From 1990 to 1999, less than a decade's time, the median age of the United States population has increased from 32.8 yr to 35.5 yr. This increase is primarily attributed to the growth of the elderly cohort, as infant and child mortality rates did not change significantly during that particular time period (*see* Fig. 3).

Table 4 is adapted from the United States Bureau of the Census and shows the absolute numbers of individuals over age 60, stratified by age group, from 1995 to 2000. Generally, over the past 5 yr, there have been upward growth patterns in nearly every age group.

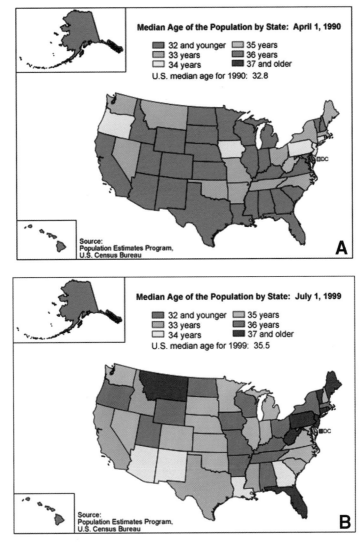

Fig. 3. (A) United States demography map in 1990 displaying median age of population by state and nationally. **(B)** Identical US demography map in 1999 displaying median age of population by state and nationally. Note the change in age composition statewide from 1990 to 1999, as well as the increase in national median age from 32.8 to 35.5 yr. From ref. *1*.

Certainly, our nation's elders have grown in number and are projected to continue to grow at an even more accelerated rate. Figure 4 depicts an exponential growth in the number of seniors in the United States from 1995 estimates to projections for 2030. The large cohort represented by the baby-boomer generation presents a highly predictive model. A typical age–sex pyramid displaying age as a variable that increases from the base to the apex demonstrates a triangular shape. With current and future trends demonstrating burgeoning of the elderly population, the age–sex pyramid becomes top heavy, essentially yielding a rectangular shape (*see* Fig. 5).

Examining overall mortality curves for the United States from 1900 to 1995, the transition to a deeper J shape is evident (*see* Fig. 6). With the decline in infant mortality, the

Table 4
Population of People (in Thousands)
in the United States over Age 60 from 1995 to 2000

Age	Year					
(yr)	2000	1999	1998	1997	1996	1995
60–64	10,757	10,514	10,263	10,061	9,997	10,046
65–69	9,414	9,447	9,592	9,777	9,901	9,926
70–74	8,758	8,771	8,798	8,751	8,789	8,831
75–79	7,425	7,329	7,215	7,083	6,891	6,700
80–84	4,968	4,817	4,732	4,661	4,575	4,478
85–89	2,734	2,625	2,554	2,477	2,415	2,352
90–94	1,196	1,148	1,116	1,078	1,043	1,017
95–99	369	343	323	304	291	268
100 +	68	59	57	54	51	48

Source: Adapted from ref. 1.

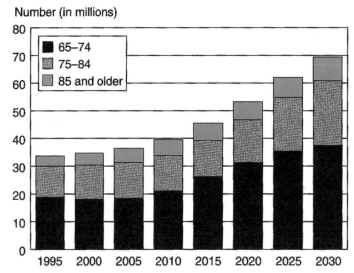

Fig. 4. United States elderly population estimates stratified by age group from 1995 to 2030. From ref. 1.

mortality curve is shifted downward on the y-axis. The plunge in death rates during childhood and adolescent years produces a deep nadir graphically. Finally, as mortality occurs at older ages and at a slower rate, the upward slope of the mortality curve is less pronounced until very old age. This trend is representative of the majority of industrialized nations.

QUALITY-OF-LIFE ISSUES

Issues surrounding quality of life are of paramount importance for the elderly. Over the past 15–20 yr, provision of health care has drifted away from the traditional, number-heavy economic model. Under the weight of expensive technologies and heavy health care use, in the 1960s administrative and economic forces began dictating how health outcomes

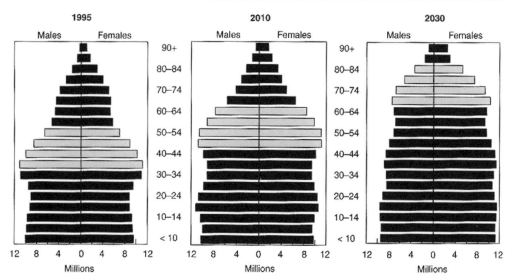

Fig. 5. Age–sex pyramids for the US population comparing 1995 rates, 2010 projections, and projections for 2030. Note how the shape of the graphic display shifts from a pyramid to a cylinder as time advances. From ref. *1*.

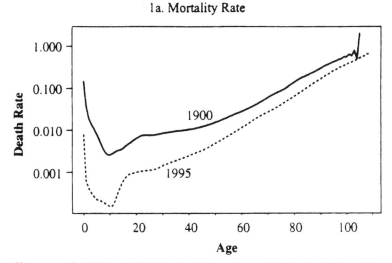

Fig. 6. Mortality curves in 1900 and 1995 in the United States. Notice the J shape. From: Office of the Chief Actuary, Social Security Administration (Bell et al. 1992; data available through ref. *9*).

weighed against cost analyses. Recently, methods such as cost analysis, which assesses direct budgetary costs to health agencies, and cost–benefit analysis, which measures costs and benefits in financial terms, have started to metamorphosize into systems of greater ethical valor, including cost-effective analyses, which measure output in terms of health and not monetary gains. Similarly, the cost–utility analysis actually gauges changes in quality of life by accounting for the patient's own perspective of his or her health status. Constructs such as the Disability Free Life Year, Health Life Expectancy, the Quality-adjusted Life Year, and the years of healthy life (YHL) system have started to replace the traditional PYL (potential years of life lost) measure *(10)*. The YHL system, alternatively the

Health Quality of Life (HQOL) index, includes an HQOL value representing various degrees of morbidity; the actual age of an individual is then multiplied by that factor, yielding an approximate number of healthy years experienced by that individual. Although many initiatives have been proposed recognizing the need to provide quality-of-life indices, support for elderly studies measuring YHLs is still lacking, as potential years lost in this age group is much smaller compared to the PYL in younger cohorts.

Many instruments have been developed to measure an elderly individual's function; these functional scales may serve as a proxy measure for quality of life. One of the most well-known and widely utilized scale is the Index of ADL (Activities of Daily Living), developed in 1963 by Katz et al. *(11)*. The ADL scale details six basic activities, including bathing, dressing, toileting, transferring, feeding, and continence *(11)*. Determining whether each of these six activities could be done independently or not is phrased in a question form and subsequently rated based on response. The sum total of the six individual scores then produces an ADL score that is intended to be highly representative of individual function, a quantity that most probably provides some reflection of life quality. Less than a decade later, the Instrumental Activities of Daily Living index (IADL) was developed by Lawton and Brody. This index incorporated slightly more complex secondary tasks of basic living, including shopping, handling family finances, food preparation, telephone use, housekeeping, laundering, transportation, and responsibility for medications *(12)*.

Several other quality-of-life measures have been developed, including the study Short Form-36 (SF-36), a 36-item questionnaire that asks specific questions regarding quality of life. The EuroQOL considers self-assessment of mood, pain, mobility, independence, primary activity and relationship maintenance as primary criteria for judging quality-of-life status *(10)*. A need for the development of more honed and comprehensive assessment tools is still pending.

REFERENCES

1. United States Bureau of the Census. http://www.census.gov/population/www/estimates/popest.html
2. Suzman R, Willis D, Manton K. The Oldest Old. Oxford University Press, New York, 1992.
3. Martin A, Camm A. Geriatric Cardiology. Wiley, Chichester, 1994.
4. Crews D. Anthropological issues in biological gerontology. In: Rubinstein R, ed. Anthropology and Aging. Kluwer, Boston, MA, 1990, pp. 11–38.
5. Albert S, Cattell M. The nature of age: biology, chronology, and culture. In: Old Age in Global Perspective: Cross-Cultural and Cross-National Views. G.K. Hall, New York, 1994, pp. 11–56.
6. Starr C. America soon to have more grandmas than grandkids. Scripps Howard News Service, November 26, 1999. http://www.bergen.com/morenews/gra199911265.htm
7. Fries J. The compression of morbidity. Milbank Mem Fund Q/Health Soc 1983;61(3):397–419.
8. Population Reference Bureau 1991: World Data Disk (World Game Institute). http://www.worldpop.org/prbdata.htm
9. Berkeley Mortality Database. http://demog.berkeley.edu/wilmoth/mortality
10. Erickson P, Wilson R, Shannon I, et al. Years of healthy life. In: Healthy People 2000: Statistical Notes No. 7. U.S. Department of Health and Human Services, Public Health Service; Centers for Disease Control National Center for Health Statistics, Atlanta, GA, 1995.
11. Katz S, Ford A, et al. Studies of illness in the aged, the index of ADL: a standardized measure of biological and psychosocial function. JAMA 1963;914–919.
12. Lawton M, Brody E. Assessment of older people: self-maintaining and instrumental activities of daily living. Gerontologist 1969;9:179–186.

2

The Evolution
of the American Health Care System

S. Brent Ridge, MD *and Christine Cassel,* MD

INTRODUCTION

The common perception of medicine in America is that we have and will continue to have the best health care in the world—the best doctors, the best hospitals, the best technology, and, likewise, every American citizen is entitled access to the best medical care. Every disease is potentially curable, and everything that can be done for a sick person must be done. In essence, where health care is concerned, there are no limits. Increasingly, however, we are confronting the fact that there are indeed limits, particularly in our ability to provide continued and equitable access to the "miracles of modern medicine."

Historically, the American health care system has operated as a "fee-for-service" enterprise. In such a system patients freely chose their providers, and along with those providers, they made all medical decisions knowing that the costs incurred were theirs to pay. Cost controls were automatic in this system, and rationing was self-imposed. For much of the nation's history, this system worked well. Doctors had little to offer in terms of effective (and expensive) therapy and patients' expectations were generally low—a critical balance.

This equilibrium began to falter by the first half of the 20th century. During the Great Depression, hospitals began to suffer from the patients' inability to pay their bills, and it was the financially stressed hospitals that prompted state legislatures to implement the insurance schemes that became known as Blue Cross.

From: *Aging, Heart Disease, and Its Management: Facts and Controversies*
Edited by: N. Edwards, M. Maurer, and R. Wellner © Humana Press Inc., Totowa, NJ

To assuage the indignation of physicians, the Blues were created as non-profit, provider-oriented insurance organizations. They did not attempt to tell physicians how to practice medicine. Physicians did what they deemed necessary, and the Blues paid the bills on a traditional fee-for-service basis. Not only did the system preserve the direct relationship between the physician and the patient, but it also paid the bills more reliably than the patients themselves. Because this system seemed flawless, there were no objections to the rather rapid formation of private health insurance companies as long as they mirrored the structure the Blues had put into place *(1)*.

The economic restructuring prompted by the Second World War brought about the next major change in the US health care system. During the wage and price controls of World War II, companies capitalized on the popularity of insurance and began offering health coverage to their employees in lieu of higher wages. By the time the war ended, this "benefit" was rapidly transforming into an "entitlement," and American labor unions began to demand that employers provide health insurance. The government encouraged the provision with lucrative tax cuts to the employers. In a short time, the majority of American workers enjoyed employer-provided health care insurance heavily subsidized by the federal government. This new tax policy represented a seminal event in the evolution of health policy. It shifted the fiscal burden of health insurance away from the consumer (and the employer) to the government.

In the 1960s, the federal government became more directly involved in supporting the nation's health care system first with the institution of Medicare and, shortly after, the Medicaid program. Prior to 1966, less than half of all elderly persons in the United States had any health insurance. For those with chronic health conditions, 70% had no insurance. With the rising costs of the time, for many elderly individuals, a hospital stay could eliminate the results of a lifetime of saving. In 1965, Congress enacted Medicare as a social health insurance program for the elderly; that is, everyone would contribute premiums while they worked and would, in turn, receive benefits when they retired, regardless of income or health history. At the time, Medicare was envisioned by many as the first stage in universalizing healthcare in the United States.

The advent of these programs, along with the tax incentives provided to employers who offered health care benefits, ushered in the "golden era" of American medicine in the second half of the 20th century. The system seemed nearly perfect. Patients had complete freedom of choice; physician decision making remained free from outside influences, and all the while, someone else was footing the bill. The result of this economic arrangement was a complete dissociation between the consumption of health care and the responsibility of paying for it. Because of the "no-limits" attitude of the system and the ability of modern society to continually provide newer, better (more expensive) therapies and interventions, the arrangement was destined to implode. The more we got, the more we wanted. The more we wanted, certainly someone was going to find a way to provide it creating an ever-intensifying positive feedback loop. It was inevitable that those paying for the escalating costs of health care (namely government and employers) would eventually reach a monetary breaking point.

During the 1950s and 1960s, the cost of hospital care nearly doubled, and as billings rose, there were increased complaints that the traditional fee-for-service method of payment was being abused. Increasingly, corporations began to integrate the hospital system (previously a decentralized structure) and many other health-related businesses, as well as consolidate control, driving a shift toward the privatization and corporatization of health care. Despite its new prominence as a media catchphrase, "managed care" is not a new concept; in fact, American companies, notably railroad and lumber, pioneered the contracting of medical services in the late 19th century. President Richard Nixon renamed prepaid group health care plans and coined the term "health maintenance organization" (HMO).

Managed care has long been a topic of discussion in academic circles frequented by health care policy experts and economists. In the latter part of the 20th century, the economically unsustainable system of health care delivery and payment that had developed encouraged the move from the classroom to the boardroom. In simplest terms, managed care aims to confer organization and accountability with the dual goal of providing adequate health care while eliminating waste and inefficiency. For the purpose of semantics, a HMO is the bureaucratic entity that applies the principles of managed care to a specific patient population. Despite the frequent association of the word "bureaucracy" with unnecessary complexity, the idea behind a HMO is simple: standardization.

The standardization of any industrial process leads to higher quality and lower cost. The health care industry, traditionally individualized and variable, should have been rife with opportunities to improve the process of delivery and do so more economically. In 1983, the federal government passed legislation that would pay the hospital's portion of Medicare patient bills based on a set fee determined by one of 467 diagnosis-related groups (DRGs). This legislation marked a major turning point in the financing of medical care. Prior to this, the government paid whatever price was billed. Many private insurers followed suit. However, there are limitations to the use of industrial management principles in medicine. In actuality, few medical processes are suitable for standardization, because they lack reproducible tasks that standardization seeks to maximize. For instance, consider the treatment pathway for congestive heart failure (CHF). CHF could be caused by coronary artery disease, valvular heart disease, or a viral infection. There are four different classes of severity of CHF and the condition can be manifest in several other organ systems. Simply knowing that a patient has CHF tells you very little about what type of treatment the patient will require. The patient could require a heart transplant or just a couple of diuretic tablets. As a result of this complexity, devising critical pathways for this and many medical illnesses has proven to be very problematic.

Attempts to make the health care industry conform to the principles of the free market have precipitated most of the problems we face with the health care system currently. The promise of greater efficiency and integration of preventative health practices are inadequately powered to overcome the strength of the bottom line, and the system that took the good part of a century to mature has devolved into one in which "cherry-picking" of patients and micromanagement of physicians are the methods employed in the avoidance of cost (2).

WHO PAYS?

Of the 1.4 trillion dollars spent on health care last year, a majority was spent on the care of patients 65 yr old and older. Approximately 10.5% of an elderly individual's household income is devoted to health care expenses, compared to 3.5% for the nonelderly (3). This proportion would be much larger were the elderly not heavily insured against health care costs. Over 95% of all Americans older than 65 are covered by Medicare. Today, Medicare pays for approx 45% of the medical expenses of the elderly. To pay for services not covered by Medicare and the deductibles and copayments associated with Medicare some individuals buy gap insurance in the private sector. Most individuals (70%) have both

Medicare and some other kind of private health insurance. Smaller but significant fractions have Medicare only (17%) or both Medicare and Medicaid (10%). Sadly, 3% of America's elderly lack any coverage at all *(4)*.

In most cases, eligiblility for Medicare begins at 65 or if one has a disability (have been receiving SSI disability income for at least 24 mo or has end-stage renal disease), regardless of income. If one is eligible for Social Security (SS) retirement benefits, one can still receive Medicare benefits regardless of age. Citizens and permanent legal aliens are also eligible for Medicare if they have lived in the United States continuously for 5 yr or more immediately preceding entitlement, or if they are 65 or older and are not eligible for other Social Security benefits. However, they generally must pay Part A premiums.

Medicare is divided into two parts: Part A and Part B. Medicare Part A covers inpatient hospital, skilled nursing facility, home health, and hospice services. Medicare Part B covers almost all reasonable and necessary medical services, including physicians' services, outpatient hospital care, durable medical equipment, laboratory tests, X-rays, therapy, mental health, and ambulance services. Medicare does not cover most preventive care, dental services, custodial or long-term nursing home care, or experimental procedures. It also does not pay for most prescription drugs.

There is no premium for Part A if you have worked more than 40 quarters (10 yr). The cost of Part B is currently around $50 per month deducted from the SS check and a $100 yearly deductible. Doctors do not have to treat Medicare patients, but if they do, they are legally bound to file claims with Medicare and to charge no more than state and federal law permits. Medicare will then pay the doctor 80% of the approved amount and the patient is responsible for the remaining 20%.

More than 80% of seniors have Original Medicare. Medicare supplemental insurance ("Medigap") can be purchased to fill gaps in Original Medicare coverage. Medigap insurance is specifically designed to supplement Medicare's benefits by paying some of the amount that Medicare does not pay for covered services and may pay for certain services not covered by Medicare. There are 10 (A–J) Medigap plans, with Plan J providing the most comprehensive (and most costly) coverage. Medicare can also be aligned with private companies in the form of Health Maintenance Organizations, Preferred Provider Organizations, Provider-Sponsored Organizations, Private Fee-for-Service Plans, and Medical Savings Account Plans. Poor seniors, those with monthly incomes less than $600 and assets less than $3600 may also be eligible for Medicaid, which fills many gaps in Medicare coverage and offers first-dollar coverage (the patient pays no out-of pocket costs).

In the 1990s, additions were made to the Medicaid program relating to eligibility. Two new categories of recipients, Qualified Medicare Beneficiaries (QMB) and Specified Low Income Medicare Beneficiaries (SLMB), were created. The income and asset limits to qualify under these programs were less strict than the limits under existing Medicaid categories. To qualify for QMB, individual assets <$4000 and monthly income less than $716 entitle individuals to coverage of Medicare premiums, deductibles, and coinsurance. SLMB participants have assets <$4000 and monthly incomes less than $855. SLMB pays for the Medicare Part B premium.

Health care financing efforts can be subdivided into three general types of health plan. Regressive plans are those in which people with increasing incomes pay a smaller percentage of income than those with lower incomes. In proportional plans the percentage of income for health care stays constant across socio-economic levels, and in progressive plans, those people with larger incomes pay a larger portion of their income than those with lower incomes. Given these basic definitions, most people would concede that regressive plans are the least reasonable. Unfortunately, the elderly are often subject to regressive plans because of their employment status or because they are unhealthy and utilize the health care system disproportionately. Most people consider the Social Security system, with its required contributions based on a flat percentage of earnings, to be a study in social progressiveness; this is not the case.

A robust history of social science research has found evidence of a widening gap between the life expectancy of high- and low-income persons, and the effect of income appears to be stronger than many other variables that impact mortality such as race and education level (5). Studies of US Life Tables comparing income level and mortality show that the highest-income retiree analyzed has a life expectancy that is about 6% longer than the lowest-income worker studied. Clearly, if Social Security contributions are a constant percentage of wages across a wide range of earnings and if high-income workers live longer, then the income distribution inherent in social security is perverse (5). All participants pay into the system at a level rate, but those with high incomes receive lifetime benefits that are worth more. A large number of variables is likely to contribute to the longevity of the well-to-do, but these aside, economic status profoundly affects use, particularly of the number of doctor visits which, in turn, may be directly related to greater purchase of private insurance (4). Wealthy individuals tend to live longer, and if they use Medicare more intensively because their supplemental insurance eliminates any co-payments, then they will receive greater lifetime benefits than the poor. Thus, the overall effect of Medicare will be regressive.

DOES HEALTH CARE MAKE US HEALTHY?

It is very easy to get mired in the discussion of health care financing and neglect the real question at hand. Do the trillions of dollars spent on health care make us healthy? Clearly, most Americans believe this to be true. However, are we correct? Without a doubt, an examination of life-expectancy patterns throughout the last century would reveal that life expectancy has nearly doubled, indicating a dramatic improvement in the general level of health over that period. However, the characteristics of "modern" medicine—new drugs, advanced technology, and more doctors—probably demonstrated only a peripheral effect on this trend. Far more important were improvements in nutrition and hygiene.

For instance, coronary artery disease is the leading cause of death in most industrialized countries. If the quantity and quality of health care was a key variable, then one would expect relatively poor countries such as Portugal to perform worse than relatively rich countries such as Norway. In fact, the opposite is true. The main variable, borne out in multiple studies, appears to be diet. Countries exhibiting the most frequent incidence of heart disease tend to be large consumers of dairy products and saturated animal fats, whereas those at the bottom of the table tend to use vegetable oils and eat large quantities of fish, fruit, and vegetables. Smoking is also a major factor. In the United States, coronary artery disease and cancers account for over half the deaths from natural causes, and both are strongly associated with tobacco abuse. Heavy smokers are four times more likely to die from coronary artery disease as are nonsmokers, and 40% of all cancer deaths are linked to smoking (6). Neither a medical degree nor an expensive test is required to intervene in the correction of these risk factors.

In fact, this misses the point of much of modern health care. Most treatment provided by doctors and hospitals is not primarily concerned with saving lives but rather with improving quality of life. Modern developments in medical technology, surgical techniques, and medicines have enabled doctors to treat many conditions that previously caused patients considerable pain and discomfort (i.e., stomach ulcers and osteoarthritis). This helps to explain why even with increased life expectancy, the demand for health care seems to be infinite and burdensome—everybody wants improvements to the quality of their life.

We are still faced with the problem of deciding how much health care we need. Some argue that we should aim for the highest level of health care. In opposition to this argument is the debate over whether or not we have a right to a certain level of health care at all. President Clinton campaigned with the slogan: "health care should be a right, not a privilege." The belief in such a right is widespread, even within the medical profession. The AMA's "Patient's Bill of Rights" includes the statement that patients have a "right to essential health care." The view that there exists some kind of right to a decent minimum of health care, or that the principle of beneficence is enough to justify a rational program of universal coverage permeates much of today's philosophical literature. Disagreement centers mainly on what constitutes a decent minimum or whether a decent minimum is, in fact, enough to discharge the implied duty of beneficence and the principle of social justice *(7)*. Policy-makers historically have made the assumption that these rights exist and quickly move the discussion forward to questions of practical implementation. Right or wrong, for the past 30 yr, the idea that people have a right to health care has led to greater and greater government control over the medical profession and the health care industry. The needs of the indigent, uninsured, and elderly, among other groups, have been put forward as claims on public resources. In that sense, public policy really dismisses the philosophical debate all together, sacrificing this intellectual endeavor to the will of the electorate.

If we accept this right to be implicit, then the answer to the question of how much health care we should provide is simple. The optimum level of health care is whatever is most efficient—the quantity where marginal cost equals marginal benefit. The questions that remain are which mixture will produce the most efficient allocation of a finite resource, and how can health care be distributed in an equitable manner?

THE BASIS OF HEALTH POLICY

In order to ration health care as fairly as possible, we need a way to measure how much good is accomplished for any given medical therapy. Treatment outcomes and other health-influencing activities have two basic components—the quantity and quality of life. Life expectancy is a traditional measure with few problems of comparison—people are either alive or not. Attempts to measure quality of life is a more recent innovation. Economists have attempted to capture both the quality and quantity elements of a health care outcome in a single measure by developing the quality-adjusted life-year (QALY).

These measurements identify public health trends for strategies to be developed, assess the effectiveness and efficiency of health care interventions, and determine the state of health in communities. QALYs offer the possibility of carrying out effective cost–benefit analysis and thus providing the information we need to make efficient decisions. Some "life-saving" treatments are unpleasant, do not extend life much, and the time remaining is full of pain and discomfort; alternative treatments may not save lives but are not expensive and may considerably improve the quality of life of the patient. An efficient allocation might shift resources from the first type of treatment to the second. QALY gives us a way to mathematically convert the amount of quality added to a person's life into a life-year equivalent. Theoretically, this allows all medical therapies to be compared to each other on an equal basis, whether or not they actually prolong life, and thus allows the numerical ranking of medical services in terms of amount of good they provide.

The basic idea of QALY is straightforward, using a scale from 0 to 1 to assess quality of life, where 1 represents a year of perfect health. Thus, an intervention that results in a patient living for an additional 4 yr rather than dying within 1 yr but where quality of life fell from 1 to 0.6 on the continuum will generate the following:

$$4 \text{ yr extra life at } 0.6 \text{ quality-of-life values} = 2.4$$

$$- \quad 1 \text{ yr at reduced quality of life } (1 - 0.6) = 0.4$$

$$\overline{\text{QALYs generated by the intervention} = 2.0}$$

Quality-adjusted life-years are a crude measurement, and although they provide the best attempt so far to solve the problem of measuring health care outcomes, they still suffer from a number of serious limitations. A key question is who should make the subjective choices that determine the QALY? Is it health professionals, the general public, politicians, or patients who have the experience of the particular medical condition and treatment? The value of a QALY can change radically according to who is making the choices. Other potential problems include the fact that the responses given are to hypothetical situations and so may not accurately reflect an individual's real decisions and the fact that valuations are influenced by the length of the illness and the way in which the questions are asked. QALYs are likely to undervalue health care, because they do not capture the wider benefits that may be gained, for example, by a patient's family, friends, and even the medical community. Nonetheless, QALYs seem to be the best measure so far for objectifying the benefit of medical therapies—a prerequisite for an ethical rationing system.

Health care decision making can take place at very high levels of abstraction or on a more individualized level. At the broadest level is the question of the most appropriate use of finite resources. It has become increasingly popular to carry out cost-effectiveness analysis in economic evaluations of health care. In cost-effectiveness analysis, costs are measured in monetary units, and health effects in non-monetary units such as life-years or the QALYs gained. The rationale for cost-effectiveness analysis is to maximize the effectiveness subject to a budget constraint. A fixed budget can be used to maximize the health effects based on information about the incremental cost-effectiveness ratios of different health programs that will implicitly yield a price per effectiveness unit or, vice versa, a price per effectiveness unit can be used to establish a budget (8). Fortunately, most physicians only see the end result of these complex economic calculations and usually in the form of clinical practice guidelines (9).

AN OUNCE OF PREVENTION

Arguably, an interest in health policy and economics is not what propelled most physicians through training. However, the implications of these two factors are inextricably woven together in the combined impact of health care and public health measures. The mortality from coronary heart disease has declined 50% in the past two decades *(10)*. Certainly part of this decline is the result of improved treatments from coronary artery bypass graft procedures, coronary care units, and better emergency response services *(11)*. On the other hand, a majority of this decline was the result of changes in lifestyle, specifically decreased smoking and serum total cholesterol levels in the general population *(12)*. If the decline in coronary heart disease continues, it will be the result of both improved treatments and improved preventive care.

The American health care system has long based its success, and rightfully so, on the introduction of new technology, but there has been increasing recognition of the potential of preventive activities to improve the health of the population. Impressive evidence supports the value of clinical preventive medicine *(11)*. Preventive medicine is defined as the maintenance and promotion of health and the reduction of risk factors that result in injury and disease. There are three main types of preventive medicine: primary prevention aims to prevent a disease from occurring (smoking cessation, diet modification); secondary prevention is the detection and treatment of asymptomatic disease before symptoms occur (antihypertensives, antilipidemics); and tertiary prevention deals with the consequences of existing disease or reduction of recurrent disease (bypass).

In 1997, cardiovascular disease (CHD) claimed nearly 1 million lives in the United States. In 1999, an estimated 1.1 million Americans had a coronary event. Of these, approx 650,000 were first events *(13)*, 25% of which presented as sudden death *(14)*. Recent evidence suggests that 12% of men and 8% of women over 45 yr of age have symptomatic CHD. In 1999, the total direct and indirect costs of CHD were estimated to be $326.6 billion *(13)*. Obviously, the goal is to reduce the incidence of coronary heart disease, not just its associated mortality. From a cost-effective standpoint alone, primary prevention is the most alluring. However, the benefits of preventive measures are often protracted. Among the American public, there is a general lack of perspective about the relative importance of preventive interventions. The public can be quick to embrace dietary supplements, miracle diets, and sophisticated screening tests without documented benefit, yet often ignore basic health behaviors known to be beneficial. Less than one in three adults consumes the recommended five servings of fruits and vegetables daily, 60% of the US population performs no regular physical activity, and 23% of the population smokes cigarettes *(11)*.

Other than the reliance on the effort of the patient, primary preventive practices face other barriers to widespread adoption. First, although evidence suggests that providing preventative services for Medicare beneficiaries would result in a modest health benefit with no additional cost *(11)*, reimbursement for primary preventive services is generally poor. The reasons for this are multifold. Most prominently, outcome data are difficult to demonstrate. Success is essentially a "non-event." For example, it is easier to recognize the effect of an antibiotic on an infection but much more difficult to document that a premature myocardial infarction was avoided because of diet and exercise counseling. Second, most benefits from primary prevention are seen only after a long period of time. Such up-front investment in the future is not enticing to insurance companies who issue short-term policies or to companies with high employee turnover rates. Finally, the training of physicians often emphasizes urgency of acute problems over chronic problems, encouraging doctors to respond to current problems rather than initiate preventive measures.

As a result, less than 5% of total annual health care expenditures in the United States is spent on primary prevention *(11)*. Far more of our health care dollars are spent on secondary and tertiary prevention; this is particularly true for coronary heart disease resulting from the proliferation of new medicines and the randomized controlled trials proving their benefit. Data from Framingham, the Multiple Risk Factor Intervention Trial, AFCAPS/TexCAPS, and WOSCOP have all shown a relative risk reduction of CHD when cholesterol levels are controlled. Multiple studies, from the SHEP trial to ALLHAT, have done the same for the management of hypertension. Despite convincing data and proven benefits, there are huge budgetary constraints on secondary prevention, and adding prescription drug plans to health benefit packages is a hot topic that brings us back to that familiar question: will health care budgets accommodate advancing technology at rising costs?

Science and technology do nothing to resolve the conflict of who pays. This conflict overshadows the entire sequence of preventive activities, from screening and risk assessment to the choice between lifestyle changes and medication, straight through to the prevention of recurrence. Although cardiovascular morbidity and mortality are problems that are predominantly associated with old age, national and international guidelines for the management of hypertension have only recently begun to include guidance that is specifically directed at the elderly or "very old" segment of the hypertensive population. Whether past neglect was a symptom of "ageism" or merely an assumption that hypertension and cardiovascular disease were conditions of old age anyway and therefore did not merit an age focus is unclear. What matters is that the special needs and problems of the elderly are now being included in guidelines.

The 1999 Guidelines of WHO (World Health Organization) International Society of Hypertension devoted a section to the "very elderly" and drew attention to the fact that there is presently very little evidence to support the health impact of anti-hypertensive treatment on patients over the age of 80. Up to that age, benefits and safety do not differ significantly between younger and older patients, "although the absolute effects are typically greater in older individuals because of their higher risk of cardiovascular events" (Guidelines Subcommittee 5, 1999). The Subcommittee considers the value of antihypertensive treatment of the over-80s as "uncertain," pending the results of new clinical trials including the very old. The absence of such evidence in today's sophisticated health care systems is both incomprehensible and inexcusable. Considering the fact that the over-85s are the fastest-growing segment of the population in the industrialized world (15), the sooner evidence is produced, the better.

The same can be said of cholesterol control. There is no evidence to suggest that atherosclerosis presents differently in the elderly. The WOSCOP trial was performed in men up to the age of 64. AFCAPS included men and women up to the age of 73. Both trials showed similar reductions with cholesterol-lowering drug therapy in all age groups studied. No outcome data exist for prevention in persons older than 73 on admission to a trial and no data are available for the very elderly. However, the Scandinavian Simvastatin Survival Study showed that the cost of a year of life gained decreased with age. Because CHD prevalence increases with age, the absolute risk reduction may be higher in the elderly than that demonstrated in the younger individuals who were included in published studies.

If primary prevention is successful, the incidence of a disease decreases. In contrast, secondary prevention does not necessarily prevent disease but, rather, delays the onset of deleterious effects. Realistically, despite our best efforts at behavior modification and medical management, coronary heart disease will likely continue to be the leading cause of death in the United States. Tertiary prevention corresponds with conventional medical care in that it can be considered treatment for an established condition. In the cardiac patient, tertiary prevention includes surgery, bypass grafting, angioplasty, and coronary care unit admissions for patients with acute events or exacerbation of chronic conditions.

Tertiary interventions, like coronary artery bypass grafting (CABG), represents a good value per QALY for younger patients, but the procedures are very costly, which warrants attention from policy-makers and economists with a special focus on whether these surgeries are cost-effective in the elderly population. The decision to provide tertiary intervention to this age group should be based on the same criteria used to make the determination in other age segments. In short, the decision that CABG should be performed in seniors depends primarily on three criteria: efficacy, effectiveness, and cost-effectiveness *(16)*. There are relatively little formal data on the use of surgical intervention in the elderly, because historically they have been considered poor surgical candidates; however, improved surgical practices and better overall health among the aging population have started to change this perception. Data are emerging that show elderly patients with coronary artery disease who undergo the surgery live longer and enjoy a better quality of life than those who are "medically managed" with drugs *(17)*. Since the mid-1980s, the number of bypass operations performed on octogenarians has increased more than 15% a year and is expected to increase even faster as the population ages and surgical techniques improve. Researchers estimate that more than 30,000 bypass surgeries will be performed on those 80 and older by the year 2050, at a cost exceeding $1.2 billion *(17)*.

With such a high cost burden, cost-effectiveness is a crucial determination. Researchers estimate that octogenarians who undergo the surgery have an average of 10.9 more years to live. The total average cost of surgery for the group they studied was $45,000. Assuming the cost of the procedure and postoperative course to be as high as $60,000, the cost per year of life saved would be roughly $5500. Because the benchmark for "cost-effectiveness" is $50,000 per year of life saved, the surgery seems to be an effective intervention *(17)*. No one would argue that preventive efforts should focus on preventing surgery-requiring conditions from developing, but with new data suggesting both efficiency and effectiveness as well as growing numbers and political influence among the older demographics, it will be increasingly more difficult to argue against surgical intervention in this age group when warranted.

BOOM OR BUST:
HEALTH CARE IN THE NEXT CENTURY

The health care system in which we currently work emerged fewer than 50 yr ago. The Medicare and Medicaid programs are barely 35 yr old, and managed care only became a significant force less than 10 yr ago. Given the brief history of the nation's health care system, the constancy of change is not surprising. We have yet to devise a solution that will ease the struggle we have encountered with advancing technology, new health care management approaches, and the perception that no matter how the numbers are crunched, there does not seem to be enough to provide everyone with the highest level of care.

The US population is both growing older and becoming more ethnically diverse. These demographic trends, especially as they relate to the "baby-boom" generation (i.e., Americans born between 1946 and 1964), will have a profound effect on the future of health care delivery. The health care industry must plan for the anticipated health care needs of the baby boomers, the fastest-growing segment of the population, as they age. Just as this cohort has transformed the workplace and government, as the boomers age and increasingly interact with the health care system, their expectations and preferences will also inevitably transform the health care industry.

The involvement of these patients in their own care may be significantly different from that of past generations of older Americans. They may accelerate the move toward self-care and wellness, dramatically changing the physician–patient relationship. With advances in health and medical technologies, boomers will experience extended longevity and may lead more active and productive lives rather than simply retiring at what is considered to be a traditional retirement age.

The full impact of the aging population will not be evident until after 2010, when the initial group of boomers reach retirement age. Indeed, it will not be until 2030, when the youngest members of the cohort reach 65 and the entire boomer population's health care will be subsidized by Medicare, that the nation's health and welfare system is expected to experience the actual social and economic impact of this large cohort.

Along with this demographic shift, the burden of disease is shifting toward chronic illnesses that emanate from our behaviors. It is projected that by the year 2010, the average life expectancy will be 86 yr for women and 76 yr for men *(18)*. Many chronic illnesses, such as cardiovascular disease, most frequently occur in the later years of life. Increases in life expectancy and the proportion of elderly people will be accompanied by an increased prevalence of chronic disease, which will need chronic management. More than ever, the expense of prescriptive medications will need to be addressed.

In 1999, the average Medicare beneficiaries spent nearly $400 out of pocket on drugs. Seniors who cannot afford to pay for their medications often neither fill the necessary prescriptions nor take their medicines irregularly. The consequences can be dangerous or even deadly. Original Medicare does not cover the cost of prescription drugs outside of the hospital, which means that more than one-third of Medicare beneficiaries lack coverage for outpatient prescriptions. The coverage gap will only grow wider as drugs grow more expensive and more important in treating the ills of old age. Drugs are more expensive in the United States than they are in any other industrialized nation because we have fragmented our purchasers so extensively. The Veteran's Administration and large HMOs pay substantially less for prescription drugs than do Medicare beneficiaries, who pay retail. Exorbitant costs paid by the American public subsidize the drugs consumed in Canada and Europe, where regulation of costs is tighter. Furthermore, the amount of money that pharmaceutical companies are spending in direct-to-consumer marketing is costing billions per year, taking therapeutic choice out of the hands of the physician and driving up both consumer demand—often without medical indications—and costs. America is the only industrialized nation with a free market for pharmaceuticals and without government restraints on drug prices. Although this is, in part, meant to provide the capital needed for innovation, it is obvious that the application of innovation will be hindered if the cost is prohibitory.

The cost of prescriptions is just one of many issues policymakers will have to tackle as they begin to address the health care needs of the growing number of elderly Americans. We will need to commit more resources to research into the diseases of aging, train more health care professionals to understand the needs of this population, make disease prevention a national priority, orient the health care system's incentives toward healthy aging, make more provisions for long-term care, correct the depletion of Medicare's Hospital Insurance Trust Fund, and establish a more humane and cost-effective approach to death and dying *(19)*.

GLOSSARY

Adjusted average per capita cost (AAPCC): The basis for HMO or Clinical Management Program (CMP) reimbursement under Medicare-risk contracts. The average monthly amount received per enrollee is currently calculated as 95% of the average costs to deliver medical care in the fee-for-service sector.

All-payer system: A system in which prices for health services and payment methods are the same, regardless of who is paying. Establishing a uniform fee bars providers from shifting costs from one payer to another.

Assignment: A process in which a Medicare beneficiary agrees to have Medicare's share of the cost of a service paid directly (assigned) to a doctor or other provider and the provider agrees to accept the Medicare-approved charge as payment in full. Medicare pays 80% of the cost and the beneficiary 20%.

Balance billing: In Medicare and private health insurance, the practice of billing patients for charges that exceed the amount that the health plan will pay. Under Medicare, the excess amount cannot be more than 15% above the approved charge.

Capitation: A method of payment for health services in which an individual or institutional provider is paid a fixed amount for each person served without regard to the actual number of nature of services provided.

Cost analysis: The direct budgetary costs to health agencies.

Cost–benefit analysis: An analytic method in which a program's cost is compared to the program's benefit for a period of time, expressed in dollars, as an aid in determining the best investment of resources.

Cost-effective analysis: A form of analysis that seeks to determine the costs and effectiveness of a medical intervention compared to similar alternative interventions to determine the relative degree to which they will obtain the desired health outcome(s). Measures output in terms of health gains (not monetary).

Cost–utility analysis: A form of analysis that measures changes in quality of life and takes into account the patient's perspective of personal quality of life.

Diagnosis Related Groups (DRGs): Groupings of diagnostic categories drawn from the International Classification of Diseases and modified by the presence of surgical procedure, patient age, comorbidities, complications, and other relevant criteria. DRGs are the case-mix measure used in Medicare's prospective payment system.

Effectiveness: A measure of the increased health benefit provided by a program or treatment.

Efficacy: The extent to which a speicific intervention, procedure, regime, or service produces a beneficial result under ideal conditions.

Efficiency: Delivering an effective intervention at the lowest possible cost.

Medicare + Choice: A Medicare program established by the 1997 Balanced Budget Act, it allows Center for Medicare and Medicaid Services (CMS) to contract with a variety of different managed care and fee-for-service entities offering greater flexibility to Medicare participants.

Medigap policy: A private health insurance policy offered to Medicare beneficiaries to cover expenses not paid for by Medicare. Medigap policies are strictly regulated by the federal government. Same as Medicare supplemental definitions are those of the Academy for Health Services Research and Health Policy.

REFERENCES

1. Cunningham R III. The Blues: A History of the Blue Cross and Blue Shield System. Northern Illinois University Press, DeKalb, IL, 1997.
2. Kuttner R. The American health care system: Wall Street and healthcare. N Engl J Med 1999;340: 664–668.
3. Yelowitz AS. Public policy and health insurance choices of the elderly. J Public Econ 2000;78:301–324.
4. Hurd MD, McGarry K. Medical insurance and the use of health care services by the elderly. J Health Econ 1997;16:129–154.
5. Brown RL. Social Security: regressive or progressive? North Am Actuarial J 1999;2:1–26.
6. Sorrentino MJ. Cholesterol reduction to prevent CAD. Postgrad Med 2000;108:40–52.
7. Veatch RM. Justice, the basic social contract and health care. In: Beauchamp TL, Walters L, eds. Contemporary Issues in Bioethics. Wadsworth, New York, 1994.
8. Johannesson M. A note on the depreciation of the societal perspective in economic evaluation of health care. Health Policy 1995;33:59–66.
9. Lohr KN, Eleazer K, Mauskopf J. Health policy issues and applications for evidence-based medicine and clinical practice guidelines. Health Policy 1998;46:1–19.
10. Healthy People 2000: National Health Promotion and Disease Prevention Objectives. US Government Printing Office, Washington, DC, 1991.
11. Hensrud DD. Clinical preventative medicine in primary care. Mayo Clin Proc 2000;75:165–172.
12. Goldman L, Cook EF. The decline in ischemic heart disease mortality rates: an analysis of the comparative effects of medical intervention and changes in lifestyle. Ann Intern Med 1984;101:825–836.
13. 2000 Heart and Stroke Statistical Update. American Heart Association, 1999.
14. Castelli W. Epidemiology of coronary heart disease: the Framingham study. Am J Med 1984;76:4.
15. Hobbs F, Damon B. 65+ in the United States. US Government Printing Office, Washington, DC, 2000.
16. Detsky AS, Naglie IG. A clinician's guide to cost-effectiveness analysis. Ann Intern Med 1990;113:147–154.
17. Sollano JA, Rose EA, Williams DL, et al. Cost-effectiveness of coronary artery bypass surgery in octogenarians. Ann Surg 1998;228:297–306.
18. Older Americans 2000: Key Indicators of Well-Being. Federal Interagency Forum on Age-Related Statistics. US Government Printing Office, Washington, DC, 1999.
19. Mechanic D. The changing elderly population and future healthcare needs. J Urban Health 1999;76: 24–38.

II   FUNDAMENTALS
OF CARING FOR THE ELDERLY

3

Nutritional Needs of the Elderly

Ashley S. Im, MS, MPH, Patrick Archdeacon, MD, and David H. Chong, MD

CONTENTS

NUTRITION AND ITS IMPORTANCE IN CHRONIC DISEASES

As the size and diversity of the elderly population increase, nutrition issues particular to this cohort assume greater significance *(1,2)*. Nutrition plays an important role in aging, which is associated with the progressive decline in energy, lean body mass, and protein intake *(3)*. A variety of physiological, psychological, economic, and social changes accompany aging that can adversely affect nutritional status. The risk of serious specific nutritional deficiencies and generalized malnutrition increases with age. Functional dependency, morbidity, mortality, and utilization of health care resources all increase with the presence of malnutrition *(4)*. Elderly individuals also demonstrate a higher prevalence of chronic disease than younger people *(5)*.

From: *Aging, Heart Disease, and Its Management: Facts and Controversies*
Edited by: N. Edwards, M. Maurer, and R. Wellner © Humana Press Inc., Totowa, NJ

There are a series of chronic diseases that are more prevalent in the elderly and are related to nutritional status and overall dietary consumption patterns. Coronary heart disease (CHD) is the number one cause of death in the United States, claiming the lives of 126.6 persons per 100,000 population *(6)*. The incidence of CHD is linked to the excess consumption of saturated fat, trans-fatty acids, cholesterol, sodium, and animal protein *(6)*. Truncal distribution of body fat and obesity also magnify the risk for coronary heart disease *(6)*. Cancer is the number two cause of death in the United States, with a cause-specific mortality rate of 123.6 persons per 100,000 population *(5)*. The incidence of cancer appears to be associated with the excess consumption of calories from fat, alcohol, red meat, nitrite-preserved meats, possibly grilled meats, and an abdominal distribution of body fat *(5,7)*. Osteoporosis afflicts more than 28 million Americans, of which 80% are women. In the United States, 10 million individuals already have the disease and 18 million more have low bone mass, which increases their risk for developing osteoporosis *(1,8)*. Excess intake of sodium, phosphorus, and protein, coupled with the inadequate intake of calcium and vitamin D, contributes to the pathogenesis of osteoporosis *(6)*.

Diabetes mellitus affects approx 18 million new persons in the United States each year. Dietary behaviors that exacerbate the disease include high caloric intake in the form of sugar, simple carbohydrate, fat, and alcohol *(6)*. Both poor choices in dietary consumption patterns and poor compliance with medical directives regarding diet and medications lead to an increased incidence of diabetes and diabetic complications in the elderly *(9)*. The exact etiology of diabetes mellitus is unknown and involves a complex interaction of genetic and environmental factors. About 39.4 million American adults are obese, with a body mass index (BMI) ≥ 30 *(10)*, and obesity is associated with the excess consumption of calories and fat *(6)*. Obese individuals are at a higher risk for coronary heart disease, diabetes, and hypertension than their non-obese counterparts.

CHANGE IN ENERGY REQUIREMENTS
AND METABOLISM WITH AGE

Both cross-sectional and longitudinal studies conducted on human subjects have demonstrated a decline in energy requirements associated with aging *(3)*. The Baltimore Longitudinal Study of Aging showed that energy intake of a sample of male subjects decreased from 2700 kcal/d at age 30 to 2100 kcal/d by age 80. Two-thirds of this reduction was attributable to a decrease in physical activity, and the rest is the result of decreased basal metabolism *(11)*. NHANES (National Health and Nutrition Examination Survey) III showed similar results. Young men and women between the ages of 20 and 29 consumed 3025 and 1959 kcal, men and women between the ages of 50 and 59 consumed 2240 and 1629 kcal, and those men and women over 80 yr or older consumed 1776 and 1329 kcal, respectively *(12)*. Thus, both a decrease in basal metabolic rate, largely the result of decline in metabolically active lean body mass, and a decrease in physical activity contribute to a decreased energy requirement with advancing age *(5)*.

The basal metabolic rate decreases almost linearly with age, concordant with a decrease in the volume of skeletal musculature and an increase in the percentage of fat tissue. Skeletal musculature consumes the largest portion of the energy produced. A decrease in lean body mass reduces basal metabolic rate by 1–2% per decade from age 20 to 75 *(13)*. The decrease in muscle mass relative to total-body mass along with atrophic changes of skeletal muscle secondary to physical inactivity may be responsible for the age-related decreases in basal metabolic rate *(14)*. Generally, this is the equivalent of a decrement in energy requirements of 20% over the life-span *(13)*.

Glucose tolerance decreases with age. Although age contributes independently to the deterioration in glucose tolerance, the decrease in glucose tolerance may be partly prevented through changes in lifestyle variables such as dietary habits, nutrition, and physical activity *(14)*. In the elderly, body fat tends to accumulate in the abdomen, a major consequence of which is a disturbance in both glucose and lipid metabolism *(14)*. With the concomitant decrease in energy requirements, there is a decrease in energy intake and a resultant decline in the intake of essential nutrients as well *(15)*. When energy intake exceeds individual energy needs, fat accumulates in the body *(14,15)*.

INTAKE

The elderly generally consume less and choose different foods than younger patients. Older adults tend to consume less calorie-dense sweets and fast-food and consume more calorie-dilute grains, vegetables, and fruits. Daily volume of food and beverages also declines as a function of age *(16)*. Low calorie intake and low nutrient density in the diet increases the risk of illnesses related to dietary deficiencies and can easily pose a serious health problem. Several factors may influence this observed decline in calorie intake. With increasing age, the senses of taste, smell, sight, hearing, and touch diminish. The onset of taste and olfactory dysfunction occurs at approximately age 60, increasing in intensity after the age of 70 *(17,18)*. Sensitivity to foods that are salty or sweet decreases with age, a change in sensory stimulation that may impair many physiologic processes. Taste and smell, in addition to increasing plasma insulin levels, induce other metabolic changes such as the stimulation of salivary, gastric acid, and pancreatic secretion *(4,19)*. Consequently, changes in gustatory and auditory sensory perception that occur with age can influence a variety of physiologic processes.

Furthermore, hearing loss, impaired vision, and loss of coordination are quite prevalent in elderly persons, possibly leading to decreased food intake because of diminished appetite, problems with food recognition, and the inability to feed oneself *(17,18)*. Because older people exhibit reduced energy requirements, satiety often occurs more readily than in younger people, and they generally seem less hungry *(20)*. Additionally, medical conditions and medications can impair the ability to recognize sweet, salty, sour, and bitter tastes *(17, 18)*. From 1994 to 1996, the majority of older persons in the United States either reported poor diets or stated that they needed improvement in their diet, which indicates that older persons would benefit from better nutritional guidance *(13)*. However, although the Recommended Daily Allowance (RDA) for calories in men and women age 51 or older is 126 kJ/ kg/d (30 kcal/kg/d), it is not stratified for age groups above the age of 51 yr to account for age-related changes *(17)*. Therefore, within the last few years, the Food and Nutritional Board standing committee on the scientific evaluation replaced RDA with dietary reference intakes (DRIs). DRI has divided older persons into those between the ages of 51 and 70 yr and those older than 70 yr for the purpose of establishing intake recommendations. However, to date, the defined DRI values in each age range have been identical to RDA, except for vitamin D, for which the level increased from 10 to 15 µg daily above age 70 *(5)*. The general caloric intake is approx 1800 kcal/d, which will provide adequate amounts of protein, calcium, iron, and vitamins—nutrient-dense food *(17)*. Table 1 shows the caloric amounts of macronutrients, carbohydrates, proteins, and fats needed for a person consum-

Table 1
Minimum Caloric Requirements for Persons 51+ Yr of Age

	Approximate caloric requirement using 1800 kcal as minimum requirement (17)
Carbohydrate (55–60%)	990–1080 kcal
Protein (14–16%) *(1)*	252–288 kcal
Fat (less than 30%)	<540 kcal

Note: Estimates are based on a 1800-kcal/d diet.
Source: ref. *17.*

ing 1800 kcal/d. Because the data on nutrient requirements for older adults are limited, the dietary guidelines have not been stratified by age to account for the dietary and nutrient needs of the growing population of elderly adults in separate groups age groups of 65–74, 75–84, and 85+ *(5).* Presently, lack of data on individuals comprising these older age groups has limited the ability to set specific guidelines for calorie requirements in this population.

CARBOHYDRATES

Currently, there is no set recommended dietary carbohydrate intake for the elderly. In general, the greatest health benefit is derived from consuming foods with a low glycemic index and high non-starch polysaccharide (fiber) content. At least 200 g of carbohydrates per day is required to sustain normal brain metabolism and muscle function in healthy, moderately active adults *(22).* Current recommendations include increasing complex carbohydrates to at least 55% of total calories, which also improves the intake of vitamins, minerals, and fiber *(23).* In middle-aged and elderly people, higher intake of carbohydrates can have a deleterious effect on blood lipids. Higher intake is only appropriate for persons engaging in a high level of physical activity who need to maintain muscle glycogen content.

In the elderly, meals with a high carbohydrate content can lead to problems of post-prandial hypotension and impaired exercise capacity in patients with angina *(22).* A reduced glucose tolerance makes the elderly more susceptible to temporary hypoglycemia, hyperglycemia, and non-insulin-dependent diabetes mellitus. To improve insulin sensitivity, use of sugar should be reduced, and the amount of complex carbohydrate and soluble fiber in the diet should be increased *(17).* Moreover, with increasing age, there is diminished lactase secretion, which can lead to lactose intolerance *(17).*

PROTEIN

With age, catabolism and synthesis rates of protein are decreased. Although the optimal amount of protein in the diet is not yet known, a recommendation is 0.8–1.0 g/kg/d, which is about 14–16% of daily caloric intake *(1).* Total-body protein in the healthy elderly is 60–70% that of young adults, which might suggest a decreased need for dietary protein. However, the need for protein among elderly still remains the same as for young adults (0.8–1.0 g/kg) *(17).* The dietary protein is closely associated with dietary energy intake; therefore, elderly persons with low dietary energy intake are at risk for insufficient protein intake *(17)*. Protein-calorie malnutrition includes symptoms of edema, pruritis, chronic eczema, fatigue, muscle weakness, and tissue wasting.

Protein deficiency is unlikely to occur in persons without debilitating disease. Types of chronic disease causing protein deficiency include infection, altered gastrointestinal function, and metabolic changes, all of which can reduce the efficiency of dietary nitrogen utilization *(17)*. Protein requirements increase in relation to the severity and duration of the disease.

FATS

The recommendation for reducing dietary fat is to decrease levels to no more than 30% of the total kilocalories *(17)*. Reducing total dietary fat, especially the amount of saturated fat and cholesterol, can lower blood cholesterol level and subsequent risk of heart disease *(17)*. The Baltimore Longitudinal Study of Aging showed that aging negatively impacted the intake of calories, fat, saturated fatty acids, and cholesterol. Studies showed that the intake of carbohydrates and cholesterol declined, whereas the intake of polyunsaturated fatty acids increased with time *(24)*.

VITAMINS

Vitamin requirements for the elderly are similar to those for the young with the exception of vitamins C, D, and B *(18)*. Vitamin C is an antioxidant that may play a role in cataract prevention *(25)*. Vitamin C intake, blood levels, and tissue levels can be low in the elderly, particular in those who either smoke or are subject to stress *(26)*. Vitamin C deficiency often presents with lassitude and fatigue. Capillary hemorrhage, bleeding from the gums, and delayed wound healing are frequent complaints in elderly who are vitamin C deficient. Intake of vitamin B_6 and folic acid in this age group is often less than two-thirds of the recommended amount for younger patients. A diet lacking in fresh, nutrient-dense foods is the most common cause of low folate levels in the non-alcoholic elderly *(17,26)*. Lower levels of $1,25 (OH)_2D_3$, the active form of 25-hydroxyvitamin D, are likely associated with both a decreased capacity of the aging kidney to convert vitamin D and a decline in skin thickness, which occurs with advancing age *(27)*. Moreover, inadequate vitamin D and calcium intake is associated with osteoporosis and osteomalacia *(17)*. Vitamin B_{12} deficiency is seen among older people as a result of either a loss of gastric intrinsic factor or hypochlorhydria/achlorhydria, which leads to pernicious anemia resulting from cobalamin malabsorption. Patients with either of these conditions may require a higher level of dietary vitamin B_{12} than the current RDA *(28)*.

There is no evidence of vitamin A deficiency among older persons. Studies of plasma retinal levels demonstrate adequate vitamin A and that these levels are sustained throughout life *(24)*. In fact, older persons taking vitamin supplements should be cognizant of hypervitaminosis A *(27)*. Vitamin E is an antioxidant that has been demonstrated to slow the aging process in animals but the data cannot be extrapolated to humans *(18)*.

ANTI-AGING ANTIOXIDANTS

Antioxidants such as vitamin A, C, and E as well as selenium are very popular in today's society as possible remedies to slow down the aging process. Thus, they may be referred to as "anti-aging" substances *(18,24,27)*. The etiology of aging is still unknown, but there are several theories that may explain why aging occurs. One theory that may elucidate the etiology of aging is the theory of free radicals (FRs) *(19,28,29)*. FRs are the substances generated constantly in living cells that lead to series of changes in the body linked to aging *(28)*. FRs are oxidizing substances that the organs and systems of the body react to in various ways and change their mechanisms because of the damage caused by FRs. FRs damage tissue through membrane lipid peroxidation, oxidation of proteins and carbohydrates, and abnormal DNA crosslinking *(28)*. The production and action of the FRs have been associated with general aging process. The substances known as antioxidants (AO) counterbalance the detrimental effects of FRs and represent an important defense against these FRs as well as show some anti-aging properties and specific protective functions for some diseases such as cancer *(28)*.

Because antioxidants are considered anti-aging substances, toxic amounts of these substances may be consumed. Hypervitaminosis A is an intake of retinoids greatly in excess of requirements and results in a toxic condition. A daily intake of more than 7.5 mg (about 30,000 IU) of retinal is not advised, and chronic use of amounts over 20 mg (100,000 IU) can result in dry, itchy skin, erythematous dermatitis, hair loss, joint pain, chapped lips, hyperostosis, headaches, anorexia, edema, and fatigue *(24)*. A dosage over 2000 mg of vitamin C per day may cause diarrhea, false-negative occult blood tests, and oxalate stones in the bladder and kidney *(25,26)*. Vitamin E is unlike other fat-soluble vitamins because the studies have failed to show a toxic dosage level, but a high dosage of vitamin E does interfere with vitamin K metabolism—increasing clotting time and interfering with arachidonic acid and prostaglandin metabolism, impairing immune function, increasing sepsis, and impairing wound healing in infants treated with high doses *(18)*. There is a growing concern over selenium toxicity—supplementation above 500 μg/d may cause toxicity *(19)*. Previous studies noted that individuals who consumed 1 mg of selenium for 2 yr experienced nail changes and garlic odor to his/her breath *(19)*. However, the elderly population is at risk of antioxidant deficiency as a result of decreased intake, inefficient absorption, diminished retention or storage capacity, or increased elimination. Because many elderly people do take supplementation without consultation of a doctor, toxic levels of these antioxidants may occur *(19)*. More studies need to be conducted to establish nutritional status, requirements, and needs of the elderly *(18)*.

SALT AND RELATED MINERALS

The Baltimore Longitudinal Study of Aging showed that 40% of men and about 50% of women consumed less than two-thirds of the recommended daily allowance of vitamins and minerals. As a result, even healthy-appearing, well-educated individuals failed to consume adequate quantities of calcium, iron, magnesium, and zinc; this was demonstrated both in individuals relying strictly upon a dietary supply of nutrients and in those taking nutritional supplements *(30)*. Various minerals serve essential roles as cofactors in enzymatic processes; they are summarized in Table 2.

It was generally presumed that malabsorption of both macronutrients and micronutrients occurred as a result of "normal" aging. This presumption has since been challenged; malabsorption of macronutrients in the elderly occurs as a consequence of disease and not of age *(33)*. For example, malabsorption may be the result of atrophic gastritis, the incidence of which increases with age and afflicts between 24% and 50% of persons over

Table 2
Trends in Essential Mineral Levels with Age

Mineral	Levels with age	Comments
Chromium	Decreases	Chromium is required to counter an increase in glucose intolerance, which tends to occur with age (27).
Calcium	Decreases	Bone loss secondary to both osteoporosis and hypochlorhydria, which causes malabsorption of certain minerals, increases the demand for a higher calcium intake (24).
Iron	Stable	Iron deficiency is not a consequence of "normal" aging. If iron-deficiency anemia is present in the elderly, suspect blood loss, often from the gastrointestinal tract. Medical attention is frequently required (32).
Zinc	Decreases	Decreased calorie intake is associated with low levels of zinc. Low plasma zinc concentration has been identified in 27% of the elderly population. Zinc deficiency is associated with impaired immune function, anorexia, delayed wound healing, and pressure sore development (31).

age 60 (29). The physiological effects of atrophic gastritis are manifest by an increased stomach pH and bacterial overgrowth of the small intestine. This can alter vitamin B_{12} absorption from the gut, potentially resulting in pernicious anemia (29). Similarly, iron deficiency is not a consequence of "normal" aging. If iron-deficiency anemia is present in the elderly, suspect blood loss, often from the gastrointestinal tract. Medical attention is frequently required (32).

Because hypertension is common in elderly individuals, recommendations include reducing sodium intake to 2–4 g/d and supplementing the diet with magnesium and potassium if on diuretics (17). Intestinal absorption of calcium decreases with age in both men and women. This may be the result of changes in several transport processes.

FLUID INTAKE

Daily fluid intake for adults is about 30 mL of water per kilogram of body weight (approx 1 mL/kcal of energy) (34). The average sedentary adult male must consume at least 2900 mL of fluid daily and the average sedentary adult female must consume at least 2200 mL of fluid daily in the form of noncaffeine, nonalcoholic beverages, soups, and food (34). About 1000 mL of water is consumed in a form of solid food (27). Dehydration is the most common cause of fluid and electrolyte disturbances in the elderly (35). Reduced thirst sensation and diminished water conservation by kidneys are important contributing factors (17,18). Metabolic stress, such as an infection, can cause dehydration by increasing fluid requirements and impairing intake (17). Dehydration can cause constipation or renal stone diseases among the elderly (17). Also, the elderly should be careful when taking laxatives and diuretics because they deplete fluids rapidly (17,18).

ADDITIONAL FACTORS
INFLUENCING NUTRITION IN THE ELDERLY

Many socio-economic and psychosocial factors specific to older individuals influence the nutritional status of this population. Food selection in the healthy elderly is affected by lifestyle, food supply, and recommendations related to diet and comorbid disease. Elderly individuals are particularly susceptible to experiencing loneliness, depression, economic concerns, frailty, and fatigue. They may also lack the dexterity for independent meal preparation. The significant number of older men and women who consume less food than required to meet energy and nutrient requirements is attributable to a combination of these and other factors *(19)*.

Socio-Economic Factors

The economic status of older people has improved over the past few decades, but major disparities are still apparent. About 11% of Americans 65 yr and older and 14% of persons age 85 and over are living below the poverty level. Characteristics associated with poverty include female gender, being unmarried, minority ethnicity, and being a female living alone. In 1998, about 19% of white older women who lived alone did so in poverty; this percentage was approx 50% for older black and Hispanic women living alone *(21)*. Social Security provides 80% of the income for elderly individuals in the lowest income bracket. In 1999, the average net worth of a household headed by an older white person was $181,000 compared to the $13,000 net worth of a household headed by an older black person *(21)*. Elderly individuals living in poverty have greater difficulty obtaining fresh, nutrient-dense foods to meet their nutritional requirements. As a result, they experience food insecurity and fail to consume sufficient calories, the consequences of which include chronic fatigue, depression, and a weakened immune system *(13)*. Food insecurity is defined as the loss of ability to acquire nutrient-dense food because of low socio-economic status *(13)*. Food-insecure elderly persons had a worse nutritional and health status as compared to the food-secure; this was consistent across three datasets, the Third National Health and Nutrition Examination Survey (1988–1994), the Nutrition Survey of the Elderly in New York State (1994), and the Longitudinal Study of Aging (1984–1990) *(36)*.

Psychosocial Factors

Because of their relatively longer life expectancies, older women are more likely to live alone than older men. In 1998, about 41% of older women lived alone, compared to 17% of the men *(21)*. Living arrangements among older women also vary by race. Approximately 41% of older white and black women, 27% of older Hispanic women, and 21% of older Asian and Pacific Islanders lived alone. The percentage of women older than 75 living alone increased from 37% in 1970 to 53% in 1998 *(21)*. Older persons typically do not live alone voluntarily; rather, living alone is often the consequence of spousal death, which also causes bereavement and depression *(37)*.

Depression is diagnosed in about 5% of people age 65 or older and is considered to be the most prevalent mental disorder affecting this age group. Because depressive symptoms may mimic those of dementia, many researchers stipulate that 5% is an underestimate *(38)*. Depressive symptoms include feelings of worthlessness, hopelessness, helplessness, inappropriate guilt, prolonged sadness or unexplained crying spells, jumpiness or irritability, poor concentration, anhedonia, withdrawal from family and friends, impaired social and work relationships, loss or increase in appetite, and loss of sexual interest. Persistent fatigue and lethargy also tend to occur, as does either insomnia or markedly increased sleeping. Depression may result from loss of a spouse. These elderly experience social isolation and often their depression may go unnoticed *(38)*. Disorganization and changes in daily routine, such as food preparation and eating occur and the psychological state may also worsen. Furthermore, aches, pains, constipation, and other physical ailments that cannot be explained organically in aging individuals can also manifest and most certainly contribute to poor oral intake *(38)*.

Oral Health

Nutrition directly impacts the dentition and thus the progression of tooth decay *(39)*. The rise in oral diseases, such as root and coronal decay in the elderly, results from a tendency for these individuals to retain more of their natural dentition. At least 60% of the elderly with teeth demonstrate decay of the root surface as well as recurrent decay around existing fillings. Untreated caries and periodontitis are major causes of tooth loss in the elderly, leading to edentulousness and the need for dentures *(40)*.

Oral manifestations of chronic diseases, such as xerostomia, medication side effects on the oral cavity, and tooth loss secondary to osteoporosis, occur more frequently in the elderly *(41)*. Xerostomia refers to a lack of salivation, a condition that affects more than 70% of the elderly and significantly alters nutrient intake *(42)*. Tooth loss and removable prostheses produce multiple negative effects, including poor eating habits, diet inadequacy, impaired masticatory function, as well as reduced sense of taste and overall gastrointestinal function *(43,44)*. Persons who wear dentures have been referred to as "oral invalids" *(39)*. Studies have shown that individuals wearing dentures have about one-sixth the chewing capacity of their dentate counterparts and generally take more drugs for gastrointestinal disorders (e.g., laxatives and antireflux agents) *(39,40,45)*. A reduced chewing capacity often leads to decreased consumption of meat, fresh fruits, and vegetables, which results in an inadequate intake of calories, iron, vitamin C, folate, and β-carotene *(43)*.

Media

The media greatly influences food choices for the elderly. Low-fat, low-cholesterol-diet messages are continuously advertised *(39,46)*. Because of concern regarding health risks for chronic diseases, many elderly individuals readily incorporate the strong fear of fat and cholesterol into their lives. Although dietary limitations on fat and cholesterol consumption are widely accepted as effective risk-reduction interventions in young and middle-aged adults, the appropriateness of such dietary restrictions on the overall health and well-being in older individuals is unknown. The suboptimal nutritional status of many older individuals is based on a lack of knowledge concerning a balanced diet. This is often complicated by a fear of certain foods and an overemphasis on single-nutrient issues *(46)*. Dietary diversity and variety promotes enjoyment and satisfaction with any particular diet *(5)*. The real issue that must be addressed is whether or not the current DRI levels for ages 51–70 and 70+ yr are appropriate for both the nutritional needs and health concerns of all the elderly *(46)*. The current DRI levels only stratify the aging groups into two: 51–70 and 70+ yr. However, within these two strata, the groups are not homogenous; and each age group specified by most gerontologist and geriatrics (51–64, 65–74, 75–84, 85+ yr) has different nutritional needs because of physiological and psychosocial changes in these groups. In light of the diverse nutritional needs based on the status of their health, as well as socio-economic and other factors mentioned, it is likely that a new approach is needed *(46)*.

MALNUTRITION AND THE CARDIAC PATIENT

Underlying comorbid disease states affect nutritional needs and can affect surgical outcomes. Postoperative organ dysfunction, gastrointestinal bleeding, prolonged ICU length of stay, an increased weaning time from mechanical ventilation, and death were more likely in patients with malnutrition (defined as a hypoalbuminemia), either alone or in association with chronic liver failure or congestive heart failure (CHF) *(47)*.

Many elderly patients undergoing cardiac surgery will experience malnutrition, the scope of which is unclear. Nutritional assessments of hospitalized patients have reported malnutrition rates as high as 50% *(48)*. Chronically ill elderly patients, at baseline, are inactive and have reduced cell mass (especially skeletal muscle); such patients are expected to have low energy requirements, but because of comorbid illnesses, they may actually have high metabolic demands *(44)*. Nutritional status is intricately linked to underlying disease processes. Cardiac cachexia, a term coined by Pittman and Cohen, is a form of malnutrition that results from heart failure *(49)*. Whereas malnutrition itself, especially in the form of protein deficiency, can be the cause of heart failure in both animals and humans, patients with congestive heart failure can become malnourished as a result of a number of different mechanisms *(50)*. Elevated venous pressure resulting in hepatic and gastrointestinal congestion can cause anorexia, diminished synthetic activity, protein-wasting nephropathy, and malabsorption *(51)*. The subsequent splanchnic congestion can also cause a protein-losing enteropathy, dyspepsia, as well as malabsorption *(52)*. Energy and caloric demands are usually increased in patients with congestive heart failure, which must be balanced carefully with fluid and sodium restriction. Thus, comorbid illnesses play a major role in determining the energy requirements for patients undergoing cardiac surgery.

COMORBIDITIES INFLUENCING NUTRITIONAL STATUS

The effects of diabetes on the nutritional status of cardiac surgery patients are complex. Glucose intolerance has increased in the general population over the past few decades. Nearly half of diabetics are aged 65 or older, making glycemic control an important issue in the elderly *(53)*. NHANES III revealed that age was not an independent risk factor for poor glycemic control, proving glucose-regulating interventions as effective in the elderly as in the young *(54)*. Aggressive glucose control may significantly reduce overall morbidity and mortality *(46,54,55)*. Evidence is now emerging that tighter individualized glucose control for surgical patients (80 mg/dL $\leq$ blood glucose $\leq$ 110 mg/dL) may significantly improve overall survival (as well as complications), particularly in critically ill patients *(56)*.

Gastrointestinal disorders such as inflammatory bowel disease and short-bowel syndrome are almost invariably associated with malnutrition *(57)*. The combination of a decreased intake of major nutrients, malabsorption of fat and vitamins, and protein-losing enteropathy produces weight loss *(57)*.

"Cancer cachexia" refers to the devastating nutritional sequelae of neoplastic disease and may be responsible for a significant percentage of prevalent malnutrition in elderly

(58). Cancer cachexia is believed to result from a host of tumor-induced cytokines, not the from tumor itself. Decreased nutrient intake secondary to loss of appetite, dysphagia, altered taste, and depression also contribute *(59)*.

There are multiple metabolic disturbances, including pancreatic dysfunction, liver disease, and renal failure, that result in a loss in body protein and fat mass and a gain in total-body water. Patient with pancreatitis often have abdominal pain, profound malabsorption, and malnutrition. Malnutrition can result directly from pancreatic inflammation. Pancreatitis patients are hypermetabolic, which is characterized by increased energy expenditure, proteolysis, gluconeogenesis, and insulin resistance *(60)*. The preferred timing, route, and composition of nutrients are still unclear. Despite the fact that the studies have failed to consistently show the impact of nutritional intervention on the natural history of pancreatitis, early enteral therapy is now encouraged for most patients *(60)*. Liver disease is associated with decreased protein synthesis, diminished anabolism, and low food intake. When dealing with the nutritional issues of patients with liver disease, particular attention should be paid to effective delivery of protein and fat and its relationship to fluid status and encephalopathy *(47)*. Guidelines call for the following: decreased protein, decreased fat nutrient delivery, strict limitations on fluids, and close monitoring of encephalopathy. Renal failure is a catabolic state with increased energy requirements. Less appreciated is the fact that vitamins and minerals, such as vitamin D, B_6, and C, calcium, and folate, are also deficient. End-stage renal disease patients on hemodialysis need to be maintained on high-calorie, high-protein, high-calcium, low-phosphate, low-volume, low-fat diets.

Finally, pulmonary disease can have a significant impact on the overall health of an elderly cardiac surgery patient. A diet high in fat calories and lower in calories from carbohydrates is recommended *(61)*. Such a diet will decrease both the patient's production of carbon dioxide and the overall demand on the work of breathing *(61)*. Unfortunately, the use of aggressive nutritional support along with anabolic steroids has yet to show a significant impact on overall patient outcome in clinical trials *(62)*. Nevertheless, nutritional support may significantly reduce the postoperative morbidity and mortality of elderly cardiac patients by improving postoperative wound healing, decreasing susceptibility to infection, and preventing the formation of decubitus ulcers *(58)*.

THERAPY

Feeding regimens emphasize repletion of calories, protein, and fat-soluble vitamins. Predigested and elemental formulas comprise the mainstays of enteral therapy.

Parenteral Nutrition

Elderly patients who fail to voluntarily consume adequate calories and/or protein should be considered candidates for enteral or parenteral feeding therapies. Parenteral nutrition should be used only if patients that cannot be fed enterally (e.g., those with necrotizing enterocolitis, short-bowel syndrome, gastrointestinal obstruction, hemorrhagic pancreatitis, and prolonged ileus) *(48)*. In the preoperative period, parenteral nutrition has only been shown to benefit severely malnourished patients fed 7–14 d prior to undergoing elective surgery *(58)*. In the postoperative period, noninfectious complications were reduced. However, patients with mild to moderate malnutrition did not benefit from parenteral nutrition secondary to the increased incidence of infection *(58)*. Benefit from short-term parenteral feeding has been demonstrated in select patient populations undergoing organ transplantation and suffering from major trauma *(44)*. In critically ill patients, postoperative patients, cancer patients, and chronically ill patients, parenteral nutrition has yet to show significant benefit and may even be harmful *(51,63)*. Total parenteral nutrition requires central venous access to accommodate the use of hypertonic solutions. The composition of the parenteral feeds depends on the calorie, fluid volume, protein, mineral, and vitamin requirements of the individual patient. Possible complications of central-line placement include pneumothorax, hemorrhage secondary to arterial puncture, hematoma at the insertion site, line-related vascular stenosis, thrombosis, and line infections. The use of aseptic technique, skin preparation with chlorhexidine, real-time ultrasound guidance, and antibiotic- and antiseptic-bonded catheters has been shown to decrease line-related complications *(64)*. Multiple randomized clinical trials have not shown the practice of routine line changes to be efficacious in decreasing the rate of line infections, but this practice may increase mechanical complication rates *(64–66)*. Elderly patients require close monitoring if placed on parenteral nutrition. Caution must be exercised in recognizing line infections, thrombosis, hyperglycemia, fluid overload, elevated liver function tests, and cholestasis *(47)*. In light of the aforementioned issues, the preferred route of feeding for most patients, including the elderly, is enteral.

Enteral

In hospitalized patients, weight loss of greater that 10% of pre-illness body weight or the inability to maintain adequate caloric and nutrient intake for 5–7 consecutive days should precipitate the use of nutrition-support therapies *(48)*. Benefits of enteral nutrition include the maintenance of bowel function, mucosal immunity and integrity, decreased infectious complications, lower cost, lower length of hospital stay, and improved overall outcomes *(47)*. The delivery of nutrition is best accomplished with a soft, small-diameter nasal feeding tube placed distal to the pylorus to minimize the risk of aspiration. If long-term feeding is considered, a percutaneous feeding-tube placement is indicated. Administration guidelines of all feeds must include the estimation of free-water needs. Basal free-water requirements are usually 1 cm^3/kcal. This estimate must be revised according to the clinical situation (i.e., diarrhea, fever, electrolyte imbalance).

Complications of enteral feeds include pulmonary aspiration with subsequent pneumonitis and pneumonia. Those at highest risk are patients with decreased level of consciousness, ventilator dependence, decreased gag reflex, gastric retention, and paralytic ileus *(67)*. Feed-related diarrhea is a common complication, occurring in 5–30% of patients *(67)*. Iatrogenic nasal skin necrosis and sinusitis secondary to excessive tape pressure should be avoided.

Types of Enteral Feeds

Feeding formulas are classified as general-use, high-calorie, high-nitrogen, fiber-enhanced, disease-specific, and elemental. Specific recommendations are beyond the scope of this review. Making decisions about what types of feeding to employ require a working knowledge of particular patient's needs and the clinical context in which the feeding is initiated. General-use formulas usually have approx 1 kcal/mL and 35–45 g/L of protein, with most of the calories derived from carbohydrates and fat. Highly stressed patients may require high-protein, calorie-dense feeds. Fiber-enhanced formulas aid in decreasing feed-related diarrhea. Patients who require less volume benefit from the calorie-dense formulas. The disease-specific formulas are more expensive and are tailored to disease-specific nutrient needs. Pulmonary and diabetic formulas rely upon fat as the major source of calories. In pulmonary patients, the reduced carbohydrate load decreases carbon dioxide production and work of breathing while delivering the high calories needed. In diabetics, decreased carbohydrates improve glucose control, ultimately either preventing or reducing diabetes-related complications. Hepatic formulas highlight the use of branch-chain amino acids and are low in aromatic amino acids in order reduce hepatic encephalopathy.

A number of formulas have been developed for critically ill patients. Some are enriched with glutamine, which, when added to enteral and parenteral feeds, has been shown to decrease infectious complications, reduce length of stay, and improve survival in major trauma and bone-marrow transplant patients *(68,69)*. Levels of glutamine, an energy source essential for the enterocyte, decrease in critical illness *(70)*. Sufficient glutamine levels are essential for adequate gut barrier function and the prevention of bacterial translocation *(71, 72)*. Although promising, immunonutrition is in its infancy *(73)*. Further study is needed to prove the efficacy and survival benefit of these new feeding therapies *(74)*.

CONCLUSIONS

Nutritional concerns can adversely impact health, function, and quality of life. Ongoing research efforts are needed to set new guidelines for the elderly, particularly those age 75 yr or older. Optimal nutrition promotes both functional health status and mental well-being.

REFERENCES

1. Hickler RB, Wayne KS. Nutrition and the elderly. Am Fam Physician 1984;29:137–145.
2. Leaf A. The aging process: lessons from observations in man. Nutr Rev 1988;46:40–44.
3. Harper EJ. Changing perspectives on aging and energy requirements: aging and energy intakes in humans, dogs and cats. J Nutr 1998;128:26,23S–26,26S.
4. McGee M, Jensen GL. Nutrition in the elderly. J Clin Gastroenterol 2000;30:372–380.
5. Drewnowski A, Warren-Mears VA. Does aging change nutrition requirements? J Nutr Health Aging 2001; 5:70–74.
6. Heimburger D. Nutrition's interface with health and disease. In: JC B, F P, eds. Cecil Textbook of Medicine, 20th ed. WB Saunders, Philadelphia, PA, 1996.
7. National Vital Statistics Report, Vol 47, No 28. National Center for Health Statistics, US Department of Health and Human Resources, Washington, DC, 1999.
8. Facts on Osteoporosis. National Institute of Health, Osteoporosis and Related Bone Diseases—National Resource Center, Washington, DC, 2000.
9. Singh I, Marshall MC Jr. Diabetes mellitus in the elderly. Endocrinol Metab Clin North Am 1995;24: 255–272.
10. Flegal K, Carroll M, Kuczmarski R, Johnson C. Overweight and obesity in the United States: prevalence and trends, 1960–1994. Int J Obes 1998;22:39–47.
11. McGandy RB, Barrows CH Jr, Spanias A, Meredith A, Stone JL, Norris AH. Nutrient intakes and energy expenditure in men of different ages. J Gerontol 1966;21:581–587.
12. Hajjar IM, Grim CE, George V, Kotchen TA. Impact of diet on blood pressure and age-related changes in blood pressure in the US population: analysis of NHANES III. Arch Intern Med 2001;161:589–593.
13. Shimokata H, Kuzuya F. Aging, basal metabolic rate, and nutrition. Nippon Ronen Igakkai Zasshi Jpn J Geriatr 1993;30:572–576.
14. Hunter GR, Weinsier RL, Gower BA, Wetzstein C. Age-related decrease in resting energy expenditure in sedentary white women: effects of regional differences in lean and fat mass. Am J Clin Nutr 2001;73: 333–337.
15. Roberts SB, Dallal GE. Effects of age on energy balance. Am J Clin Nutr 1998;68:975S–979S.
16. Drewnowski A, Shultz JM. Impact of aging on eating behaviors, food choices, nutrition, and health status. J Nutr Health Aging 2001;5:75–79.

17. Shuman J. Nutrition in elderly. In: Escott-Stump S, ed. Krause's Food, Nutrition, and Diet Therapies. WB Saunders, Philadelphia, PA, 1996, pp. 287–310.
18. Williams M. The American Geriatic Society's Complete Guide to Aging and Health. Harmony Books, New York, 1995.
19. Steen B. Preventive nutrition in old age—a review. J Nutr Health Aging 2000;4:114–119.
20. Clarkston W, Pantano M, Morley J, Horowitz M, Littlefield J, Burton F. Evidence for anorexia of aging: gastrointestinal transit and hunger in healthy elderly vs. younger adults. Am J Physiol 1997;272: R243–R248.
21. Older Americans 2000: Key Indicators of Well-Being. Federal Interagency Forum on Aging Related Statistics. Hyattsville, 2000.
22. Macdonald IA. Carbohydrate as a nutrient in adults: range of acceptable intakes. Eur J Clin Nutr 1999; 53(Suppl 1):S101–S106.
23. Hallfrisch J, Muller D, Drinkwater D, Tobin J, Andres R. Continuing diet trends in men: the Baltimore Longitudinal Study of Aging (1961–1987). J Gerontol 1990;45:M186–M191.
24. Elahi VK, Elahi D, Andres R, Tobin JD, Butler MG, Norris AH. A longitudinal study of nutritional intake in men. J Gerontol 1983;38:162–180.
25. Troisi RJ, Heinold JW, Vokonas PS, Weiss ST. Cigarette smoking, dietary intake, and physical activity: effects on body fat distribution—the Normative Aging Study. Am J Clin Nutr 1991;53:1104–1111.
26. Bjorkegren K, Svardsudd K. Serum cobalamin, folate, methylmalonic acid and total homocysteine as vitamin B12 and folate tissue deficiency markers amongst elderly Swedes—a population-based study. J Intern Med 2001;249:423–432.
27. Haveman-Nies A, de Groot LC, Van Staveren WA. Fluid intake of elderly Europeans. J Nutr Health Aging 1997;1:151–155.
28. Vitale S, West S, Hallfrisch J, et al. Plasma antioxidants and risk of cortical and nuclear cataract. Epidemiology 1993;4:195–203.
29. Wood SM, Watson RR. Antioxidants and cancer in the aged. In: Watson RR, ed. Handbook of Nutrition in the Aged, 2nd ed. CRC, Ann Arbor, MI, 1994, pp. 282–291.
30. Herbert P. Principles of nutritional support in adult patients. In: Andreoli T, Carpenter C, Griggs R, Loscalzo J, eds. Cecil Essentials of Medicine. WB Saunders, New York, 2001, pp. 522–525.
31. Hallfrisch J, Muller DC. Does diet provide adequate amounts of calcium, iron, magnesium, and zinc in a well-educated adult population? Exp Gerontol 1993;28:473–483.
32. Koehler KM, Hunt WC, Garry PJ. Meat, poultry, and fish consumption and nutrient intake in the healthy elderly. J Am Diet Assoc 1992;92:325–330.
33. Lee JS, Frongillo EA Jr. Understanding needs is important for assessing the impact of food assistance program participation on nutritional and health status in U.S. elderly persons. J Nutr 2001;131: 765–773.
34. de Castro JM. Age-related changes in natural spontaneous fluid ingestion and thirst in humans. J Gerontol 1992;47:P321–P330.
35. Russell RM. Factors in aging that effect the bioavailability of nutrients. J Nutr 2001;131:1359S–361S.
36. Fact Sheet: Depression in the Elderly. US Department of Health and Human Services, Public Health Service, Alcohol, Drug Abuse and Mental Health Administration, Rockville, MD, 2000.
37. Brodeur J, Laurin D, Vallee R, Lachapelle D. Nutrient intake and gastrointestinal disorder related to masticatory performance in edentulous elderly. J Prosthet Dent 1993;70:468–473.
38. Rudney JD. Does variability in salivary protein concentrations influence oral microbial ecology and oral health? Crit Rev Oral Biol Med 1995;6:343–367.
39. Dolan T, Atchison K. Implications of access, utilization and need for oral health care by the nonnstitutionalized and institutionalized elderly on the dental delivery system. J Dent Educ 1993;57:876–885.
40. Davis J, Sherer K. Applied nutrition and diet therapy for nurses. WB Saunders, Philadelphia, PA, 1994.
41. Kapur K, Soman S. Masticatory performance and efficiency in denture wearers. J Prosthet Dent 1964;14: 687–694.
42. Martin W. Oral health in elderly. In: Chernoff R, ed. Geriatric Nutrition: The Health Professional's Book. Aspen, Gaithersburg, MD, 1991.
43. Harris MI, Flegal KM, Cowie CC, et al. Prevalence of diabetes, impaired fasting glucose, and impaired glucose tolerance in U.S. adults: NHANES III. Diabetes Care 1998;21:518–524.
44. Brennan MF. Total parenteral nutrition in the cancer patient. N Engl J Med 1981;305:375–382.
45. Briley ME, Owens MS, Gillham MB, Sharplin SW. Sources of nutrition information for rural and urban elderly adults. J Am Diet Assoc 1990;90:986–987.

46. Shorr RI, Franse LV, Resnick HE, DiBari M, Johnson KC, Pahor M. Glycemic control of older adults with type 2 diabetes: findings from NHANES III, 1988–1994. J Am Geriatr Soc 2000;48:264–267.
47. Clarck NG, Rappaport JI, DiScala C, Lamothe PA, Blackburn GL. Nutritional support of the chronically ill elderly female at risk for elective or urgent surgery. J Am Coll Nutri 1988;7:17–26.
48. Veterans Affairs Total Parenteral Nutrition Cooperative Study Group: perioperative total parenteral nutrition in surgical patients. N Engl J Med 1991;325:525–532.
49. Ware AJ. The liver when the heart fails. Gastroenterology 1978;74:627–628.
50. Watanabe S, Bruera E. Anorexia and cachexia, asthenia, and lethargy. Hematol/Oncol Clin North Am 1996;10:189–206.
51. Davidson JD, Goodman DS, Waldman TA, et al. Protein-losing gastroeneropathy in congestive heart failure. Lancet 1961;1:899–902.
52. Webb JG, Kiess MC, Chan-Yan CC. Malnutrition and the heart. CMAJ 1986;135:753–758.
53. Wallace JI, Schwartz RS. Involuntary weight loss in elderly outpatients. Clin Geriatr Med 1997;13: 717–735.
54. Agner E, Thorsteinsson B, Eriksen M. Impaired glucose tolerance in diabetes mellitus in elderly subjects. Diabetes Care 1982;5:600–604.
55. Pittman JC, Cohen P. The pathogenesis of cardiac cachexia. N Engl J Med 1964;271:403–409.
56. Malhi-Chowla N, Scolapio JS, Ukleja A. Nutrition supplementation in patients with acute and chronic pancreatitis. Gastroenerol Clin North Am 1999;28:695–707.
57. Silk BA, Payne-James JO. Complications of enteral nutrition. Enteral and Tube Feeding. WB Saunders, Philadelphia, PA, 1990, p. 510.
58. Jones RV. Fat malabsorption in congestive cardiac failure. Br Med J 1961;1:1276–1278.
59. Jensen GL, McGee M, Binkley J. Nutrition and the elderly. Gastroenterol Clin North Am 2001;30: 313–334.
60. Hambrecht R, Hilbrich L, Erbs S, et al. Correction of endothelial dysfunction in chronic heart failure: additional effects of exercise training and oral L-arginine supplementation. J Am Coll Cardiol 2000;35: 706–713.
61. Leaf A. Dietary prevention of coronary heart disease: the Lyon Diet Heart Study. Circulation 1999;99: 733–735.
62. Lavie CJ, Milani RV. Cardiac rehabilitation and preventive cardiology in the elderly. Cardiol Clin 1999; 17:233–242.
63. Ferreira IM, Brooks D, Lacasse Y, Goldstien RS. Nutritional Intervention COPD Chest 2001;117: 672–678.
64. Cobb DK, High KP, Sawyer RG, et al. A controlled trial of scheduled replacement of central venous and pulmonary catheters. N Engl J Med 1992;327:1062–1068.
65. Bauer P, Charpentier C, Bouchet C, Nace L, Raffy F, Goconnet N. Parenteral with eneral nutrition in the critically ill. Intensive Care Med 2000;26:893–900.
66. Berghe GV, Wouters P, Weekers F, et al. Intensive insulin therapy in critically ill patients. N Engl J Med 2001;345:1359–1367.
67. Christie PM, Hill GL. Effect of intravenous nutrition on nutrition and function in acute attacks of inflammatory bowel disease. Gastroenterology 1990;99:730–736.
68. Ng PK, Ault MJ, Ellrodt AG, Maldonado L. Peripherally inserted central catheters in general medicine. Mayo Clin Proc 1997;72:225–230.
69. Foitzik T, Kruschewski M, Kroesen AJ, Hotz HG, Eibl G, Bhur HJ. Does glutamine reduce bacterial translocation? A study in two animal models with impaired gut barrier. Int J Colorectal Dis 1999;14:143–149.
70. Houdijk APJ, Rijinsburger ER, Jansen J, Wesdorp RI, Weiss JK, McCamish MA, et al. Randomized trial of glutamine-enriched enteral nutrition on infectious morbidity in patients with multiple trauma. Lancet 1998;352:1–5.
71. The Hospital Infection Control Practices Advisory Committee. Draft Guideline for Prevention of Intravascular Device-Related Infections. MMWR 1995;44:757–804.
72. McAndrew, Lloyd DA, Rintala R, van Saene HKF. Intravenous glutamine or short-chain fatty acids reduce central venous catheter infection in a model of total parenteral nutrition. J Pediatr Surg 1999;34: 281–285.
73. Griffiths RD, Andrews F. Glutamine: a life-threatening deficiency in the critically ill? Intensive Care Med 2001;27:12–15.
74. Beale RJ, Bryg DJ, Bihari DJ. Immunonutrition in the critically ill: a systematic review of clinical outcome. Crit Care Med 1999;27:2799–2805.

4

Pharmacological Management of the Older Patient

Rudina M. Odeh-Ramadan, PHARMD
and Tami L. Remington, PHARMD

CONTENTS

INTRODUCTION

Nearly one-third of all the prescription medications used in this country today is consumed by Americans aged 65 and older *(1–3)*. In the community setting, this patient population receives, on average, two to six prescription medications at one time; this does not include the multiple over-the-counter and herbal medications *(3)*. The number of drug exposures increases with age and tends to be higher in patients treated in long-term care facilities or nursing homes, compared to community-dwelling elders. The prescription rate in nursing facilities is, on average, five to eight medications per patient, not including medicines dispensed on an "as needed" basis *(4)*. Not surprisingly, pharmacologic management was ranked as the number one target for quality improvement by experts in geriatric care from a list of 78 conditions common among vulnerable older adults *(5)*. In persons 65 yr and older, the combination of complex medication regimens, altered pharmacodynamics, and multiple prescription and nonprescription medications places this patient population at high risk for adverse drug events, drug–drug interactions, and noncompliance.

One of the greatest threats to the health and well-being of the elderly patient is that of adverse drug events (ADEs). Approximately 28% of hospital admissions for patients over age 60 are drug induced *(6,7)*. A variety of factors may predispose elderly patients to ADEs. These factors include polypharmacy, concomitant disease states, altered pharmacokinetics

From: *Aging, Heart Disease, and Its Management: Facts and Controversies*
Edited by: N. Edwards, M. Maurer, and R. Wellner © Humana Press Inc., Totowa, NJ

and pharmcodynamics, inappropriate prescribing, and poor compliance. In addition, the type of medication prescribed has been identified as a major contributing factor to the incidence of ADEs in the elderly. The medications most commonly associated with undesired effects are cardiovascular medications (e.g., antihypertensives, diuretics, digoxin, antiarrhythmics, and antianginals) and medications that act on the central nervous system—primarily psychotropics (e.g., antipsychotics, anxiolytics, antidepressants, stimulants, and anticonvulsants). Other prescription medications commonly associated with adverse drug reactions include warfarin, nonsteroidal anti-inflammatory agents, corticosteroids, respiratory agents, and antimicrobials *(7–13)*.

It has been shown that drug-induced adverse events result in substantial morbidity and mortality and significantly increase health care costs and lengths of stay *(14,15)*. In 1995, it was estimated that drug-related morbidity and mortality in the ambulatory setting in the United States cost approx $76.6 billion and result in 79,000–199,000 deaths annually *(16)*. Since 1995, the cost of drug-associated mortality and morbidity has more than doubled, to an estimated $177.4 billion in 2000 *(17)*. Unfortunately, it is the elderly patient who is the most vulnerable to drug-related morbidity and mortality, a trend that is associated with immense health care costs. It has been reported that for every dollar spent in a nursing facility, approx $1.33 is spent on health care resources for the treatment of drug-related problems *(18)*. The high incidence of drug-related problems in the elderly population has produced a tremendous economic and health care burden. To appropriately manage the elderly patient pharmacologically and to reduce the incidence of drug-related morbidity and mortality, we must first understand the various factors influencing drug therapy in this patient population. This chapter will explore the many factors influencing the pharmacological management of disease in the older patient.

NONPHARMACOLOGIC FACTORS INFLUENCING DRUG THERAPY

When considering the pharmacologic management of the older patient, we tend to focus primarily on age-related alterations in pharmacokinetic and pharmacodynamic parameters. However, understanding the nonpharmacologic factors that influence drug therapy in the elderly is imperative to achieving a safe and successful response. Because of features unique to the elderly patient, the nonpharmacologic factors are often more essential to effective drug therapy than are age-related pharmacologic changes. There are multiple nonpharmacologic factors that can interfere with the appropriate management of the elderly patient. These factors include inaccurate diagnoses, inaccurate medication records, noncompliance, and economic constraints.

Accurate Diagnosis

It is often difficult to recognize disease and make accurate diagnoses in the elderly patient. Geriatric patients tend to have multiple comorbidities, which may either be exacerbated by or alter drug therapy. Unfortunately, many of these illnesses may progress undetected. It has been reported that four out of every five elderly patients have at least one chronic illness and demonstrate a vast array of symptoms *(19)*. The Dunedin study found that more than 40% of the study subjects had 4–7 comorbid states and reported approx 3.7 symptoms per person *(20)*. These symptoms often present atypically in the elderly and are frequently underreported. In addition, some of the reported symptoms may be iatrogenic. The complexity involved in interpreting symptoms reported by the older patient can lead to inaccurate diagnoses. Often, the clinician may overlook an iatrogenic cause for a complaint and, instead, treat the reported symptoms with additional medications. Hence, prescribing drugs for symptoms should be avoided. Instead, a thorough examination and evaluation of the symptoms should be conducted to make a correct diagnosis and create a minimal yet rational drug regimen.

Medication Records

One of the hallmarks of good pharmaceutical care is a thorough medication history. A complete medication record is essential in assessing total drug use and determining an accurate diagnosis. The medication record should include all prescription, over-the-counter (OTC), herbal, and complementary (or alternative) medicines the patient may be taking. An exhaustive medication history should be obtained at every medical appointment and be an integral part of the medical record. This can serve as an effective strategy in reducing polypharmacy and noncompliance among the elderly patient population. To obtain a comprehensive medication history, it is imperative to inquire about the occurrence of undesired or intolerable side effects, compliance, and the use of nonprescription medications. The increasing trend toward OTC, herbal, and complementary medication use has mandated the thorough assessment of using such agents. Because these agents are obtainable without a prescription, the patient may fail to disclose the use of such medicines.

Bedell et al. *(21)*, who examined the incidence of medication discrepancies among outpatients, compared patients' medication bottles and their reported use of medications to the physicians' records. The study sample included 312 patients with a mean age of 62 yr, with follow-up care by either an internist or a cardiologist. Discrepancies were identified in 76% of patients and they were reported more frequently in patients over age 60 (82%). In addition, they were more likely to occur in patients treated by cardiologists (82%) as compared to internists (65%). Most of the discrepancies (51%) were attributable to patients taking non-recorded medications. An important finding was that of all the medications implicated in the medication record discrepancies, OTC medicines comprised the single largest category. Thus, medication record discrepancies are common and the most significant predictors of discrepancies are age, number of medications the patient is taking, and the involvement of another physician in the patient's care.

Because the most commonly reported predictors of medication discrepancies occur more frequently in the elderly, it is especially important for the clinician to view and maintain the medication record of the older patient in a meticulous and systematic manner. An accurate medication record should be able to identify any prescription and nonprescription additions or deletions, dose changes, and noncompliance. In addition, patients should be given a pocket medication record that includes the name, dose, frequency, purpose, and any special instructions (i.e., take on an empty stomach). The patient should be instructed to keep this record with them at all times and bring it to all medical appointments to prevent the prescribing of overlapping or interacting medicines.

Clinicians tend to treat elderly patients with multiple medicines, leading to polypharmacy and a higher probability of undesirable effects such as drug–drug interactions and medication nonadherance. A thorough and well-kept medication record can help combat such problems. In addition, the clinician must be cognizant of the use of medicines to self-treat. The addition of such medicines to a patient's complex drug regimen can result in overlapping therapy or antagonistic effects. It must also be stressed that, in addition to the primary care physician, all subspecialists and clinicians treating the patient must accurately communicate any medication changes to maintain optimal accuracy of the medical record.

Medication Noncompliance and Improvement Strategies

An inability to comply with long-term medication use can hinder successful drug therapy among all age groups. It has been reported that a third of patients always comply, a third never comply, and a third sometimes comply (22). Noncompliance among the elderly has been categorized as either intentional or nonintentional (23). The most common reasons cited for intentional noncompliance include discontinuing medications prematurely because of intolerable side effects, an inability to afford prescription drugs, or because the patient "feels better" (23–27). Physiologic barriers such as slowing of cognitive processes, impaired vision, and diminished hearing, most often contribute to nonintentional noncompliance. Such debilitations can inhibit prescriber-to-patient or pharmacist-to-patient communication.

Cognitive impairment can result in medication nonadherance either as a result of a failure to understand the necessity of the medication or simply forgetfulness (28). The elderly tend to experience a notable decline in memory for learning, particularly in situations requiring a high level of attention. Hence, in communicating with the elderly, the clinician should categorize information as it is being provided, use short, simple sentences, and avoid a condescending attitude. Other tactics that can be employed to enhance communication in patients with decreased cognitive function include the following: providing written educational materials, communicating only essential information, allowing the patient time to process the information and respond, and highlighting and emphasizing important points (29–32). In addition, innovative techniques like dosage calendars and pill boxes that dispense a week's supply of medication serve to remind patients to take their medications, thus preventing missed doses.

Communication techniques that can be employed to overcome visual barriers include using large bold type for prescription or warning labels and written educational materials. Providing the package insert should be avoided. The package insert is often printed in small lettering on a glossy background, making it difficult to read. Additional methods to aid the visually impaired patient in distinguishing prescription bottles include varying the size or color code prescription containers and labels. When color coding, it is best to use bright colors like yellow, orange, or red because the older patient may find it difficult to distinguish subtle differences in color. Darker colors like blue, violet, or green are most difficult to distinguish from one another (33–36).

Hearing loss is prevalent among the elderly population, affecting one in four people over 65 (37). Techniques that may facilitate communication between the clinician and the hearing impaired include maintaining eye contact and speaking in a slow and distinct manner. It is also helpful to supplement verbal communication with written and visual aides. Most importantly, the health care professional should elicit a response from the patient to ensure that the information was received correctly.

Another potential physical barrier to compliance is reduced manual dexterity. Joint stiffness and weak hands may impede the ability of the older patient to open "child-proof" medication containers or tamper-resistant packaging. When appropriate, the clinician should ask the patient to request that the pharmacist dispense medications in easy-open prescription containers and nontamper-resistant packaging. The pharmacist can make a note of this request on the patient's medication profile to ensure that refills are dispensed in the same manner.

A lack of social support and limited access to transportation may also contribute to medication non-adherence. Providing medication education to a family member or caregiver and using mail-order pharmacy services can assist in these circumstances. In addition, potential economic constraints should be explored and identified when noncompliance is evident.

Ultimately, one of the most effective strategies to improve compliance in the elderly is to avoid prescribing multiple medications and create a drug regimen that is simple to both follow and maintain. This can be accomplished by prescribing medications on the same dosage schedule as often as possible and using once-daily dosing when clinically appropriate. Medication administration should correspond to a daily routine to enhance consistency and aid compliance.

In summary, we must recognize and overcome the physiologic barriers that hamper medication compliance. It is imperative to regularly review the patients' medication knowledge, their ability to comply, and the occurrence of undesired effects. Overall, the risk of noncompliance can be reduced by simplifying the drug regimen, avoiding polypharmacy, and maintaining an accurate drug profile.

Prescription Costs

Escalating prescription drug costs represent a serious problem that threatens successful health maintenance in the elderly. In 1997, prescription drug expenditures rose to 14.1% at a time when the total national health expenditures decreased *(38)*. This trend of increasing drug costs most significantly impacts the elderly patient population. In 1992, it was reported that the per capita health care costs for those under 65 was approx $2000, as compared to $9000 in those older than 65 *(39)*. The greatest per capita spending on prescription medications is seen in the elderly patient population *(38,40)*. Unfortunately, a declining income typically accompanies increasing age. For approximately two-thirds of the nation's elderly, Social Security comprises at least 50% of their income. In the remaining 30% of elders, approx 90–100% of their income comes from Social Security. The average household income for more than 50% of people over 75 who live alone is less than $10,000, and more than half of married couples over 75 report a household income of less than $20,000. Furthermore, the overall poverty rate among the elderly was reported at approx 12% (approx 4 million people) in 1990 *(41)*.

Medicaid covers the cost of medications for patients suffering from severe economic constraints. However, those elderly who do not have Medicaid or a Medigap plan may incur a large out-of-pocket expense for prescription drugs. This out-of-pocket expense has been reported to be as high as $170 per month *(42)*. As discussed previously, an inability to afford costly prescriptions can result in medication noncompliance. As a result, the elderly have been forced into devising self-management strategies to cope with the rising costs of medications. Self-management strategies include a failure to fill or to partially fill required prescriptions, taking less than the recommended dosage, hoarding medications, sharing prescription medications with others, prematurely discontinuing medications, and replacing one medication with another. It has been reported that as many as 44% of older patients use at least one of these strategies to manage the high cost of prescription medicines *(43)*. Unfortunately, such strategies may interfere with achieving the desired pharmacotherapeutic effect and can result in a deleterious outcome. The health

care professional can assist the elderly patient with prescription drug expenditures by prescribing generic medications when possible, streamlining the patient's medication profile
to only necessary medicines, and avoiding high-cost prescriptives when a less expensive alternative is available. In addition, financially disadvantaged patients may qualify
to receive specific medications free of charge or at reduced cost through special patient
assistance programs offered by the pharmaceutical manufacturer. Other means of obtaining medications at lower cost include state assistance programs like the Elderly Pharmaceutical Insurance Coverage (EPIC) in New York State or Medicare supplemental insurance
like American Association for Retired Persons (AARP) and Blue Cross Blue Choice.

CHANGES IN BODY
COMPOSITION AND ORGAN FUNCTION

Generally speaking, the elderly are more sensitive to the effects of medications. They
often exhibit therapeutic responses at lower doses than younger patients and can experience adverse events at lower doses as well. The full therapeutic and adverse effects of
a given dose may not be seen for a longer than expected period of time. These changes are
associated with age-related changes in the pharmacokinetics and pharmacodynamics of
drugs. Safe and effective use of medications in the elderly population requires an appreciation of these differences.

Pharmacokinetic Changes

Pharmacokinetic parameters describe the absorption, distribution, metabolism, and
excretion of drugs. These properties are determined by drug and formulation characteristics, body composition, and organ function. Age-related changes in body composition and
organ function affect the pharmacokinetic properties of many drugs, which is often clinically relevant. Historically, pharmacokinetic differences in the elderly population were not
quantified. More recently, however, efforts have been made to measure pharmacokinetic
properties of medications in elders. Understanding documented and potential differences
in pharmacokinetics of drugs in the elderly is essential to promoting safe and rational use
of drug therapy in this vulnerable population.

ABSORPTION

Absorption of oral dosage forms is influenced by gastric pH, gastrointestinal motility,
splanchnic blood flow, liver function (first-pass extraction), and active transport processes involved in absorption from the gastrointestinal tract. Although the incidence of
hypochlorhydria and achlorhydria increases with age, changes in gastric pH most often
do not significantly alter drug absorption. Age-related changes in physiology that may
influence drug absorption include reduced hepatic extraction and reduced active transport for some drugs. Reductions in active transport across intestinal epithelium result in
reduced rate of absorption, but the extent of absorption is usually unchanged. However,
most often, these differences are clinically unimportant. Reduced hepatic extraction produces meaningful increases in bioavailability for drugs that are highly extracted during
a first pass through the liver. Such drugs include propranolol, morphine, verapamil, desi-
pramine, and imipramine. Elderly patients may require lower than expected doses of such
medications as compared to younger patients.

Skin integrity, skin hydration, skin thickness, temperature, and cutaneous blood flow affect absorption of transdermal dosage forms. Age-related changes in the physiology of the skin include decreased skin hydration, epidermal and dermal thinning, and wrinkling. There is little evidence examining the clinical importance of these age-related changes on absorption of medications through the skin. The possibility that transdermal absorption of drugs in the elderly is different from younger populations should be considered when prescribing such medications.

DISTRIBUTION

Distribution of medications in the body is dependent on body composition, plasma protein binding, and blood flow. Aging produces reductions in lean body mass (including muscle mass), total-body water and serum proteins, and an increase in body fat. Despite these measurable changes, drug distribution in the elderly is not altered significantly. A notable exception to this, however, is digoxin. Digoxin has a lower volume of distribution in older adults, owing to reductions in muscle mass. This results in a reduction in dosing requirements to produce a desired therapeutic blood level.

METABOLISM

A reduction in hepatic metabolic capacity is one of the most important age-related changes that affects the pharmacokinetics of drugs. Although phase II metabolism (conjugation, acetylation, sulfation) is essentially unchanged in older adults, phase I metabolism (hydroxylation, deamination, oxidation) is slowed, primarily the result of reductions in liver mass.

Medications that exhibit important slowing of hepatic metabolism in the elderly include warfarin, theophylline, phenytoin, diazepam, and naproxen. As a result of slowed hepatic metabolism, these medications will exhibit longer elimination half-lives, prolonged durations of action, longer times to achieve steady state, and higher serum drug concentrations in the elderly. Doses of such medications often must be adjusted to accommodate these differences. Utilization of lower doses, longer titration schedules, and longer dosing intervals are maneuvers that can be employed.

EXCRETION

Drugs are eliminated from the body principally through fecal and renal routes. Although changes in fecal elimination are not important in this population, decreases in renal elimination are very significant. With age, renal blood flow and nephron mass decline, producing reductions in glomerular filtration rates. Methods that estimate renal function based on serum creatinine may be inaccurate in the elderly because of reduced muscle mass and because tubular secretion of creatinine remains largely intact despite concurrent reductions in glomerular filtration. However, these estimations are still clinically useful, as long as the user considers that the estimation is likely to be an overrepresentation of the patient's actual renal function.

Similar to age-related changes in hepatic metabolism, changes in renal excretion of drugs can produce longer elimination half-lives, prolonged durations of action, longer times to achieve steady state, and higher serum drug concentrations in the elderly. Consequently, doses of many drugs must be adjusted to avoid toxicity. Once again, lower doses, slower titration schedules, and longer dosing intervals can be employed to accommodate changes in renal excretion of drugs.

Table 1
Age-Related Changes in the Pharmacodynamics of Medications

Drug	Change
Narcotics	Increased sensitivity to analgesic effects
Benzodiazepines	Increased sensitivity to sedative properties and effects on balance
Warfarin	Increased sensitivity to anticoagulant effects
Isoproterenol	Decreased sensitivity to effects on heart rate, atrioventricular conduction, cardiac contractility, and vasodilatation
β-Blockers	Increased sensitivity to slowing heart rate during exercise or stress
β-Agonists	Decreased sensitivity to effects on heart rate
Vasodilators	Decreased sensitivity to effects on heart rate
Nondihydropyridine calcium channel blockers	Increased sensitivity to atrioventricular nodal blocking characteristics Increased sensitivity to blood-pressure-lowering effects
Anticholinergic medications	Increased sensitivity to effects of urinary retention, constipation, and and central nervous system effects (delirium). Decreased sensitivity to effects on heart rate
Furosemide	Decreased diuretic response

Pharmacodynamics

Pharmacodynamics describes the relationship between blood concentration of a drug and its clinical responses at the level of the target tissues. It can be thought of as the body's "sensitivity" to a drug. Pharmacodynamics of drugs is not as well characterized as pharmacokinetic characteristics. However, age-related changes in the pharmacodynamics of certain drugs have been documented, and it is likely that others exist as well (*see* Table 1).

Age-related differences in pharmacodynamics can occur as a result of changes at either the cellular level (changes in production or activity of intracellular messengers) or the tissue level (changes in number or affinity of receptors for a drug). They can also occur as a result of changes in normal compensatory or homeostatic mechanisms. There are several age-related changes in homeostatic mechanisms that involve the cardiovascular system that may alter the pharmacodynamics of medications (*see* Table 2). For example, many elderly persons develop reduced baroreceptor sensitivity, resulting from increased circulating catecholamines, decreased parasympathetic tone, and downregulation of peripheral adrenergic receptor function and vasomotor responsiveness. This physiologic change predisposes patients to postural hypotension from drugs with anticholinergic or antihypertensive action, especially when volume depleted from diuretics.

GENERAL PRINCIPLES
FOR PRESCRIBING IN THE ELDERLY

Differences in drug response resulting from changes in pharmacokinetics or pharmacodynamics can include longer onset of action, longer duration of action, longer time to achieve maximum response (steady state), and exaggerated (or blunted) responses to medications. These differences warrant initiating therapy at lower than usual starting doses, titrating doses more slowly, and considering longer dosing intervals.

Table 2
Age-Related Physiologic Changes in the Cardiovascular System
that Impact the Pharmacodynamics of Medications

Physiologic characteristic	Age-related change
Baroreceptor response	↓
Intrinsic heart rate	↓
Change in heart rate in response to exercise or stress	↓
Diastolic function	↓
Atrial and ventricular ectopy	↑
AV conduction times	↑
Repolarization times	↑
Elasticity of the aorta and large vessels	↓
Vascular endothelium-mediated function	↓

The elderly population is at increased risk of experiencing ADEs for reasons other than pharmacodynamic/pharmacokinetic. In one study, patients taking more than 12 medication doses daily, 9 or more different medications daily, or who had 6 or more active chronic diagnoses were at an increased risk for drug-related morbidity and mortality (44). Another study documented ADEs in the previous year in 35% of patients taking five or more medications (45). Certain classes of medications may be more problematic in the elderly population. Cardiovascular drugs were the leading cause of ADEs in one study, causing 33% of all events observed. Cardiovascular events comprised 15% of all observed ADEs and were second only to gastrointestinal effects in frequency (9). Although differences in pharmacokinetics and pharmacodynamics may partially explain the excess risk associated with these factors, much of the risk may be attributable to drug–disease interactions, additive drug toxicities, drug use without indication, and so forth.

In an effort to improve prescription patterns in the elderly population, explicit recommendations for avoidance of certain drugs thought to represent excess risk if used in the elderly have been proposed (11). These recommendations were generated by the consensus of a panel of experts and include general recommendations for use in any geriatric population (see Table 3) as well as disease-specific recommendations (see Table 4) (11). Despite clear recommendations for avoidance of these medications, it is clear that these warnings often go unheeded, and medications that are likely to be harmful in the elderly continue to be prescribed (46,47). Critics of the use of Beers' criteria to judge appropriateness of prescribing point out that these criteria were not generated through review of clinical trials but rather through consensus of opinions of experts. However, because elderly patients are underrepresented in many clinical trials, expert opinions may be the best evidence available to guide prescribing. In addition, some of these recommendations are substantiated in observational studies that identify certain medications or medication classes as being of higher risk for causing drug-related morbidity or mortality in the elderly population (9,44). Although evidence demonstrating improved patient outcomes when such criteria are followed is lacking, these recommendations are being used by some regulatory agencies to judge the appropriateness of prescribing and to mandate intervention by clinical pharmacists in nursing facilities when certain criteria are violated (48).

Table 3

Recommendations for Avoidance of Specific Medications in the Elderly: Independent of Diagnoses

Summary of prescribing concern	Applicable medications[a]	High severity
Propoxyphene should generally be avoided in the elderly. It offers few analgesic advantages over acetaminophen, yet has the side effects of other narcotic drugs.	Propoxyphene and combination products	No
Of all available nonsteroidal, anti-inflammatory drugs, indomethacin produces the most central nervous system side effects and should, therefore, be avoided in the elderly.	Indomethacin (Indocin, Indocin SR)	No
Phenylbutazone may produce serious hematological side effects and should not be used in elderly patients.	Phenylbutazone (Butazolidin)	No
Pentazocine is a narcotic analgesic that causes more central nervous system side effects, including confusion and hallucinations, more commonly than other narcotic drugs. Additionally, it is a mixed agonist and antagonist. For both reasons, its use should generally be avoided in the elderly.	Pentazocine (Talwin)	Yes
Trimethobenzamide is one of the least effective antiemetic drugs, yet it can cause extrapyramidal side effects. When possible, it should be avoided in the elderly.	Trimethobenzamide (Tigan)	No
Most muscle relaxants and antispasmodic drugs are poorly tolerated by the elderly leading to anticholinergic side effects, sedation, and weakness. Additionally, their effectiveness at doses tolerated by the elderly is questionable. Whenever possible, they should not be used by the elderly.	Methocarbamol (Robaxin), carisoprodol (Soma), oxybutynin (Ditropan) chlorzoxazone (Paraflex), metaxalone (Skelaxin), and cyclobenzaprine (Flexeril)	No
Benzodiazepine hypnotic has an extremely long half-life in the elderly (often days), producing prolonged sedation and increasing the incidence of falls and fractures. Medium- or short-acting benzodiazepines are preferable.	Flurazepam (Dalmane)	Yes
Because of its strong anticholinergic and sedating properties, amitriptyline is rarely the antidepressant of choice for the elderly.	Amitriptyline (Elavil), chlordiazepoxide-amitriptyline (Limbitrol), and perphenazine-amitriptyline (Triavil)	Yes
Because of its strong anticholinergic and sedating properties, doxepin is rarely the antidepressant of choice for the elderly.	Doxepin (Sinequan)	Yes
Meprobamate is a highly addictive and sedating anxiolytic. Avoid in elderly patients. Those using meprobamate for prolonged periods may be addicted and may need to be withdrawn slowly.	Meprobamate (Miltown, Equanil)	Yes if recently started[b]

Because of increased sensitivity to benzodiazepines in the elderly, smaller doses may be effective as well as safer. Total daily doses should rarely exceed the following suggested maximums.	Lorazepam (Ativan), 3 mg; oxazepam (Serax), 60 mg; alprazolam (Xanax), 2 mg; temzepam (Restoril), 15 mg; zolpidem (Ambien), 5 mg; triazolam (Halcion), 0.25 mg	No
Chlordiazepoxide and diazelpam have a long half-life in the elderly (often several days), producing prolonged sedation and increasing the risk of falls and fractures. Short- and intermediate-acting benzodiazepines are preferred if a benzodiazepine is required.	Chlordiazepoxide (Librium), chlordiazepoxide-amitriptyline (Limbitrol), clidinium-chlordiazepoxide (Librax), and diazepam (Valium)	Yes
Disopyramide, of all antiarrhythmic drugs, is the most potent negative inotrope and therefore may induce heart failure in the elderly. It is also strongly anticholinergic. When appropriate, other antiarrhythmic drugs should be used.	Disopyramide (Norpace, Norpace CR)	Yes
Because of decreased renal clearance of digoxin, doses in the elderly should rarely exceed 0.125 mg daily, except when treating atrial arrhythmias.	Digoxin (Lanoxin)	Yes if recently started[b]
Dipyridamole frequently causes orthostatic hypotension in the elderly. It has been proven beneficial only in patients with artificial heart valves. Whenever possible, its use in the elderly should be avoided.	Dipyridamole (Persantine)	No
Methyldopa may cause bradycardia and exacerbate depression in the elderly. Alternate treatments for hypertension are generally preferred.	Methyldopa (Aldomet); methyldopa/hydrochlorothiazide (Aldoril)	Yes if recently started[b]
Reserpine imposes unnecessary risk in the elderly, inducing depression, impotence, sedation, and orthostatic hypotension. Safer alternatives exist.	Reserpine (Serpasil); reserpine hydrochlorothiazide (Hydropres)	No
Chlorpropamide has a prolonged half-life in the elderly and can cause prolonged and serious hypoglycemia. Additionally, it is the only oral hypoglycemic agent that causes SIADH. Avoid in the elderly.	Chlorpropamide (Diabinese)	Yes
Gastrointestinal antispasmodic drugs are highly anticholinergic and generally produce substantial toxic effects in the elderly. Additionally, their effectiveness at doses tolerated by the elderly is questionable. All these drugs are best avoided in the elderly, especially for long-term use.	Dicyclomine (Bentyl); hyoscyamine (Levsin, Levsinex); propentheline (Pro-Banthine); belladonna alkaloids (Donnatal and others); and clidinium-chlordiazepoxide (Librax)	Yes
All nonprescription and many prescription antihistamines have potent anticholinergic properties. Many cough and cold preparations are available without antihistamines, and these are safer substitutes in the elderly.	Examples include single and combination preparation containing chlorpheniramine (Chlor-Trimeton), diphenhydramine (Benadryl), hydroxyzine (Vistaril, Atarax), cyproheptadine (Periactin), promethazine (Phenergan), tripelennamine, and dexchlorpheniramine (Polaramine)	No

Table 3 (Continued)

Summary of prescribing concern	Applicable medications[a]	High severity
Diphenhydramine is potently anticholinergic and usually should not be used as a hypnotic in the elderly. When used to treat or prevent allergic reactions, it should be used in the smallest possible dose and with great caution.	Diphenhydramine (Benadryl)	No
Hydergine (ergot mesyloids) and the cerebral vasodilators have not been shown to be effective, in the doses studied, for the treatment of dementia or any other condition.	Ergot mesyloids (Hydergine), cyclospasmol	No
Iron supplements rarely need to be given in doses exceeding 325 mg of ferrous sulfate daily. When doses are higher, total absorption is not substantially increased, but constipation is more likely to occur.	Iron supplements, >325 mg	No
Barbiturates cause more side effects than most other sedative or hypnotic drugs in the elderly and are highly addictive. They should not be started as new therapy in the elderly except when used to control seizures.	All barbiturates except phenobarbital	Yes if recently started[b]
Meperidine is not an effective oral analgesic and has many disadvantages to other narcotic drugs. Avoid in the elderly.	Meperidine	Yes
Ticlopidine has been shown to be no better than aspirin in preventing clotting and is considerably more toxic. Avoid in the elderly.	Ticlopidine	Yes

It is important to note that most package circulars produced by drug manufacturers do not include language identical to the statements presented herein. Although the adverse effects that these drugs can produce are generally listed in the package circulars, these as well as warnings and contraindications must be approved by regulatory agencies and in general are not based on consensus or surveys. SIADH indicates syndrome of inappropriate antidiuretic hormone.

[a]Dose limits are total daily dose.

[b]Panelists believed that the severity of adverse reaction would be substantially greater when these drugs were recently started. In general, the greatest risk would be within about a 1-mo period.

Table 4
Recommendations for Avoidance of Specific Medications in the Elderly: Considering Diagnoses

Disease and condition	Drug[a]	Alert	High severity
Heart failure	Disopyramide	Negative inotrope. May worsen heart failure.	Yes
	Drugs with high sodium content (such as sodium alginate. bicarbonate, biphosphate, citrate, phosphate, salicylate, and sulfate)	Large sodium load, leading to fluid retention. May worsen heart failure.	No
Diabetes	β-Blockers (limited to people with diabetes taking oral hypoglycemics or insulin)	May block hypoglycemic symptoms in people with diabetes receiving treatment.	No
	Corticosteroids (limited to recently started use)	May worsen diabetic control.	No
Hypertension	Diet pills; amphetamines	May elevate blood pressure.	Yes
Chronic obstructive pulmonary disease	β-Blockers	May worsen respiratory function in persons with chronic obstructive pulmonary disease.	Yes
	Sedative/hypnotics	May slow respirations and increase carbon dioxide retention in persons with severe chronic obstructive pulmonary disease.	Yes
Asthma	β-Blockers	May worsen respiratory function in persons with chronic obstructive pulmonary disease.	Yes
Ulcers	NSAIDs	May exacerbate ulcer disease, gastritis, and GERD.	Yes
	Aspirin (>325 mg)	May exacerbate ulcer disease, gastritis, and GERD.	No
	Potassium supplements (all)	May cause gastritic irritation with symptoms similar to ulcer disease.	No
Seizures or epilepsy	Clozapine, thorazine, thioridazine, and chlorprothixene	Lower seizure threshold.	No
	Metoclopramide		Yes
Peripheral vascular disease	β-Blockers	May worsen peripheral arterial blood flow and precipitate claudication.	Yes
Blood-clotting disorders, limited to those receiving anticoagulant therapy	Aspirin	May worsen peripheral arterial blood flow and precipitate disease claudication.	Yes
		May cause bleeding in those using anticoagulants.	
	NSAIDs	May cause bleeding in those using anticoagulants.	Yes
	Dipyridamole and ticlopidine	May cause bleeding in those using anticoagulants.	Yes

Table 4 (Continued)

Disease and condition	Drug[a]	Alert	High severity
BPH	Anticholinergic antihistamines	Anticholinergic drugs may impair micturation and cause obstruction in persons with BPH.	Yes
	Gastrointestinal antispasmodic drugs	Anticholinergic drugs may impair micturation and cause obstruction in persons with BPH.	Yes
	Muscle relaxants	Anticholinergic drugs may impair micturation and cause obstruction in persons with BPH.	No
	Narcotic drugs (including propoxyphene)	Narcotic drugs may impair micturation and cause obstruction in persons with BPH.	No
	Flavoxate, oxybutynin	Bladder relaxants may cause obstruction in persons with BPH.	No
	Bethanechol	Anticholinergic bladder relaxants may cause obstruction in persons with BPH.	No
	Anticholinergic antidepressant drugs	Anticholinergic drugs may impair micturation and cause obstruction in persons with BPH.	Yes
Incontinence	α-Blockers	α-Blockers relax the external bladder sphincter and may cause incontinence.	No
Constipation	Anticholinergic drugs	Will worsen constipation.	No
	Narcotic drugs	Will worsen constipation.	No
	Tricyclic antidepressant drugs	May worsen constipation.	Yes
Syncope or falls	β-Blockers	Negative chronotrope and inotrope. May precipitate syncope in susceptible persons.	No
	Long-acting benzodiazepine drugs	May contribute to falls.	Yes
Arrhythmias	Tricyclic antidepressant drugs	May induce arrhythmias.	Yes if started recently[b]
Insomnia	Decongestants	May cause or worsen insomnia.	No
	Theophylline	May cause or worsen insomnia.	No
	Desipramine, SSRIs, methylphenidate, and MAOIs	May cause or worsen insomnia.	No
	β-Agonists	May cause or worsen insomnia.	No

It is important to note that most package circulars produced by drug manufacturers do not include language identical to the statements presented herein. Although the adverse effects that these drugs can produce are generally listed in the package circulars, these as well as warnings and contraindications must be approved by regulatory agencies and in general are not based on consensus or surveys. NSAIDs indicates nonsteroidal anti-inflammatory drugs; GERD, gastroesophageal reflux disease; BPH, benign prostatic hyperplasia; SSRIs, selective serotonin reuptake inhibitors; and MAOIs, monoamine oxidase inhibitors.

[a]Dose limits are total daily dose.

[b]Panelists believed that the severity of adverse reaction would be substantially greater when these drugs were recently started. In general, the greatest risk would be within about a 1-mo period.

Overprescribing is another phenomenon related to drug use in the elderly that can increase the risk of adverse events. Overprescribing occurs when an adverse effect of a drug is misinterpreted as a new medical problem requiring additional medical therapy rather than modification of current medication regimens. It can also occur when drug therapy is used for nonspecific minor complaints that could be managed nonpharmacologically or when the benefits of pharmacotherapy are questionable.

The antithesis to overprescribing medications known to be associated with excess risk in the elderly is underuse of medications with known benefit. Underuse of several types of beneficial therapies in the elderly population has been documented; these therapies include the following: anticoagulation *(49–52)*; β-blockers *(53–59)*, ACE inhibitors *(60–62)* or aspirin after myocardial infarction *(51,57,58,63)*; thrombolytics *(57,64)*; lipid-lowering therapy *(58)*; ACE inhibitors for left ventricular dysfunction *(51,60)*; and anti-hypertensives *(65,66)*.

Several factors may contribute to the phenomenon of underutilization of therapies with known benefit. In one trial, patients with a chronic illness like emphysema were less likely to receive drug therapy with known benefit for another chronic illness, such as hyperlipidemia *(67)*. Fear of adverse effects from therapy is another reason treatments with documented benefits may be underutilized. Concerns about iatrogenic bleeding complications from warfarin therapy lead to uncertainty about its role in preventing stroke in patients with atrial fibrillation *(68)*. Use of β-blockers after myocardial infarction was less prevalent in patients with diabetes, obstructive pulmonary disease, heart failure, and chronic renal insufficiency, despite evidence that these populations still derive clinical benefit from such therapy *(55)*. Although avoiding beneficial therapy can be appropriate under certain circumstances, in many cases it is unintended or unnecessary and contributes to suboptimal outcomes from drug therapy.

Based on these data, recommendations for prescribing in the elderly are as follows:

1. Obtain an accurate and complete medication history prior to evaluating and amending treatment regimens. Include scheduled and as-needed prescription drugs, over-the-counter remedies, herbal products, and non-oral dosage forms such as eye drops, inhalers, and topical preparations.
2. Initiate new drug therapy judiciously. Use nonpharmacologic measures, when possible, to reduce the need for drug therapy. Try to avoid using medications for minor complaints or when evidence for benefit of a therapy is ambiguous. When possible, make definitive diagnoses rather than treating symptoms empirically.
3. Simplify drug therapy whenever possible. Regularly review drug therapy and discontinue drugs that are no longer indicated, are poorly tolerated, or have not produced the desired treatment outcomes.
4. Employ strategies to improve the safety of medication use. Based on age-related changes in physiology and pharmacokinetics and pharmacodynamics of drugs, initiate treatment with lower than usual doses, and titrate upward slowly to the target dose. Avoid medications that are thought to represent excess risk in the elderly population.
5. Achieve treatment goals. Prospectively identify monitoring parameters for safety and efficacy of therapy; titrate drug therapy slowly to achieve desired outcomes of treatment.
6. Involve patients in their drug therapy. Consider patients' preferences regarding drug therapy when designing regimens. Inquire about barriers to adherence with medications (financial constraints, low vision, etc.), and address them or adjust treatment plans accordingly. Clearly communicate the name, dose, and purpose of each medication, appropriate dosing sched-

ules, desired effects, possible untoward effects and their management, and duration of treatment verbally and in writing.

THE ROLE OF THE PHARMACIST

High-quality medication therapy for the elderly clearly demands extensive skill, knowledge, and commitment from the health care provider, particularly the geriatric pharmacist. The role of the pharmacist in the management of the older patient is of vital importance. As a provider of pharmaceutical care, the clinical pharmacist must assess, monitor, initiate, and modify medication use to assure the safety and efficacy of the medication regimen. A comprehensive review of studies revealed that in the geriatric patient population, 44–90% of medications are misused, which included errors in dosing, frequency, route, duration, and monitoring. In addition, 7–37% of medicines were prescribed to treat the wrong illness or no illness at all *(69)*. Inappropriate prescribing can result in life-threatening adverse events, increased length of hospital stay, unnecessary hospital admissions, unpleasant side effects, and patient noncompliance. Drug-induced illnesses result in higher rates of morbidity and mortality and have been estimated to cost $4.5–7 billion dollars annually *(70)*. Involvement of the clinical pharmacist on the multidisciplinary health care team has been shown to improve patient care, reduce the incidence of adverse events, and decrease drug costs *(71–73)*. Leape et al. evaluated the impact of clinical pharmacist participation on physician rounds in the intensive care unit. The interventions of the clinical pharmacist resulted in a reduction of preventable ADEs by 66% at a cost of $4685 per preventable ADE *(73,74)*. Pharmacist interventions have also been shown to have a significant financial impact on health care. Pharmacist-initiated interventions reduced drug costs by 41% in patients treated at a large university hospital *(72)*.

Heart failure is the most common discharge diagnosis among patients over 65 *(75)*. Recently, the Pharmacist in Heart Failure Assessment Recommendation and Monitoring (PHARM) Study was conducted to evaluate the effect of a clinical pharmacist on outcomes in outpatients with heart failure. Patients in the intervention group received evaluations from the clinical pharmacist, including medication assessments, therapeutic recommendations, patient education, and follow-up telemonitoring. The control group received usual care. The results of this study revealed that patients in the intervention group were closer to target angiotensin-converting enzyme (ACE)-inhibitor doses at 6 mo follow-up. Furthermore, of patients who were not receiving ACE inhibitors in the intervention group, 75% were receiving an alternative vasodilator as compared to only 26% of patients in the control group. As a result, patients who received clinical pharmacist intervention had a significantly lower incidence of heart failure events and all-cause mortality as compared to the control group. The results of this study revealed that the addition of a clinical pharmacist on the multidisciplinary heart failure team significantly reduced the incidence of clinical events and improved patient outcomes *(71)*.

As a result of their specialized background and training, pharmacists contribute a unique skill set to the management of the geriatric patient. The pharmacist's role includes the following: the selection and optimization of appropriate and cost-effective drug therapy, pharmacokinetic and pharmacodynamic monitoring, assessment of the patients' response to drug therapy, and providing clinical drug information. In addition, the clinical and the community pharmacist have a vital role in patient follow-up and evaluation of drug therapy. The pharmacist is responsible for monitoring patient compliance, identifying ADEs and intolerable side effects, and preventing unnecessary therapeutic duplication. In addition, the pharmacist thoroughly monitors the patient's medication records to prevent and identify drug–drug and drug–food interactions and to evaluate the use of OTC and alternative medicines. Finally, the pharmacist has an important role as the patient educator.

THE FUTURE DIRECTION OF GERIATRIC CLINICAL RESEARCH

Approximately 24 million Americans over the age of 65 obtain prescription medications each year *(76)*. Unfortunately, most of the prescription medications used to treat the elderly are tested on younger patient populations or on healthy elderly volunteers. There is clearly a need for conducting clinical trials in the elderly who suffer from the disease that a particular drug is intended to treat. To ensure sufficient representation of elderly patients in such studies, randomized, double-blind, placebo-controlled trials are needed. Proper clinical research in the elderly must be scientifically valid, medically important, and ethically sound *(77)*. In addition, clinical trials should address the need for improving existing therapies by increasing efficacy and decreasing toxicity of current drug regimens. Unfortunately, achieving such goals in the geriatric population can be an arduous task. Obtaining an adequate number of volunteers to participate in a study may be problematic *(77)*. Elderly people tend to avoid risks and, therefore, are less likely to volunteer for a study, particularly if it may involve discomfort, like venipuncture. Also, many family members, legal guardians, members of institutional review boards, and nursing home policies will prohibit the elderly person from participating in a research study as an act of "protecting" the elderly *(78,79)*. In addition, there may be difficulty in obtaining informed consent for fear of signing a legal-appearing document *(77)*. Commonly, elderly people may suffer from some degree of cognitive impairment, making them particularly vulnerable to enrollment in a clinical trial. Other factors contributing to vulnerability in this population include an eagerness to enroll in a clinical trial with unreasonable expectations for cure of a disease state that they may have suffered from for a prolonged period of time *(80,81)*.

A problem with extrapolating data from current randomized trials to the elderly is achieving external validity or generalizability. Most often, results of a trial may not be generalizable because the trial did not include a sufficient number of participants or did not adequately represent the population at large with the specific disease to be treated *(80)*. This is especially difficult in the elderly because of the heterogenous nature of the population. Hence, it is important that the research question asked is specific, so that the degree of generalizability is known. In addition, clinical trials conducted in the elderly require a large sample size to obtain valid results. A large sample size can reduce the risk of obtaining a false-negative conclusion and account for the variability associated with the heterogeneous geriatric population *(82)*. Variability is much more pronounced in the elderly as compared to the younger patient population. For instance, the rate of decline of cardiovascular function with increasing age varies dramatically *(83)*. This variability is compounded by the physical condition of the patient and by various concomitant disease states.

In designing future clinical trials for medications to be used in the elderly, proper patient selection must be considered. When considering which patients should participate in a clinical trial, the selection must include subjects who have the disease the drug is intended to treat. Also, it is necessary to recruit subjects whose projected life expectancy will likely overlap with the intended duration of the study. Currently, very few studies extend enrollment to include those over 70, particularly the oldest old (those 85 yr of age and older). Clinical trials involving the elderly must also have sufficient numbers of females. This is especially true because among those over 75, women outnumber men by a ratio of 2:1 and maybe as high as 3:1 *(80)*. It is also of great importance to include a sufficient number of minorities in clinical trials to account for the racial variability in drug disposition and response. Often, the proportion of African-Americans included in studies is less than the proportion in the general population *(84–86)*.

As previously noted, pharmacokinetic and pharmacodynamic changes in the elderly can modify the pharmacologic effect of a drug; this highlights the importance of individualization of drug therapy. One of the most prominent differences between the elderly and the younger patients is the rate of drug elimination. The decline in renal function with increasing age is most prominent. This alteration in renal function significantly impacts the rate of drug excretion, which holds true for drug metabolism as well. Generally, drug metabolism in the older patient is significantly slowed as compared to the younger patient. Nevertheless, in agents that are used to treat both younger and elderly patients, these pharmacokinetic parameters are most often only studied in the younger population. Because most pharmacokinetic studies are conducted in patients less then 70 yr of age, the clinician is forced to extrapolate pharmacokinetic data from the younger patient to the older patient.

Extrapolation of data generated in healthy volunteers under the age of 70 to the elderly patient population can be perilous and misleading. In addition to altered pharmacokinetic and pharmacodynamic parameters, the older patient will commonly experience more drug–drug and drug–disease interactions, a poorer nutritional status, and decreased cognitive function *(87)*. Other confounding variables include decreased body size with age, concomitant chronic disease states, polypharmacy, and the possibility of pronounced genetic effects in the elderly. All of these factors can alter the safety and efficacy of a medication *(88)*.

Areas of geriatric research that are in need of further investigation include the influence of increased age on adverse drug effects, identifying the effects of age-related changes in body composition and function on medication outcomes, and determining mechanisms of altered receptor sensitivity with increasing age *(89)*.

In summary, despite the meticulous scrutiny and the stringent requirements enforced by the Food and Drug Administration on research and development, a critical need remains for additional investigation in geriatric pharmacotherapy. Too often drug therapy in the elderly patient is based on assumptions extrapolated from clinical trials conducted in the patient under 65 or in young, healthy volunteers. Well-designed trials in the elderly patient population should be sure to include those over 70, an appropriate number of female and minority patients, and, most importantly, those who suffer from the disease state that the agent is intended to treat. It is clear that designing clinically relevant trials involving the elderly is associated with a greater degree of complexity. However, more randomized, double-blind, well-controlled trials involving the older patient can provide important safety, efficacy, pharmacokinetic, and pharmacodynamic data that are not available today.

REFERENCES

1. US Bureau of the Census. Population Projections of the United States by Age, Sex, Race, and Hispanic Origin: 1995–2000. http://www.census.gov/population/projections/nation/nas/npas0105.txt.
2. US Bureau of the Census. Population Projections of the United States by Age, Sex, Race, and Hispanic Origin: 2000–2005. http://www.census.gov/population/projections/nation/nas/npas0105.txt.
3. Kohn LT, Corrigan JM, Donaldson MS, eds. To Err is Human: Building a Safer Health System. National Academy Press, Washington, DC, 2000, pp. 26–48.
4. Monette J, Gurwitz JH, Avorn J. Epidemiology of adverse drug events in the nursing home setting. Drugs Ageing 1995;7:203–211.

5. Sloss EM, Solomon DH, Shekelle PG, et al. Selecting target conditions for quality of care improvement in vulnerable older adults. J Am Geriatr Soc 2000;48:363–369.

6. Beard K. Adverse reactions as a cause of hospital admission in the aged. Drugs Ageing 1992;2:356–367.

7. Kraajj DJW, Haagsma CJ, Go IH, et al. Drug use and adverse drug reactions in 105 elderly patients admitted to a general medical ward. Neth J Med 1994:44:166–173.

8. Cooper JW. Probable adverse drug reactions in a rural geriatric nursing home population: a four-year study. J Am Geriatr Soc 1996;44:194–196.

9. Hanlon JT, Schmader KE, Koronkowski MJ, et al. Adverse drug events in high risk older outpatients. J Am Geriatr Soc 1997;45:945–948.

10. Lindley CM, Tully MP, Paramsothy V, et al. Inappropriate medication is a major cause of adverse drug reactions in elderly patients. Age Ageing 1992;21:294–300.

11. Beers MH. Explicit criteria for determining potentially inappropriate medication use by the elderly. Arch Intern Med 1997;157:1531–1536.

12. Beers MH, Ouslander JG, Fingold SF, et al. Inappropriate medication prescribing in skilled-nursing facilities. Ann Intern Med 1992;117:684–689.

13. Chrischilles EA, Segar ET, Wallace RB. Self-reported adverse drug reactions and related resource use. Ann Intern Med 1992;117:634–640.

14. Classen DC, Pestontnik SL, Evans S, et al. Adverse drug events in hospitalized patients. J Am Med Assoc 1997;277:301–306.

15. Bates DW, Spell N, Cullen DJ, et al. The costs of adverse drug events in hospitalized patients. J Am Med Assoc 1997;277:307–311.

16. Johnson JA, Bootman JL. Drug-related morbidity and mortality. Arch Intern Med 1995;155:1949–1956.

17. Ernst FR, Grizzle AJ. Drug-related morbidity and mortality: updating the cost-of-illness model. J Am Pharm Assoc 2001;41:192–199.

18. Bootman JL, Harrison DL, Cox E. The health care cost of drug-related morbidity and mortality in nursing facilities. Arch Intern Med 1997;157:2089–2096.

19. Stewart RB. Polypharmacy in the elderly: a fait accompli? DICP Ann Pharmacother 1990;24:321–323.

20. Hale WE, Perkins L, May FE, et al. Symptom prevalence in the elderly: an evaluation of age, sex, disease, and medication use. J Am Geriatr Soc 1986;34:333–340.

21. Bedell SE, Jabbour S, Goldberg R, et al. Discrepancies in the use of medications. Arch Intern Med 2000; 160:2129–2134.

22. Hogarty GE, Goldberg SC. Drug and sociotherapy in the after care of schizophrenic patients. Arch Gen Psychiatry 1973;28:54.

23. Cooper J, Love D, Rafoul P. Intentional prescription nonadherance (noncompliance) by the elderly. J Am Geriatr Soc 1982;30:329–333.

24. Rafoul P. Drug misuse among older people: focus for interdisciplinary efforts. Health Social Work 1986; 11:197–203.

25. McGrath JM. Physicians' perspectives on communicating prescription drug information. Qual Health Res 1999;9:731–745.

26. Bazargan M, Barbre AR, Hamm V. Failure to have prescriptions filled among black elderly. J Aging Health 1993;5:264–282.

27. Levit K, Cowan C, Braden B, et al. National health expenditures in 1997: more slow growth. Health Affairs (Millwood) 1998;17:99–110.

28. Hanlon JT, Landerman LR, Wall WE, et al. Is medication use by community-dwelling elderly people influenced by cognitive function? Age Ageing 1996;25:190–196.

29. Svarstad B. Patient–practitioner relationships and compliance with prescribed medical regimens. In: Aiken LH, Mechanic D, eds. Applications of Social Science to Clinical Medicine and Health Policy. Rutgers University Press, New Brunswick, NJ, 1986, pp. 438–459.

30. Dreher BB. Communication skills for working with elders. Springer-Verlag, New York, 1987.

31. Bradshaw PW, Ley P, Kincey JA, Bradshaw J. Recall of medical advice: comprehensibility and specificity. Br J Soc Clin Psychol 1975;14:55–62.

32. Ley P. What the patient forgets. Med Opin Rev 1966;1:71–73.

33. Tindall WN. The elderly patient: communicating with compassion. Patient Counc Commun Pharm 1983; 1:3–5.

34. Berardo DH. Identifying the elderly patient who needs counseling. Patient Counc Commun Pharm 1984; 2:3–11.

35. Carroll K, ed. Compensating for Sensory Loss. Ebenezer Center for Aging and Human Development, Minneapolis, MN, 1978.

36. Kline DW, Schieber F. Vision and aging. In: Birren JE, Schaie KW, eds. Handbook of the Psychology of Aging. 2nd ed. Van Nostrand Reinhold, New York, 1985, pp. 296–331.

37. National Health Interview Survey. US National Center for Health Statistics, Hyattsville, MD, 1981.

38. Copeland C. Prescription drugs: issues of cost, coverage, and quality. Employee Benefit Research Institute (EBRI) Issue Brief. 1999;208:1–21.

39. American Federation for Aging Research and the Alliance for Aging Research. Putting aging on hold: delaying the diseases of old age. An official report to the White House Conference on Aging. American Federation for Aging Research, Washington, DC, 1995, p. 9.

40. Mueller C, Schur C, O'Connell J. Prescription drug spending: the impact of age and chronic disease status. Am J Public Health 1997;87:1626–1629.

41. US Bureau of the Census. Current Population Reports, Special Studies, P-23-190. 65+ in the United States. US Government Printing Office, Washington, DC, 1996.

42. Ives TJ. Pharmacotherapeutics. In: Ham RJ, Sloane PD, eds. Primary Care Geriatrics: A Case-Based Approach, 3rd ed. Mosby, St. Louis, MO, 2002, pp. 137–148.

43. Mitchell J, Mathews HF, Hunt LM, et al. Mismanaging prescription medications among rural elders: the effects of socioeconomic status, health status, and medication profile indicators. 2001;41:348–356

44. Fouts M, Hanlon J, Pieper C, et al. Identification of elderly nursing facility residents at high risk for drug-related problems. Consult Pharm 1997;12:1103–1111.

45. Hanlon JT, Shimp LA, Semla TP. Recent advances in geriatrics: drug-related problems in the elderly. Ann Pharmacother 2000;34:360–365.

46. Hanlon JT, Fillenbaum GG, Schmaker KE. Inappropriate drug use among community-dwelling elderly. Pharmacotherapy 2000;20:575–582.

47. Zhan C, Sangl J, Bierman AS, Miller MR, Friedman B, Wickizer SW, et al. Potentially inappropriate medication use in the community-dwelling elderly–findings from the 1996 medical expenditure panel survey. JAMA 2001;286:2823–2829.

48. American Society of Consultant Pharmacists. Nursing Facility Survey Briefing Room. http://www.ascp.com/public/pr/may_hcfa_PDFs.shtml.

49. McCrory DC, Matchar DB, Samsa G, et al. Physician attitudes about anticoagulation for nonvalvular atrial fibrillation in the elderly. Arch Intern Med 1995;155:277–281.

50. Mendelson G, Aronow WS. Underutilization of warfarin in older persons with chronic nonvalvular atrial fibrillation at thigh risk for developing stroke. J Am Geriatr Soc 1998;46:1423–1424.

51. Ganz DA, Lamas GA, Orav EJ, Goldman L, Gutierrez PR, Mangione CM, for the Pacemaker Selection in the Elderly (PASE) Investigators. Age-related differences in management of heart disease: a study of cardiac medication use in an older cohort. J Am Geriatr Soc 1999;47:145–150.

52. Gurwitz JH, Field TS, Avorn J, et al. Incidence and preventability of adverse drug events in nursing homes. Am J Med 2000;109:87–94.

53. Soumerai SB, McLaughlin TJ, Spiegelman D, et al. Adverse outcomes of underuse of beta-blockers in elderly survivors of acute myocardial infarction. JAMA 1997;277:115–121.

54. Krumholz HM, Radford MJ, Wang Y, et al. National use of effectiveness of beta-blockers for the treatment of elderly patients after acute myocardial infarction—National Cooperative Cardiovascular Project. JAMA 1998;280:623–629.

55. Gottlieb SS, McCarter RJ, Vogel RA. Effect of beta-blockade on mortality among high-risk and low-risk patients after myocardial infarction. N Engl J Med 1998;339:489–497.

56. Barakat K, Wilkinson P, Deaner A, et al. How should age affect management of acute myocardial infarction? a prospective cohort study. Lancet 1999;353:955–959.

57. McLaughlin TJ, Soumerai SB, Willison DJ, et al. Adherence to national guidelines for drug treatment of suspected acute myocardial infarction: evidence for undertreatment in women and the elderly. Arch Intern Med 1996;156:799–805.

58. McCormick K, Gurwitz JH, Lessard D, et al. Use of aspirin, beta-blockers, and lipid-lowering medications before recurrent acute myocardial infarction. Arch Intern Med 1999;159:561–567.

59. Mendelson G, Aronow WS. Underutilization of beta-blockers in older patients with prior myocardial infarction or coronary artery disease in an academic, hospital-based geriatrics practice. J Am Geriatr Soc 1997;45:1360–1361.

60. Mendelson G, Aronow WS. Underutilization of angiotensin-converting enzyme inhibitors in older patients with Q-wave anterior myocardial infarction in an academic hospital-based geriatrics practice. J Am Geriatr Soc 1998;46:751–752.

61. Chin MH, Wang JC, Zhang JX, et al. Utilization and dosing of angiotensin-converting enzyme inhibitors for heart failure. Effect of physician specialty and patient characteristics. J Gen Intern Med 1997;12: 563–566.
62. Croft JB, Giles WH, Roegner RH, et al. Pharmacologic management of heart failure among older adults by office-based physicians in the United States. J Fam Practice 1997;44:382–390.
63. Krumholz HM, Radford MJ, Ellerbeck EF, et al. Aspirin for secondary prevention after acute myocardial infarction in the elderly: prescribed use and outcomes. Ann Intern Med 1996;124:292–298.
64. Gurwitz JH, Gore JM, Goldberg RJ, Rubison M, Chandra N, Rogers WJ, for the Participants in the National Registry of Myocardial Infarction. Recent age-related trends in the use of thrombolytic therapy in patients who have had acute myocardial infarction. Ann Intern Med 1996;124:283–291.
65. Berlowitz DR, Ash AS, Hickey EC, et al. Inadequate management of blood pressure in a hypertensive population. N Engl J Med 1998;339:1957–1963.
66. Mendelson G, Ness J, Aronow WS. Drug treatment of hypertension in older persons in an academic hospital-based geriatrics practice. J Am Geriatr Soc 1999;47:597–599.
67. Redelmeier DA, Tan SH, Booth GL. The treatment of unrelated disorders in patients with chronic medical diseases. N Engl J Med 1998;338:1516–1520.
68. Monette J, Gurwitz JH, Rochon PA, et al. Physician attitudes concerning warfarin for stroke prevention in atrial fibrillation: results of a survey of long-term care practitioners. J Am Geriatr Soc 1997;45: 1060–1065.
69. Brooke RH, Kamberg CJ, Mayer-Oakes A, et al. Appropriateness of acute medical care for the elderly. Health Policy 1990;14:225–242.
70. Kusserow RP. Medicare drug utilization review. Office of the Inspector General, Washington, DC, 1989.
71. Gattis WA, Hasselbald V, Whellan DJ, et al. Reduction in heart failure events by the addition of a clinical pharmacist to the heart failure management team. Arch Intern Med 1999;159:1939–1945.
72. McMullin ST, Hennenfent JA, Ritchie DJ, et al. A prospective, randomized trial to assess the cost impact of pharmacist-initiated interventions. Arch Intern Med 1999;159:2306–2309.
73. Leape LL, Cullen DJ, Clapp MD, et al. Pharmacist participation on physician rounds and adverse drug events in the intensive care unit. JAMA 1999;282:267–270.
74. Bates DW, Leape LL, Cullen DJ, et al. Effect of computerized physician order entry and a team intervention on prevention of serious medication errors. JAMA 1998;280:1311–1316.
75. Graves EJ. 1993 Summary: National Hospital Discharge Survey: Advance Data from Vital and Health Statistics No. 264. National Center for Health Statistics, Hyattsville, MD, 1995.
76. Koch H. Highlights of drug utilization in office practice: National Ambulatory Medical Care Survey, 1985. U.S. Department of Health and Human Services Publication 87-1250. Public Health Service, Washington, DC, 1987.
77. Reidenberg MM. Drug therapy in the elderly: the problem from the point of view of a clinical pharmacologist. Clin Pharmacol Ther 1987;42:677–680.
78. Zimmer AW, Calkins E, Hadley E, et al. Conducting clinical research in geriatric populations. Ann Intern Med 1985;103:276–283.
79. Levine RJ, ed. Selection of subjects. In: Ethics and Regulation of Clinical Research, 2nd ed. Urban & Schwarzenberg, Baltimore, MD, 1986, pp. 84–86.
80. Kitler ME. Clinical trials in the elderly. Clin Geriatr Med 1990;6:235–255.
81. Sundram CJ. Informed consent for major medical treatment of mentally disabled people. N Engl J Med 1988;318:1368–1373.
82. Pocock SJ, ed. The size of a clinical trial. In: Clinical Trials: A Practical Approach. Wiley, New York, 1983, p.188.
83. Wenger NK, O'Rourke A, Marcus FI. The care of elderly patients with cardiovascular disease. Ann Intern Med 1988;109:425–428.
84. Kalow W. Ethnic differences in drug metabolism. Clin Pharmacokinet 1982;7:373–400.
85. Hiller R, Kahn H. Blindness from glaucoma. Am J Opthalmol 1975;80:62–69.
86. Svensson CK. Representation of american blacks in clinical trials of new drugs. JAMA 1989;267:263–265.
87. Azarnoff DL. Physiologic factors in selecting human volunteers for drug studies. Clin Pharmacol Ther 1972;13:796–802.
88. Lamy PP. Geriatric drug therapy. Am Fam Physician 1986;34:118–124.
89. Ouslander JG. Drug therapy in the elderly. Ann Intern Med 1981;95:711–722.

5

Psychiatric Issues in the Care of the Elderly Cardiothoracic Surgery Patient

Edward T. Kenny, MD, *Philip R. Muskin,* MD, *and Peter A. Shapiro,* MD

Contents

INTRODUCTION

Psychological and psychiatric issues that arise in the setting of major surgery for the elderly patient are both challenging and complex. The psychological implications of cardiothoracic surgery, the meaning of the operation in the context of the patient's life, will vary from person to person. There are numerous potential complications caused by normal age-related changes in physiology that may affect the patient's mental status and cause or exacerbate psychiatric conditions. The patient's social environment, including how he or she affects and is affected by interpersonal exchanges with family and staff, will also impact on the preoperative and postoperative phases. This chapter will focus on common influences on geriatric patients' mental health, including social relations, character structure and coping methods, vulnerability to the emotional and cognitive sequelae of surgery, underlying psychiatric conditions, and adverse responses to medication. In addition to the discussion of diagnoses, therapeutic interventions will be suggested, including psychotherapeutic, systems-oriented, and pharmacological treatments.

From: *Aging, Heart Disease, and Its Management: Facts and Controversies*
Edited by: N. Edwards, M. Maurer, and R. Wellner © Humana Press Inc., Totowa, NJ

THE STRESS OF HOSPITALIZATION
AND THE PSYCHOLOGICALLY HEALTHY PATIENT

There are predictable stressors that each patient must experience during hospitalization for surgery. These include separation from the patient's home environment and all of the usual visual and other sensory clues that aid in orientation and provide reassurance through stability. The hospital environment is disorienting for the elderly patient not only because of its physical appearance but also because of the disruption of the patient's daily routine. The patient's everyday life is now replaced by the disruptive hospital routine: The intercom is on 24 h a day; vital signs are recorded when ideal for the nursing staff (early in the morning); the food is served on hospital time, not when the patient normally eats; and familiar faces (visitors) can only be present during the day. The patient may have to share quarters with a roommate who may be noisy or have noisy visitors. In the postoperative period, the disorienting effects of anesthesia, pain medications, the possible discontinuation of habitual medications, and pain itself all tend to alter the patient's sensorium. In addition, the patient will have at least temporary loss of function postoperatively as compared to his or her baseline, including physical limitations and possible cognitive changes of which the patient may be aware.

Cardiothoracic surgery and hospitalization place a major strain on the psyche. Ideally, the patient will traverse the hospital stay and deal effectively with the anxiety, sadness, and other difficult emotions that are generated. Many people endure these events well and only a few develop psychological or psychiatric illness. In part, these differences are the result of the patient's ability to cope and adapt to the challenges. Some are able to employ flexible coping skills, whereas others decompensate. This section will focus on healthy adaptational styles, to be contrasted later in the chapter with more maladaptive responses.

The psychologically healthy patient demonstrates a number of attributes and resources. She or he has good function in several domains, including intellectual and cognitive functioning, intact reality testing, and relationships with family and friends (1). Intellectual functioning can be gauged informally by the patient's educational level and level of achievement in work. Although staff members naturally form an impression of the patient through brief spontaneous conversations in the course of the day-to-day clinical routine, such impressions can be misleading. Social skills may function adequately even when other cognitive functions are impaired, such as memory and abstract thinking, which may adversely impact the patient's postoperative course. Family reports of the patient's cognition should be considered with a degree of skepticism, as family members may be unaware of the patient's deficits and are not trained in formal assessment. When the patient is living alone, he or she may have a routine that conceals cognitive deficits from others. More extensive formal neuropsychological testing is not routinely performed preoperatively, but in selected cases, it can be invaluable in helping the team decide whether the patient is sufficiently cognitively intact to undergo surgery. The patient's intellectual functioning must be differentiated from his or her ability to test reality. It is possible, for example, for a patient to have intact cognitive function (e.g., memory, abstract reasoning, calculation, etc.) but nonetheless have a distorted world view that may become a significant obstacle in surgical care. Sometimes, such distortions or delusions are immediately apparent to staff, but they often require formal psychiatric evaluation.

Clinical sketch: Mr. S was an 85-yr-old man who ran a large business with other family members. He had become lost driving himself to work on several occasions. Although he retained the ability to perform rapid mathematical calculations, he quoted prices to customers that were from a previous decade. When interviewed, he responded appropriately to every question, including questions about orientation. The interviewer noticed the daily newspaper was carefully placed so that Mr. S could see the date. Nurses reported he was pleasant and charming. However, careful probing revealed that he did not know why he was in the hospital; nor did he have an understanding of his serious illness that required surgical intervention.

The psychosocial supports available to the patient and visible to staff are another sign of the patient's psychological health and resilience. Having a host of family and friends who are interested in the patient's care indicates that the patient is able to form and maintain meaningful interpersonal relationships. This gives an immediate clue that personality problems are either not present in the person or are not severe enough to alienate other people. If such social connections are established, then it is likely that significant others will visit the patient in the hospital postoperatively. The therapeutic effects of such visits should not be underestimated. Visits will aid the patient in becoming reoriented postoperatively, reduce the effects of an unfamiliar hospital environment, attenuate the loneliness of hospitalization, and allow the patient access to better food. Visits by members of other social groups, such as church members, can also improve the morale of the patient.

The patient's accomplishments in recruiting others to affiliate with him in his private life are likely predictive of his ability to recruit support from the hospital team, including aides, nurses, social workers, physical and occupational therapists, surgeons, and other medical personnel. Bluntly stated, if the team comes to like the patient, it follows that its members will tend to pay more attention and pursue the workup and treatment of more reported symptoms; likeability is an important prognostic factor *(2)*. Even if the medical care preoperatively and postoperatively is technically the same for two patients, if one is well-liked and the other is not, it is likely that the relative harmony with the well-liked patient will contribute to his mental health in the recovery period and to a generally better outcome. However, what is important in the patient's recovery is not just what objectively measurable social supports are in place (e.g., number of family/friends involved in the care, frequency of visits) but is also the patient's perceived sense of social support. Instruments have been developed to measure this, such as Blumenthal's perceived social support scale *(3)*. One study has demonstrated that a high level of perceived social support moderates the negative impact that depression has on survival following myocardial infarction *(4)*. The relationship with reality of the patient's life is not always congruent with the person's objective experience. Patients with ample support from family and staff may, nonetheless, feel isolated and be subject to depressed mood and anxiety, whereas those who have few visitors and limited staff interaction may feel connected to others, remain euthymic, and fare better medically. Psychologically healthy patients adapt better to the stresses imposed upon them by illness, surgery, and recovery. The most appealing and psychologically mature strategy is the use of humor *(5)*. The prospect of having one's chest cut open and vital organs altered or removed is frightening to most people. Humor acknowledges the reality of the procedure but also deflects its impact by making light of it. Patients who use humor effectively reduce their own anxiety and attract the support of staff. Another high-level coping mechanism is sublimation. In the context of major surgery, sublimation might refer to the patient's conceptualization of the operation as a way to live longer or in better health, thus achieving a larger goal beyond his or her own personal well-being; for example, earning the opportunity to participate more in the raising of grandchildren. Healthy narcissism is another adaptive way to cope. A patient may brag about him or herself in a manner that appropriately draws admiration from the staff. Such narcissism is healthy if it does not entail the kind of anger, inconsiderate treatment of others, or demanding entitlement that alienates other people. Compulsive ways of coping can also be adaptive for dealing with the stress and anxiety of surgery. This is the type of patient who wishes to remain in control of all the facts. The patient may have a long daily list of concerns regarding laboratory results, the stage of healing of the wound, the reasons for medication changes, the timing of planned examinations or rehabilitation exercises, or a list of minor complaints that he or she wishes addressed. Clearly, this patient requires more work on behalf of the staff compared to the one who can laugh, ask a question or two, and feel comfortable giving up some control of life to the staff in order to recover. If the compulsive patient is able to ally with the staff after the many questions have been patiently answered and does not derail the care with excessive concerns and demands, he or she also too counts as a healthy patient. Another indication of health is the patient who uses adaptive denial, minimizing the importance of the operation or subsequent complications but cooperating fully with the team's plan. This is in contrast to the patient in denial who refuses to comply with medical recommendations (6).

More problematic coping styles will be discussed in the section on Personality Disorders.

DIAGNOSIS AND MANAGEMENT
OF VARIOUS PSYCHIATRIC DISORDERS

Adjustment Disorders

Partly as a result of the combined effect of stressors in the hospital setting, new or recurrent psychiatric problems may appear. Along the spectrum of severity, the adjustment disorders tend to be the most mild of the affective disorders. According to the diagnostic manual published by the American Psychiatric Association, an adjustment disorder entails the development of emotional or behavioral symptoms in response to a recent identifiable stressor; typically, an anxious or depressed mood is present (7). Symptoms occur within 3 mo of the stressor, do not last more than 6 mo, and do not meet the criteria for another disorder such as major depression or generalized anxiety disorder. Treatment may consist of periodic assessment and supportive care. If the mood or anxiety symptoms seem more severe or chronic, medication treatment, similar to that discussed next, should be considered.

Anxiety Disorders

Anxiety can take many forms; it may manifest as fear, apprehensiveness, hypervigilance, or an exaggerated startle and autonomic response to unexpected stimuli. New anxiety symptoms can become evident in the immediate postoperative period, even while the patient is still intubated. Patients with a history of chronic obstructive pulmonary disease (COPD) are especially at risk for developing panic attacks when intubated (8), which may complicate attempts at weaning from the ventilator. A common practice in some surgical intensive care units is to administer a short-acting benzodiazepine such as alprazolam (Xanax) when a panic attack occurs. In general, benzodiazepines should be avoided in the treatment of the elderly because they are more likely to cause paradoxical agitation in addition to side effects, including memory impairment and the potential for addiction (9). Very short-acting benzodiazepines such as midazolam (Versed), which are often given in intensive care units as an intravenous infusion, have the potential of causing rebound agitation and anxiety.

If a benzodiazepine is to be used, one with an intermediate half-life such as lorazepam (Ativan) is preferable. Benzodiazepines with long half-lives, such as diazepam (Valium) and especially flurazepam (Dalmane), should be avoided, as they have the potential to cause lethargy and mental status changes in the elderly patient. These effects can complicate the diagnosis and treatment of a patient with mental status changes, particularly if there is an unknown medical reason for altered mental status (infection, electrolyte disturbance, etc.).

Treatment of the anxious patient who cannot be weaned off of the ventilator often requires both pharmacological and behavioral interventions. Low doses of haloperidol or a second-generation antipsychotic (e.g., olanzapine, quetiapine, risperidone, ziprasidone) can be useful in treating acute anxiety in the intensive care unit.

In addition to psychopharmacological management of anxiety and panic in the intubated patient, behavioral techniques can be an effective adjunct. If the clinician can engage the anxious patient who is taking rapid and shallow breaths, it may be possible to influence him to take deeper, slower, abdominal breaths. Encouraging the patient to concentrate on this type of breathing helps move dead-space air and provides a focus that itself can be calming. Most patients are not able to learn abdominal breathing in a single session; usually, several sessions of training over consecutive days are necessary. Anxious patients constrict their chest walls and take quick shallow breaths from their chests. One method of teaching deep abdominal breathing is for the physician to place a hand on the chest wall and the other hand on the abdomen, instructing the patient to relax the chest and keep it still while expanding the abdomen fully with each inspiration and pulling it in forcefully on expiration. The patient can place his hands over or under the physician's to progressively gain mastery of these movements.

> **Clinical sketch:** Mr. M was a 77 yr-old man with a history of hypertension, cerebrovascular accident (CVA) with residual left hemiparesis, and COPD secondary to cigarette smoking. Following his CVA years earlier, he developed chronic dysphoria but refused psychiatric care at the time. He was admitted to the hospital for mitral valve repair. His postoperative course was complicated by a sternal wound dehiscence, a respiratory infection, and panic attacks during weaning attempts from the ventilator. A psychiatry consult was called. After numerous medication trials and dosage adjustments, the patient was stabilized on 15 mg mirtazapine, 20 mg citalopram, and 5 mg olanzapine, all administered at night. In addition, he was taught deep abdominal breathing. After several weeks of an up-and-down course, with near-daily attention from his cardiologist, pulmonologist, and psychiatrist, he was successfully weaned, underwent rehabilitation, and was discharged from the hospital. His mood improved markedly and both the patient and his wife agreed that it was better than at preoperative baseline. After he was able to speak, he remarked that despite his initial skepticism, he found the deep breathing effective in enabling him to calm himself and to greatly diminish the sensation of suffocation.

Major and Minor Depressive Disorders

Symptoms of depression include marked depressed mood, loss of interest in those activities or relationships that the individual formerly was involved with, troubled sleep characterized by difficulty falling asleep, frequent awakenings, and/or early-morning awakening, feelings of guilt, worthlessness or hopelessness, fatigue or low energy, diminished ability to concentrate or make decisions, increased or decreased appetite or weight, psychomotor agitation or retardation, and thoughts of death or suicide. Patients who complain of only a few symptoms may not meet the criteria for a major depressive disorder and might not be considered as candidates for treatment with an antidepressant. However, in a study of patients with hypertension who had subthreshold depression, it was found that they resembled, both demographically and clinically, patients who had affective illness *(10)*. Such patients have a 25% risk of developing a major depression within the ensuing two years *(11)*.

RISKS OF DEPRESSION AND GENERAL MEDICAL ILLNESS

Depression confers an increased risk of morbidity and mortality on patients with a variety of medical illnesses. In a recent study, 47% of depressed patients with acute, life-threatening medical illness died, a mortality rate five times higher than that in similar patients without depression *(12)*. Symptoms of anhedonia, hopelessness, worthlessness, indecisiveness, and insomnia are predictors of death in hospitalized patients *(13)*.

In the first 10 yr following a stroke, depressed patients are 3.4 times more likely to die than are patients without depression *(14)*. Because most patients do not react with sadness to medical problems, and because depression typically has a somatic component, depression should be considered in every patient who presents with sadness. Conversely, a depressive or anxiety disorder should be considered as one possible cause of symptoms in patients with undiagnosed somatic complaints.

RISKS OF DEPRESSION AND CARDIAC DISEASE

There now exists a substantial body of evidence indicating that depression of any severity is associated with adverse cardiac health, even in the absence of known pre-existing coronary artery disease *(15)*. The risk of death in the 6–18 mo following a myocardial infarction is increased fourfold in patients with depression *(16,17)*.

Based on a recent study of 309 patients, risk factors for depression after coronary artery bypass graft (CABG) surgery included a prior history of depression, combined CABG and valve repair/replacement surgery or reoperation, NYHA Class IV congestive heart failure symptoms (which include resting shortness of breath, fatigue, and chest pain), and length of hospital stay greater than 5 d *(18)*. Low ejection fraction and history of myocardial infarction were not risk factors for depression in this study.

The prevalence of depression after CABG surgery has been estimated at 20–40% *(18,19)*. Table 1 summarizes the findings of several studies *(15–17,20–29)*. There have been several mechanisms proposed to explain the connection between depression and coronary artery disease (CAD). Of the mechanisms proposed, perhaps the most intuitive is evidence for decreased compliance with medical treatment for CAD *(30)*. Another candidate mechanism is a generalized vascular disease process that affects both the heart and the central nervous system. Evidence for this includes white-matter hyperintensities on brain magnetic resonance images, which suggest microvascular disease seen frequently in geriatric patients with depression *(31)*. Other evidence indicates enhanced platelet aggregation in depression, possibly resulting in increased incidence of thrombus formation. Another well-documented association is decreased beat-to-beat variability on the electrocardiogram, a manifestation of decreased vagal tone relative to sympathetic tone; this results in increased vulnerability to arrhythmias, including sudden death from ventricular tachycardia. The additional proposed mechanism points to the altered inflammatory processes in depression, such that plaque formation is increased and plaque stability is decreased. It may be that all of these mechanisms—possibly in addition to other undiscovered mechanisms—combine synergistically to increase the risk of adverse cardiac events *(30,32–34)*.

Table 1
Depression and Risk of CAD

Condition (ref.)	Population	Outcome	Odds ratio or relative risk
Depressive symptoms (15,20–23)	Community samples	Incident CAD	1.5–2.0
Depressive symptoms (24)	Unstable angina patients	Nonfatal myocardial infarction (MI) or death	6.7
Depressive symptoms (16,17)	Post-MI patients	Cardiac death at 18 mo	6.6
Major depressive disorder (15,20–23)	Community samples	MI	4.0
Major depressive disorder (25–27)	CAD patients	Acute coronary syndromes	1.5–4.0
Major depressive disorder (16,17)	Post-MI patients	Cardiac death, (6 mo follow-up)	3.6
Major depressive disorder (28,29)	Post-CABG patients	Recurrent cardiac events (12 mo follow-up)	3.2

UNCOVERING DEPRESSION IN THE MEDICALLY ILL

Making the diagnosis of depression is especially challenging in patients with disease in whom the illness or the treatment causes symptoms that resemble the somatic component of depression. A variety of medical disorders or their treatments can cause fatigue, decreased appetite, muscular aches, or headaches. Pain, nausea, nocturnal urination, and concerns about one's health and about stressful life events may interrupt normal sleeping patterns. When people feel unwell, they lose interest in activities that they usually find appealing. They may also lose interest in sexual activity. Numerous medical disorders can produce some of the vegetative symptoms of depression. The physician may facilitate the diagnostic evaluation by inquiring about the psychological symptoms of depression (e.g., indecisiveness, dissatisfaction with medical care, a feeling of failure, feeling "punished" by the illness, hopelessness, frequent crying, and thoughts about dying) (35). Inquiry about previous episodes of depression, a family history of depression, or substance abuse can be helpful in reaching a decision about the current psychiatric state of the patient. Women have consistently been found to show a higher incidence of depression than men (2:1); therefore, the physician should have a higher index of suspicion (36). Another clue that a patient is depressed and is not just unhappy about his or her illness is a mismatch of the medical course and the patient's emotional state. A patient whose mood does not improve in concert with his or her medical illness may be suffering from a depressive disorder.

Time constraints sometimes make obtaining a full psychiatric history difficult. In keeping with the general principle that simple is better, the question "Are you depressed?" has been shown to be a valid screen, as good as a more time-consuming screening instrument, in terminally ill patients (37).

In considering treatment of a depressive episode in the postoperative patient, it is important to determine whether the patient has had prior episodes and what treatments (pharmacological and/or psychotherapeutic) have been successful or unsuccessful in the past. Information obtained from family members or outpatient mental health providers can aid in planning treatment.

PHARMACOLOGICAL TREATMENT OF DEPRESSION

Serotonin reuptake inhibitors (SSRIs) have replaced tricyclic antidepressants (TCAs) as first-line pharmacologic agents in the treatment of depression. The primary reason for this shift is not an efficacy difference but a difference in safety and tolerability of side effects. Although TCAs have type 1A antiarrhythmic effects (they can become proarrhythmic in the setting of myocardial ischemia), the most common cardiovascular side effect of TCAs is orthostatic hypotension, which increases the risk of falling, a serious threat for elderly individuals. Nortriptyline is the least likely TCA to cause orthostatic hypotension in geriatric patients. In contrast to the TCAs, serotonin reuptake inhibitors have demonstrated minimal adverse hemodynamic effects and minimal electrocardiographic effect in patients with heart disease *(38,39)*. SSRIs are even considered safe in patients with severely compromised cardiac function and with most arrhythmias. Preliminary data suggest reasonable safety in acute myocardial infarction (MI) patients. There is some evidence that SSRIs may improve ejection fraction in patients with impaired left-ventricular function *(38–40)*.

Initial side effects of SSRIs include gastrointestinal effects such as frequent bowel movements and nausea. Although these side effects are usually transient, they may persist in some cases and preclude the use of this class of agents. Another aspect of SSRI action to be taken into consideration is the relative potential for these agents to cause either sedation or activation. Citalopram, fluoxetine, and sertraline tend to be activating and, for many elderly patients, can cause agitation and insomnia. Treatment should typically be initiated at a low dose and be titrated up as needed. Paroxetine tends to be the most sedating of the SSRIs and may cause oversedation.

In postoperative patients who are taking multiple medications, an important point of consideration in antidepressant selection is the effect on the hepatic cytochrome P450 (CYP) system (*see* Table 2). Fluoxetine, paroxetine, bupropion, and sertraline (in this order) have the greatest potential effect of altering drug levels of medications that are metabolized by the CYP2D6 enzyme system. Numerous antiarrythmics, narcotics, antidepressants, β-blockers, as well as codeine and dextromethorphan are metabolized by the CYP2D6 system.

Nefazodone and fluvoxamine have the greatest effects on the CYP3A4 system. Drugs that inhibit the hepatic cytochrome P450 3A4 isoenzyme will reduce metabolism and increase blood levels of other drugs such as calcium-channel blockers, certain benzodiazepines, and many of the new antihistamines (most of which are no longer on the market). Drugs such as ketoconazole, itraconazole, macrolide antibiotics, and antiretroviral agents are also potent CYP3A4 inhibitors. Elevated levels of some 3A4-metabolized drugs lead to QT prolongation and increased risk of ventricular tachycardia or fibrillation. Some drugs, such as rifampin, induce the CYP2D6 system, increasing clearance and decreasing the serum level of other drugs. In a similar manner, St. John's Wort induces the CYP3A4 system.

Data concerning the use of antidepressant agents in elderly cardiac patients are sparse. Bupropion has no known adverse hemodynamic side effects. It can be activating, which may be problematic in some patients. Venlafaxine increases the levels of synaptic norepinephrine as well as serotonin in doses above 225 mg/d. At doses above 225 mg daily, it has been associated with a small increase in blood pressure in up to 10% of patients. Nefazodone is a mild serotonin reuptake inhibitor, but it also blocks the effects of serotonin on one of the postsynaptic receptors. It may cause orthostatic hypotension in some patients. It can be sedating, which is advantageous for some patients who have insomnia, but some patients may not tolerate the sedative effect.

Table 2
Pharmacokinetic Profiles of Selected Antidepressants

					Feature				
	Half-life	Metabolite	Metabolite half-life	Steady state	Dose-proportional plasma levels	Protein binding	Dose reduction in elderly	CYP enzyme inhibition	Dose range
Sertraline	1 d	20–30%	2–4 d	1–2 wk	Yes	98%	No	Dose related p2D6, 3A4	50–250
Fluoxetine	2–3 d	Equal	7–9 d	4–6 wk	No	95%	No	2D6 +++ 34A +++ 2C19 +++	20–80
Paroxetine	1 d	No	—	5 d	No	95%	No	2D6 +++	20–50
Mirtazapine	20–40 h	10%	30–40 h	5–7 d	Yes	85%	No	Minimal	15–45
Nefazodone	2–4 h	Variable activity	1.5–18 h	<5 d	No	99%	No	3A4+++	300–600
Bupropion	14 h	Yes	20 h	5–8 d	Yes	84%	No	2D6 ++	300–450
Venlafaxine	5 h	Equal activity	11 h	<5 d	Yes	20–30%	No	Minimal	75–375
Citalopram	35 h	Low activity	49 h	1 wk	Yes	80%	No	Minimal	20–60

The most troubling side effects of the newer antidepressants are the effect on sexual function and the potential for weight gain. Although not an immediate problem for the patient postoperatively, these side effects are disconcerting and lead to noncompliance. An open rapport with the patient and inquiry about side effects during outpatient follow-up will typically reveal the problem if present. Consulting a psychiatric colleague about alternative treatments or referring the patient to a psychiatrist are a worthwhile consideration.

The psychostimulants are underutilized agents in the treatment of depression in the elderly. They are useful in elderly patients who demonstrate apathy, withdrawal, and loss of appetite, sometimes without other signs of major depression *(41)*. In this state, recovery from surgery can be compromised if the patient is not motivated to comply with rehabilitation efforts or if oral food intake is inadequate. Although other antidepressant agents can be initiated, the time-course of onset of action can be weeks. In contrast, psychostimulants can take effect within a few days and often have the additional benefit of mild cognitive enhancement. Treatment with a psychostimulant can be initiated in the same time frame as starting an SSRI (perhaps with staggering treatment for a few days to observe for any initial side effects from either agent). If effective, psychostimulants can either be continued or tapered off after symptoms have resolved and adequate time has been allowed for other antidepressants to take effect. Many surgical and medical teams are reluctant to allow use of these medications because of a concern regarding the development of hypertension and tachycardia. However, with careful initial dosing (e.g., methylphenidate started at 2.5 mg in the morning [qam]) and monitoring, these effects need not be limiting. In fact, in the post-MI setting, such hemodynamic effects can easily be managed through adjusting other components of the patient's medication regimen. For example, patients who have suffered myocardial infarction are treated routinely with β-blockers, which lower both heart rate and blood pressure. Adverse hemodynamic effects from psychostimulants are rare *(42)*, but if they occur, one strategy for alleviating them is to adjust the dose of the β-blocker.

PSYCHOTHERAPEUTIC TREATMENT OF DEPRESSION

Taking the time and effort to ensure a solid therapeutic alliance with the elderly surgical patient is perhaps even more important for the psychiatrist than for the surgeon. In most traditional societies, mental health problems were considered shameful and, hence, were concealed, denied, or reformulated as somatic problems that could then legitimately be treated by medical means. It is only in the last few decades in the United States that mental health treatment has begun to be accepted by the general public as having comparable legitimacy as surgical and medical treatment. The majority of elderly patients today are from a generation in which where mental illness and its treatment carry the same stigma as in most traditional societies. A multinational study of depression revealed that 69% of patients with depression present with a somatic, not a psychological, complaint *(43)*. This supports the view that most patients consider it acceptable to seek help for medical or somatic complaints but not for mental health problems. If the physician requests a psychiatric consultation for a patient, it should be expected that the patient might be thinking, "does my doctor think I am crazy?" Changing this perception is essential for the successful treatment of depression, including compliance with medication. This needs to be overtly addressed, even if it remains unspoken by the patient.

The surgeon or internist should always inform the patient ahead of time when a consultation with a psychiatrist is necessary. The phrasing of this communication can either facilitate or impede the initial consultation. If the surgeon says, "I would like a psychiatrist to come and speak with you, is that alright with you?," this approach invites patient refusal. A suggested alternative statement is the following:

"You seem depressed to me and I am concerned this may adversely affect your recovery. Because I need help with this, I have asked one of our psychiatrists to come speak with you in order to assist me in understanding you better and improving our care."

This formulation was recommended by Jennifer Downey, MD. Communicating the request for the psychiatric consultation in this way makes it more acceptable to the patient, because it is formulated as a need of the surgeon or internist, rather than of the patient.

Controlled trials have demonstrated that psychotherapy in addition to psychiatric medication is more effective than medication alone *(44,45)*.

Bipolar Disorder

Bipolar disorder tends to be less common than unipolar major depressive disorder in the elderly preoperative patient. Patients with bipolar disorder often experience depressive episodes and also suffer from varying degrees of mania. Manic symptoms include unnaturally elevated mood, irritability, racing thoughts, increased level of activity (which may be organized and productive or disorganized), and abnormally and uncharacteristically impulsive behavior, such as increased spending or sexual activity. The decision whether or not to proceed with a major cardiothoracic operation in an elderly patient with bipolar disorder will be based in part on the preoperative psychiatric stability of the patient. Factors to consider include the frequency of manic and depressive episodes (the degree of cycling), the time since the last manic or depressive episode, and the degree to which psychosis and behavioral dyscontrol have been present. In addition, the patient's response to medications, especially mood stabilizers (e.g., lithium, valproic acid), antipsychotic drugs, and antidepressants should be taken into account, as should response to electrical convulsive therapy (ECT), including the degree of cognitive loss resulting from ECT. Routine preoperative assessment should include a thorough review of these issues with the patient, his family, and the patient's psychiatrist. Studies should include a complete blood count (in particular, to determine the platelet count in patients on valproate), a chemistry panel including BUN/Cr and a urinalysis (to gauge kidney function in patients on lithium), liver function tests (for patients on valproate), and thyroid function tests (for patients on lithium). At the time of surgery, there are often marked fluid shifts; hence, lithium should probably be withheld to avoid the risk of lithium toxicity. Postoperatively, analgesics are routinely used to reduce postoperative pain, including opioid drugs, which often alter mental status. In this setting, adjustment of mood-stabilizing drugs may be necessary to limit oversedation. There is conflicting evidence regarding whether abrupt discontinuation of lithium may reduce its effectiveness *(46,47)*; in patients who may need to discontinue lithium temporarily for medical reasons in the perioperative period, a planned tapering off of lithium prior to the operation is advised.

MENTAL STATUS CHANGES AFTER CARDIOTHORACIC SURGERY

Postoperative mental status changes can manifest as agitation, confusion, and cognitive impairment. Anxiety as a potential cause has already been discussed. Encephalopathy is cerebral dysfunction with impaired cognition or confusion. It may be acute or chronic (static encephalopathy) and may or may not meet criteria for delirium. Withdrawal from alcohol, benzodiazepines, or other substances should always be considered. Other common causes of mental status changes, including dementia, delirium, and psychosis, will be discussed in detail in this section.

Delirium

Delirium is a disturbance of consciousness that usually develops acutely, over the course of hours or days. It is manifested by changes in consciousness and cognition. Typically, it involves fluctuation in the level of consciousness during the course of the day. Hallmarks of delirium also include waxing and waning levels of alertness, reduced ability to focus, sustain or shift attention, disorientation, memory and language deficits, and hallucinations. A final criterion is that there must be direct evidence that delirium is the physiological consequence of a general medical condition *(7)*.

The other primary diagnostic possibility from which delirium must be differentiated is a worsening or evolving dementia. Delirium can occur in patients with pre-existing dementia. It is important to recognize the presence of delirium in these cases, because improved mental status can result from discovering its cause and properly directing treatment. Diagnosis is more difficult if an acute delirium is superimposed on a more chronic dementing process. Diagnosing delirium in a patient with pre-existing dementia is particularly important to avoid prematurely attributing the patient's change in mental status to a chronic degenerative disease about which little can be done. Clues to the diagnosis of dementia include a history of slow, progressive cognitive decline and a more constant level of alertness and attention that does not fluctuate.

There are multiple common causes of delirium in the elderly surgical patient, which may act singly or in combination. These include the effects of general anesthesia, which can persist for several days after the operation, causing disorientation, behavioral dyscontrol, and hallucinations. The effects tend to recede spontaneously over the course of a few days. If the patient requires a stay in the intensive care unit, pharmacologic agents in common use in many units can contribute to delirium. These include opioid medications (e.g., fentanyl), benzodiazepines (e.g., midazolam [Versed]), and barbiturates (e.g., propofol [Diprivan]). Of these, the benzodiazepines and barbiturates deserve special note: both administration of and withdrawal from these medications may precipitate delirium. The term "ICU psychosis" has come into common usage among medical and surgical teams and refers to the delirium that often occurs in the intensive care setting. It is important to note that "ICU psychosis" is usually caused by medical disorders or medication side effects. Thus, a thorough workup for treatable causes of mental status changes must be initiated and continued while treatment is started. In addition to possible physiologic causes of delirium, aspects of the ICU environment itself may contribute to the development of delirium, including frequent interruptions for monitoring, blood draws, sleep-disrupting noises such as beeping sounds from ventilators and other equipment, and disruption of day–night cycles. It is clear that the current typical ICU environment creates extraordinary psychophysiological stress, particularly for the elderly.

After the patient is beyond the initial postoperative recovery period, ongoing use of opioid analgesic agents is a frequent contributor to altered mental status and delirium. A variety of other medications can cause confusion in elderly patients, including anticholinergics, anti-Parkinson medications, antibiotics, antihistamines, and nonsteroidal anti-inflammatory drugs (NSAIDs) *(48)*. It is important to keep in mind that patients on multiple medications may be particularly at risk for developing a medication-induced delirium.

Infectious causes of delirium are common, including sternal wound infections and urinary tract infections (UTIs). Although more frequent in women than men, UTIs become a greater concern as a potential cause of delirium in both genders with advancing age. It should be noted that certain antibiotics used to treat UTIs can also cause delirium, notably ciprofloxacin. There are multiple other causes of delirium in the elderly, including electrolyte imbalances and endocrinologic disorders.

TREATMENT

In addition to addressing the underlying causes of delirium, physical restraint, use of antipsychotic agents, and other environmental supports comprise the basic treatment of delirium. Safe and effective physical restraints include vest restraints (Poseys) and two- or four-point restraints. Family members need to be informed of both the safety and necessity of these restraints. The use of bed rails alone is contraindicated, as they constitute a fall risk. Almost every delirious patient could benefit from having a 24-h aide at bedside to provide surveillance, reassurance, frequent verbal reorientation, and some degree of mild physical restraint if necessary, which, in some cases, would obviate the need for Poseys and other restraints. However, the use of aides is extremely expensive for the hospital. The family can assist by providing a private-duty nurse or by taking turns staying with the patient.

The short-term use of antipsychotic medication helps attain behavioral control, causes necessary sedation during the day and at night, improving quality of sleep, and helps control psychosis, including hallucinations. The typical antipsychotic agent, haloperidol, is in wide use, has minimal risk side effects at low doses when used transiently, and can safely be administered by all routes (orally, intramuscularly, and intravenously). It is the only antipsychotic now available for intravenous use. In a study of agitated cardiac patients at the Massachusetts General Hospital, high-dose intravenous haloperidol was found to be safe *(49)*, although there have been reports linking haloperidol with torsade de pointes *(50–52)*.

Chlorpromazine, a more sedating antipsychotic agent, can be given orally or intramuscularly, but it can cause problematic orthostatic hypotension, an effect even more pronounced when the drug is co-administered with benzodiazepines. However, in the low doses typically required by medical patients, a sedating antipsychotic such as chlorpromazine may be quite efficacious and avoids the need to combine a nonsedating antipsychotic with a benzodiazepine *(53)*.

In general, the use of benzodiazepines should be avoided in the elderly, as this class of medication can paradoxically cause agitation and aggravate confusion. If the patient can be administered medication orally, we favor the use of second-generation antipsychotic drugs. Of these, risperidone may be used as a first-line agent for the following reasons: it is at least as effective as haloperidol, has negligible risk for side effects such as extrapyramidal symptoms, tardive dyskinesia, and akathisia, and has the least anticholinergic effect of this class of drugs. In our clinical experience, olanzapine (typically at doses of 5 mg qd or bid) or quetiapine (at doses of 50 mg bid) are also safe and effective agents for use during episodes of delirium, despite an increased potential for anticholinergic side effects as compared to risperidone *(54)*. Data are limited for the use of the newest antipsychotic, ziprasidone (Geodon); this medication should probably be avoided in elderly cardiac patients until further data are available because of the potential for Q-T prolongation.

Psychosis

Psychosis includes both changes in perception, such as hallucinations, and aberrations in thinking, such as delusions. A delusion can be defined as a fixed, false belief that is not culturally shared and not subject to reality testing. The presence of psychosis is not in itself diagnostic, as psychosis can be associated with a wide variety of psychiatric conditions such as affective disorders (depression and mania), delirium, dementia, brief reactive psychosis, schizophrenia, and schizoaffective disorder. As in any psychiatric condition, diagnosis can be greatly aided by collateral history from the patient's significant other and outpatient caregivers. The most important aspect of treatment for any psychotic disorder is the administration of antipsychotic medication.

Dementia

In general, dementia is differentiated from delirium by its chronic, progressive course (subacute onset) of decline in cognitive functions and the preservation of the level of alertness. Multiple cognitive deficits are seen in dementia, including memory impairment and one or more of the following: aphasia, apraxia, agnosia, or impaired executive function. There is a clinically significant impairment in function—a decline from the patient's previous level of ability—and these deficits do not occur exclusively in the setting of acute delirium. Fifteen million people worldwide are affected by Alzheimer's disease (55), which is the most prevalent type of dementia, followed by vascular dementia (formerly multi-infarct dementia). Although the progression of Alzheimer's tends to be gradual, cognitive deficits in vascular dementias tend to be stepwise, associated with adverse intracerebral vascular events such as cerebrovascular accidents.

It is particularly important to assess the degree of dementia in the surgical candidate because of the risk of significant further cognitive impairment as a result of cardiopulmonary bypass (56). Although collateral history may be helpful, the clinician must be alert to the possibilities of subjective distortion by family members based on their wish that the patient is thinking and functioning on a higher level than he actually is. Similarly, casual conversations with the patient do not suffice; she may have preserved social skills and may appear quite bright and reactive but may have hidden memory or other cognitive deficits that would increase her risk of postoperative cognitive morbidity.

If confusion occurs in the postoperative setting in a patient known to suffer from dementia, it is important to consider the possibility of the co-occurrence of other psychiatric disorders, notably delirium and depression. Being diagnostically thorough is necessary to avoid the risk of attributing all abnormal mental status findings to dementia, which would deprive the patient of potentially helpful laboratory examinations and treatment.

A tool that is useful in initial screening for dementia is the Mini-Mental State Examination (MMSE), which tests for orientation, short-term memory, attention, constructional ability, and verbal skills (57). This test takes only a few minutes to perform and does not have to be administered by a psychiatrist. It will help differentiate patients who are in the normal range from those who clearly suffer from significant cognitive deficits. In cases where the MMSE score is borderline and other evidence of the patient's mental state is equivocal, more extensive neurologic assessment and neuropsychological testing can be undertaken if needed.

See Table 3 for a summary of management suggestions for postoperative confusion and agitation.

Table 3
Summary of Management of Postoperative Confusion and Agitation

Identify and treat correctable contributors
Use antipsychotics, not benzodiazepines
Avoid antipsychotics that can prolong the QT interval and increase the risk of torsade de pointes
Improve the environment:
  Maximize orienting stimuli
    Increase human contact through the presence of family members and 24-h aides, if possible
    Institute frequent checks by nursing staff
    Foster day–night cycles of activity

Adverse Cerebral Outcomes after CABG

The risks of developing adverse cognitive function following coronary artery bypass surgery are significant. One study found that the incidence of adverse cerebral outcomes after CABG was 6.1%; the percentage of patients with focal injury or stupor–coma at discharge was 3.1%; the rate of deterioration of intellectual function or seizures was 3.0%. Those patients who suffered adverse cerebral outcomes had a higher in-hospital mortality rate, longer hospital stays, and a higher rate of discharge to assisted-living facilities. Predictors of focal injury or stupor–coma at discharge included proximal aortic atherosclerosis, history of neurologic disease, and older age. Predictors of deterioration in intellectual function or seizures included older age, systolic hypertension on admission, pulmonary disease, or alcohol abuse *(56)*.

In a longitudinal study, 261 patients who had CABG underwent neurocognitive testing preoperatively, before discharge, and after surgery at 6 wk, 6 mo, and 5 yr. The incidence of cognitive decline was 53% at discharge, 36% at 6 wk, 24% at 6 mo, and 42% at 5 yr. It was found that early improvement followed by a later decline in cognitive function was predicted by early postoperative cognitive decline; cognitive function at discharge was found to be a significant predictor of long-term function *(58)*. It is important to note that this study was done without age-matched controls.

Risk factors for postoperative confusion include age, alcohol use, prior cerebrovascular disease, prior head injury, prior cognitive impairment, prolonged sedation, hepatic dysfunction, renal insufficiency, and the use of narcotics *(56,58–60)*.

Assessing the patient's preoperative cognitive level and risk factors for cognitive decline is essential for weighing the risks and benefits of the operation. Quality-of-life improvements after CABG, expected from improved cardiac function, may be vitiated by neurocognitive decline. This may be especially so if there is a threshold effect for patients who show only mild cognitive impairment preoperatively but who become more profoundly cognitively impaired following cardiopulmonary bypass. Other factors associated with poor improvement or decline in quality of life after cardiac surgery in elderly patients include diabetes, COPD, female gender, and reoperation *(61)*.

PERSONALITY DISORDERS

The character style of the patient has a major influence on his or her experience of illness and hospitalization. Character style does not mean character pathology but rather is the characteristic manner in which an individual will experience the world and behave in it. We all have a personality with certain typical features. Although there can be pathological concomitants for each personality type, we should try not to overemphasize a "diagnosis." Instead, we should try to understand how the patient's typical reactions are shaded by personality. Recognizing the character styles on each side in a particular patient–doctor dyad helps the psychiatrist clarify the extent to which the treating doctor is engaged positively or negatively by the patient's character.

Kahana and Bibring conceptualized seven personality types *(62)*. These are not psychiatric disorders, but styles. Keeping in mind that both patients and physicians have personality styles will allow greater flexibility in helping patients cope with the psychological stress of serious illness and surgery.

Patients Who Are Dependent and Overdemanding (Oral)

The overdemanding individual seems to need special attention and has an urgency about his needs. Such people can be impulsive, appear naive about their demands, and be insistent upon care without limitations from their doctors. There is the potential for anger, depression, and inappropriate use of medications or drugs, as these people often have a low tolerance for frustration. The individual fears abandonment and wishes for unlimited care. Illness reawakens the desire to exist in a secure, infantile state where another provides for all of the person's needs. Acute illness is perceived as the result of a failure of protection and caring by others. The physician needs to structure interactions to convey the intent to care for the patient as is necessary (i.e., make it clear *what* the physician will do to help the patient recover). The inevitable setting of limits should be presented neither as punishment for the patient's inexhaustible demands nor as the doctor's withdrawal, but as thoughtfully considered realities.

Patients Who Are Orderly and Controlled (Compulsive)

"Knowledge is power" might best describe these people, who seek to control their anxiety by finding out as many "facts" as are possible. Orderly, neat, and conscientious patients may be quite obstinate in dealings related to their health. Physical illness strains the person's psychological defenses against unconscious impulses to soil, to be aggressive, or to act hedonistically. This increases his or her insistence on being orderly and containing emotions. It may result in the person behaving in a ritualized manner or in behavior that is odd and intensely formal. In an effort to gain control through knowledge, such patients ask questions repeatedly. Never satisfied that they have "enough information," they may become indecisive when required to make decisions regarding their care. "Informed consent" can become a caricature with such patients. By providing details of the medical/surgical plan, addressing why a procedure is required, and reviewing the science of the medical approach, the physician can reassure these patients. When given adequate, but not overwhelming detail, such patients can use psychological defenses such as intellectualization to calm their anxiety. When feasible, these patients benefit from active participation in treatment planning and in carrying out appropriate components of their treatment.

Patients Who Are Dramatic and Captivating (Hysterical)

These patients are often charming, interesting, and pleasurably challenging. They act toward the physician in a warm and personal manner. The physician may wonder if the patients are malingering, given the contrast between their way of relating and their claims to be ill. The dramatic, sometimes teasing, or seductive manner of the patient and the tendency to form idealized and intimate relationships with doctors is this person's typical style of coping with stress. To these people, being ill is equated with being weak, unattractive, and unloved. They experience illness as a threat to their masculinity or femininity. Attempts to master these fears and regain psychological control may result in inappropriate displays of strength, power, and sexuality. Such attempts at re-establishing control typically frighten, anger, and distance doctors and nurses from the patient. These reactions by the medical care team, particularly responses to the patient's seductiveness, are an effort to control the impulses that are aroused by the patient. Establishing a comfortable degree of appreciation for the patient's attractiveness and strength while remaining aware of the possibility of the need to seek intense emotional involvement is the ideal way for the physician to treat such patients. The often quoted clinical pearl of the physician telling the counterphobic body builder with a recent myocardial infarction that he has to be "strong enough" to lie in bed doing "specialized" finger and toe exercises, as opposed to vigorous calisthenics, is the insightful comment that should be applied to the anxious patient with a hysterical character style.

Patients Who Are Long-Suffering and Self-Sacrificing (Masochistic)

This personality style is perplexing to medical staff that cannot understand how unfortunate events seem to "happen" to the patient. There is often the suspicion that the patient plays some role in his or her misfortunes and there is often "evidence" that this is the case. These are not malingering patients or patients with factitious disorder, as the motivation for causing unfortunate events to happen to themselves is unconscious. They are exhibitionist about their suffering, in contrast to their otherwise humble demeanor. The need to psychologically "pay" in advance for pleasure, or pay for real or fantasized pleasure, fuels this patient's experience and behavior. They wish to be loved and cared for, but they feel unworthy and guilty. Thus, they expect to either fail to get what they want or to be punished for having their wishes gratified. Such patients can cause great frustration in their doctors if they show emotional deterioration in the face of positive medical advancement. Acknowledgment by the physician of the patient's difficulties and suffering and a demonstration of understanding of the patient's "burden" will help the patient move forward. If the physician structures his communications to the patient about recovery as a tough ordeal or as necessary to benefit others for whom the patient feels responsible, this may enable the patient to more adaptively master the psychological conflicts stirred up when he receives attention from the medical staff.

Patients Who Are Guarded and Querulous (Paranoid)

The suspicious, watchful individual who reacts to the most minimal of slights is easily recognized. The patient overreacts to any criticism and seems to expect an attack at any moment. Everything is externalized (i.e., nothing is their fault). This can be particularly problematic in the hospital setting, where there is much in the way of bad news, unexpected discomfort, lost laboratory results, incorrect meals, and so forth. It follows from this that these patients have a tendency to blame others for their illness. Their fears of being harmed intensify when they are ill, which increases their aggressive impulses, intensifying anxiety. The anxiety is controlled by an increase in the guardedness, suspiciousness, and need to control others, principally the doctors and nurses who are responsible for the patient's care. These are patients for whom care needs to be taken that they not be surprised by what happens in the hospital. Particular attention needs to be paid to inform them regarding what the physician expects to happen at each step of the diagnostic and therapeutic process. There should be an attempt to acknowledge how the patient feels rather than a hostile confrontation of the person's "perceptions." This can be particularly challenging for an exhausted intern or resident. It is sometimes possible to ally with the patient and enlist his cooperation in "putting up" with the realities of the hospital, thus gaining cooperation in staying in the hospital and in the recovery phase of the illness.

Patients Who Have a Feeling of Superiority (Narcissistic)

These people see themselves as being powerful and important, whether or not their station in society substantiates this feeling. Overtly, they may appear quite humble or modest, but others see through this facade. Relating to a doctor on whom the patient must depend can be a difficult task, especially if the doctor does not have a "special" status that reinforces the patient's "special" status. Illness threatens this patient's need to be perfect and invulnerable. The patient's increased grandiosity and entitlement is a defensive maneuver. He or she easily finds fault with others but fears the doctor might not be able to help. The fantasy that the patient must be seen by the "great professor" can be demoralizing for the intern or resident who may feel devalued. The tactful, not defensive, assertion of one's knowledge, training, and abilities is reassuring to the patient. This allows the patient to idealize the doctor and contain the overwhelming anxiety.

Patients Who Appear Aloof and not Involved (Schizoid)

These patients seem eccentric or odd in their behavior on the ward, uninvolved with the doctors and nurses, and seemingly "too calm" regarding their illness. They do not seem easily swayed by things and appear quite independent. This external calm conceals a fragile interior that requires a withdrawal from everyday life to manage otherwise overwhelming anxiety. Although they may apparently function well in their regular lives and may have VIP status as a result of their accomplishments, their illness and hospitalization present a stress with which they cannot cope. This may result in the denial that they are ill, in spite of hard evidence to the contrary, as illness disrupts their carefully balanced system. Although the impulse to "break through" to the patient may be strong, a better management technique acknowledges the need to remain safe, with the physician and family doing a large portion of the decision making.

Physician Responses to Patients and Systems Issues

The patient who is difficult because of personality traits will elicit a number of reactions from the staff. Some of these reactions may adversely impact patient care and so deserve mention. For example, patients who tend to polarize their own feelings intra-psychically (especially patients with borderline traits) often produce division in the team. Some staff members may feel intensely sympathetic toward the patient and his/her plight, whereas others who are vilified by the patient will either engage the patient angrily or avoid the patient. This constellation must be recognized before it can be defused. Groves points out that there is little discussion in the medical and surgical literature of what he terms "the hateful patient"—one who evokes intensely negative feelings in most caregivers (63). Rather than disavowing negative feelings, these must be assessed as data *about the patient*. When these feelings are recognized, accepted, and examined, they may be used constructively in the patient's care. For example, if the patient or a family member irrationally criticizes one member of the team, it is often useful and time-effective to plan a meeting including different members of the team and the patient. The addition of a psychiatrist to the team, particularly one with expertise in group issues, can greatly facilitate the meeting. One of the goals is to demonstrate that the team functions together as a unit for the patient's well-being and is not divided or in conflict. Another goal is to confront the patient with the reality of limits to the care the team is able to provide and that perfect care is not possible. Identifying who the patient is and how he or she functions in other social settings will improve the effectiveness of the meeting; issues to consider are whether the patient is isolated or is the matriarch/patriarch of a family and whether the patient is accustomed to making decisions herself or to having decisions made for her. Such meetings are also particularly helpful to diffuse the anger of family members who are either caught up in the patient's struggles or are driven by their own psychopathology, independent of the patient.

Sexuality and the Elderly

A frequently neglected area of concern for the physician is the issue of the elderly patient's sexual functioning after surgery. Too often it is assumed that the elderly have no interest in sex. Because patients may be embarrassed by such difficulties, they may remain silent. To address this issue, the physician should actively inquire about the patient's sexual function in an open-ended way, thus enabling the patient to explore any sexual difficulties.

Specific Management Issues

PAIN

Careful assessment and treatment of pain that the individual is experiencing will help limit mental status changes caused by analgesics, especially narcotics. In general, there is underdiagnosis of pain in patients who are cognitively impaired and unable to express themselves clearly. Conversely, there may be overdiagnosis and overtreatment of pain in anxious patients. Antidepressants may be utilized adjunctively in the treatment of refractory pain *(64,65)*. Of the available tricyclic antidepressants, amitriptyline (Elavil) has been demonstrated to ameliorate neuropathic pain; it also has a potential role as a sleep aid. Nortriptyline (Pamelor) has not been as extensively studied as amitriptyline for its analgesic properties but tends to cause less orthostatic hypotension in the elderly. Gabapentin (Neurontin) can be used in conjunction with other medications for headache and neuropathic pain, has few side effects, and offers mild sedating effects as well as mood stabilization. In addition to various forms of pain control through pharmacotherapy, frequent reassurance will also help reduce pain, especially in many anxious patients. For those who seem to be responsive to this kind of supportive psychotherapeutic intervention, hypnosis can also be considered as an adjunct in pain management *(66)*.

SLEEP

The quality of the elderly patient's sleep postoperatively is extremely important, as sleep influences mood and mental status, level of energy, and willingness to participate in rehabilitation. The differential diagnosis of insomnia is vast and includes pain, environmental stressors (e.g., loud intercoms in patients' rooms), depression, anxiety, and agitation resulting from either primary psychiatric processes (e.g., dementia) or medical problems (e.g., hypoxia). Assuming that the insomnia is not caused by a general medical condition, we recommend the following agents for the treatment of insomnia:

1. Olanzapine at starting doses of 2.5–5 mg is sedating, in part as a result of its effects at the H_1 histamine receptors. It also functions as an antipsychotic agent, making it useful for insomnia from agitation secondary to dementia or delirium.
2. Risperidone at a starting dose of 0.5–2 mg at bedtime (qhs) is also useful as a first-line agent in insomnia resulting from agitation.
3. Mirtazapine at a starting dose of 7.5 mg, up to 15 mg, works well in a number of patients where anxiety is a component of insomnia. Because it post-synaptically blocks the serotonin $5-HT_2$ receptors, which may be involved in nausea caused by SSRIs, it can be combined with SSRIs and may help alleviate gastrointestinal side effects. Residual sedation may be limiting, although many patients accommodate in a few days.
4. Trazodone at doses of 50–100 mg is effective for many patients. However, residual sedation may be limiting.
5. Doxepin, as a TCA, carries the potential for prominent anticholinergic effects as well as the potential for cardiac arrhythmias. However, at very low doses (1–10 mg), these risks are minimal and the medication can be very effective, especially for patients who wake multiple times during the night (67).

ANXIETY

Treatment of anxiety in the elderly postoperative patient will be guided by the cause. We reiterate that benzodiazepines should, in general, be avoided except in special, carefully monitored cases. The main diagnostic categories to consider are affective disorders (postoperative depression, anxiety disorders, adjustment disorders, etc.), dementia, and delirium, which may include iatrogenic causes. For many conditions, low-dose antipsychotics are useful. If the cause of the anxiety is a new depressive or anxiety disorder or the recurrence of an underlying affective disorder, then the treatment is as discussed for these disorders—pharmacologic approaches (especially SSRIs, newer agents such as nefazadone and mirtazapine, low-dose antipsychotics) and psychotherapeutic approaches. Anxiety, like agitation, may be a symptom of dementia; careful adjustment of antipsychotic dosages is usually effective. Iatrogenic causes of anxiety include commonly used medications. Of the many possible medications that cause delirium, special mention should be made of steroids used in the postcardiac transplantation patient; treatment involves adjustment of the dose of the medication and antipsychotics.

AGITATION AND AGGRESSION

The differential diagnosis of agitation and aggression includes medical causes resulting in delirium (e.g., hypoxia, infection, adverse medication reactions, endocrinologic abnormalities, hepatic dysfunction, and other metabolic causes), independent psychotic disorders, dementia, and mood disorders. More rarely seen in the elderly is agitation and aggression caused by personality disorders (with borderline and/or antisocial traits). The most urgent management interventions must be directed at preventing injury to the patient or staff. Often, physical and chemical restraint of the patient is necessary. Recommended physical restraints include the use of vests and two- or four-point restraints; bed rails should be avoided, as they constitute a fall risk. Chemical restraint consists of oral or parenteral administration of antipsychotics. Rarely in the elderly if a personality disorder is the cause of agitation, is the threat of using restraint sufficient to help the patient remain in behavioral control. In most cases of agitation and aggression, the use of a personal attendant is indicated to monitor the patient, redirect and reorient the patient if he or she is not in restraint but becomes intermittently agitated, and report to the nursing staff.

REFERENCES

1. Druss RG. The Psychology of Illness. American Psychiatric Association, Washington, DC, 1995.
2. Stone MH. Abnormalities of Personality. WW Norton, New York, 1993.
3. Blumenthal JA, Burg M, Barefoot J, Williams RB, Haney T, Zimet G. Social support, type A behavior, and coronary artery disease. Psychosom Med 1987;49:331–340.
4. Frasure-Smith N, Lesperance F, Gravel G, Masson A, Juneau M, Talajic M, et al. Social support, depression, and mortality during the first year after myocardial infarction. Circulation 2000;101:1919–1924.
5. Vaillant GE. Ego mechanisms of defense. American Psychiatric Association, Washington, DC, 1992.
6. Muskin PR, Feldhammer T, Gelfand JL, Strauss DH. Maladaptive denial of physical illness: a useful new diagnosis. Int J Psychiatry Med 1998;28:503–517.
7. Diagnostic and Statistical Manual of Mental Disorders, 4th ed. text rev. American Psychiatric Association, Washington, DC, 2000.
8. Pollack MH, Kradin R, Otto MW, Worthington J, et al. Prevalence of panic in patients referred for pulmonary function testing at a major medical center. Am J Psychiatry 1996;153:110–113.
9. Markovitz PJ. Treatment of anxiety in the elderly. J Clin Psychiatry 1993;54(5 Suppl):64–68.
10. Sherbourne CD, Wells KB, Hays RD, et al. Subthreshold depression and depressive disorder: clinical characteristics of general medical and mental health specialty outpatients. Am J Psychiatry 1994;151: 1777–1784.
11. Wells KB, Burnam MA, Rogers W, et al. Course of depression for adult outpatients: results from the Medical Outcomes Study. Am J Psychiatry 1992;49:788–794.
12. Silverstone PH. Depression increases mortality and morbidity in acute life threatening medical illness. J Psychosom Res 1990;34:651–657.
13. Furlanetto LM, et al. Association between depressive symptoms and mortality in medical inpatients. Psychosomatics 2000;41:426–432.
14. Morris PL, Robinson RG, Andrzejewski P, et al. Association of depression with 10 year post-stroke mortality. J Clin Psychiatry 1993;54:119–126.
15. Barefoot J, Schroll M. Symptoms of depression, acute myocardial infarction, and total mortality in a com-munity sample. Circulation 1996;93:1976–1980.
16. Frasure-Smith N, Lesperance F, Talajic M. Depression following myocardial infarction: impact on 6-month survival. JAMA 1993;270:1819–1825.
17. Frasure-Smith N, Lesperance F, Talajic M. Depression and 18-month prognosis following myocardial infarction. Circulation 1995;91:999–1005.
18. Connerney I, Shapiro PA, McLaughlin JS, Bagiella E, Sloan RP. Relation between depression after coronary artery bypass surgery and 12-month outcome: a prospective study. Lancet 2001;358:1766–1771.
19. Shapiro PA, DePena M, Lidagoster L, Woodring S, Pierce DW, Glassman A. Depression after coronary artery bypass graft surgery. Psychosom Med 1998;60:108 (abstract).
20. Pratt LA, Ford DE, Crum RM, Armenian HK, Gallo JJ, Eaton WW. Depression, psychotropic medication and risk of myocardial infarction. Prospective data from the Baltimore ECA follow-up. Circulation 1996;94:3123–3129.
21. Ariyo AA, Haan M, Tangen CM, Rutledge JC, Cushman M, Dobs A, et al., for the Cardiovascular Health Study Collaborative Research Group: depressive symptoms and risks of coronary heart disease and mortality in elderly americans. Circulation 2000;102:1773–1779.
22. Ford DE, Mead LA, Chang PP, Cooper-Patrick L, Wang N-Y, Klag MJ. Depression is a risk factor for coronary artery disease in men. Arch Intern Med 1998;158:1422–1426.
23. Penninx BWJH, Beekman ATF, Honig A, Deeg DJH, Schoevers RA, van Eijk JTM, et al. Depression and cardiac mortality. Results from a community-based longitudinal study. Arch Gen Psychiatry 2001; 58:221–227.
24. Lesperance F, Frasure-Smith N, Juneau M, Theroux P. Depression and 1-year prognosis in unstable angina. Arch Intern Med 2000;160:1354–1360.
25. Carney RM, Rich MW, Freedland KE, Saini J, TeVelde A, Simeone C, et al. Major depressive disorder predicts cardiac events in patients with coronary artery disease. Psychosom Med 1988;50:627–633.
26. Barefoot JC, Helms MJ, Mark DB, Blumenthal JA, Califf RM, Haney TL, et al. Depression and long term mortality risk in patients with coronary artery disease. Am J Cardiol 1996;78:613–617.
27. Ahern DK, Gorkin L, Anderson JL, Tierney C, Hallstrom A, Ewart C, et al., for the CAPS Investigators. Biobehavioral variables and mortality or cardiac arrest in the cardiac arrhythmia: pilot study (CAPS). Am J Cardiol 1990;66:59–62.

28. Connerney I, Shapiro PA, McLaughlin JS, Sloan RP. In-hospital depression after CABG surgery predicts 12-month outcome. Psychosom Med 2000;62:107(abstract).

29. Connerney I. The impact of post operative depression on cardiac events after coronary artery bypass surgery. Doctoral dissertation, Columbia University, New York, NY, 1999.

30. Ziegelstein RC, Fauerbach JA, Stevens SS, Romanelli J, Richter DP, Bush DE. Patients with depression are less likely to follow recommendations to reduce cardiac risk during recovery from a myocardial infarction. Arch Intern Med 2000;160:1818–1823.

31. Krishnan KR, Hays JC, Blazer DG. MRI-defined vascular depression. Am J Psychiatry 1997;154(4): 497–501.

32. Musselman DL, Tomer A, Manatunga AK, Knight BT, Porter MR, Kasey S, et al. Exaggerated platelet reactivity in major depression. Am J Psychiatry 1996;153:1313–1317.

33. Musselman DL, Evans DL, Nemeroff CB. The relationship of depression to cardiovascular disease. Arch Gen Psychiatry 1998;55:580–592.

34. Sloan RP, Shapiro PA, Bagiella E, Myers MM, Gorman JM. Cardiac autonomic control buffers blood pressure variability responses to challenge: a psychophysiological model of coronary artery disease. Psychosom Med 1999;61:58–68.

35. Cavanaugh S. Depression in the medically ill: critical issues in diagnostic assessment. Psychosomatics 1994;36:48–59.

36. Myers JK, Weissman MM, Tischler GL, et al. Six-month prevalence of psychiatric disorders in three communities: 1980–1982. Arch Gen Psychiatry 1984;41:959–967.

37. Chochinov HM, Wilson KG, Enns M, et al. Desire for death in the terminally ill. Am J Psychiatry 1995; 152:1185–1191.

38. Roose SP, Glassman AH, Attia E, Woodring S, Giardina EGV, Bigger JT. Cardiovascular effects of fluoxetine in depressed patients with heart disease. Am J Psychiatry 1998;155:660–665.

39. Shapiro PA, Lesperance F, Frasure-Smith N, O'Conner C, Jiang JW, Baker BPD, et al. An open label preliminary trial of sertraline treatment of major depression after acute myocardial infarction (the "SADHAT" study). Am Heart J 1999;137:1100–1106.

40. Roose SP, Laghrissi-Thode F, Kennedy JS, Nelson JC, Bigger JT Jr, Pollock BG, et al. Comparison of paroxetine and nortriptyline in depressed patients with ischemic heart disease. JAMA 1998;279:287–291.

41. Arana GW, Rosenbaum JF. Handbook of Psychiatric Drug Therapy. Lippincott Williams & Wilkins, Philadelphia, PA, 2000, pp. 215–216.

42. Masand PS, Tesar GE. Use of stimulants in the medically ill. Psychcol Clin North Am 1996;19(3): 515–547.

43. Simon GE, Vonkorff M, Piccinelli M, Fullerton C, Ormel J. An international study of the relation between somatic symptoms and depression. N Engl J Med 1999;341:1329–235.

44. Keller MB, McCullough JP, Klein DN, et al. A comparison of nefazodone, the cognitive behavioral-analysis system of psychotherapy, and their combination for the treatment of chronic depression. N Engl J Med 2000;342:1462–1470.

45. Reynolds CF, Miller MD, Pasternak RE, Frank E, et al. Treatment of bereavement-related major depressive episodes in later life: a controlled study of acute and continuation treatment with nortriptyline and interpersonal psychotherapy. Am J Psychiatry 1999;156:202–208.

46. Maj M, Pirozzi R, Magliano L. Nonresponse to reinstituted lithium prophylaxis in previously responsive bipolar patients: prevalence and predictors. Am J Psychiatry 1995;152:1810–1811.

47. Coryell W, Solomon D, Leon AC, Akiskal HS, et al. Lithium discontinuation and subsequent effectiveness. Am J Psychiatry 1998;155:895–898.

48. Anon. Drugs that may cause cognitive disorders in the elderly. Med Lett 2000;40(1093):111–112.

49. Tesar G, Murray G, Cassem N. Use of high-dose intravenous haloperidol in the treatment of agitated cardiac patients. J Clin Psychopharmacol 1985;5:344–347.

50. Wilt J, Minnema A, Johnson R, et al. Torsade de pointes associated with the use of intravenous haloperidol. Ann Intern Med 1993;119:391–394.

51. Sharma ND, Rosman HS, Padhi D, Tilsdale JE. Torsades de pointes with intravenous haloperidol in critically ill patients. Am J Cardiology 1998;81(2):238–240.

52. Jackson T, Ditmanson L, Phibbs B. Torsade de pointes and low-dose oral haloperidol. Arch Intern Med 1997;157:2013–2015.

53. Muskin PR, Mellman LA, Kornfeld DS. A "new" drug for the treatment of agitation in the general medical setting: chlorpromazine. Gen Hosp Psychiatry 1986;8:404–410.

54. Arana GW, Rosenbaum JF, eds. Antipsychotic drugs. In: Handbook of Psychiatric Drug Therapy. Lippincott Williams & Wilkins, Philadelphia, PA, 2000, pp. 35–36.
55. Mayeux R, Sano M. Drug therapy: treatment of Alzheimer's disease. N Engl J Med 1999;341(22): 1670–1679.
56. Roach GW, Kanchuger M, Mangano CM, Newman M, et al. Multicenter Study of Perioperative Ischemia Research Group, Ischemia Research and Education Foundation Investigators. Adverse cerebral outcomes after coronary bypass surgery. N Engl J Med 1996;335:1857–1863.
57. Folstein MF, Folstein SE, McHugh PR. "Mini-Mental State": a practical method for grading the cognitive state of patients for the clinician. J Psychiatr Res 1975;12:189–198.
58. Newman MF, Kirchner JL, Phillips-Bute B, Gaver V, et al. Longitudinal assessment of neurocognitive function after coronary artery bypass surgery. N Engl J Med 2001;344:395–402.
59. Lipowski Z. Delirium in the elderly patient. N Engl J Med 1989;320:578–582.
60. Bergeron N, Dubois MJ, Dumont M, Dial S, Skrobik Y. Delirium in an intensive care unit: a study of risk factors. Eur J Intensive Care Med 2001;27:1297–1304.
61. Yun KL, Sintek CF, Fletcher AD, Pfeffer TA, Kochamba GS, Mahrer PR, et al. Time related quality of life after elective cardiac operation. Ann Thorac Surg 1999;68(4):1314–1320.
62. Kahana RJ, Bibring GL. Personality types in medical management. In: Zinberg N, ed. Psychiatry and Medical Practice in a General Hospital. International Universities Press, New York, 1964, pp. 98–123.
63. Groves JE. Taking care of the hateful patient. N Engl J Med 1978;298(16):883–887.
64. Sindrup SH, Jensen TS. Efficacy of pharmacologic treatments of neuropathic pain: an update and effect related to mechanism of action. Pain 1999;83:389–400.
65. Ansari A. The efficacy of newer antidepressants in the treatment of chronic pain: a review of the literature. Harvard Rev Psychiatry 2000;7:257–277.
66. Spiegel H, Spiegel D. Trance and Treatment. American Psychiatric Association, Washington, DC, 1978.
67. Moran MG, Stoudemire A. Sleep disorders in the medically ill patient. J Clin Psychiatry 1992;53:29–36.

6   Neurological Aspects of Caring for the Aged

Mitchell S. V. Elkind, MD, MS

CONTENTS

INTRODUCTION
NERVOUS SYSTEM CHANGES ASSOCIATED WITH AGING
DEMENTIA
STROKE
CONTROVERSIES
REFERENCES

INTRODUCTION

The human brain changes as it ages, and the elderly are increasingly susceptible to many neurological diseases and symptoms. Neurological disorders are the leading source of serious disability among the elderly and one of the major reasons for institutionalization of elderly individuals. As many as 90% of institutionalized elderly persons have disabilities caused by neurological disease, and as many as 50% of the elderly living in the community have neurological problems. This burden of age-related neurological disease in the population is only expected to increase as the population ages.

To a great extent, advances in medical and cardiac care have made the neurological ravages of aging more apparent. As medicine has become better able to handle diseases of the heart and other organ systems, patients are living longer, into the age when neurological diseases are more common. Simultaneously, the complexities of the brain and nervous system have only recently begun to yield their secrets to the neuroscientific community. Therapies for the most common neurological ailments, including Alzheimer's disease and stroke, as discussed in this chapter, have only just become available within the past decade, trailing therapeutic advances in medicine by many years. Because neurologic disorders are so frequently found in elderly patients undergoing cardiac evaluation and management, it is imperative for those who treat these patients to have some understanding of the aging nervous system and its most common afflictions.

This chapter will review some of what is known about how the nervous system changes as it ages and then consider two of the most common age-related neurological problems:

From: *Aging, Heart Disease, and Its Management: Facts and Controversies*
Edited by: N. Edwards, M. Maurer, and R. Wellner © Humana Press Inc., Totowa, NJ

Table 1
Changes in the Nervous System Associated with Aging

Central nervous system changes
   Gross pathological changes
      Decrease in brain weight
      Decrease in brain volume
      Atrophy, particularly in frontal lobes and caudate nucleus
   Microscopic changes
      Neuronal loss
         Locus ceruleus
         Substantia nigra
         Inferior olive
         Raphe nuclei
         Cerebellar Purkinje cells
         Cortical pyramidal neurons
         Subiculum of hippocampus
      Loss of axons in cerebral white matter
      Loss of myelin in cerebral white matter
      Loss of synaptic density
      Iron deposition
   Functional changes
      Decrease in levels of neurotransmitters (?)
Peripheral nervous system changes
   Loss of anterior horn cells of spinal cord (motor neurons)
   Loss of muscle tissue
   Loss of myelin in peripheral nerves

dementia and cerebrovascular disease. Finally, the chapter will discuss several controversies relevant to the care of the elderly patient, particularly with regard to cardiovascular disease.

NERVOUS SYSTEM CHANGES ASSOCIATED WITH AGING

The biological processes of aging in the nervous system may be divided, both in fundamental scientific terms and in clinical terms, into those processes that are generally considered "normal" aging and those that are considered pathological, or the result of some underlying disease process (*see* Table 1). However, in practice, it can be hard to tell normal and pathological processes apart. At the most gross level, brain shrinkage, or atrophy, occurs with normal aging. In the elderly, brain weight is decreased on average by approx 8% compared with peak adult weight *(1)*. Brain volume loss also occurs at a rate of about 2–3% per decade after the age of 50 *(2)*. This atrophy reflects a loss of neurons as well as white matter, and a reduction in synaptic density *(3)*. The neuronal loss, however, is not a generalized process. Selective neuronal loss appears to occur in the locus ceruleus of the brainstem, the substantia nigra, the inferior olive, and the raphe nuclei of the brainstem, regions of the brainstem responsible for widespread connections to cortical and other areas of the brain *(4)*. In addition, Purkinje cells in the cerebellum and large pyramidal neurons in the cortex are lost *(4)*. In the hippocampus, the brain region in the medial temporal lobe most closely associated with memory, normal aging has been asso-

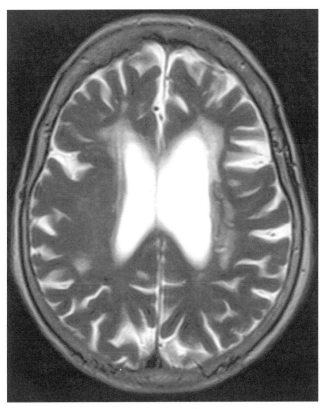

Fig. 1. Leukoaraiosis. Axial T2-weighted brain MRI scan of an 84-yr-old woman with a history of aphasia and right hemiparesis, showing bilateral hyperintensity in the periventricular white matter. Other levels of the MRI showed an old left basal ganglia infarction.

ciated with loss of neurons in the subiculum, but not in other areas. Reasons for this selective vulnerability of certain neuronal populations to aging are not clear.

The white matter is also affected by the aging process, although the causes of this and its functional consequences remain uncertain. Both primary axon loss and reduction in myelin covering the axons may contribute to the rarefaction of white matter often seen on magnetic resonance imaging (MRI) scans as periventricular white matter changes, also termed leukoaraiosis (*see* Fig. 1). Many neurologically normal elderly individuals, however, may also have this kind of rarefaction of the deep cerebral white matter, making clinical–pathological correlation difficult *(5)*. The cause of this white-matter loss over time is unclear, but it may reflect decreased perfusion in the deep white matter of the brain related to thickening of cerebral arterioles, often in association with hypertension and diabetes mellitus. In addition to these apparent structural changes, which occur in normal aging, it remains unclear whether there are substantial changes in levels of neurotransmitters in the healthy aging brain. Methodological limitations, including possible inclusion of subjects with preclinical dementing illness and small sample sizes, have obscured results of some earlier studies that suggested such changes occurred.

The radiographic changes on brain imaging associated with aging include white-matter signal abnormalities seen best on a MRI, sulcal and ventricular enlargement related to atrophy, and the accumulation of iron in certain brain regions (*see* Table 2) *(6)*. Atrophy

Table 2
Radiographic Correlates of Aging

Brain atrophy
Periventricular white-matter signal abnormalities ("leukoariosis")
Enlarged perivascular spaces
T2 signal decrease on MRI as a result of iron deposition
Calcification of basal ganglia

and white-matter rarefaction, when prominent, may also be seen on computed tomography (CT) scans. Punctate hyperintensities seen on T2-weighted MRIs occur in up to 65% of elderly individuals (7). Pathologically these regions of abnormal signal correspond to enlarged perivascular spaces, perivascular demyelination, and, less commonly, frank infarction (8). Prospective cohort studies have shown progression in these white-matter abnormalities with aging, without clear clinical correlates (9). Brain atrophy as seen on imaging, like neuronal loss, occurs selectively, with more rapid atrophy in the frontal lobes (10) and the caudate nucleus (11). Atrophy may occur more rapidly in men than women (12). Iron deposition causing T2 signal hypointensity on brain MRI is commonly seen in the putamen in patients over the age of 60, without clinical significance (6). More specialized imaging studies, such as positron-emission tomography (PET) scanning may reveal subtle changes in cerebral metabolism associated with aging, such as decreased glucose metabolism in temporal lobes and other areas of the brain (13). The functional consequences of changes in brain structure have been assessed using electroencephalography (EEG) as well. Although it has been commonly held that there are EEG changes associated with normal aging, such as temporal lobe slowing, investigators have recently questioned this notion, suggesting that abnormalities seen on EEG are, in fact, usually a sign of neurologic disease (14).

In addition to changes in the central nervous system, alterations in peripheral nerve and muscle also occur with aging. Anterior horn cells, the "lower motor neurons," in the spinal cord, like the pyramidal cells, or "upper motor neurons" in the cortex, decrease with age. Muscle wasting occurs and there is reduced myelination of the sensory nerves. Functional consequences of these peripheral nervous system changes include a loss of vibratory, touch, and pain sensation, as well as autonomic dysfunction affecting pupillary reactivity, temperature regulation, and heart and peripheral vascular control.

Aging is commonly associated with some degree of cognitive impairment relative to younger individuals, even in the absence of any functional impairment. As many as two-thirds of the healthy elderly have some decrease in performance on neuropsychological testing compared with younger subjects (15). However, it is difficult to say for certain that these subtle deficits are not related to the early onset of pathological processes, such as Alzheimer's disease, because many of the studies are limited by their cross-sectional design and consequent lack of longitudinal data (16). Nonetheless, several investigators have found evidence that certain cognitive realms are affected in presumably normal elderly subjects. It is notable that the cognitive changes associated with normal aging are not generalized; that is, not all areas are equally affected. The specific domains of cognition that tend to be affected in the healthy elderly include the speed of cognitive processing, problem-solving skills ("fluid intelligence"), and short-term memory *(17)*. Identification of more pronounced focal cognitive abnormalities, such as language or praxis disturbances, for example, should suggest a primary neurologic condition, such as Alzheimer's disease or stroke.

In summary, aging is associated with myriad structural, functional, and clinical effects on the central and peripheral nervous systems. Even in the absence of identifiable disease, elderly individuals manifest changes compared with younger individuals. In the clinical realm, when encountering elderly patients with neurological complaints, important differences in the radiological appearance of brain structures must be considered. However, much research is needed to determine which radiological and other findings are "normal" and which are pathological.

DEMENTIA

Dementia is classically defined as an impairment in memory and at least one other area of cognitive function—for example, aphasia, apraxia, agnosia, or a disturbance in executive functioning. Although isolated memory loss (i.e., amnestic syndrome) may be the initial manifestation of dementia, it may result from focal brain disease affecting structures crucial to memory, such as the medial temporal lobes or hippocampus, and it should not be construed as dementia. For these deficits to qualify as dementia, they must also be severe enough to preclude normal social and occupational functioning and they must represent a decline in the individual's previous level of functioning. Recent guidelines from the American Academy of Neurology (AAN), based on comprehensive reviews of the relevant literature, have been published regarding detection *(16)*, diagnosis *(18)*, and treatment *(19)* of dementia.

Some cognitive decline, as noted above, is common in normal, healthy, fully independent elderly individuals when compared with younger individuals. Complaints of memory loss are also common. Cross-sectional studies of cognitive function in the elderly discloses three primary groups of individuals with different degrees of cognitive function: the demented, the nondemented, and an intermediate group with some decline relative to their age cohort but without frank functional impairment. These latter individuals have been variously categorized as having mild cognitive impairment, isolated memory impairment, incipient dementia, and dementia prodrome. All of these terms refer to a similar constellation of findings: memory complaints (ideally corroborated by an informant such as a family member), evidence of memory loss on exam, normal general cognitive function, and preserved independent function. One of the critical questions for clinicians caring for the elderly—not to mention for their patients—is whether the presence of this mild cognitive impairment predicts eventual frank dementia. Most data suggest that these patients do, in fact, go on to develop dementia, at rates of approx 6–25% per year *(16)*. In a longitudinal study from the Mayo Clinic, among patients with initial evidence of subtle memory loss (mean age 81), 80% had developed Alzheimer's disease by 6 yr *(16,20)*. General cognitive screening instruments, such as the Mini Mental State Examination (MMSE), are useful for the detection of progression to dementia in patient populations with an increased prevalence of cognitive impairment as a result of age. Studies are ongoing in these populations to determine whether therapeutic interventions, such as those already shown to be effective in patients with established dementia (discussed in this section), can reduce incidence of conversion to dementia.

Table 3
Differential Diagnosis of Dementia

Reversible causes
   Structural
      Chronic subdural hematoma
      Hydrocephalus
      Tumors (meningioma, craniopharyngioma, etc.)
   Endocrine: hypothyroidism
   Metabolic: hypocalcemia
   Deficiencies: vitamin B_{12} deficiency, thiamine deficiency
   Psychiatric: depression ("pseudodementia")
   Paraneoplastic
   Medication toxicity
   Infectious: syphilis, chronic meningitis, others
   Epilepsy
  Treatable
   Alzheimer's disease
   Vascular dementia
   Parkinson's disease
   Paraneoplastic
   Infectious: HIV
   Drug or alcohol abuse
  Untreatable
   Huntington's disease
   Pick's disease
   Frontotemporal dementia
   Diffuse Lewy body disease
   Prion diseases (Creutzfeldt–Jakob disease and others)
   Head trauma

Age is the most important factor predictive of dementia. The overall annual incidence of dementia increases from 0.1% at ages 60–64 to 1.82% at ages 75–79 to 8.68% above age 95. Of note, although the incidence of dementia increases sharply with age, there appears to be some leveling off in this increase in risk among the oldest old *(21)*. Other risk factors for dementia include family history *(22)*, head injury *(23)*, and lower educational level *(24)*.

The differential diagnosis of dementia is broad and includes fully reversible causes, as well as those that are treatable to some degree and those that are not treatable at all (*see* Table 3). The importance of recognizing and treating the reversible causes of dementia cannot be overestimated, as failure to do so consigns the individual to a state of significant disability. In some cases, such as when structural lesions like subdural hematoma are present, failure to promptly treat may lead to permanent cognitive dysfunction. In all cases evaluation for reversible causes of dementia should include at a minimum structural brain imaging, thyroid function tests, and vitamin B_{12} levels. Testing for neurosyphilis or human immunodeficiency virus (HIV) may be appropriate in individuals with a history of exposure or a compatible clinical history. Structural brain imaging can include noncontrast CT or MRI to exclude conditions such as subdural hematoma or neoplasm (*see* Fig. 2).

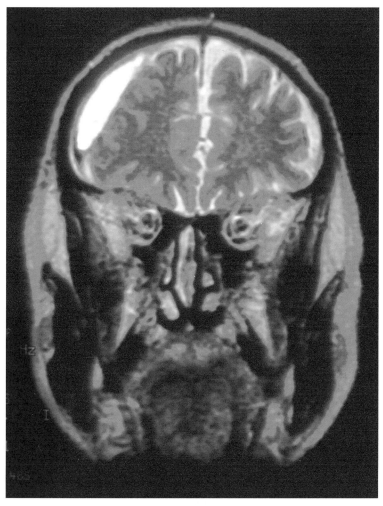

Fig. 2. Subdural hematoma causing dementia. Coronal T1-weighted brain MRI scan of a 78-yr-old man with a 1-mo history of mild memory loss and confusion. He had bumped his head on a door frame 1 mo prior to presentation. The right-sided lenticular hyperdensity is a subdural hematoma with moderate mass effect. Surgical evacuation and treatment with steroids led to a resolution of symptoms.

Approximately 5% of patients may have an abnormality detected on imaging that would not have been anticipated on the basis of clinical history alone *(25)*. Screening for depression, if necessary with a validated instrument such as the Hamilton Depression Scale *(26)* or the Geriatric Depression Scale short form *(27)*, is appropriate, particularly because many elderly individuals may not present with classical symptoms of depression, such as depressed mood and anhedonia.

Among the elderly, the most common causes of dementia are Alzheimer's disease (AD) and vascular dementia. Clinical criteria for a diagnosis of "probable AD" generally achieved either good sensitivity (average 81% across several studies) or specificity (average 70%), but not both, when compared with neuropathological criteria *(28)*. This presumably reflects the fact that many of the manifestations of AD are similar to those of other forms of dementia.

Vascular dementia is even more difficult to definitively diagnose on clinical grounds alone. Some vascular pathology is quite common in the elderly, even in the absence of clinical stroke; vascular abnormalities are present in 29–41% of patients undergoing autopsy in population-based studies (29). Pure vascular pathology, uncontaminated by evidence of other diseases, is present in only approx 10% of cases (25,26). In a cohort of 453 stroke survivors in northern Manhattan, 26% developed dementia, of which 57% had vascular dementia and 39% AD with concomitant stroke (30). Only 4.2% had dementia for other reasons.

Certain specific features of some other, less common causes of primary degenerative dementia can help to distinguish them from AD and vascular dementia, although specificity is again rarely perfect. For example, in diffuse Lewy body disease, in which the pathological hallmark of Parkinson's disease, the Lewy body, is seen not only in the substantia nigra and deep nuclei but also in the cerebral cortex, visual hallucinations and delusional misidentification are seen, as well as prominent deficits in attention, profound deficits in visuo-constructional skills, and relative sparing of memory. In fronto-temporal dementia, early loss of personal and social awareness, hyperorality, and stereotyped, perseverative behavior may be seen.

Despite more than a decade of research into neuroimaging, genetic and other biomarker correlates of AD, and other forms of dementia, there are no ancillary tests that provide improved accuracy of diagnosis over expert clinical diagnosis. There is simply too much overlap among the different forms of dementia to provide definitive information. The only exception is the exciting discovery that a specific neuronal degradation product called 14-3-3 protein, which can be measured in cerebrospinal fluid, has excellent sensitivity (96%) and specificity (99%) for the presence of Creutzfeldt–Jakob disease (CJD) (31). Other common (stroke) and rare (paraneoplastic) conditions, however, may also be positive on this assay. However, because the incidence of CJD is exceptionally rare, on the order of 1 per million, and its course nearly pathognomonic in its rapidity of development and the features of myoclonus and amyotrophy, it is unlikely to pose a diagnostic dilemma in the vast majority of cases of dementia in the elderly.

The management of the reversible causes of dementia will depend on the specific causes. Less than a decade ago, there were no treatments proven efficacious for the treatment of AD, the most common form of dementia in the elderly. In the past 10 yr, however, basic and clinical research have demonstrated the key role of loss of cholinergic neurons in the basal forebrain in the pathophysiology of AD. Consequent to these insights, cholinesterase inhibitors have been shown in several randomized controlled trials to reduce the decline of cognitive function and slow progression to functional dependence in patients with AD. Although these treatments do not cure AD, they do provide some important benefits to patients and their caregivers. Benefits have generally been found in those with mild to moderate disease, again emphasizing the importance of early diagnosis and treatment. Effective cholinesterase inhibitors that have been shown effective in clinical trials include tacrine, donepezil, rivastigmine, and galantamine. Tacrine, the first agent approved for the treatment of AD, may slow the progression of cognitive decline in up to 25% of patients, but it has been associated with unacceptable rates (as high as 50%) of elevation of transaminases (32–34). Donepezil has produced benefits in neuropsychological tests and global functional scores at doses of 5–10 mg daily with a more favorable side-effect profile (35,36). Rivastigmine tartrate produced benefits in cognition, global assessments of function and activities of daily living in patients in a dose-dependent fashion. Higher doses, 6–12 mg daily, were associated with weight loss in up to 50% of subjects and led to drug discontinuation in approx 25% *(37,38)*. Galantamine, a newer cholinesterase inhibitor that also modulates activity at the nicotinic acetylcholine receptor, has been associated with improvement in cognitive function, global function, activities of daily living, and behavior. Doses are between 16 and 32 mg daily, with an acceptable side-effect profile *(39,40)*. The consistent benefits across trials and using different agents in the cholinesterase inhibitor class in a disease even recently considered untreatable is encouraging. However, patients do eventually progress, and improved therapies are sorely needed.

Additional therapies that have been shown to be of benefit in slowing functional decline, despite an absence of effect on cognition, include vitamin E (1000 IU bid) and selegiline (5 mg bid), a monoamine oxidase inhibitor expected to increase brain levels of catecholamines. These agents were tested in a factorial design in a 2-yr trial *(41)*. Although each agent was effective in prolonging the time to a composite end point of death, institutionalization, loss of the ability to perform basic activities of daily living, or severe dementia, there was no additive benefit to the use of both agents together. Trials of other agents, including hormone therapy, prednisone, and nonsteroidal agents, have been negative thus far, despite epidemiologic data suggesting protective benefits *(19,42)*. Gingko biloba, although safe, has not been shown to be effective *(19)*. Because depression, agitation, hallucinations, and psychosis frequently complicate dementias of several types, treatment of these behavioral disturbances also plays an important role in the management of these patients. Both typical antipsychotic agents, such as haloperidol, and atypical agents, such as risperidone, may reduce agitation; resperidone is better tolerated generally *(43)*. Tricyclic agents and serotonin reuptake inhibitors may be used for symptoms of depression *(19)*. More detailed reviews of pharmacotherapy of AD have been published recently *(44)*.

Studies of pharmacologic treatment of other types of dementia, most notably vascular dementia, have suffered from small sample sizes and uncertain diagnostic criteria. No specific therapeutic recommendations can be made in these cases, although treatment directed at behavioral problems can be employed, as indicated earlier. In addition, although no definite conclusions can be drawn regarding the benefits on cognition of treatments directed at vascular risk factors, it is plausible that treatments that reduce the risk of stroke will reduce the likelihood of developing vascular dementia *(45)*.

The implications of dementia for cardiovascular therapy in general have been incompletely determined. The relative risks and benefits of thrombolytic therapy in elderly patients and in patients with dementia, both in the setting of myocardial infarction and in stroke, are addressed in the Controversies section. The importance of the presence of dementia in the decision-making process regarding coronary artery bypass surgery or other procedures is less clear.

STROKE

Stroke is one of the oldest recognized diseases of human beings, but remains one of the least understood. There is a pervasive sense, for example, that stroke is a sudden, unpredictable, irretrievable event. Most lay people, and many physicians, believe that a stroke occurs like a bolt out of the blue, without warning, and that once it has occurs, the damage to the brain is final and complete. The last two decades of neuroscience research, however, have suggested that stroke is neither unpredictable nor irreversible.

It is difficult to overestimate the public health impact of stroke. Stroke is the third leading cause of death and the leading cause of chronic serious disability in the United States. Moreover, recent epidemiological studies have provided evidence that previous estimates

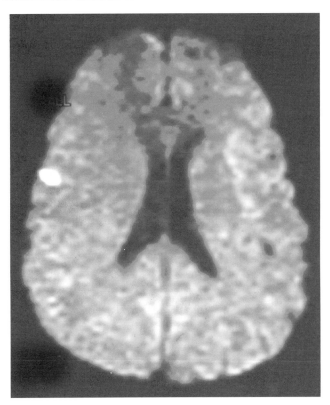

Fig. 3. Abnormal diffusion-weighted MRI with 5 min of symptoms. Diffusion-weighted MRI scan in a 54-yr-old man with a history of atrial fibrillation who presented with 5 min of dysarthria. Neurological examination was completely normal. The MRI shows a small focus of diffusion signal abnormality in the right frontal operculum, consistent with acute ischemia or infarction.

of stroke incidence have underestimated the burden of disease. Although earlier data based on the Framingham study have suggested that there are 500,000 strokes annually in the United States, these data fail to take into account the racial and ethnic heterogeneity of the country and the fact that minority groups are at higher risk of stroke than the predominantly white population studied in the Framingham study are. Estimates based on data from the incidence of stroke in the Cincinnati/Northern Kentucky area *(46)*, which appears to more closely approximate that of the United States as a whole, indicates that there may be as many as 750,000 strokes annually—an upward revision of 50% over previous estimates.

The generally accepted definition of stroke dates to 1980 and originates with the World Health Organization: "rapidly developing clinical signs of focal (at times global) disturbance of cerebral function, lasting more than 24 hours or leading to death with no apparent cause other than that of vascular origin" *(47)*. A transient ischemic attack, or TIA, is generally accepted as consisting of the same symptoms, but lasting less than 24 h. Although this definition has served clinical and research purposes fairly well for the past two decades, it has become clear with the advent of improved imaging technologies, such as diffusion-weighted MRI, which is exquisitely sensitive to the earliest changes of ischemia, that changes consistent with infarction may be seen on MRIs in patients whose symptoms last much less than 24 h (*see* Fig. 3). In fact, in systematic studies, as many as one-third of patients with symptoms lasting as little as up to 1 h have MRI evidence of brain injury *(48)*. The artificial distinction between stroke and TIA has therefore been called into question. From the neurologist's point of view, more important than the duration of the symptoms is the cause of the event and what can be done to prevent a future, perhaps more serious or even fatal, event.

Stroke comes in two major varieties, hemorrhagic and ischemic. Approximately 15–20% of strokes are hemorrhagic, divided roughly evenly between subarachnoid hemorrhage and primary intracerebral hemorrhage. The former is classically related to the rupture of a berry aneurysm at the base of the brain, whereas the latter is the result of bleeding from "microaneurysms" of smaller blood vessels weakened by hypertension. Although the elderly can be affected by either type of hemorrhage, subarachnoid hemorrhage affects people at all ages of life.

One increasingly recognized cause of intracerebral hemorrhage in the elderly is cerebral amyloid angiopathy, which is caused by the accumulation in the walls of cerebral vessels of the same amyloid β-protein that accumulates in the senile plaques of Alzheimer's disease *(49)*. Amyloid angiopathy is important because of the high rate of recurrent hemorrhage, approx 10% per year *(50)*. Subclinical hemorrhages, detected by special gradient echo sequences on MRI scanning (*see* Fig. 4), may occur even more frequently *(51)*. Patients with amyloid angiopathy may present with seizures, focal deficits, dementia, or transient attacks not unlike TIAs *(52)*. Additional causes of cerebral hemorrhage include vascular malformations (arteriovenous malformations and cavernous angiomas), coagulopathies and blood dyscrasias, and neoplasms.

The majority of strokes, roughly 80%, are ischemic. Within the category of ischemic strokes, however, there are several major subtypes (*see* Table 4 and Fig. 5). Unlike myocardial infarction, which is usually the result of large-artery atherosclerosis, only approx 20% of ischemic strokes are the result of large-cerebral-vessel atherosclerosis. Importantly, this is further subdivided into extracranial atherosclerosis ("surgical disease"), affecting the carotid or vertebral arteries, and intracranial atherosclerosis, affecting the distal carotid arteries and the vessels of the circle of Willis. Another roughly 20% of ischemic strokes are the result of cardiac embolism from a well-defined source of cardiac disease such as valvular heart disease, atrial fibrillation, or post-MI mural thrombus. Approximately 20–30% of strokes are considered "lacunar," because of small-vessel disease affecting the threadlike penetrating arteriolar branches of the vessels of the circle of Willis. These are the infarcts that typically result in loss of elementary neurological function, such as weakness, sensory loss, or unsteadiness, but spare the higher-level cortical functions such as language and praxis—functions that localize, for the most part, to the surface gray matter of the hemispheres. Less than 5% of ischemic strokes are the result of a gamut of other unusual causes, including arteritis, dissections, and hypercoagulable states. Finally, about 30–40% of ischemic strokes remain unexplained even after a thorough investigation, and these are usually termed "cryptogenic" (although "cryptogenous" might be the more correct term). Many of these strokes may, in fact, be emboli from less well-recognized cardiovascular sources, such as patent foramen ovale and aortic arch atheroma *(53)*.

Determination of the type of stroke depends on the results of a thorough diagnostic evaluation. At a minimum, all stroke patients should undergo diagnostic imaging of the brain (CT or MRI), noninvasive evaluation of the blood vessels of the neck and brain (duplex Doppler ultrasound, transcranial Doppler ultrasound, MR angiography, or CT angiography), and echocardiographic evaluation (transthoracic echocardiogram or trans-

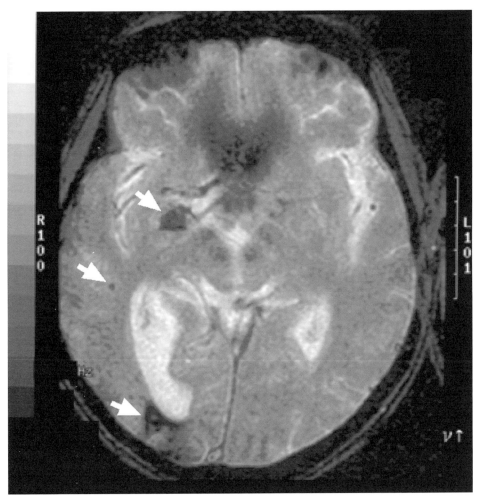

Fig. 4. Imaging appearance of cerebral amyloid angiopathy. Gradient echo MR imaging of a 78-yr-man with a history of headache, mild dementia, right superior quadrantanopia, and difficulty recognizing faces (prosopagnosia). The arrows indicate several separate foci of hypointensity on this sequence representing old blood products in the right medial temporal and occipital lobes, consistent with multiple small hemorrhages. Brain pathology on biopsy demonstrated congophilic angiopathy. Other images showed the left occipital infarction, explaining the right quadrantic defect and the higher-order visual processing disturbance as a result of bilateral lesions.

esophageal echocardiogram), in addition to routine blood tests and electrocardiography (54,55). The advantages of MRI scanning include visualization of the location and extent of ischemia at the very earliest stages, and the ability to detect smaller infarcts particularly in brainstem regions, which are often difficult to see on CT scans. MRIs may also show additional infarcts not seen on CT scans, aiding in the differential diagnosis of the cause of stroke and potentially altering management (see Fig. 6). Noninvasive vascular imaging is usually adequate to answer most questions about the presence and degree of stenosis in major cerebral vessels, but occasionally conventional angiography is required when noninvasive tests are equivocal. The role of additional further diagnostic imaging depends on the results of the initial evaluation and the clinical scenario.

Table 4
Stroke Subtypes and Causes

Hemorrhagic strokes
  Subarachnoid hemorrhage
    Traumatic
    Aneurysmal
    Other
  Intracerebral hemorrhage
    Traumatic
    Hypertensive
    Cerebral amyloid angiopathy
    Hemorrhagic conversion of infarction
    Coagulopathy
    Neoplasm
    Vascular malformation
      Cavernous angioma
      Arteriovenous malformation
Ischemic strokes
  Lacunar
  Extracranial atherosclerosis
  Intracranial atherosclerosis
  Cardioembolic
  Cryptogenic
  Other (dissection, vasculitis, etc.)

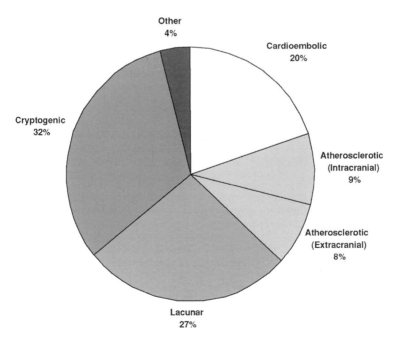

Fig. 5. Distribution of ischemic stroke subtypes in the Northern Manhattan Stroke Study.

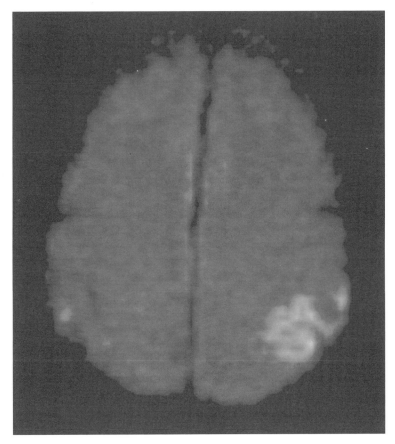

Fig. 6. Bilateral infarcts in setting of MI. Diffusion-weighted brain MRI scan in a 72-yr-old man who presented with acute aphasia and fluctuating right hemiparesis. He had had chest pain for the first time 2 d prior. Emergency echocardiography disclosed anterior wall MI with mural thrombus. Intra-arterial thrombolysis and clot retraction of the angular branch of the left middle cerebral artery was performed with excellent angiographic and clinical result. The follow-up MRI shows abnormal signal in the left parietal region consistent with infarction, as well as an additional focus of diffusion signal abnormality in the right parietal region. These bilateral superficial infarcts are most consistent with a cardiogenic "shower" of emboli.

Strokes after cardiac surgery are generally ischemic infarcts related to embolization of particulate matter, particularly from an atherosclerotic aorta, during the procedure, and, less often, the result of hypoperfusion. The general imaging appearance of postoperative infarcts from emboli is of a superficial cortical infarction. Most emboli go to the middle cerebral arteries (MCAs), which supply the bulk of the cerebral hemispheres, but other large vessels may also be affected. Approximately 20% of cerebral blood flow goes to the posterior circulation, so as many as one-fifth of infarcts may be expected to occur in these vessels. It is important to remember that not all cerebral infarctions cause weakness; an overreliance on symptoms or signs of weakness may underestimate the frequency of stroke. Common stroke syndromes that do not involve weakness are fluent (or Wernicke's) aphasia and cortical visual loss. Because the inferior division of the MCA supplies the lateral temporal lobe and parietal lobes, including Wernicke's area, infarcts in that vessel may cause a prosodic, fluent speech with multiple paraphasic errors and poor comprehension, while sparing the motor strip in the frontal lobe. Emboli traveling up the basilar artery may cause significant infarction in bilateral posterior cerebral arteries, causing complete blindness, sometimes without awareness of the deficit on the part of the patient, resulting from infarction of both occipital lobes (the "top of the basilar syndrome"). Behavioral abnormalities are common, and memory loss and eye movement abnormalities may also occur, resulting from the involvement of the medial temporal lobe structures and the midbrain eye movement centers, respectively. Emboli may be of any size; small emboli to branches of the superior division of the middle cerebral artery may cause limited weakness of the hand, particularly fine finger movements, which may be mistaken for a compression neuropathy as a result of placement of the patient while under anesthesia. Watershed infarction, because of decreased perfusion pressure, sometimes through vessels already narrowed because of intracranial atherosclerosis, also occurs in approximately one-quarter of patients. These appear on imaging as more or less broad swaths of infarction over the surface of the brain extending from the frontal to occipital lobes, along the borders between the middle cerebral and anterior and posterior cerebral arteries (see Fig. 7). Infarcts need not be limited to the cortical surface, and small deep infarcts resulting from embolic obstruction of deep penetrating arterioles may also be seen.

The impact of ischemic stroke on the population differs according to age, gender, and race –ethnicity, factors generally considered to be risk "markers" for stroke. Age, for instance, has been consistently identified as the most important determinant of stroke. For every 10 yr after age 55, the stroke rate more than doubles in both men and women (56,57). Men have a slightly greater stroke incidence than women, but the absolute number of women suffering stroke each year is greater because women live longer than men; therefore, in the elderly population, women stroke victims outnumber men significantly. Thus, stroke should not be considered simply a disease of men.

Race and ethnicity are also related to stroke incidence and mortality rates. Stroke incidence among blacks in the Cincinnati region is two to four times as high as among whites in Rochester, Minnesota (46). In the Northern Manhattan Stroke Study, blacks and Hispanics each had elevated annual age-adjusted relative risks of ischemic stroke compared with whites (2.0 and 3.2 for black men and women, and 1.9 and 2.3 for Hispanic men and women, respectively) (58). Several studies have shown increased stroke-related mortality rates among blacks and other minority groups; overall, blacks are more than twice as likely as whites to die of stroke (59). There is some evidence that the increased mortality among blacks is related to socio-economic and environmental factors, although as much as 50% of the difference in mortality remains unexplained (60).

Although about 30–40% of strokes remain unexplained, the majority of strokes occur in people with well-established risk factors (see Table 5) and in those in whom a first stroke could be prevented with the appropriate medications (see Table 6). Antihypertensive medications can reduce the risk of stroke in hypertensive patients by about 30% (61), and warfarin can reduce the risk in patients with atrial fibrillation by about 60–70% (62). Treatment of hyperlipidemia reduces the risk of a first stroke, although not to the same degree that it reduces the risk of a first myocardial infarction, reflecting the heterogeneity of causes of stroke compared with those of MI (63). In diabetics, treatment with angiotensin-converting-enzyme (ACE) inhibitors can reduce the risk of stroke by about 20% (64), and there is also limited data supporting the use of metformin for stroke prevention among obese type II diabetics (65).

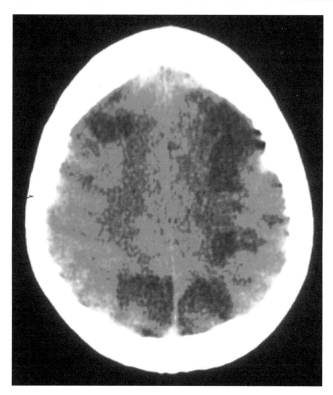

Fig. 7. Bilateral border-zone infarcts in a patient with thoracic aneurysm surgery. A head CT scan of a 78-yr-old woman with a subacute thoracic aortic aneurysm who underwent surgical repair. The wide swaths of hypodensity in both hemispheres is consistent with infarction in the "border zone" supplied by both the middle and anterior cerebral arteries. These are generally attributed to decreased cerebral perfusion, which would be expected to affect the distal fields of the cerebral vessels first, but may also be caused by multiple microemboli to the most distal branches.

Surgical carotid endarterectomy reduced the risk of a first stroke among patients with asymptomatic carotid stenosis of at least 60% in the Asymptomatic Carotid Atherosclerosis Study (ACAS) *(66)*. The benefit is of moderate clinical significance however, reducing the incidence of stroke from about 2% to 1% annually, reflecting the low rate of stroke in the asymptomatic patient. Complication rates were higher among women than men (3.6% vs 1.7%), and an independent clinically significant benefit was not found in women. It should be noted that patients age 80 and older and those with symptomatic cardiac disease were not eligible for the study, so caution must be exercised in applying these results to elderly cardiac patients. In addition, the procedure should only be performed by experienced surgeons with a demonstrated perioperative complication rate below 3%. The role of carotid angioplasty and stenting in this population also remains unproven. Table 6 shows the many interventions that have been proven in randomized, clinical trials in recent years to prevent a first ischemic stroke.

Once a stroke has occurred, many of the same risk-factor-modifying therapies shown to be effective in primary prevention are likely to continue to be of benefit in preventing recurrence. Investigators have recently suggested that among patients with a first stroke or TIA, even in the absence of documented hypertension, treatment with antihypertensive

Table 5
Stroke Risk Factors

Nonmodifiable risk markers
   Age
   Male gender
   Race and ethnicity
   Genetic factors
Potentially modifiable risk factors
   Cardiac risk factors (well accepted)
      Atrial fibrillation
      Myocardial infarction
      Left-ventricular thrombus
      Valvular heart disease
   Hypertension
   Hyperlipidemia
   Cigarette smoking
   Diabetes mellitus
   Physical inactivity
   Heavy alcohol consumption
   Drug abuse (especially cocaine)
   Carotid artery stenosis
   Transient ischemic attack
Postulated stroke risk factors under further investigation
   Cardiac risk factors (less well accepted)
      Patent foramen ovale
      Atrial septal aneurysm
      Mitral annular calcification
      Mitral valve strands
      Aortic arch atheroma
   Antiphospholipid antibodies
   Homocysteine
   Infection (*Chlamydia pneumoniae,* periodontal infection)
   Obstructive sleep apnea

therapy may reduce the risk of a recurrent event. In the PROGRESS trial, an international randomized, double-blind, placebo-controlled trial of antihypertensive therapy among 6105 patients with a history of stroke (hemorrhagic or ischemic) or transient ischemic attack within the past 5 yr, patients were enrolled independent of hypertension status, and 52% were considered non-hypertensive (i.e., systolic BP <160 mm Hg and diastolic BP <90 mm Hg) *(67)*. The mean blood pressure among non-hypertensives was 136/79 at baseline. Active treatment with the combination of the ACE inhibitor, perindopril 4 mg daily, and the diuretic, indapamide 2.5 mg daily, led to a reduction in blood pressure of 12/5 mm Hg compared with placebos, and a statistically significant 43% reduction in stroke risk. The combination therapy provided a benefit of a similar magnitude among both hypertensive and nonhypertensive patients. These results are also supported by the HOPE (Heart Outcomes Prevention Evaluation) trial, noted earlier, which also enrolled patients with a history of stroke independent of blood pressure status and randomized patients to the ACE inhibitor ramipril or placebo *(64)*. In that study, despite a very small mean blood pressure

Table 6
Primary Prevention of Stroke

Risk factor	Treatment	Trial
Hypertension	Antihypertensives	HDFP,[a] MRC,[b] SHEP,[c] STOP-H,[d] others
Myocardial infarction	HMGCoA reductase inhibitors	4S[e], CARE,[f] LIPID[g]
Hyperlipidemia	HMGCoA reductase inhibitors	WOSCOPS[h]
Atrial fibrillation	Warfarin; aspirin	AFASAK1,[i] SPAF1,[j] BAATAF,[k] SPINAF[l]
DM, Type II, obesity	Metformin	UK-PDS[m]
DM/vascular disease	Ramipipril (ACE inhibitor)	HOPE[n]
Aymptomatic carotid stenosis	Carotid endarterectomy	ACAS[o]

[a] Hypertension Detection and Follow-up Program Cooperative Group. Five-year findings of the Hypertension Detection and Follow-up Program. III. Reduction in stroke incidence among persons with high blood pressure. JAMA 1982;247:633–638.

[b] Medical Research Council Working Party. MRC trial of treatment of mild hypertension: principal results. Br Med J 1985;291:97–104.

[c] SHEP Cooperative Research Group. Prevention of stroke by antihypertensive drug treatment in older persons with isolated systolic hypertension. JAMA 1991;265:3255–3264.

[d] Dahlöf B, Lindholm LH, Hansson L, Scherstén B, Ekbom T, Wester P-O. Morbidity and mortality in the Swedish Trial in Old patients with Hypertension (STOP-Hypertension). Lancet 338:1281–1284.

[e] Scandinavian Simvastatin Survival Study Group: Randomized trial of cholesterol-lowering in 4444 patients with coronary heart disease: the Scandinavian Simvastatin Survival Study (4S). Lancet 1994;344:1383–1389.

[f] Sacks FM, Pfeffer MA, Moye LA, et al. The effect of pravastatin on coronary events after myocardial infarction in patients with average cholesterol levels. Cholesterol and Recurrent Events Trial Investigators. N Engl J Med 1996;335:1001–1009.

[g] The Long-Term Intervention with Pravastatin in Ischaemic Disease (LIPID) Study Group. Prevention of cardiovascular events and death with pravastatin in patients with coronary heart disease and a broad range of initial cholesterol levels. N Engl J Med 1998;339:1349–1357.

[h] Shepherd J, Cobbe SM, Ford I, et al. Prevention of coronary heart disease with pravastatin in men with hypercholesterolemia. N Engl J Med 1995;333:1301–1307.

[i] Petersen P, Boysen G, Gotfredsen J, Andersen ED, Andersen B. Placebo-controlled, randomised trial of warfarin and aspirin for prevention of thromboembolic complications in chronic atrial fibrillation: the Copenhagen AFASAK Study. Lancet 1989;1:175–179.

[j] Stroke Prevention in Atrial Fibrillation (SPAF) Investigators: stroke prevention in atrial fibrillation study, final results. Circulation 1991;84:527–539.

[k] Boston Area Anticoagulation Trial in Atrial Fibrillation Investigators. The effect of low dose warfarin on the risk of stroke in patients with non-rheumatic atrial fibrillation. N Engl J Med 1990;323:1505–1511.

[l] Ezekowitz MD, Bridgers SL, James KE, et al. Warfarin in the prevention of stroke associated with non-rheumatic atrial fibrillation. N Engl J Med 1992;327:1406–1412.

[m] UK Prospective Diabetes Study (UKPDS) Group. Effect of intensive blood-glucose control with metformin on complications in overweight patients with type 2 diabetes (UKPDS 34). Lancet 1998;352:854–865.

[n] The Heart Outcomes Prevention Evaluation Study Investigators. Effects of an angiotensin-converting-enzyme inhibitor, ramipril, on cardiovascular events in high-risk patients. N Engl J Med 2000; 342:145-153.

[o] Executive Committee for the Asymptomatic Carotid Atherosclerosis Study. Endarterectomy for asymptomatic carotid artery stenosis. JAMA 1995;273:1421–1428.

Abbreviations: DM = diabetes mellitus; HMG CoA = 3-hydroxy-3-methylglutaryl–coenzyme A; HDFP = Hypertension Detection and Follow-up Program; MRC = Medical Research Council; SHEP = Systolic Hypertension in the Elderly Prevention Trial; STOP-H = Swedish Trial in Old Patients with Hypertension; 4S = Scandinavian Simvastatin Survival Study; CARE = Cholesterol and Recurrent Events Trial; LIPID = Long-Term Intervention with Pravastatin in Ischaemic Disease; WOSCOPS = West of Scotland Coronary Prevention Study; AFASAK = Atrial Fibrillation, Aspirin and Anticoagulation Study; SPAF = Stroke Prevention in Atrial Fibrillation; BAATAF = Boston Area Anticoagulation Trial in Atrial Fibrillation; SPINAF = Veterans Affairs Stroke Prevention in Nonrheumatic Atrial Fibrillation Study; UK-PDS = HOPE = Heart Outcomes Prevention Evaluation.

reduction of 3/2 mm Hg, there was a 22% risk reduction in vascular events. Trials are currently ongoing to determine whether lipid-lowering therapy with statins can reduce the risk of recurrent stroke in patients with normal or near-normal lipid levels (and free of concomitant heart disease) in the same way that such treatment reduces the risk of recurrent cardiac disease.

In patients with symptomatic carotid stenosis, carotid endarterectomy can substantially reduce the risk of a recurrent stroke. In the North American Symptomatic Carotid Endarterectomy Trial (NASCET), surgery reduced the risk of recurrent stroke at 2 yr from 26% to 9% compared with medical management alone (68). Again, the role of angioplasty and stenting in this setting is uncertain. The available data suggest that there is no advantage to angioplasty and stenting over carotid surgery for the symptomatic patient either (69,70). Unlike the situation in the coronary vessels, in which coronary angioplasty allows the patient to avoid a sternum-splitting procedure, obtaining surgical access to the carotid artery involves a small incision and minimal dissection in the neck. Patients do not have significant pain, do not require prolonged rehabilitation, and may leave the hospital the day after the procedure. Carotid endarterectomy may even be performed under local anesthesia in some patients. Until large randomized trials demonstrate its value, angioplasty and stenting should be considered experimental procedures and endarterectomy the procedure of choice. In certain select settings, however, angioplasty offers advantages over end-arterectomy. In patients with surgically inaccessible disease because of a high carotid bifurcation or intracranial atherosclerosis, angioplasty may be the only option. Angioplasty may also be the only option in patients with symptomatic disease at other inaccessible sites, such as the basilar artery (see Fig. 8A,B).

In addition to management of medical and behavioral risk factors, antiplatelet therapy has been shown to reduce the risk of a recurrent stroke after a first event. Traditionally, aspirin had been used for stroke patients, but the past decade has witnessed the development of several newer agents with alternative mechanisms of action, which can be used in place of or in addition to aspirin. These include ticlopidine, clopidogrel, and dipyridamole (see Table 7).

Studies among patients with cerebrovascular disease have consistently demonstrated the benefit of aspirin (71–74). The best dosage of aspirin remains controversial, although recent trial data provide support for doses of 50–325 mg (75,76). Gastrointestinal side effects are generally less with lower aspirin doses. In a meta-analysis (74) of randomized data among more than 10,000 patients with cerebrovascular disease, investigators found that 37 future vascular events per 1000 patients treated could be prevented ($p < 0.000005$) with aspirin. The relative odds reduction was similar for those presenting with completed stroke (23%) vs TIA (22%), again demonstrating the artificiality of strict distinctions between these two related conditions.

Ticlopidine and clopidogrel, related thienopyridine derivative compounds that inhibit adenosine diphosphate-induced platelet aggregation, are alternative antiplatelet agents (77). Ticlopidine was more effective than aspirin at preventing stroke among those with TIA or minor stroke, although its benefit in reducing the composite end point of stroke, MI, or vascular death is less clear (78). The use of ticlopidine is limited by side effects, which include diarrhea in over 10% and worrisome neutropenia in approx 1% of patients. Clopidogrel, a related compound approved by the Food and Drug Administration (FDA) in 1998, is comparable to aspirin among patients with cerebrovascular disease (79). Clopidogrel is generally well tolerated, although recent reports of thrombotic thrombocytopenic

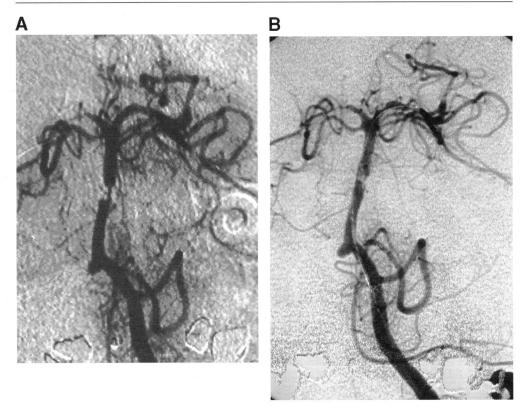

Fig. 8. Angioplasty of symptomatic intracranial basilar artery stenosis. Basilar artery angiograms before and after angioplasty in a 65-yr-old man with a history of recurrent transient episodes of diplopia and loss of consciousness. (**A**) Tight stenosis of the basilar artery. This lesion would not be accessible to surgical endarterectomy. (**B**) After angioplasty, the stenosis is improved. Transcranial Doppler velocity profiles show marked improvement.

purpura have led many to suggest routine monitoring of platelet levels after initiating therapy *(80)*. Combination therapy with two antiplatelet agents has been tested in the European Stroke Prevention Study 2 (ESPS 2), which utilized a factorial design comparing placebo, aspirin 25 mg twice daily, a new extended release formulation of dipyridamole 200 mg twice daily, and the combination of aspirin and dipyridamole at the same doses *(76)*. The combined therapy arm demonstrated the greatest benefit with reduction in risk that was essentially additive of the single-treatment arms (risk reduction of 37% with combined treatment). The combination of antiplatelet agents with different mechanisms of action is currently being tested in other studies and may play an increasing role in the future.

The role of warfarin in secondary-stroke prevention among patients without definite cardioembolism has recently been revised to some extent on the basis of the Warfarin Aspirin Recurrent Stroke Study (WARSS) *(81)*. The WARSS study was designed to test whether warfarin (International Normalized Ratio [INR] 1.4–2.8) is more effective than aspirin (325 mg) in preventing recurrent stroke. The study was a randomized, blinded trial in patients who, without severe carotid stenosis or cardioembolic stroke, had an ischemic stroke within 30 d of randomization. There was no benefit of warfarin over aspirin among patients, nor among the different subgroups of patients defined by stroke etiologic sub-

Table 7
Comparison of Antiplatelet Therapies for Secondary Stroke Prevention

Agent	Estimated efficacy[a] (RRR,%)	Side effects	Dosing	Cost
Aspirin	10–20	Bleeding	qd	Low
Ticlopidine	20–25	Rash, GI, neutropenia, TTP	bid	High
Clopidogrel	10–20	Rash, GI, TTP (?)	qd	High
Dipyridamole	10–20	Headache, GI	tid–qid	Moderate
ER-DP	10–20	Headache, GI	bid	N/A in United States
Aspirin/ER-DP	30–40	Headache, GI, bleeding	bid	High

[a]Estimated efficacy versus placebo for end-point stroke, MI, death.

Abbreviations: RRR = relative risk reduction. GI = gastrointestinal upset. TTP = thrombotic thrombocytopenic purpura. ER-DP = extended release dipyridamole. N/A = not available.

type. Of equal importance, however, was the fact that warfarin was nearly as safe as aspirin (annual risk of major hemorrhage 2.2% on warfarin and 1.5% on aspirin, $p = 0.10$). Warfarin is still indicated for secondary stroke prevention among patients with atrial fibrillation or other high risk sources of cardiac embolism, such as valvular heart disease and left-ventricular thrombus.

Recent basic science work and clinical evidence has also demonstrated that stroke is not an immediate and irreversible event. Rather, a stroke evolves over a period of time, with the time required for irreversible neuronal injury dependent on the degree of the reduction in blood flow to the brain. In other words, the longer that blood flow is impaired and the lower the blood flow, the more likely that irreversible brain injury will occur. Thus, the sooner blood flow can be restored, the more likely brain tissue will be salvaged. Therapies designed to restore blood flow, such as tissue plasminogen activator, should therefore be given as quickly as possible. The pivotal trial that demonstrated the benefit of recombinant tissue plasminogen activator (rt-PA) for acute ischemic stroke was the NINDS trial, which showed that there was a statistically significant benefit in favor of rt-PA over placebo for patients treated within 3 h of symptom onset *(82)*. The proportion of patients achieving functional independence in activities of daily living at 3 mo after stroke was 50% in the group treated with rt-PA compared with 38% in the placebo group. The earlier that thombolytic therapy was administered in the pivotal NINDS rt-PA study, the more likely patients were to have a favorable outcome, a point which was not recognized at the time TPA was first approved for stroke *(83)*. A second consequence of the recognition of the dynamic process of stroke and its dependence on cerebral blood flow is that low blood pressure levels must be avoided in the setting of acute ischemic stroke. Although the healthy brain is able to maintain cerebral blood flow across a relatively wide spectrum of blood pressure because of the process of autoregulation, the injured brain cannot. Collateral blood flow through the circle of Willis and other routes is therefore heavily dependent on systemic blood pressure in the setting of stroke. Thus, attempts to reduce blood pressure may actually exacerbate brain ischemia and worsen the infarct. Recent studies have even suggested a benefit of induced hypertension in patients with acute ischemic stroke, although large randomized clinical trials of this therapy have not yet been conducted *(84)*.

CONTROVERSIES

Neurological Complications of Cardiac Surgery: How Common Is It and Why Does It Occur?

Adverse neurological outcomes are among the most feared and controversial complications after cardiac surgery. Neurological complications have been divided into acute complications, including stroke and coma, and long-term neurological problems such as cognitive decline. Estimates of the frequency of strokes after coronary artery bypass surgery have ranged over an order of magnitude, from approx 0.5–5.2%, depending on the population studied, study design, and the methods used to detect the stroke *(85–87)*. Patients who suffer stroke have a greater mortality, which may be as high as 38% *(88–91)*. Valvular surgery and combined valvular and bypass surgery are associated with a higher risk of stroke than coronary artery bypass graft (CABG) alone *(92–94)*.

Cognitive decline in the absence of an acute focal insult occurs even more commonly than stroke: A recent meta-analysis of cohort and interventional trials among coronary artery surgery patients indicated an incidence of cognitive deficit on neuropsychological testing of 22.5% at 2 mo postoperatively *(95)*. Consistent with this, longitudinal data with repeated testing of a single cohort suggest that about 50% of patients have some cognitive deficit at discharge after surgery, and roughly 25% still have a deficit after 6 mo *(96)*. Cognitive decline was defined as a decrease by at least one standard deviation in performance on at least one of four cognitive function tests. Late cognitive decline, at 5 yr, occurred in 42% of patients, a rate much greater than would be expected in similar patients who do not undergo surgery, and was predicted by early cognitive decline *(96)*. Controversy surrounds these data, particularly because definitions of cognitive decline differ, and many of these changes are asymptomatic. The functional consequences of these cognitive changes remain uncertain. Among elderly, retired individuals, in particular, it may be argued that mild decrements in cognitive status may be less important than similar decrements in younger, working persons. In addition, depression may also occur after cardiac surgery, and it is possible that this may contribute to reversible cognitive dysfunction, although at least some data suggest that depression and cognitive decline occur independently of each other after surgery *(97)*.

Several investigators have attempted to identify factors associated with risk of stroke after CABG, with largely concordant results. A history of prior stroke or TIA has been identified as a predictor of stroke after CABG in most studies *(91,98–105)*. Carotid stenosis, similarly, has been found to be a predictor of stroke in most, but not all studies *(85,104, 106–108)*. The controversy regarding the role of carotid stenosis in the prognosis and management of the cardiac surgery patient is discussed in the following subsection. Additionally, some investigators have suggested that women are at higher risk than men are *(109)*. Of note, although age does not necessarily increase the risk of cardiac complications of heart surgery, it does appear to consistently increase risk of neurological injury. Nonetheless, emerging data indicate that even among those over age 80, the age group expected to be at highest risk of neurological complications after surgery, most patients can have an excellent outcome, with resolution of symptoms and an improved quality of life *(110)*. As older patients continue to be referred for cardiac revascularization procedures, it has become increasingly important to identify factors predictive of neurologic injury and ways in which to prevent it.

Prospective studies using multivariate regression techniques may be expected to provide the most robust data on the relation of various risk factors to stroke after surgery. McKhann and others (88) identified five preoperative factors associated with an increased risk of stroke after CABG: age, prior stroke, hypertension, diabetes mellitus, and presence of carotid bruit. The only intraoperative factor of importance was duration of cardiopulmonary bypass. Using these factors in combination, the authors were able to stratify patients into low-, medium-, and high-risk groups for stroke. Roach et al. (104) reviewed data on 2108 patients undergoing CABG and found a 6.1% incidence of neurological complications, of which 3.1% could be classified as Type I injuries (focal cerebral injury or stupor) and 3% as Type II outcomes (cognitive decline or seizures). Not surprisingly, mortality, length of stay, and likelihood of discharge to an institution for long-term care were greater among those who suffered adverse neurological outcomes. Older age was associated with an increased risk of both types of adverse outcomes, with a 75% increase in risk per decade for Type I outcomes and more than a doubling of risk per decade for a Type II outcome. Additional risk factors for a Type I outcome in multivariate analysis included, in declining order of importance, proximal aortic atherosclerosis, a history of "neurological disease," use of an intra-aortic balloon pump, hypertension, diabetes mellitus, pulmonary disease, and unstable angina. Neurological disease was not carefully defined, and it is unclear whether this included history of dementia as well as stroke. All operations analyzed in this study were elective, and other investigators have shown that neurological outcomes after urgent or emergent surgery are worse (98,110).

The importance of proximal aortic atherosclerosis has been increasingly recognized as the major determinant of stroke and encephalopathy after bypass surgery (88,111,112). Recent data suggest that hypoperfusion during bypass is probably not the usual mechanism of adverse neurologic outcome (113). Pathological and transcranial Doppler studies have demonstrated the importance of microemboli as a cause of neurocognitive sequelae of CABG (114). Autopsy studies have demonstrated small capillary and arteriolar dilatations (or SCADs) in patients dying after CABG but not in patients dying for other reasons. These SCADs stain for fat and are thought to be microembolic in nature. The best method for detection of aortic atherosclerosis is intraoperative echocardiography (111,112). Surgeon awareness of significant aortic atheroma may allow a change in technique designed to decrease the risk of embolization. For patients with mobile or protruding plaque, or with aortic plaque >3 mm in thickness, a more proximal cannulation or clamping site or a fibrillatory arrest approach may be used (115). The use of off-pump CABG procedures has been suggested to reduce the occurrence of neurological complications after coronary surgery (116). The technique remains promising but as yet unproven (117). Randomized trials thus far have shown feasibility but no significant difference in terms of mortality, quality of life, or cognitive outcome (118).

Although investigators continue to debate the relative magnitude and clinical significance of the cognitive changes after CABG, it remains clear that stroke and neurologic dysfunction are among the most important complications of cardiac surgery. Improved methods of prediction and prevention are sorely needed.

Carotid Stenosis and CABG

Several investigators have suggested, as indicated earlier, that the presence of carotid stenosis predicts a worse outcome after cardiac surgery. The absolute rates of stroke associated with carotid stenosis vary across studies, depending on patient populations, surgical techniques, and degree of stenosis considered. Based on overviews *(119,120)*, the mean stroke rate may be as high as 4% among patients with asymptomatic stenosis >50% and approx 8% among patients with symptomatic stenosis >50%. Among patients with higher degrees of stenosis (e.g., >80%) the risk may be higher, approaching 15% in earlier studies *(111,120–122)*. Despite this apparent increase in risk, it remains less clear what to do about carotid stenosis in this setting. No randomized trial has established that carotid endarterectomy in the neurologically asymptomatic patient prior to cardiac surgery reduces the risk of perioperative stroke or cognitive deterioration. The magnitude of the problem is significant, as a substantial proportion of patients with coronary disease have cerebrovascular disease. Nearly a quarter of patients undergoing elective CABG have moderate carotid stenosis (>50%) and approx 9% have severe stenosis (>80%) *(121,122)*.

Options for the patient with combined coronary and cerebrovascular disease include (1) performing cardiac surgery without carotid surgery, (2) carotid endarterectomy in a separate operation prior to the cardiac surgery, (3) CABG prior to carotid surgery, and (4) a combined operation, with carotid surgery conducted first, followed by cardiac surgery. Several authors have advocated performing carotid surgery prior to CABG in a staged or single procedure on the assumption that correcting the cerebral hemodynamic impairment first will prevent cerebral ischemic complications *(123,124)*. It must be remembered, however, that most strokes occurring in the setting of open heart surgery are the result not of hemodynamic impairment but rather of embolic phenomena *(125,126)*. The cardiac complication rate of carotid endarterectomy is also not insignificant; the postoperative MI rate in the NASCET trial was 0.9%, and the overall stroke or death rate was 5.8% *(68)*. The MI and mortality rates of endarterectomy are much higher in patients with active cardiac disease *(127)*. Therefore, although there is intuitive appeal to the approach of correcting the carotid disease prior to the cardiac intervention, there are equally strong theoretical reasons to avoid this approach. Unfortunately, there are no reliable randomized or controlled multicenter trials to address the merits of these different approaches. Attempts to synthesize the many published series indicate that, consistent with the theoretical concerns just discussed, carotid endarterectomy performed prior to cardiac surgery may reduce the risk of stroke but increase mortality *(120)*. Combined procedures have no clear benefit in reducing the risk of stroke or mortality and should not be advocated in most patients. Overall, considering the combined risk of stroke and death, there was no benefit to either staged approach over CABG without endarterectomy. This conclusion does not eliminate the potential role of staged procedures in selected subgroups of patients.

A rational approach to the problem of the patient with combined coronary artery and carotid disease is to take into account the presence and type of symptoms and the degree of severity of the carotid disease, as well as the severity of the coronary disease. The benefits of carotid surgery for asymptomatic carotid disease are not as clear as they are for symptomatic disease. In the ACAS, for example, asymptomatic patients had only a 2% annual risk of stroke *(66)*. Given the low stroke risk, it seems likely that many of these patients could tolerate cardiac surgery without complications. When patients have both symptomatic coronary and carotid disease, the severity of neurological symptoms should be considered. For example, medically treated patients with carotid stenosis with transient monocular blindness have a 3-yr stroke rate half that of patients with hemispheric TIAs *(128)*. It may also be important to take into account not only the degree of stenosis at the level of the extracranial carotid artery but also the severity of hemodynamic impairment in the intracerebral vessels. Measurement of cerebrovascular reserve using techniques such as oxygen extraction fraction on PET scanning or CO_2 reactivity on transcranial Doppler testing have been used to predict risk of stroke in patients with carotid occlusion or stenosis *(129)*. There are no good, large-scale studies demonstrating the predictive role of these tests for patients undergoing CABG. Nonetheless, a more aggressive approach to correction of the carotid lesion could be entertained in patients with distal hemodynamic impairment who are likely to be at higher risk of stroke.

Should rt-PA Be Used for the Treatment of MI and Ischemic Stroke in the Elderly?

Trials of thrombolytic therapy for MI found that hemorrhagic stroke was a rare complication, on the order of 0.3–1% *(130–132)*. Characteristics of the hemorrhages were varied: these included single and multifocal hemorrhages, as well lobar and deep locations. Most occurred within 24 h. Mortality was high, approx 50% *(132)*. Because of the rarity of the event, it has been difficult to identify predictors of hemorrhage, although some have suggested advanced age, hypertension, and prior stroke as risk factors for hemorrhage. Moreover, some have suggested that amyloid angiopathy and dementia may put patients at higher risk for hemorrhage after thrombolytic therapy for MI *(133)*. There is no systematic data to show that patients with a history of dementia should not receive thrombolytic therapy for MI.

The use of rt-PA for acute ischemic stroke has encountered greater resistance in some quarters as a result of the increased risk of hemorrhagic conversion associated with rt-PA use after ischemic stroke (*see* Fig. 9). In the NINDS trial, there was a 6.4% risk of symptomatic hemorrhage within 36 h among those treated with rt-PA, compared with a 0.6% risk among those treated with placebo *(82)*. Not surprisingly, this 10-fold increase in risk has scared many away from rt-PA use in ischemic stroke. It is important to remember, however, that the overall rate of neurologic worsening in 36 h was, in fact, similar between the two groups (17.4% in the rt-PA group and 18.3% in the placebo group). This perhaps surprising result is attributed to the fact that other adverse consequences of having a stroke —brain swelling and herniation, recurrent ischemia, seizures, and so forth—occurred more frequently in those who did not receive rt-PA. In other words, hemorrhage is not the only bad thing that can happen after a stroke. In addition, those patients who suffered symptomatic hemorrhages were those with large strokes; these were patients who were likely to go on to hemorrhage or a poor prognosis even in the absence of rt-PA. Several phase IV studies have since confirmed the generalizability of the benefits of rt-PA to the community at large *(134)*.

The reluctance to use rt-PA is particularly strong when patients are elderly, as it is believed that they are at higher risk of hemorrhage after thrombolysis than are younger patients. Elderly patients are more likely to have amyloid angiopathy or other brain pathology. Older patients also have a worse overall prognosis after stroke than do younger patients. A secondary analysis of the pivotal NINDS thrombolysis trial found that although elderly patients do have a higher risk of converting to symptomatic hemorrhage, on average they demonstrate the same benefit from rt-PA compared to those who did not receive it as do younger patients *(135)*. There is, therefore, no *a priori* reason to exclude the elderly patient from thrombolytic treatment on the basis of age alone, much as there would be no reason to exclude from cardiac surgery the elderly but otherwise healthy cardiac patient. Because the benefit of treatment is primarily in increasing the long-term likelihood of

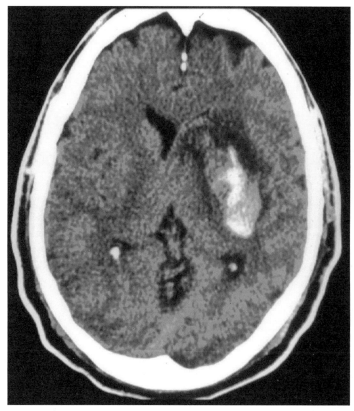

Fig. 9. Symptomatic hemorrhagic conversion of ischemic infarction after thrombolysis. A head CT scan in a 53-yr-old man after thrombolytic treatment with rt-PA for an acute left hemispheric stroke. The initial CT prior to thrombolytic treatment was normal. He initially improved after thrombolysis, but at 12 h, he developed worsening right hemiparesis and aphasia. The hyperdensity on the left side represents hemorrhage into a large deep basal ganglia infarction. He eventually recovered, but was left with mild right hemiparesis and dysarthria.

independence, it would not be unreasonable to limit treatment to those who were previously independent. The elderly, demented nursing home resident, for instance, will not be restored to independence by thrombolytic therapy, and in this situation, it may be reasonable to withhold treatment.

Should all Ischemic Stroke and TIA Patients Receive Statin Therapy?

Over the past decade HMG-CoA reductase inhibitors (statins) have come to play an increasingly important role in the management of patients with elevated cholesterol and heart disease. The scope of their use has expanded significantly, with clinical trials demonstrating their value in reducing the risk of heart disease and cardiac mortality among hypercholesterolemic patients with coronary artery disease, nonhyperlipidemic cardiac patients, and hypercholesterolemic patients without heart disease (63,136–138). There are even data to suggest that among those with average cholesterol levels, these agents may prevent a first cardiac event (139). In most of these studies, reductions were also seen for cerebrovascular disease end points, although the magnitude of benefit was generally smaller and the level of statistical significance less *(63,136–138)*. The more moderate impact of these agents on stroke risk is probably because of both of the following: (1) among heart patients stroke is less common than recurrent ischemic cardiac disease and (2) the greater heterogeneity of stroke compared with heart disease. Nonetheless, the recognition of the importance of statin therapy in ischemic heart disease and the similar, if lesser, benefits seen for stroke prevention has led to the suggestion that stroke patients without heart disease should also receive statin therapy *(140)*. In addition, an expanding literature on the anti-inflammatory and neuroprotective effects of statins has suggested that there may be additional benefits in stroke patients beyond those involved in cholesterol reduction *(140,141)*. The data indicating a role of elevated cholesterol levels in development of vascular dementia further lead to the speculation that statin therapy may also have a role to play in reducing cognitive decline in some patients *(45)*.

It would be incorrect to simply assume that what benefits patients with other forms of vascular disease, such as peripheral arterial disease or coronary artery disease, must also benefit stroke patients. Each of these disorders, although sharing many features, may also behave differently in important ways. There is preclinical scientific evidence of the differences in the biology of these different vascular beds *(142)*. More importantly, clinical data also indicate different natural histories for each of these disorders. In the Antiplatelet Trialists Collaborative analysis *(74)*, stroke patients went on to have further strokes at much higher rates than they had MIs, and, similarly, MI patients were much more likely to have a future MI than stroke. Stroke also tends to occur, on average, in patients at older ages than MI. Clinical trials also provide evidence that therapies thought to act similarly across all patient subgroups actually demonstrate heterogeneity of effect among peripheral, coronary, and cerebral artery disease patients *(79)*. A stroke is, therefore, not simply a "heart attack of the brain." Thus, the appeal of statins for heart disease does not necessarily entail a benefit for all stroke patients.

The latest guidelines of the National Cholesterol Education Program *(143)* indicate that patients at high risk of myocardial infarction and vascular death, defined as a 10-yr risk of 20% or more, should have a target low-density lipoprotein (LDL) level <100 and receive statin therapy if needed to achieve this goal. Included in this high-risk group are those who have already suffered a first MI or angina, those with diabetes mellitus, those with peripheral vascular disease, and those with "symptomatic carotid artery disease." Because large-vessel atherosclerosis accounts for only 10–20% of ischemic stroke, it remains unclear whether other stroke patients—those with lacunar disease or cryptogenic infarcts, for example, who together account for as many as 60% of patients—should similarly be treated with statins. The answer, it would appear, depends on the absolute risk of suffering MI or vascular death among these different subgroups of patients. The benefit provided by targeting low levels of LDL or by using statins, in other words, depends not as much on the specific underlying disease that brings the patient to attention as it does on the patient's future risk of a cardiac event, for which statins are already proven effective. Data from several clinical trials among stroke patients indicates that rates of MI after all ischemic stroke subtypes combined, although lower than rates of recurrent stroke, is on the order of 1–2% per year *(76–79,144)*. Preliminary data from the observational Northern Manhattan Stroke Study, in which ischemic stroke subtypes were determined, indicate that absolute rates of MI and sudden death after a first ischemic stroke are, indeed, on the order of 2% annually for cardioembolic and extracranial atherosclerotic subtypes, but may be 1% or less among patients with intracranial atherosclerosis, lacunar infarcts, and cryptogenic strokes. Longer follow-up of this and other observational studies, as well as ongoing randomized clinical trials of statins in stroke patients, may provide additional information to help determine which, if not all, stroke patients should be treated with statins.

An Aspirin a Day:
Is Aspirin Indicated for the Primary Prevention of Stroke?

There has been increasing recognition among the lay public of the benefits of aspirin therapy in the prevention of cardiovascular disease. Many patients are keenly aware of the advisability of taking an aspirin at the earliest sign of chest pain to prevent a myocardial infarction. Many assume that there is probably good reason to take aspirin every day to prevent cardiac disease in the first place, and many also know that aspirin may have benefits in preventing stroke as well. Many healthy individuals, not unreasonably, wonder whether they should be taking aspirin to stave off that first event as well.

Although aspirin has an extremely important role to play in the care of the cardiac and stroke patient, as discussed earlier, it is less clear that aspirin should be routinely given to patients without cardiovascular disease or risk factors. The relative risk reduction with antiplatelet treatment for nonfatal stroke among patients in the "high-risk" groups in the ATC meta-analysis was 31%, comparable to that for myocardial infarction (35%) (74). High risk was not specifically defined, but included patients with a wide range of medical conditions and risk factors generally felt to lead to vascular disease. The risk of fatal stroke was not significantly decreased, however, possibly because aspirin increases the risk of hemorrhagic strokes, which are more often fatal. Overall mortality was still, however, significantly reduced among high-risk patients (odds ratio 17%). Among "low-risk" participants in trials (i.e., those without established vascular disease or vascular disease risk factors), the role of aspirin as primary prevention for stroke has not been established. Although aspirin provides a small but significant benefit in reducing the risk of myocardial infarction among those at low risk, it also causes a slight increase in risk of hemorrhagic stroke. In the Physicians' Health Study, aspirin was also associated with a slight increase in risk of ischemic stroke, although for unclear reasons (145). Other studies have similarly shown no effect or an increase in total stroke with aspirin in primary prevention (146,147). A recent meta-analysis (148) of four primary prevention trials suggested that there may be a small but not statistically significant increase (6%) in risk of overall stroke with aspirin therapy. There was no significant impact on overall mortality. Aspirin can also cause life-threatening gastrointestinal and other types of major hemorrhage in the elderly.

As is the case for decisions about the use of statins, the decision to use aspirin for primary prevention will, therefore, generally depend more on absolute cardiac risk than stroke risk. For those with an absolute cardiac risk of 1.5% per year, the benefits of aspirin may outweigh the risks (148). For those with event rates likely to be less than 0.5% (i.e., the low-risk group), the complications of stroke and other forms of bleeding are likely to outweigh any benefits. Aspirin, therefore, should not be routinely recommended for patients without existent cardiovascular disease or risk factors for cardiovascular disease.

REFERENCES

1. Creasey H, Rapoport SI. The aging human brain. Ann Neurol 1985;17:2–10.
2. Esri MM, Hyman BT, Beyreuther K, et al. Ageing and the dementias. In: Graham DI, Lantos PL, eds. Greenfield's Neuropathology, 6th ed. Oxford University Press, New York, 1997, vol 1, pp. 153–233.
3. Masliah E, Mallory M, Hansen L, et al. Quantitative synaptic alterations in the human neocortex during normal aging. Neurology 1993;43:192–197.

 4. Schochet SS. Neuropathology of aging. Neurol Clin 1998;16:569–580.
 5. Pantoni L, Garcia JH. The significance of cerebral white matter abnormalities 100 years after Bins-wanger's report: a review. Stroke 1995;26:1293–1301.
 6. Ketonen LM. Neuroimaging of the aging brain. Neurol Clin 1998;16:581–598.
 7. Fazekas F. Magnetic resonance signal abnormalities in asymptomatic individuals: their incidence and functional correlates. Eur Neurol 1989;29:164–168.
 8. Awad I, Johnson P, Spetzler R, et al. Incidental subcortical lesions identified on magnetic resonance imaging in the elderly. I. Postmortem pathological correlation. Stroke 1986;17:1090–1097.
 9. Yue NC, Arnold AM, Longstreth WT, et al. Sulcal, ventricular, and white matter changes at MR imaging in the aging brain: data from the cardiovascular health study. Radiology 1997;202:33–39.
10. Coffey CE, Wilkinson WE, Parashos IA, et al. Quantitative cerebral anatomy of the aging human brain: a cross-sectional study using magnetic resonance imaging. Neurology 1992;42:527–536.
11. Jernigan T, Archibald S, Berhow M, et al. Cerebral structure on MRI, part I: localization of age-related changes. Biol Psychiatry 1991;29:55–67.
12. Cowell PE, Turetskky BI, Gur RC, et al. Sex differences in aging of the human frontal and temporal lobes. J Neurosci 1994;14:4748–4755.
13. Eberling JL, Nordahl TE, Kusubov N, et al. Reduced temporal lobe glucose metabolism in aging. J Neuro-imaging 1995;5:178–182.
14. Shigeta M, Julin P, Almkvist O, et al. EEG in successful aging: a 5 year follow-up study from the eighth to ninth decade of life. Electroencephal Clin Neurophysiol 1995;95:77–83.
15. Albert MS. Predictors of cognitive change in older persons: MacArthur studies of successful aging. Psychol Aging 1995;10:578–589.
16. Petersen RC, Stevens JC, Ganguli M, Tangalos EG, Cummings JL, DeKosky ST. Practice parameter: early detection of dementia: mild cognitive impairment (an evidence-based review): Report of the Quality Standards Subcommittee of the American Academy of Neurology. Neurology 2001;56:1133–1142.
17. Keefover RW. Aging and cognition. Neurol Clin 1998;16:635–648.
18. Knopman DS, DeKosky ST, Cummings JL, Chui H, Corey-Bloom J, Relkin N, et al. Practice param-eter: diagnosis of dementia (an evidence-based review): Report of the Quality Standards Subcommit-tee of the American Academy of Neurology. Neurology 2001;56:1143–1153.
19. Doody RS, Stevens JC, Beck C, Dubinsky RM, Kaye JA, Gwyther L, et al. Practice parameter: man-agement of dementia (an evidence-based review): Report of the Quality Standards Subcommittee of the American Academy of Neurology. Neurology 2001;56:1154–1166.
20. Petersen RC, Smith GE, Waring SC, et al. Mild cognitive impairment: clinical characterization and out-come. Arch Neurol 1999;56:303–308.
21. Perls TT, Morris JN, Ooi WL, et al. The relationship between age, gender, and cognitive performance in the very old: the effect of selective survival. J Am Geriatr Soc 1993;41:1193–1201.
22. Van Duijn C, Clayton D, Chandra V, et al. Familial aggregation of Alzheimer's disease and related disorders: a collaborative re-analysis of case control studies. Int J Epidemiol 1991;20(Suppl):13–20.
23. Mortimer J, van Duijn C, Chandra V, et al. Head trauma as a risk factor for Alzheimer's disease: a collaborative re-analysis of case control studies. Int J Epidemiol 1991;20(Suppl):28–35.
24. Stern Y, Gurland B, Tatemichi T, et al. Influence of education and occupation on the incidence of Alzheimer's disease. JAMA 1994;271:1004–1010.
25. Chui H, Zhang Q. Evaluation of dementia: a systematic study of the usefulness of the American Academy of Neurology's practice parameters. Neurology 1997;49:925–935.
26. Hamilton M. A rating scale for depression. J Neurol Neurosurg Psychiatry 1960;23:56–62.
27. Burke WJ, Roccaforte WH, Wengel SP. The short form of the Geriatric Depression Scale: a comparison with the 30-item form. J Geriatr Psychiatry Neurol 1991;4:173–178.
28. Holmes C, Cairns N, Lantos P, et al. Validity of current clinical criteria for Alzheimer's disease, vascular dementia and dementia with Lewy bodies. Br J Psychiatry 1999;174:45–50.
29. Lim A, Tsuang D, Kukull W, et al. Clinico-neuropathological correlation of Alzheimer's disease in a community-based case series. J Am Geriatr Soc 1999;47:564–569.
30. Desmond DW, Moroney JT, Paik MC, Sano M, Mohr JP, Aboumatar S, et al. Frequency and clinical determinants of dementia after ischemic stroke. Neurology 2000;54:1124–1131.
31. Hsich G, Kenney K, Gibbs CJ, et al. The 14-3-3 brain protein in cerebrospinal fluid as a marker for transmissible spongiform encephalopathies. N Engl J Med 1996;335:924–930.
32. Knapp M, Knopman D, Solomon P, et al., for the Tacrine Study Group. A 30-week randomized con-trolled trial of high-dose tacrine in patients with Alzheimer's disease. JAMA 1994;271:985–991.

33. Watkins P, Zimmerman H, Knapp M, et al. Hepatotoxic effects of tacrine administration in patients with Alzheimer's disease. JAMA 1994;271:992–998.

34. Davis K, Thal L, Gamzu E, et al. A double-blind, placebo-controlled multicenter study of tacrine for Alzheimer's disease. N Engl J Med 1992;327:1253–1259.

35. Rogers S, Doody R, Mohs R, et al., and the Donepezil Study Group. Donepezil improved cognition and global function in Alzheimer's disease. Arch Intern Med 1998;158:1021–1031.

36. Rogers S, Farlow M, Doody R, et al., and the Donepezil Study Group. A 24-week, double-blind, placebo-controlled trial of donepezil in patients with Alzheimer's disease. Neurology 1998;50:136–145.

37. Forette F, Anand R, Gharabawi G. A phase II study in patients with Alzheimer's disease to assess the preliminary efficacy and maximum tolerated dose of rivastigmine (Exeloninfinity). Eur J Neurol 1999; 6:423–429.

38. Rosler M, Anand R, Cicin-Sain A, et al. Efficacy and safety of rivastigmine in patients with Alzheimer's disease: international randomised controlled trial. Br Med J 1999;318:633–638.

39. Raskind M, Peskind E, Wessel T, et al., and the Galantamine Study Group. Galantamine in AD. A 6-month randomized, placebo-controlled trial with a 6-month extension. Neurology 2000;54:2261–2268.

40. Tariot P, Solomon P, Morris J, et al., and the Galantamine Study Group. A 5-month, randomized, placebo-controlled trial of galantamine in AD. Neurology 2000;54:2269–2276.

41. Sano M, Ernesto C, Thomas RG, et al. A controlled trial of selegiline, alpha-tocopherol, or both as treatment for Alzheimer's disease. N Engl J Med 1997;336:1216–1222.

42. 't Veld BA, Ruitenberg A, Hofman A, Launer LJ, van Duijn CM, Stijnen T, et al. Nonsteroidal antiinflammatory drugs and the risk of Alzheimer's disease. N Engl J Med 2001;345:1515–1521.

43. De Deyn P, Rabheru K, Rasmussen A, et al. A randomized trial of risperidone, placebo, and haloperidol for behavioral symptoms of dementia. Neurology 1999;53:946–955.

44. Mayeux R, Sano M. Drug therapy: treatment of Alzheimer's disease. N Engl J Med 1999;341:1670–1679.

45. Moroney JT, Tang MX, Berglund L, Small S, Merchant C, Bell K, et al. Low-density lipoprotein cholesterol and the risk of dementia with stroke. JAMA 1999;282(3):254–260.

46. Broderick J, Brott T, Kothari R, Miller R, Khoury J, Pancioli A, et al. The Greater Cincinnati/Northern Kentucky Stroke Study. Preliminary first-ever and total incidence rates of stroke among blacks. Stroke 1998;29:415–421.

47. Aho K, Harmsen P, Hatano S, Marquardsen J, Smirnov WE, Strasser T. Cerebrovascular disease in the community: results of a WHO collaborative study. Bull WHO 1980;58:113–130.

48. Kidwell CS, Alger JR, Di Salle F, Starkman S, Villablanca P, Bentson J, et al. Diffusion MRI in patients with transient ischemic attacks. Stroke 1999;30(6):1174–1180.

49. Sacco RL. Lobar intracerebral hemorrhage. N Engl J Med 2000;342:276–279.

50. O'Donnell HC, Rosand J, Knudsen KA, Furie KL, Segal AZ, Chiu RI, et al. Apolipoprotein E genotype and the risk of recurrent lobar intracerebral hemorrhage. N Engl J Med 2000;342:240–245.

51. Greenberg SM, O'Donnell HC, Schaefer PW, Kraft E. MRI detection of new hemorrhages: potential marker of progression in cerebral amyloid angiopathy. Neurology 1999;53:1135–1138.

52. Greenberg SM, Vonsattel JP, Stakes JW, Gruber M, Finklestein SP. The clinical spectrum of cerebral amyloid angiopathy: presentations without lobar hemorrhage. Neurology 1993;43:2073–2079.

53. Sacco RL, Ellenberg JH, Mohr JP, Tatemichi TK, Hier DB, Price TR, et al. Infarcts of undetermined cause: the NINCDS Stroke Data Bank. Ann Neurol 1989;25:382–390.

54. Adams HP Jr, Brott TG, Crowell RM, Furlan AJ, Gomez CR, Grotta J, et al. Guidelines for the management of patients with acute ischemic stroke. A statement for healthcare professionals from a special writing group of the Stroke Council, American Heart Association. Stroke 1994;25:1901–1914.

55. Feinberg WM, Albers GW, Barnett HJ, Biller J, Caplan LR, Carter LP, et al. Guidelines for the management of transient ischemic attacks. From the Ad Hoc Committee on Guidelines for the Management of Transient Ischemic Attacks of the Stroke Council of the American Heart Association. Stroke 1994; 25:1320–1335.

56. Brown RD, Whisnant JP, Sicks RD, O'Fallon WM, Wiebers DO. Stroke incidence, prevalence, and survival: secular trends in Rochester, Minnesota, through 1989. Stroke 1996;27:373–380.

57. Wolf PA, D'Agostino RB, O'Neal MA, Sytkowski P, Kase CS, Belanger AJ, et al. Secular trends in stroke incidence and mortality: the Framingham Study. Stroke 1992;23:1551–1555.

58. Sacco RL, Boden-Albala B, Gan R, Chen X, Kargman DE, Shea S, et al. Stroke incidence among white, black, and Hispanic residents of an urban community: the Northern Manhattan Stroke Study. Am J Epidemiol 1998;147:259–268.

59. Howard G, Anderson R, Sorlie P, Andrews V, Backlund E, Burke GL. Ethnic differences in stroke mortality between non-Hispanic whites, Hispanic whites, and blacks: the National Longitudinal Mortality Study. Stroke 1994;25:2120–2125.

60. Giles WH, Kittner SJ, Hebel JR, Losonczy KG, Sherwin RW. Determinants of black–white differences in the risk of cerebral infarction. Arch Intern Med 1995;155:1319–1324.

61. MacMahon S, Rodgers A. Blood pressure, antihypertensive treatment and stroke risk. J Hypertens 1994; 12(Suppl 10):S5–S14.

62. Laupacis A, Albers G, Dalen J, Dunn MI, Jacobson AK, Singer DE. Antithrombotic therapy in atrial fibrillation. Chest 1998;114:579S–589S.

63. Shepherd J, Cobbe SM, Ford I, et al. Prevention of coronary heart disease with pravastatin in men with hypercholesterolemia. N Engl J Med 1995;333:1301–1307.

64. The Heart Outcomes Prevention Evaluation Study Investigators. Effects of an angiotensin-converting-enzyme inhibitor, ramipril, on cardiovascular events in high-risk patients. N Engl J Med 2000;342: 145–153.

65. UK Prospective Diabetes Study (UKPDS) Group. Effect of intensive blood-glucose control with metformin on complications in overweight patients with type 2 diabetes (UKPDS 34). Lancet 1998;352: 854–865.

66. Executive Committee for the Asymptomatic Carotid Atherosclerosis Study. Endarterectomy for asymptomatic carotid artery stenosis. JAMA 1995;273:1421–1428.

67. PROGRESS Collaborative Group. Randomised trial of a perindopril-based blood-pressure-lowering regimen among 6105 individuals with previous stroke or transient ischaemic attack. Lancet 2001;358: 1033–1041.

68. North American Symptomatic Carotid Endarterectomy Trial Collaborators. Beneficial effect of carotid endarterectomy in symptomatic patients with high-grade carotid stenosis. N Engl J Med 1991;325: 445–453.

69. Endovascular versus surgical treatment in patients with carotid stenosis in the Carotid and Vertebral Artery Transluminal Angioplasty Study (CAVATAS): a randomised trial. Lancet 2001;357:1729–1737.

70. Sacco RL. Extracranial carotid stenosis. N Engl J Med 2001;345:1113–1118.

71. The Canadian Cooperative Study Group. A randomized trial of aspirin and sulfinpyrazone in threatened stroke. N Engl J Med 1978;299:53–59.

72. The SALT Collaborative Group. Swedish Aspirin Low-dose Trial (SALT) of 75 mg aspirin as secondary prophylaxis after cerebrovascular ischemic events. Lancet 1991;338:1345–1349.

73. Farrell B, Godwin J, Richards S, Warlow C. The United Kingdom Transient Ischaemic Attack (UK-TIA) Aspirin Trial: final results. J Neurol Neurosurg Psychiatry 1991;54:1044–1054.

74. Antiplatelet Trialists' Collaboration. Collaborative overview of randomised trials of antiplatelet therapy —I: prevention of death, myocardial infarction, and stroke by prolonged antiplatelet therapy in various categories of patients. Br Med J 1994;308:81–106.

75. The Dutch TIA Trial Study Group. A comparison of two doses of aspirin (30 mg vs. 283 mg a day) in patients after a transient ischemic attack or minor ischemic stroke. N Engl J Med 1991;325:1261–1266.

76. Diener HC, Cunha L, Forbes C, et al. European Stroke Prevention Study 2. Dipyridamole and acetylsalicylic acid in the secondary prevention of stroke. J Neurolog Sci 1996;143:1–13.

77. Gent M, Blakely JA, Easton JD, Ellis DJ, Hachinski VC, Harbison JW, et al. The Canadian American Ticlopidine Study (CATS) in thromboembolic stroke. Lancet 1989;i:1215–1220.

78. Hass WK, Easton JD, Adams HP Jr, Pryse-Phillips W, Molony BA, Anderson S, et al. A randomized trial comparing ticlopidine hydrochloride with aspirin for the prevention of stroke in high-risk patients. N Engl J Med 1989;321:501–507.

79. CAPRIE Steering Committee. A randomised, blinded, trial of clopidogrel versus aspirin in patients at risk of ischaemic events (CAPRIE). Lancet 1996;348:1329–1339.

80. Bennett CL, Connors JM, Carwile JM, Moake JL, Bell WR, Tarantolo SR, et al. Thrombotic thrombocytopenic purpura associated with clopidogrel. N Engl J Med 2000;342:1773–1777.

81. Mohr JP, Thompson JLP, Lazar RM, Levin B, Sacco RL, Furie KL, et al., for the Warfarin–Aspirin Recurrent Stroke Study Group. A comparison of warfarin and aspirin for the prevention of recurrent ischemic stroke. N Engl J Med 2001;345:1444–1451.

82. The National Institute of Neurological Disorders and Stroke rt-PA Stroke Study Group. Tissue plasminogen activator for acute ischemic stroke. N Engl J Med 1995;333:1581–1587.

83. Marler JR, Tilley BC, Lu M, Brott TG, Lyden PC, Grotta JC, et al. Early stroke treatment associated with better outcome: the NINDS rt-PA stroke study. Neurology 2000;55:1649–1655.

84. Rordorf G, Koroshetz WJ, Ezzeddine MA, Segal AZ, Buonanno FS. A pilot study of drug-induced hypertension for treatment of acute stroke. Neurology 2001;56:1210–1213.

85. Gardner TJ, Horneffer PJ, Manolio TA, et al. Stroke following coronary artery bypass grafting: a ten-year study. Ann Thorac Surg 1985;40:574–581.

86. Coffey CE, Massey EW, Roberts KB, Curtis S, Jones RH, Pryor DB. Natural history of cerebral complications of coronary artery bypass graft surgery. Neurology 1983;33:1416–1421.

87. Breuer AC, Furlan AJ, Hanson MR, et al. Central nervous system complications of coronary artery bypass graft surgery: prospective analysis of 421 patients. Stroke 1983;14:682–687.

88. McKhann GM, Goldsborough MA, Borowicz LM, Mellits ED, Brookmeyer R, Quaskey SA, et al. Predictors of stroke risk in coronary artery bypass patients. Ann Thorac Surg 1997;63:516–521.

89. Parker FB, Marvasti MA, Bove EL. Neurological complications following coronary artery bypass. The role of atherosclerotic emboli. Thorac Cardiovasc Surg 1985;33:207–209.

90. Faggioli GL, Curl GR, Ricotta JJ. The role of carotid screening before coronary artery bypass. J Vasc Surg 1990;12:724–731.

91. John R, Choudhri AF, Weinberg AD, Ting W, Rose EA, Smith CR, et al. Multicenter review of preoperative risk factors for stroke after coronary artery bypass grafting. Ann Thorac Surg 2000;69:30–35.

92. Ricotta JJ, Faggioli GL, Castilone A, Hassett JM. Risk factors for stroke after cardiac surgery: Buffalo Cardiac–Cerebral Study Group. J Vasc Surg 1995;21:359–364.

93. Wolman RL, Nussmeier NA, Aggarwal A, Kanchuger MS, Roach GW, Newman MF, et al. Cerebral injury after cardiac surgery: identification of a group at extraordinary risk. Stroke 1999;30:514–522.

94. Svedjeholm R, Hakanson E, Szabo Z, Vanky F. Neurological injury after surgery for ischemic heart disease: risk factors, outcome and role of metabolic interventions. Eur J Cardiothorac Surg 2001;19:611–618.

95. van Dijk D, Keizer AMA, Diephuis JC, Durand C, Vos LJ, Hijman R. Neurocognitive dysfunction after coronary artery bypass surgery: a systematic review. J Thorac Cardiovasc Surg 2000;120:632–639.

96. Newman MF, Kirchner JL, Phillips-Bute B, Gaver V, Grocott H, Jones RH, et al., for The Neurological Outcome Research Group and the Cardiothoracic Anesthesiology Research Endeavors Investigators. Longitudinal assessment of neurocognitive function after coronary–artery bypass surgery. N Engl J Med 2001;344:395–402.

97. Tuman KJ, McCarthy RJ, Najafi H, Ivankovich AD. Differential effects of advanced age on neurological and cardiac risks of coronary artery operations. J Thorac Cardiovasc Surg 1992;104:1510–1517.

98. Almassi GH, Sommers T, Moritz TE, Shroyer ALW, London MJ, Henderson WG, et al. Stroke in cardiac surgical patients: determinants and outcome. Ann Thorac Surg 1999;68:391–397.

99. Stamou SC, Hill PC, Dangas G, Pfister AJ, Boyce SW, Dullum MKC, et al. Stroke after coronary artery bypass: incidence, predictors, and clinical outcome. Stroke 2001;32:1508–1513.

100. Puskas JD, Winston AD, Wright CE, Gott JP, Brown WM, Craver JM, et al. Stroke after coronary artery operation: incidence, correlates, outcome, and cost. Ann Thorac Surg 2000;69:1053–1056.

101. Beall AC Jr, Jones JW, Guinn GA, Svensson LG, Nahas C. Cardiopulmonary bypass in patients with previously completed stroke. Ann Thorac Surg 1993;55:1383–1385.

102. Redmond JM, Greene PS, Goldsborough MA, et al. Neurological injury in cardiac surgical patients with a history of stroke. Ann Thorac Surg 1996;61:42–47.

103. Rorick MB, Furlan AJ. Risk of cardiac surgery in patients with prior stroke. Neurology 1990;40:835–837.

104. Roach GW, Kanchuger M, Mangano CM, Newman M, Nussmeier N, Wolman R, et al., The Multicenter Study of Perioperative Ischemia Research Group and the Ischemia Research and Education Foundation Investigators. Adverse cerebral outcomes after coronary bypass surgery. N Engl J Med 1996;335:1857–1864.

105. McKhann GM, Borowicz LM, Goldsborough MA, Enger C, Selnes OA. Depression and cognitive decline after coronary artery bypass grafting. Lancet 1997;349:1282–1284.

106. Breslau PJ, Fell G, Ivey TD, Bailey TD, Miller DW, Strandness DE. Carotid arterial disease in patients undergoing coronary artery bypass operations. J Thorac Cardiovasc Surg 1981;82:765–767.

107. Gerraty RP, Gates PC, Doyle JC. Carotid stenosis and perioperative stroke risk in symptomatic and asymptomatic patients undergoing vascular or coronary surgery. Stroke 1993;24:1115–1118.

108. Brenner BJ, Bried DK, Alpert A, Goldenkranz RJ, Parsonnet V. The risk of stroke in patients with asymptomatic carotid stenosis undergoing cardiac surgery: a follow-up study. J Vasc Surg 1987;5:269–279.

109. Hogue CW Jr, Murphy SF, Schechtman KB, Davila-Roman VG. Risk factors for early or delayed stroke after cardiac surgery. Circulation 1999;100:642–647.

110. Fruitman DS, MacDougall CE, Ross DB. Cardiac surgery in octogenarians: can elderly patients benefit? Quality of life after cardiac surgery. Ann Thorac Surg 1999;68:2129–2135.

111. Wareing TH, Davila-Roman VG, Daily BB, et al. Strategy for the reduction of stroke incidence in cardiac surgical patients. Ann Thorac Surg 1993;55:1400–1408.
112. Katz ES, Tunick PA, Rusinek H, Ribakove G, Spencer FC, Kronzon I. Protruding aortic atheromas predict stroke in elderly patients undergoing cardiopulmonary bypass: experience with intraoperative transesophageal echocardiography. J Am Coll Cardiol 1992;20:70–77.
113. Borger MA, Ivanov J, Weisel RD, Rao V, Peniston CM. Stroke during coronary bypass surgery: principal role of cerebral macroemboli. Eur J Cardiothorac Surg 2001;19:627–632.
114. Moody DM, Bell MA, Chall VR, et al. Emboli occur at the initiation of bypass and during aortic cross-clamping and release brain microemboli during cardiac surgery or aortography. Ann Neurol 1990;28:477–486.
115. Eagle KA, Guyton RA, Davidoff R, Ewy GA, Fonger J, Gardner TJ, et al. ACC/AHA guidelines for coronary artery bypass graft surgery: executive summary and recommendations: a report of the American College of Cardiology/American Heart Association Task Force on Practice Guidelines (Committee to Revise the 1991 Guidelines for Coronary Artery Bypass Graft Surgery). Circulation 1999;100:1464–1480.
116. Stump AD, Rorie KD, Jones TJJ. Does off-pump coronary artery bypass surgery reduce the risk of brain injury? Heart Surg Forum. 2001;4(Suppl 1):S14–S20.
117. Hart JC, Spooner TH, Pym J, et al. A review of 1,582 consecutive Octopus off-pump coronary bypass patients. Ann Thorac Surg 2000;70:1017–1020.
118. van Dijk D, Nierich AP, Jansen EWL, Nathoe HM, Suyker WJL, Diephuis JC, et al. Early outcome after off-pump versus on-pump coronary bypass surgery: results from a randomized study. Circulation 2001;104:1761–1766.
119. Rizzo RJ, Whittemore AD, Couper GS, et al. Combined carotid and coronary revascularisation; the preferred approach to the severe vasculopath. Ann Thorac Surg 1992;54:1099–1108.
120. Das SK, Brow TD, Pepper J. Continuing controversy in the management of concomitant coronary and carotid disease: an overview. Int J Cardiol 2000;74:47–65.
121. Schwartz LB, Bridgman AH, Kieffer RW, et al. Asymptomatic carotid stenosis and stroke in patients undergoing cardiopulmonary bypass. J Vasc Surg 1995;21:146–153.
122. Salasidis GC, Latter DA, Steinmetz OK, Blair J, Graham AM. Carotid artery duplex scanning in preoperative assessment for coronary artery revascularisation. J Vasc Surg 1995;21:154–161.
123. Gott JP, Thourani VH, Wright CE, Brown WM, Adams AB, Skardasis GM, et al. Risk neutralization in cardiac operations: detection and treatment of associated carotid disease. Ann Thorac Surg 1999;68:850–856.
124. Youssuf AM, Karanam R, Prendergast T, Brener B, Hertz S, Saunders CR, et al. Combined off-pump myocardial revascularization and carotid endarterectomy: early experience. Ann Thorac Surg 2001;72:1542–1545.
125. Johnsson P, Algotsson L, Ryding E, Stahl E, Messeter K. Cardiopulmonary perfusion and cerebral blood flow in bilateral carotid artery disease. Ann Thorac Surg 1991;51:579–584.
126. Hise JH, Nipper ML, Schnitkev JC. Stroke associated with coronary artery bypass grafting. Am J Neuroradiol 1991;12:811–814.
127. Riles TS, Kopelman I, Imparato AM. Myocardial infarction following carotid endarterectomy: a review of 683 operations. Surgery 1979;85:249–253.
128. Benavente O, Eliasziw M, Streifler JY, Fox AJ, Barnett HJM, Meldrum H, the North American Symptomatic Carotid Endarterectomy Trial Collaborators. Prognosis after Transient Monocular Blindness Associated with Carotid-Artery Stenosis. N Engl J Med 2001;345:1084–1090.
129. Grubb RL Jr, Derdeyn CP, Fritsch SM, Carpenter DA, Yundt KD, Videen TO, et al. Importance of hemodynamic factors in the prognosis of symptomatic carotid occlusion. JAMA 1998;280:1055–1060.
130. Kase CS, Pessin MS, Zivin JA, del Zoppo GJ, Furlan AJ, Buckley JW, et al. Intracranial hemorrhage after coronary thrombolysis with tissue plasminogen activator. Am J Med 1992;92:384–390.
131. Gebel JM, Sila CA, Sloan MA, Granger CB, Mahaffey KW, Weisenberger J, et al. Thrombolysis-related intracranial hemorrhage: a radiographic analysis of 244 cases from the GUSTO-1 trial with clinical correlation. Global Utilization of Streptokinase and Tissue Plasminogen Activator for Occluded Coronary Arteries. Stroke 1998;29:563–569.
132. Sloan MA, Sila CA, Mahaffey KW, Granger CB, Longstreth WT Jr, Koudstaal P, et al. Prediction of 30-day mortality among patients with thrombolysis-related intracranial hemorrhage. Circulation 1998;98:1376–1382.
133. Leblanc R, Haddad G, Robitaille Y. Cerebral hemorrhage from amyloid angiopathy and coronary thrombolysis. Neurosurgery 1992;31:586–590.

134. Albers GW, Bates VE, Clark WM, Bell R, Verro P, Hamilton SA. Intravenous tissue-type plasminogen activator for treatment of acute stroke: the Standard Treatment with Alteplase to Reverse Stroke (STARS) study. JAMA 2000;283:1145–1150.

135. The NINDS t-PA Stroke Study Group. Generalized efficacy of t-PA for acute stroke. Subgroup analysis of the NINDS t-PA Stroke Trial. Stroke 1997;28:2119–2125.

136. Scandinavian Simvastatin Survival Study Group: randomized trial of cholesterol-lowering in 4444 patients with coronary heart disease: the Scandinavian Simvastatin Survival Study (4S). Lancet 1994; 344:1383–1389.

137. Sacks FM, Pfeffer MA, Moye LA, et al. The effect of pravastatin on coronary events after myocardial infarction in patients with average cholesterol levels. Cholesterol and Recurrent Events Trial Investigators. N Engl J Med 1996;335:1001–1009.

138. The Long-Term Intervention with Pravastatin in Ischaemic Disease (LIPID) Study Group. Prevention of cardiovascular events and death with pravastatin in patients with coronary heart disease and a broad range of initial cholesterol levels. N Engl J Med 1998;339:1349–1357.

139. Downs JR, Clearfield M, Weis S, Whitney E, Shapiro DR, Beere PA, et al., for the AFCAPS/TexCAPS Research Group. Primary prevention of acute coronary events with lovastatin in men and women with average cholesterol levels: results of AFCAPS/TexCAPS. JAMA 1998;279:1615–1622.

140. Hess DC, Demchuk AM, Brass LM, Yatsu FM. HMG-CoA reductase inhibitors (statins). A promising approach to stroke prevention. Neurology 2000;54:790–796.

141. Alberts MJ. Suppression of recurrent transient ischemic attacks by a statin agent. Neurology 2001;56: 531–532.

142. Rosenberg RD, Aird WC. Vascular-bed-specific hemostasis and hypercoagulable states. N Engl J Med 1999;340:1555–1564.

143. Expert Panel on Detection, Evaluation, and Treatment of High Blood Cholesterol in Adults. Executive Summary of the Third Report of the National Cholesterol Education Program (NCEP) Expert Panel on Detection, Evaluation, and Treatment of High Blood Cholesterol in Adults (Adult Treatment Panel III). JAMA 2001;285:2486–2497.

144. Albers GW. Choice of endpoints in antiplatelet trials. Which outcomes are most relevant to stroke patients? Neurology 2000;54:1022–1028.

145. Steering Committee of the Physicians' Health Study Research Group. Final report on the aspirin component of the ongoing Physicians' Health Study. N Engl J Med 1989;321:129–135.

146. Manson JE, Stampfer MJ, Colditz GA, et al. A prospective study of aspirin use and primary prevention of cardiovascular disease in women. JAMA 1991;266:521–527.

147. Peto R, Gray R, Collins R, et al. Randomised trial of prophylactic daily aspirin in British male doctors. Br Med J 1988;296:313–316.

148. Sanmuganathan PS, Ghahramani P, Jackson PR, Wallis EJ, Ramsay LE. Aspirin for primary prevention of coronary heart disease: safety and absolute benefit related to coronary risk derived from meta-analysis of randomised trials. Heart 2001;85:265–271.

7

Cardiac Rehabilitation in the Older Patient

Marjorie L. King, MD, FACC, FAACVPR

CONTENTS

INTRODUCTION

Cardiac rehabilitation is a multidisciplinary treatment that includes exercise, education, and behavior modification to improve functional capacity, decrease recurrent cardiac events, and improve quality of life *(1)*. Heart disease is the most common cause of mortality and morbidity in persons 65 yr of age and older, with the loss of functional capacity from heart disease more significant in older compared to younger individuals—most notably in women *(2,3)*. Over the past decade, meta-analyses and randomized trials have supported the efficacy of cardiac rehabilitation in younger patients to decrease mortality, morbidity, and disability *(1,4)*. More recently, it has become clear that many of these benefits extend to the elderly, although the exact mechanisms and extent of benefit remain unclear *(5–11)*. In addition, older individuals, especially women, are referred to cardiac rehabilitation less often than younger patients *(12–15)*, although this is rapidly changing *(16)*. This chapter will review aspects of cardiac rehabilitation unique to older patients, recognized standards of care, and current controversies in this population.

WHAT IS DIFFERENT?

Participation

Although the current generations of older patients have a strong work ethic related to their experiences during the Depression and World War II, performance of regular aerobic exercise for health benefit is a foreign concept to the majority of these individuals. These patients often do not approach their physicians about rehabilitation, and if they are referred for an exercise program, they may not understand the potential benefits. Confounding this, it has been shown that the most important factor influencing participation in cardiac rehabilitation is physician referral, with only 2% of patients participating without

From: *Aging, Heart Disease, and Its Management: Facts and Controversies*
Edited by: N. Edwards, M. Maurer, and R. Wellner © Humana Press Inc., Totowa, NJ

physician recommendation compared with a 66% participation rate with strong physician recommendation for participation *(17)*. Unfortunately, older coronary patients are less likely to be referred to cardiac rehabilitation than their younger counterparts (21% vs 42% in one study), contributing significantly to the low participation rates in older patients *(12)*.

Exercise culture in America favors the young and fit, and many older individuals feel uncomfortable exercising in a traditional gymnasium-like environment with younger individuals. Lack of transportation and issues related to caring for an elderly spouse also interfere with participation in rehabilitation programs. Special sensitivity is needed when dealing with older patients during the referral and enrollment processes to encourage patients to begin the behavioral changes needed for a regular exercise and lifestyle modification program.

Exercise Prescription

The typical cardiac rehabilitation program uses a treadmill stress test to determine exercise prescription. The ideal stress test for exercise prescription lasts between 8 and 12 min; however, many elderly patients are unable to achieve this time using a standard Bruce treadmill protocol. Exercise testing modalities such as low-level stationary biking, modified treadmill protocols, and adapted equipment are less intimidating, and the workloads can be chosen to allow peak exercise to be reached within 6–12 min. Nuclear and echocardiographic imaging can be added to increase diagnostic accuracy, regardless of exercise modality *(18)*.

Exercise Programming

Creative programming and modification of the exercise environment for older patients is necessary. It is important to determine a patient's specific functional goals beyond general increased endurance and strength and to design the rehabilitation program to meet these goals. Maximum functional capacity in the elderly varies from the master's level athlete to a patient whose exercise reserve is limited to light household activities. Unfortunately, maximal aerobic power, muscular strength, and explosive power decline even with healthy aging *(19)*. This decline is exacerbated by deconditioning and muscle loss associated with chronic illness and inactivity. Simple activities of daily living, such as leisurely walking, may require a high percentage of an elderly individual's maximum cardiopulmonary function. For example, the oxygen cost of walking at 3 mph is approx 12.5 mL/kg/min, and at 2 mph, it is approx 9 mL/kg/min. To comfortably sustain walking, the oxygen cost should be less than 50% of an individual's aerobic power-to-weight ratio (maximum oxygen consumption corrected for body weight). In the English National Fitness Survey, 35% of men and 80% of women aged 70–74 had an aerobic power-to-weight ratio less than 25 mL/kg/min, making it difficult for them to comfortably sustain a 3-mph walk *(19)*.

Fortunately, regular exercise training has been shown to increase maximum oxygen consumption (VO_{2max}) by 15–50% in the elderly *(5,6,8–10)* and can make community-level ambulation a realistic goal for many of these patients. Older patients may respond to aerobic conditioning with significant improvements in submaximal endurance capacity, out of proportion to the more modest gains in maximal exercise performance *(11)*. The most limited patients achieve the highest percent improvement in functional capacity after a rehabilitation program *(20)*, and cardiac rehabilitation can mean the difference between a home-bound lifestyle and return to independent community-level functioning *(11)*.

Treadmill and standard bicycle exercise may not be appropriate as initial exercise modalities for patients with significantly decreased maximum exercise capacity. Use of newer modalities such as seated arm/leg ergometry is often more appropriate for older patients. Interval training, with shorter periods of low-level exercise interspersed with rest periods, may be needed at the start of the rehabilitation program. Exercises should target postural and pelvic floor muscles, develop body awareness and balance skills, and emphasize safety techniques to avoid falls (21,22). In addition to exercise training, referral to other professionals such as occupational therapists for specific home and food management retraining may be needed.

Response to Training

The cardiovascular response to exercise in elderly individuals is influenced by the decreased compliance of the aging ventricle, with increased dependence on diastolic filling, particularly during late diastole, to maintain cardiac output (21). During dynamic exercise, elderly individuals demonstrate lower submaximal and peak cardiac output, higher systemic vascular resistance, and higher submaximal arteriovenous oxygen difference as compared to younger individuals. Despite these differences in exercise physiology, regular exercise training improves functional capacity in elderly individuals primarily because of peripheral training mechanisms such as a redistribution of cardiac output to the exercising limbs, a decrease in arterial stiffness, and changes in muscle fiber type (10,11,19,23–25), although there is some evidence that central mechanisms may also play a role (26–28).

Special attention must be given to the cool-down phase of exercise in elderly individuals. Cool-down allows the heat load of exercise to gradually dissipate and peripheral vasodilation to decrease. Elderly patients are at higher risk for venous pooling and post-exercise hypotension, possibly the result of age related decrease in baroreceptor responsiveness. Therefore, increased duration of the cool-down phase of exercise is needed for elderly individuals. Similarly, the efficiency of sweating and temperature regulation is decreased in the elderly, and the exercise environment should be controlled to avoid hot or humid conditions (29).

Comorbidities such as osteoarthritis, obesity, osteoporosis, diabetes, hypertension, peripheral vascular disease, and neurological disease are more prevalent in elderly patients. Special attention should be given to exercise modalities, avoiding joint trauma in patients with osteoarthritis, high-impact activities in osteoporosis, and skin trauma in diabetics. Swimming may be an appropriate exercise modality for patients with arthritis or osteoporosis. Referral for more specific cognitive retraining or physical therapy may be needed in patients with neurological dysfunction.

Most of the benefits of regular exercise, such as increased functional capacity and changes in insulin resistance, are lost if regular exercise is not continued (30,31). Referral to appropriate community-based programs, supervised unmonitored cardiac rehabilitation, or home exercise is important to maintain these gains. This may require liaison with community groups to assure that appropriate exercise programs are available for older individuals.

Patient Education

Older patients, especially those who are recently retired, are becoming more sophisticated in their ability to assess information related to health issues, including rapidly growing use of the Internet. Many patients, however, have not been exposed to principles of

Table 1
Components of Cardiac Rehabilitation

Exercise therapy
    Exercise testing/prescription
    Monitored and/or supervised exercise
    Physical activity counseling
Nutritional counseling
    Weight loss
    Lipid-lowering nutrition
    Diabetic dietary education
    Sodium intake
Risk-factor education and management
    Hypertension
    Diabetes mellitus
    Dyslipidemias
    Smoking cessation
Psychosocial support and management
    Anxiety
    Depression
    Anger

secondary prevention of cardiovascular disease and need basic information to understand why changes in diet and lifestyle are important. Others have auditory, visual, or cognitive problems limiting their ability to participate in standard group teaching. Again, flexibility and creativity by the rehabilitation staff is important to individualize patient education and secondary-risk-factor modification.

STANDARDS OF CARE

Cardiac rehabilitation standards of care are clearly stated in the Agency for Health Care Policy and Research (AHCPR) Clinical Practice Guidelines *(1)*, American Heart Association (AHA)/American Association for Cardiovascular and Pulmonary Rehabilitation (AACVPR) Scientific Statement *(32)*, and other AHA, AACVPR, and American College of Sports Medicine (ACSM) policy statements *(18,33–35)*. All of these documents stress the multidisciplinary nature of the treatment, including exercise therapy, nutritional counseling, lipid, hypertension, and diabetes education and management, smoking cessation, weight management, psychosocial management, and physical activity counseling (*see* Table 1). Specific details for programming are covered in the AACVPR Guidelines for Cardiac Rehabilitation and Secondary Prevention Programs *(36)*.

Rationale for Exercise as Therapy

The relationship between regular exercise and decreasing risk of cardiac events has been well established over the past decade *(37)*. In 1996, the American Heart Association Statement on Exercise Benefits stated that "there is a direct relation between physical inactivity and cardiovascular mortality, and physical inactivity is an independent risk factor for the development of coronary artery disease (CAD)" *(18)*. This statement is confirmed by data from multiple sources, including the Harvard Alumni Health Study *(38–40)* and the Honolulu Heart Program *(41)*. The latter specifically evaluated the effect of regular exercise (walking) on the development of coronary heart disease in physically capable elderly individuals (71–93 yr of age) over a 2- to 4-yr period. The risk of cardiac events significantly decreased with increased distance walked per day, confirming that regular exercise is an important adjunct to primary prevention in the elderly. Recent studies have also evaluated the beneficial effect of regular exercise on cardiovascular events in individuals with established risk factors for CAD, including smoking *(42)* and diabetes *(43)*.

The benefit of regular exercise has also been well established in older men with diagnosed coronary heart disease. The British Regional Heart Study evaluated cardiovascular and all-cause mortality in 7735 men (average age: 63 yr) with CAD 12–14 yr after initial screening. Compared to a persistent sedentary lifestyle, light or moderate physical activity was associated with a significantly lower risk of all-cause mortality. More importantly, when sedentary men began at least light activity, their relative risk for mortality was decreased, compared to those who remained inactive (relative risk: 0.58, $p = 0.06$) *(44)*.

Although the mechanisms for the decrease in mortality rate with physical activity have not been fully elucidated, increased physical fitness has been clearly associated with improvements in lipid profile *(5,6,31,45,46)*, blood pressure *(46)*, fasting glucose *(46–48)*, and body composition *(5,6,46)*. Lavie et al. *(5)* evaluated the effect of cardiac rehabilitation and exercise training on exercise capacity, obesity indices, and lipids in 92 elderly patients (mean age: 70.1 ± 4.1 yr) compared to 182 younger patients (mean: 53.9 ± 7.4 yr). Both groups demonstrated similar statistically significant improvements in all three areas, confirming that elderly patients should not be categorically denied the benefits of cardiac rehabilitation and exercise training.

Several mechanisms have been suggested to explain the beneficial effect of exercise therapy as treatment in primary and secondary prevention of cardiovascular disease. In addition to the favorable effects on risk factors such as lipid levels, blood pressure, and glucose metabolism, exercise has also been shown to modify triggers for acute coronary syndromes and factors involved in the progression of cardiac disease *(37)*. Thrombosis and endothelial dysfunction contribute to acute coronary syndromes and restenosis following angioplasty, stenting, or bypass surgery. Acute physical exercise may lead to a prothrombotic state related to an acute increase in fibrinogen, generation of thrombin, activation of platelets, and hemoconcentration, which is counterbalanced by a rapid rise in fibrinolytic activity in healthy individuals. Elderly patients with CAD often exhibit disturbances in the balance between procoagulatory and fibrolytic parameters. Regular exercise training favorably effects the hemostatic system, including a reduction in fibrinogen and plasminogen activator and modulation of platelet activation following acute exercise *(37,49)*.

Endothelial dysfunction also plays an important role in the evolution and clinical expression of coronary artery disease. Alterations in endothelial function caused by oxidative or hemodynamic stressors can lead to inappropriate vasoconstriction, thrombosis, or intimal growth. Conditions resulting in endothelial dysfunction include advanced age, cardiovascular risk factors, and coronary artery disease *(50)*. Regular aerobic exercise helps prevent and restore age-related declines in endothelium-dependent vasodilation in athletic *(51)*, healthy *(52,53)*, and hypertensive *(54)* men. This may also explain the improvement in hyperemic myocardial blood flow (flow reserve) seen in patients following a short-term cardiovascular conditioning and low-fat diet program *(55,56)*.

Improvements in autonomic function may partially explain the increased survival demonstrated in a meta-analysis of exercise rehabilitation studies following myocardial infarction *(4)*. Exercise training has been shown to increase parasympathetic tone in patients with congestive heart failure *(57)* or following a myocardial infarction *(58)*. Regular aerobic exercise has also been shown to modify heart rate variability in a favorable direction in low- to intermediate-risk elderly patients recovering from a recent coronary event *(59)*. Autonomic dysfunction is associated with an increased risk of sudden death *(60)*, and endurance training may be cardioprotective in patients with coronary artery disease *(61)*. Hambrecht et al. showed that chronic physical exercise accompanied by multifactor risk reduction may slow the progression of coronary artery disease *(62–65)*. Long-term physical activity during leisure time has also been shown to be directly associated with the degree of collateral coronary artery flow *(66)*. Both of these mechanisms may contribute to the improved cardiovascular outcomes seen following cardiac rehabilitation.

Exercise training for patients with congestive heart failure improves peripheral endothelial function and oxygen delivery to exercising muscle, contributing to the improvement in functional capacity seen in these patients *(67)*. Other factors that improve with exercise training in patients with congestive heart failure include extraction of oxygen by exercising muscles, change in muscle fiber type, improvement in ventilatory parameters, and enhanced parasympathetic tone *(68)*. In addition, regular exercise does not exacerbate left-ventricular remodeling following myocardial infarction or in patients with left-ventricular dysfunction, with recent studies confirming significant functional and physiological benefit from regular exercise in patients with congestive heart failure *(68–76)*.

Exercise training and cardiac rehabilitation have also been shown to improve functional capacity *(10,45,77,78)* and quality of life in many patient populations, including those with congestive heart failure *(71–76)* as well as elderly *(10,45)*, female *(45,77)*, and obese patients *(78)* with cardiac disease. These effects are mediated by the physiological mechanisms described here as well as by other central and peripheral adaptations and psychosocial support.

During the past decade, resistance exercise has been shown to be safe and effective for healthy individuals, patients with coronary artery disease, and select elderly patients with cardiac disease *(79–81)*. Resistance training increases muscular strength, endurance, and mass, may prevent decrease in bone mineral density, and assists in the maintenance of basal metabolic rate *(79)*. Because of these effects, the addition of resistance exercises to an aerobic exercise program may decrease falls and fractures, increase independence, and improve body composition in elderly patients. Moderate- to-high-level-intensity resistance training performed two to three times per week for 3–6 mo has been shown to increase muscular strength and endurance by 25–100%, depending on the training stimulus and baseline status *(79)*. It was initially felt that resistance training would generate high-pressure rate products and myocardial stress, with adverse outcomes in patients with cardiac disease. However, many studies have now shown that the systolic blood pressure and left ventricular (LV) wall stress is actually lower during properly performed resistance exercise compared to aerobic training, despite similar Borg Rating of Perceived Exertion (RPE) and heart rate *(79,82)*. As a result, most professional and government organizations now include resistance exercise in their recommendations for exercise therapy *(1,21,32,37,79)*.

The standards of care for exercise training in cardiac rehabilitation have evolved over the past two decades in response to studies that have confirmed the safety and efficacy of properly applied exercise therapy for the majority of patients following cardiac events, including post-myocardial infarction, open heart surgery, and catheter-based interventions *(1,5,49,83)*. Traditionally, cardiac rehabilitation begins with low-level ambulation and self-care activities in the inpatient setting, followed by referral to a supervised outpatient setting. Alternatives include intensive inpatient rehabilitation in an acute or subacute rehabilitation facility or home exercise *(36)*.

Exercise Testing and Prescription

Exercise prescription for both aerobic and resistance exercise specifically addresses intensity, frequency, duration, and mode of activity. Ideally, the prescription is written following clinical assessment, including review of past cardiac records, history and physical exam, and a maximal stress test using oxygen consumption parameters and cardiac imaging techniques.

Significant details in an elderly patient's cardiac history include (1) angina, (2) bypass surgery, (3) risk of future coronary events, (4) proximity to recent cardiac events, (5) arrhythmia history, and (6) heart failure symptoms. Screening should include contraindications to exercise, such as unstable angina, severe valvular stenosis or insufficiency, uncontrolled hypertension, or worsening congestive heart failure symptoms. The general medical history should include other comorbidities and risk factors such as diabetes, hypertension, hypercholesterolemia, cigarette use, arthritis, peripheral vascular disease, osteoporosis, history of falls or prior orthopedic injury, and history of neurological events. The entrance physical examination should include assessment of postoperative wounds as well as a standard cardiovascular and medical examination.

Stress testing should be individualized, designed to minimize anxiety and risk of injury in elderly individuals and to maximize the peak workload. It should also simulate the exercise conditions that will be present during the exercise sessions, including use of chronic medications and exercise modality. The most accurate way to set exercise intensity prescriptions is to measure gas exchange utilizing indirect calorimetry, which measures minute ventilation (VE), oxygen uptake (VO_2), and carbon dioxide output (VCO_2) during exercise. Most elderly patients can tolerate the newer and lighter combination mouthpiece and pneumotach devices used for gas-exchange analysis, but not all facilities have the equipment and personnel to add this measurement to prerehabilitation stress testing. Standard stress testing includes baseline blood pressure and electrocardiogram (ECG), followed by continuous multilead rhythm monitoring, 12-lead ECG during each stage of exercise, and frequent blood pressure determination. The Borg RPE scale is another useful tool, which asks the patient to subjectively rate his or her level of exercise during each stage of exercise using either a 6- to 20-point scale or 0 to 10 scale (modified RPE).

When gas-exchange analysis is used to set exercise intensity, the ideal test should last between 8 and 12 min. This requires an accurate estimate of exercise capacity prior to testing. In our laboratory, we frequently utilize bicycle ergometry protocols in our frail elderly patients, using 5- or 10-W workloads and 2-min stages. Patients who can ambulate on the 6-min walk test for more than 250 ft without an assistive device are often tested using a Bruce, modified Bruce, or Naughton treadmill protocol, depending on their exercise history. We have also used adaptive cycle ergometry for patients following stroke or amputation to set exercise guidelines.

Exercise testing must include some measure of inducible myocardial ischemia. For patients without historical evidence of exercise-induced ischemia, ECG and symptom monitoring during exercise is generally sufficient. However, when ischemia is suspected, the ideal method is to add a cardiac imaging modality to the test, such as echocardiography

Table 2
Exercise Prescription for Patients
Without Exercise-Induced Myocardial Ischemia on Stress Testing

	VT detected	VT not detected but maximal effort*	VT not detected and not maximal effort*	VT not detected, not maximal effort, and cannot use RPE scale	Pulmonary limitation to exercise
Set target training zone at:	HR, RPE, and WL at VT	HR, RPE, and WL corresponding to 60–70% VO$_{2max}$	HR and WL corresponding to RPE 13	20 Beats above resting HR, not to exceed 85% age predicted HR or 70–85% HR$_{max}$ on test	HR, RPE and WL at 75% MVV

*Criteria for valid maximal effort: At least two of the following levels are reached: RER $\geq$ 1.10, maximal HR $\geq$ 85% age predicted, RPE $\geq$ 17, or plateau in VO$_2$ $\leq$ 2.5 mL/kg over the last two workloads.

Definitions: VT, ventilatory threshold; HR, heart rate; RPE, rating of perceived exertion; WL, workload; VO$_{2max}$, maximal oxygen consumption; HR$_{max}$, maximal heart rate; RER, respiratory exchange ratio; MVV, maximum voluntary ventilation.

or nuclear imaging. In our laboratory, we use concomitant gas-exchange analysis and upright bicycle exercise echocardiography, acquiring echocardiogram images prior to exercise, during each stage of the exercise test and immediately postexercise to determine the ischemic threshold. Other programs use nuclear cardiac imaging to determine the presence and extent of exercise-induced ischemia. However, this only reflects conditions at peak exercise and, in the absence of symptoms or electrocardiographic changes, and does not indicate the onset of ischemia, which is useful when determining the exercise prescription.

The basic principle of aerobic exercise prescription is to recommend a target intensity of exercise, which will stress the peripheral oxygen delivery and utilization system so that an adaptive training effect is begun without inducing excess fatigue or myocardial ischemia. For patients without exercise-induced myocardial ischemia, gas-exchange analysis alone can be used to set the prescription, using either ventilatory threshold or maximum oxygen consumption measurements (see Table 2). Ventilatory threshold is defined as the point at which the VE/VO$_2$ shows a distinct and sustained rise without a concomitant rise in the VE/VCO$_2$. The heart rate ($\pm$5 bpm) and workload at the ventilatory threshold can be used as the target-training zone. If the ventilatory threshold cannot be detected and the subject meets the criteria for a valid maximal effort (at least two of the following levels are reached: respiratory exchange ratio (RER) $\geq$ 1.10; maximal heart rate [HR] $\geq$ 85% age predicted; RPE $\geq$ 17; plateau in VO$_2$ $\geq$ 2.5 mL/kg over the last two workloads), then the target training zone should be set at the heart rate ($\pm$5 bpm) and workload corresponding to 60–70% of the maximal oxygen consumption. If the ventilatory threshold cannot be detected and criteria for a maximal test are not met, then the exercise intensity can be set at the heart rate and workload corresponding to an RPE of 13. In the rare patient who cannot accurately use an RPE scale, the target heart rate zone can be set at 20 beats above resting, as not to exceed 85% of the age-predicted heart rate (or 70–85% maximal heart rate on the test).

Table 3
Exercise Prescription for Patients
with Exercise-Induced Myocardial Ischemia on Stress Testing

	If ischemia is detected using ECG tracings	*If ischemia is detected by immediate post-exercise imaging*	*If ischemia is detected using submaximal echocardiographic imaging*
Set target training zone at:	HR and RPE at two WL prior to onset of significant ST segment depressions or symptoms.	Infer onset of ischemia by symptoms, signs, or ECG changes. Set prescription as HR and RPE at two WL prior to onset of ischemia.	HR and RPE achieved one WL prior to onset of wall motion abnormalities.

Definitions: ECG, electrocardiographic; HR, heart rate; RPE, rating of perceived exertion; WL, workload.

If the patient has exercise-induced myocardial ischemia (Table 3), the exercise prescription should be written so that the training zone is lower than the amount of work that induces myocardial ischemia (*see* Table 3). If ischemia is detected using submaximal echocardiographic imaging, then the exercise prescription can be set at the heart rate and RPE can be achieved one workload prior to the onset of wall-motion abnormalities. If myocardial ischemia is detected using ECG tracings alone (because ECG changes and symptoms occur later than wall-motion abnormalities during the ischemic cascade), the heart rate and RPE at two workloads prior to the onset of significant ST-segment depression and/or symptoms should be used for prescription. If myocardial ischemia is detected by only immediate postexercise imaging (using either echocardiography or nuclear imaging), other submaximal parameters such as symptoms, ST-segment changes, arrhythmias, or blood pressure changes can be used to infer the onset of ischemia, and the exercise prescription can be set based on these data.

Some patients also have significant pulmonary disease, which limits their exercise capacity, rather than cardiovascular factors or deconditioning. Pulmonary limitation to exercise is defined as achieving peak VE >75% maximum ventilatory volume in a nonathletic patient or O_2 saturation < 90%. In these patients (in the absence of myocardial ischemia), the exercise prescription can be set at the heart rate and workload at 75% maximum voluntary ventilation (MVV).

Empiric exercise prescription is often used for frail elderly patients who are in acute or subacute rehabilitation settings or in outpatient settings less than 4–6 wk after open heart surgery. Maximal stress testing is often limited by wound discomfort or arrhythmias in early postoperative patients, but exercise rehabilitation is an important therapeutic tool soon after surgery. For an elderly patient without suspected exercise-induced ischemia, a prudent exercise prescription is to set the target heart rate zone at 20 beats above the resting heart rate, not exceeding 120 bpm (for patients in sinus rhythm) or 130 bpm (for patients in atrial fibrillation), corresponding to a RPE of 12–13. Anchoring the target heart rate to the resting rate corrects for β-blocker use, changes in medication doses or administration times, and conduction system disease. Most patients without significant cognitive dysfunction can use the RPE scale appropriately, given sufficient instruction and encouragement.

Finally, exercise-intensity prescription is as much an art as a science. Intensity-training guidelines drafted by professional organizations such as the American Heart Association, American Association for Cardiovascular and Pulmonary Rehabilitation, Center for Disease Control and the American College of Sports Medicine vary, and include "moderate" (CDC); 50% minimum oxygen consumption (VO_{2min}) (AACVPR); 50–60% VO_{2max} or HR_{max} reserve (AHA); 55–90%HR_{max} or 40/50–85% VO_{2max} or HR_{max} reserve (ACSM) *(84)*. In practice, most professionals use a combination of the exercise-intensity prescription written from the stress test, the patient's symptomatic response to their exercise session, and a large measure of clinical common sense.

Exercise Sessions

Improvement in aerobic capacity is related to both the frequency and the amount of work accomplished, as well as the initial level of fitness, with most graduates of cardiac rehabilitation programs improving by 15–50% in maximum VO_2 or workload *(5,6,8–10)*. The amount of work performed is related to the intensity as well as the duration of training. Activities performed at a lower intensity but for a longer duration provide the same fitness benefit as those done at higher intensity for a shorter duration, as long as the total energy requirements are the same *(37)*, although there has been some recent evidence that a central training effect also occurs at higher-intensity training *(26–28)*. The duration of aerobic training can range from 20 to 45 min, often accompanied by a warm-up phase for 5–15 min, including stretching, low-level calisthenics, and walking or range of motion, as well as a cool-down phase with low-level aerobic exercise and stretching lasting 5–15 min. Low-impact exercise, stretching, gentle range of motion, and longer warm-up and cool-down sessions are important for elderly individuals to decrease the risk of orthopedic injuries and postexertional hypotension *(29,84)*.

Cardiac rehabilitation begins during the inpatient period, continues at home or an inpatient rehabilitation facility, and then moves to a supervised and/or monitored outpatient program. During inpatient and early home programs, an empiric exercise prescription is used, including RPE monitoring during range-of-motion exercises, walking, and exercises using light weights. A slow, gradual increase in intensity and duration allows adequate time for adaptation and maximizes health benefits. The goal is to reverse deconditioning, maintain range of motion, and begin to improve strength, balance, and endurance. Attention should be paid to both upper and lower extremity exercise and range of motion. Selected patients may also need cognitive evaluation and retraining, specific gait retraining and orthoses, and dysphagia therapy.

Regular aerobic exercise improves the ability of the cardiovascular system to transport and provide oxygen to exercising muscles, resulting in a lower heart rate and blood pressure needed to generate a specific workload. This is known as the "training effect" and occurs during a patient's cardiac rehabilitation program, necessitating progression of the training stimulus to continuously overload and stimulate the system *(33,34,36,85)*. Many elderly patients begin exercise using interval training, which consists of short periods of aerobic exercise at the training heart rate or RPE, interspersed with brief rest periods. The duration of the exercise periods are gradually increased until the patient can perform the aerobic portion of their exercise session for 20–45 min continuously. Beginning with relatively low-level exercise minimizes soreness and injury, avoiding discouragement and withdrawal from the program. When the patient has successfully performed a steady workload for more than a week, the workload intensity can be gradually increased, carefully monitoring that the patient remains within the prescribed target heart rate/RPE zone. This gradual progression in workload can continue for up to a year in elderly deconditioned patients and is followed by a period of exercise known as the maintenance phase, during which the training stimulus remains constant (given no intercurrent medical events) and emphasis is placed on maximizing compliance.

Exercise modalities for aerobic exercise should be chosen to maximize long-term compliance and minimize injury for an individual patient. Elderly patients are often comfortable with the standard treadmills and bicycles used in cardiac rehabilitation programs, given low-level workloads as well as proper training and supervision. Some patients require trunk support to stay within their target heart rate zone, and seated ergometers are ideal for these individuals. Others prefer aerobic exercise to music in a group session. Low-impact exercise is generally recommended to avoid injury, and sessions should include both lower- and upper-body aerobic training. Use of different exercise modalities employing various muscle groups minimizes overuse syndrome in joints and muscles. For patients with a recent sternotomy incision, range of motion exercises are encouraged. Exercise sessions should be designed to facilitate both the general goals of increasing endurance, range-of-motion, and strength for activities of daily living, as well as specific individual goals such as recreation, fall prevention, or return to work.

Resistance training is an important component of an exercise program to increase muscular strength and endurance. Because injuries are more likely to occur in a previously injured area, it is important to screen for old injuries prior to designing the program. Resistance training can be safely started as early as 4–6 wk after myocardial infarction (85,86), although most programs wait to add resistance training until the patient has been participating in aerobic exercise for 2–4 wk. Properly performed resistance exercise has also been shown to be safe (87) and effective (88) in patients with congestive heart failure. Poststernotomy patients should be carefully screened for sternal wound stability before beginning resistance exercise, and most programs wait until 6 wk poststernotomy to begin these exercises.

Resistance training uses the principle of progressive overload to increase muscle mass and strength, employing exercises that increase, to more than normal, the resistance to movement or frequency and duration of activity. Any amount of overload will result in strength development, but near-maximal effort elicits the greatest training effect. However, injury rate and pressure rate product increase with maximal effort. The intensity and volume of overload can be manipulated by varying the weight load, number of repetitions and sets completed, and the rest period between exercises. Exercise prescription can be determined using a one repetition maximum (RM) test for various muscle groups, then recommending 30–40% of 1 RM intensity for the upper body and 50–60% of 1 RM for the hips and legs as the starting weight for the initial session. Alternatively, a trial-and-error method can be used to set the initial resistance, aiming for a weight or resistance that allows the participant to achieve the proper repetition range at an RPE of 13–15 (79).

It is important to include both upper- and lower-body exercises as well as competing muscle groups around a joint in the exercise set, concentrating on muscles used for balance and daily activities. Exercises should be rhythmical, at a slow to moderate controlled speed, through a pain-free range of motion, and using normal breathing patterns. From a practical perspective, many patients will not be compliant if their combined aerobic and resistance exercise session lasts longer than 60 min, so most recommend 1 set of 10–15 repetitions for 8–10 exercises, 2–3 times per week for elderly and/or frail persons *(79–81)*. Rest periods of approx 48 h between resistive exercise sessions are recommended to allow for muscle recuperation without deconditioning. Variable-resistance equipment is recommended to maximize benefits and safety because of its known resistance, the ability to control and titrate the progression of exercise, the presence of proper skeletal support, and the ability to double-pin the machine to restrict movement to a pain-free range of motion *(79)*.

Monitoring during cardiac rehabilitation exercise sessions generally includes continuous ECG rhythm and heart rate monitoring, blood pressure monitoring (at rest, peak exercise, and postexercise), and symptom monitoring. Supervision is generally provided by physical therapists, registered nurses, and exercise physiologists who have experience treating patients with cardiovascular disease. One member of the team should be trained in advanced cardiac life support, and emergency equipment and medications should be in the exercise area *(36)*. A physician with expertise in cardiac rehabilitation provides medical supervision for the program. Duration of monitoring and supervision should be individualized and is somewhat controversial, so this topic will be discussed in the final section of this chapter.

Most cardiac rehabilitation sessions are scheduled 3 times per week for 8–12 wk, although many programs encourage their patients to supplement their exercise training at home with walking or other low- to moderate-level aerobic exercise on 1 to 3 additional days. Following completion of monitored cardiac rehabilitation, all programs encourage their patients to continue regular exercise to maintain their functional and aerobic gains.

Nonexercise Components of Cardiac Rehabilitation

The core components of cardiac rehabilitation/secondary prevention programs not only include assessment, physical activity counseling, and exercise training but also lipid management, nutritional counseling, hypertension management, smoking cessation, diabetes management, and psychosocial management *(32)*. Many of these topics are thoroughly covered in other chapters of this book, but standards of care specific to cardiac rehabilitation programs will be highlighted here as well.

Lipid Management and Nutritional Counseling

Multiple studies have shown a significant benefit of lipid-lowering therapy on cardiovascular morbidity and mortality including in the elderly *(89–91)*. As a result, the National Cholesterol Education Program (NCEP) Adult Treatment Panel III recommended that age restrictions are no longer appropriate when consider lipid-lowering pharmacological therapy in older adults (men > 65 yr, women > 75 yr) *(92)*.

Cardiac rehabilitation programs provide the ideal setting to screen patients for dyslipidemias and to begin the lifestyle modifications necessary to complement pharmacological therapy. Specific programmatic details range from comprehensive coronary risk reduction such as the SCRIP *(93)* or Multicenter Lifestyle Demonstration projects *(94)* to group counseling and education provided by cardiac rehabilitation staff members.

Exercise has been shown to favorably affect serum lipids (especially high-density lipoprotein [HDL] cholesterol) and body composition *(1,34,37)* in both younger and elderly individuals engaged in vigorous physical activity *(95)*. However, the independent effect of exercise during a cardiac rehabilitation program, without nutritional intervention, is only modest. Following a 3-mo exercise training program in 82 coronary patients (aged

61.2 ± 12.2 yr), Brochu et al. demonstrated no overall effects on body weight, total cholesterol, LDL cholesterol, triglycerides, glucose, or insulin levels, and only an 8% (3 ± 8 mg/dL) increase in HDL cholesterol *(96)*. This group also reported low caloric expenditure (270 ± 112 kcal) during a typical outpatient cardiac rehabilitation session *(97)*, which may partially explain these results. In contrast, Lavie et al. demonstrated that a comprehensive cardiac rehabilitation program can significantly impact body composition and lipid profile in elderly individuals (mean age: 70.1 ± 4.1 yr) *(5)*. Compared to baseline measures, study subjects demonstrated significant improvements in body mass index (26.0 ± 3.9 vs 25.6 ± 3.8 kg/m², $p < 0.01$), percent body fat (24.4 ± 7.0 vs 22.9 ± 7.2%, $p < 0.0001$), and HDL cholesterol (40.4 ± 12.1 vs 43.0 ± 11.4 mg/dL, $p < 0.001$), a trend toward significance in triglycerides (141 ± 55 vs 130 ± 76 mg/dL, $p = 0.14$), but no significant improvement in total cholesterol or LDL *(5)*. None of these patients were treated with lipid-lowering medications. In a more recent study involving 481 patients (age: 64.4 ± 10.6 yr), Yu et al. showed a significant decrease in LDL cholesterol (3.2 ± 1.0 vs 2.7 ± 0.7 mmol/L, $p < 0.001$) following an intensive cardiac rehabilitation program *(98)*. This Hong Kong-based program included aerobic exercise, two 1-h education classes per week for 8 wk that focused on secondary prevention issues, and continued community-based exercise and clinic follow-up for at least 18 mo. Fifty percent of these patients were on lipid-lowering agents (44% statins) on entry into the study, at least partially explaining these results but also confirming the need to combine medical management with exercise and nutritional counseling.

Standards for nutritional screening in cardiac rehabilitation include (1) baseline estimates of total daily caloric intake and dietary content of fat, cholesterol, sodium, and other nutrients, (2) assessment of eating habits, including number of meals, snacks, frequency of dining out, and alcohol consumption, and (3) assessment of target areas for nutrition intervention related to weight, hypertension, diabetes, heart failure, kidney disease, and other comorbidities *(32)*. Specific dietary modifications are aimed to at least attain the saturated fat and cholesterol content limits of the American Heart Association Step II diet, individualizing the diet plan to target specific comorbidities and incorporating behavior modification models and compliance strategies into the counseling sessions. Recent NCEP guidelines add the inclusion of plant sterols and increased viscous fiber to these recommendations and stress the need to limit saturated fats and trans fatty acids *(92)*. A modified Step I, Mediterranean-style diet can also be used and will be discussed in more depth later in this chapter.

Weight management is another core component of cardiac rehabilitation *(32)*. Baseline evaluation includes measurement of weight, height, and waist circumference and calculation of body mass index (BMI). Those patients with BMI > 25 kg/m² and/or waist > 40 in. in men and > 35 in. in women are referred for specific intervention. A combined diet, exercise, and behavioral program is designed to reduce total caloric intake, increase energy expenditure, and maintain appropriate intake of nutrients and fiber, aiming for an energy deficit of 500–1000 kcal/d *(32)*.

Hypertension

Cardiac rehabilitation sessions are ideal for monitoring the effect of therapy on blood pressure, and close communication between cardiac rehabilitation staff and a patient's physicians can facilitate optimal control. Group and individual education sessions are ideal opportunities to reinforce dietary management of hypertension, including the reduction of sodium and alcohol intake. In patients with mild hypertension, chronic aerobic exercise, weight loss, and dietary changes may lower blood pressure sufficiently to reduce medication use *(85)*.

Diabetes Mellitus

Patients who have both coronary artery disease and diabetes mellitus have significantly increased cardiac morbidity and mortality compared to those without diabetes. This finding includes patients who are enrolled in cardiac rehabilitation *(98)*, suggesting the need for increased surveillance and appropriate intervention in this group. Cardiac rehabilitation sessions are ideal for monitoring glycemic control, addressing other secondary prevention issues, and educating patients about subtle signs and symptoms of worsening cardiac disease.

Regular glycemic monitoring during cardiac rehabilitation sessions can be performed either by the patient or by the rehabilitation staff. The acute effects of exercise on plasma glucose levels are variable, depending on the intensity of exercise, severity of insulin deficiency, and medications. Brief intense bouts of exercise may cause transient hyperglycemia if glycogenolysis exceeds the rate of glucose utilization. More commonly, however, there is an exaggerated decrease in plasma glucose concentration in insulin-treated diabetics following prolonged moderate exercise. This is related to depot insulin suppressing the physiological fall in insulin levels during exercise, resulting in relative hyperinsulinemia. In addition, exercise of skeletal muscle underlying an insulin injection site may accelerate the absorption of insulin and disturb a patient's usual glycemic pattern. Some patients may also have disturbances in the secretion of epinephrine or glucagon, contributing to exercise-induced hypoglycemia. Although exercise-related hypoglycemia occurs most frequently 30–45 min after the start of moderate-intensity exercise, it can also occur between 6 and 10 h after an exercise session *(99)*. The reason for late hypoglycemia is not clear, but patients should be counseled to monitor for this effect and to modify their medications or caloric intake if appropriate.

Smoking Cessation

It is unusual for an elderly patient enrolled in cardiac rehabilitation at our facility to continue to smoke. However, in those who do resume cigarette use after a cardiac event, smoking cessation is often difficult. Older age, longer education, and higher occupational level are favorably associated with smoking cessation *(100)*. Cardiac rehabilitation standards stress screening for past, recent, and current tobacco use, assessment of confounding psychosocial issues, and use of readiness to change models to determine timing for intervention *(32)*. Minimal interventions should include individual education and counseling by program staff, supplemented by self-learning materials and family support, with referral to the primary physician for pharmacological intervention if needed. Optimally, formal smoking cessation programs are offered using group and/or individual counseling, pharmacological support, and supplemental strategies such as acupuncture and hypnosis *(32)*.

Psychosocial Interventions

Depression, anger, and anxiety are associated with an increased risk for cardiac events *(101–105)*. Psychological and cognitive dysfunction must also be considered during screening and program design for elderly cardiac rehabilitation patients. In fact, cardiac rehabilitation professionals are uniquely positioned to identify patients who would benefit from psy-chosocial intervention beyond the group support occurring during exercise and educa-tion sessions. Depression is a prevalent finding in elderly patients following a major cardiac event *(106)*, and few of these patients are treated or referred for treatment by their primary physicians. Appropriate use of screening tools such as the Geriatric Depression Scale *(107)* can facilitate appropriate referral and treatment.

All elderly patients can benefit from an age-specific approach to program design, includ-ing additional time spent gathering historical information and answering questions, use of gentle, philosophical language that explains aging processes yet provides hope for func-tional improvement with rehabilitation, recognition of the wisdom accumulated with aging, linkage of rehabilitation goals to tangible functional activities, and bolstering a patient's sense of self-worth *(107)*. Economic realities, family obligations, spiritual beliefs, and the presence of other disabilities can also influence an elderly patient's response to exercise and educational sessions.

Cardiac rehabilitation can have a significant impact on depression, anxiety, and quality of life. Milani et al. studied depressive symptoms and other behavioral and quality of life parameters in 338 patients who completed 36 outpatient cardiac rehabilitation sessions, without additional referral for psychosocial intervention *(108)*. Depression was present in 20% of these patients, and after rehabilitation, depressed patients had marked improve-ments in depression scores, other behavioral parameters (anxiety, somatization, and hostil-ity), and quality of life (all $p < 0.001$). Two-thirds of the patients who were initially depressed resolved their symptoms by study completion. These authors also evaluated 268 consecu-tive elderly (>65 yr) patients referred to cardiac rehabilitation and found an 18% preva-lence of depression among this group. Compared to nondepressed patients, these patients had significantly reduced exercise capacity ($p = 0.02$), lower levels of HDL ($p = 0.08$), more symptoms of anxiety ($p < 0.001$), hostility ($p < 0.001$), and somatization ($p < 0.001$), as well as a reduction in all quality-of-life measures ($p < 0.005$). Cardiac rehabilitation signifi-cantly improved all measures of quality of life ($p < 0.001$) in these patients as well as the mean scores for depression ($-57\%, p < 0.0001$), anxiety ($-53\%, p < 0.0001$), hostility (-36%, $p < 0.004$), and somatization ($-39\%, p < 0.0001$). In addition, depressed patients dem-onstrated statistically significant improvements in these parameters compared to nonde-pressed patients. After completion of cardiac rehabilitation, 63% of these elderly patients were no longer depressed.

CONTROVERSIES IN CARDIAC REHABILITATION

Less than a decade ago, it was not clear whether elderly patients should routinely be included in cardiac rehabilitation programs. Many of the early studies excluded patients over age 70 and only recently have researchers evaluated outcomes in patients over age 75 *(7)*. As a result of these more recent studies, it has finally become clear that elderly patients derive benefits from cardiac rehabilitation in terms of improvement in maximal exercise capacity, training effect at submaximal workloads, body composition, lipid profile, and quality of life *(5,6,8,10,45,87)*. However, referral to cardiac rehabilitation programs remain low for elderly patients, and there continues to be a paucity of studies specifically evaluating optimal program design for subsets of this age group. This section will discuss current controversies in exercise programming, dietary management, and psychological/

cognitive issues in cardiac rehabilitation with emphasis on what needs to be learned about these issues for elderly patients.

Controversies in Exercise Programming

Current controversies in exercise programming include the selection of appropriate patients for rehabilitation, the degree of supervision and monitoring needed during exercise, and the evaluation of the intensity/type of exercise to maximize functional capacity. Very few studies have specifically addressed these issues in the elderly, although more recent work in these areas has not excluded older patients.

Most cardiac rehabilitation professionals consider patients to be appropriate for an exercise and risk-factor-modification program if they (1) have decreased functional capacity compared to either their peers or their own recent baseline, (2) have either chronic heart disease or a recent cardiac event, (3) are cognitively and physically able to participate in rehabilitation, and (4) do not have contraindications to exercise such as class IV symptoms, severe valvular stenosis, or uncontrolled hypertension. However, not all health insurance carriers recognize these criteria despite recent evidence that cardiac rehabilitation has been shown to be safe and effective in a variety of conditions including congestive heart failure, post-myocardial-infarction, stable angina, post-coronary-artery-bypass or valve replace-ment, and following percutaneous revascularization *(1,5,49,82)*. As a result, rehabilitation programs have developed alternative methods for program delivery, including home exercise, community-based programs, unmonitored hospital-based programs, and hybrid models involving several locations for the rehabilitation sessions.

The safety of supervised exercise sessions for patients with heart disease is well documented in the literature, with rates of myocardial infarction or cardiac arrest ranging from 1 per 49,315 to 1 per 120,000 patient exercise hours *(109)*. The heightened surveillance during cardiac rehabilitation may lead to earlier detection of progressive coronary artery disease, with appropriate intervention. Vongvanich and Merz evaluated the frequency of medical problems detected during supervised exercise in 666 patients during a 1-yr period and found that 17% had problems detected which prompted calls to referring physicians, with 55% of these calls resulting in patient care alteration and 5% resulting in a major alteration such as revascularization *(110)*. Patients with events were more likely to be older (mean age 70 ± 12 vs 67 ± 11 yr, $p = 0.03$) than those without events.

Structured, unmonitored home-based cardiac rehabilitation has been proposed as an alternative for some patients, although this is not currently widely employed in the United States and large-scale trials have not been performed. Oka et al. studied the impact of a home-based walking and resistance training program in 40 patients with stable congestive heart failure, aged 30–76 *(111)*. Compared to a usual care control group, the exercise intervention decreased fatigue and improved emotional function, and mastery, but there was no significant difference in peak exercise capacity between the two groups. No training-related cardiac events occurred and there were no musculoskeletal injuries. Brubaker et al. studied home-based maintenance exercise as an alternative to either maintenance exercise in a center-based supervised program or unstructured discharge to usual care ($n = 48$ patients, age 62 ± 11 yr) *(112)*. Exercise testing, fasting blood analysis, and body composition were assessed at baseline, 3 mo, and at 12 mo post-entry into rehabilitation. The home-based program was as effective as the center-based program at improving/maintaining functional capacity, blood lipids, and body weight/composition.

Another approach is to use an abbreviated (4 wk) traditional cardiac rehabilitation program, followed by an off-site exercise regimen with continued education and group support. This approach facilitates continued independent exercise, reduces costs and has been shown to be as effective as a traditional (12 wk) program in improving physiologic outcomes such as maximal oxygen uptake, blood lipids, and hemodynamic measurements *(113)*. In addition, patients participating in the reduced-cost modified program (age 59 ± 10 yr) had higher rates of exercise adherence and program participation.

Questions remain about the applicability of home-based and community exercise for elderly cardiac rehabilitation patients. Large-scale studies evaluating the safety and effectiveness of home and community exercise for elderly cardiac patients need to be completed before these approaches can be universally applied.

Most recent studies demonstrating the effectiveness of cardiac rehabilitation in the elderly have used traditional programming, including resistance exercise *(114–116)*. These studies have confirmed that elderly patients, including those older than 75 yr *(117)*, make significant improvements in functional capacity, body composition, quality of life, and serum lipids following a rehabilitation program *(118–120)*. However, cardiac rehabilitation professionals are just beginning to evaluate specific program issues such as duration and frequency of exercise *(118)*, intensity of exercise *(118)*, interval training *(119)*, and timing of resistance exercise following cardiac events *(85,86)*. None of these studies are specific to elderly patients, and few articles exist concerning optimal exercise programming in the frail elderly, obese elderly, patients with class III symptoms, and patients with significant arthritis or neurological disability. Future clinical research will be needed to address optimal exercise programming for these patients.

Inpatient cardiac rehabilitation for frail elderly patients, generally aged 75 or older, and for younger patients with complicated, prolonged acute care following myocardial infarction or open-heart surgery can be a bridge to independence at home, followed by outpatient cardiac rehabilitation. These programs vary from inpatient acute rehabilitation units dedicated to cardiac patients with telemetry monitoring and medical care by a cardiologist to subacute rehabilitation in a skilled nursing facility. Outcomes measures reflecting independence scores show significant improvement in these patients *(119)*, but no controlled studies have been performed to confirm that these programs prevent rehospitalization and accelerate return to independence in elderly patients. However, as the volume of invasive cardiac procedures and surgery in elderly individuals continues to grow, cost-effective programs to return these patients home will become even more important.

Controversies in Psychosocial and Cognitive Programming

One of the challenges in cardiac rehabilitation is to provide each patient with the full range of services shown to improve function and decrease the risk of future cardiac events and to do this in a timely and cost-effective manner. There is no doubt that psychosocial issues, including anger, anxiety, and depression, play a large role in disability from cardiac disease. However, reimbursement options for treatment of these conditions are limited for many patients, especially if their impairment is mild. Some programs incorporate behavior modification and stress-reduction sessions into their cardiac rehabilitation programs for all patients, whereas others offer these on a self-pay basis. Many programs only offer referral to mental health professionals for services. The literature concerning the impact of stress-reduction techniques on secondary prevention of cardiac disease is sparse but compelling *(120–123)*. Blumenthal et al. *(120)* studied 117 patients (58.5 ± 8.4 yr) with coronary artery disease and myocardial ischemia induced by mental stress, randomly assigning them to either a 4-mo exercise or stress-reduction program. A usual care comparison group was selected from patients living at a distance from the facility. Stress management was associated with a relative risk of 0.26 compared to controls for recurrent cardiac events and was associated with reduced ischemia induced by mental stress or ambulation. The relative risk for the exercise group was also lower than controls (0.68) but did not reach statistical significance. The authors postulated that the decrease in ischemia and cardiac events in the stress-reduction group was related to decreased expression of hostility and anger following stress management training.

Subsequent studies have confirmed the benefits of relaxation therapy for patients with cardiac disease *(121,122)*. Van Dixhoorn et al. randomized 156 patients to either exercise training plus relaxation therapy or exercise training alone *(121)*. At 5-yr follow-up, 15 (20%) of the relaxation plus exercise group and 26 (33%) of the exercise alone group had experienced at least one cardiac event (adjusted odds ratio for the relaxation group: 0.52, 95% confidence interval: 0.28–0.99). In addition, the total number of hospitalizations was reduced by 31% as a result of relaxation exercise. After 5 yr, 70% of the patients were still performing the relaxation techniques regularly. However, further studies are needed to generalize these results to elderly patients, and creative programming will be needed to incorporate stress reduction into cardiac rehabilitation in a cost-effective manner.

Unfortunately, many elderly patients have neurocognitive deficits, often exacerbated by recent open heart surgery. These deficits need to be recognized to optimize learning during rehabilitation and to avoid injury or misunderstanding. A structured cardiac rehabilitation program is the ideal setting to screen for deficits, use simple cognitive retraining techniques, and refer to other professionals for more intensive testing and retraining. However, many cardiac rehabilitation professionals are not aware of the extent of this problem and are unfamiliar with cognitive screening and training.

Cognitive decline following coronary artery bypass has been recognized for several years *(124–126)*, and the time-course of cognitive changes was recently documented by Newman et al. *(127)*. Neurocognitive tests were performed preoperatively in 261 patients (age: 60.9 ± 10.6 yr) who underwent CABG, then repeated before discharge, at 6 wk, 6 mo, and 5 yr post-CABG. Decline in postoperative function was defined as a drop of one standard deviation or more in the scores of any one of four cognitive tests, which corresponded to approx 20% decline in function. Cognitive function declined in 53% of patients at discharge, 36% at 6 wk, 24% at 6 mo, and 42% at 5 yr. Function improved gradually up to 6 mo, both in patients with early postoperative cognitive decline and those without early cognitive decline. Cognitive testing in patients without early decline returned to near-baseline values. However, in patients with early postoperative cognitive impairment, by the fifth postoperative year cognitive function declined below baseline levels to a level similar to that seen at discharge. Predictors of late cognitive decline included older age, less education, and higher degrees of baseline impairment. This study, although it may have significant implications for cardiac rehabilitation personnel (who are in a unique position to help with screening and treatment of these patients), lacked a control group in its evaluation. Despite promising data, the impact of early aggressive treatment on later cognitive function is not known; neither are the indicated treatment techniques. Elderly cardiac patients are particularly vulnerable to cognitive decline, which makes this topic an important area for future research.

Summary

Although most cardiac rehabilitation is done in group sessions, it is important that the cardiac rehabilitation program for an individual elderly patient be individualized, selecting exercise modalities, psychosocial and cognitive screening/treatment, and educational approaches that are best suited to this particular patient. Assessment tools, program details, and outcomes measures should be age-specific and should take into account any coexisting medical, psychological, or neurological conditions.

REFERENCES

1. Wenger NK, Froelicher ES, Smith LK, et al. Cardiac Rehabilitation: Clinical Practice Guideline No. 17. AHCPR Publication No. 96-0672. US Dept of Health and Human Services, Public Health Service, Agency for Health Care Policy and Research, Public Health Service, Agency for Health Care Policy and Research, National Heart, Lung, and Blood Institute, Rockville, MD, 1995, pp. 1–202.
2. Pinsky JL, Jette AM, Branch LG, et al. The Framingham Disability Study: relationship of various coronary heart disease manifestations to disability in older persons living in the community. Am J Public Health 1990;80:1363–1368.
3. Mosca L, Manson JE, Sutherland SE, et al. Cardiovascular disease in women: a statement for healthcare professionals from the American Heart Association. Circulation 1997;96:2468–2482.
4. O'Connor GT, Buring JE, Usuf S, et al. An overview of randomized trials of rehabilitation with exercise after myocardial infarction. Circulation 1989;80:234–244.
5. Lavie CJ, Milani RV, Littman AB. Benefits of cardiac rehabilitation and exercise training in secondary coronary prevention in the elderly. J Am Coll Cardiol 1993;22:678–683.
6. Lavie CJ, Milani RV. Benefits of cardiac rehabilitation and exercise training in elderly women. Am J Cardiol 1997;79:664–666.
7. Oldridge J. Cardiac rehabilitation in the elderly. Aging Clin Exp Res 1998;10:273–283.
8. Lavie CJ, Milani RV. Disparate effects of improving aerobic exercise capacity and quality of life after cardiac rehabilitation in young and elderly coronary patients. J Cardiopulmonary Rehabil 2000;20: 235–240.
9. Balady GJ, Jette D, Scheer J, et al. Changes in exercise capacity following cardiac rehabilitation in patients stratified according to age and gender. J Cardiopulmonary Rehabil 1996;16:38–46.
10. Ades PA, Waldmann ML, Poehlman ET, et al. Exercise conditioning in older coronary patients: submaximal lactacte response and endurance capacity. Circulation 1993;88:572–577.
11. Ades PA, Waldman ML, Meyer WL, et al. Skeletal muscle and cardiovascular adaptations to exercise conditioning in older coronary patients. Circulation 1996;94:323–330.
12. Ades PA, Waldmann ML, Polk DM, et al. Referral patterns and exercise response in the rehabilitation of female coronary patients aged ≥ 62 years. Am J Cardiol 1992;69:1422–1425.
13. Thomas RJ, Houston Miller N, Lamendola C, et al. National survey on gender differences in cardiac rehabilitation programs. J Cardiopulmonary Rehabil 1996;16:402–412.
14. Evenson KR, Rosamond WD, Luepker RV. Predictors of outpatient cardiac rehabilitation utilization: the Minnesota heart survey registry. J Cardiopulmonary Rehabil 1998;18:192–198.
15. Blackburn GG, Foody JM, Sprecher DL. Cardiac rehabilitation participation patterns in a large, tertiary care center: evidence for selection bias. J Cardiopulmonary Rehabil 2000;20:189–195.
16. Richardson LA, Buckenmeyer PJ, Bauman BD, et al. Contemporary cardiac rehabilitation: patient characteristics and temporal trends over the past decade. J Cardiopulmonary Rehabil 2000;20:57–64.
17. Ades PA, Waldmann ML, McCann W, et al. Predictors of cardiac rehabilitation participation in older coronary patients. Arch Intern Med 1992;152:1033–1035.
18. Fletcher GF, Balady G, Froelicher V, et al. Exercise standards: a statement for healthcare professionals from the American Heart Association. Circulation 1992;86:340–344.
19. Malbut-Shennan K, Young A. The physiology of physical performance and training in old age. Coronary Artery Dis 1999;10:37–42.
20. Ades PA, Maloney A, Savage PS, et al. Determinants of physical functioning in coronary patients. Arch Intern Med 1999;159:2357–2360.
21. Mazzeo RS, Cavanagh P, Evans WJ, et al. Exercise and physical activity for older adults. Med Sci Sports Exerc 1998;30:992–1008.

22. Ades PA. Cardiac rehabilitation in older coronary patients. J Am Geriatr Soc 1999;47:98–105.
23. Coggan AR, Spina RJ, King DS, et al. Skeletal muscle adaptations to endurance training in 60- to 70-yr-old men and women. J Appl Physiol 1992;72:1780–1786.
24. Beere PA, Russell SD, Morey M, et al. Aerobic exercise training can reverse age-related peripheral circulatory changes in healthy older men. Circulation 1999;100:1085–1094.
25. Vaitkevicius PV, Fleg JL, Engel JH, et al. Effects of age and aerobic capacity on arterial stiffness in health adults. Circulation 1993;88(Part 1):1456–1462.
26. Levy WC, Cerqueira MD, Abrass IB, et al. Endurance exercise training augments diastolic filling at rest and during exercise in healthy young and older men. Circulation 1993;88:116–126.
27. Ehsani AA, Ogawa T, Miller TR, et al. Exercise training improves left ventricular systolic function in older men. Circulation 1991;83:96–103.
28. Seals DR, Hagberg JM, Spina RJ, et al. Enhanced left ventricular performance in endurance trained older men. Circulation 1994;89:198–205.
29. Wenger NK. Elderly coronary patients. In: Wenger NK, ed. Rehabilitation of the Coronary Patient, 3rd ed. Churchill Livingstone, New York, 1992, pp. 415–420.
30. Dorn J, Naughton J, Imamura D, et al. Results of a multicenter randomized clinical trial of exercise and long-term survival in myocardial infarction patients: the National Exercise and Heart Disease Project (NEHDP). Circulation 1999;100:1764–1769.
31. Brubaker PH, Warner JG, Rejeski WJ, et al. Comparison of standard- and extended-length participation in cardiac rehabilitation on body composition, functional capacity, and blood lipids. Am J Cardiol 1996;78:769–773.
32. Balady GJ, Ades PA, Comoss P, et al. Core components of cardiac rehabilitation/secondary prevention programs: a statement for healthcare professionals from the American Heart Association and the American Association of Cardiovascular and Pulmonary Rehabilitation. Circulation 2000;102:1069–1073.
33. Balady GJ, Fletcher BJ, Froelicher ES, et al. Cardiac rehabilitation programs: a statement for healthcare professional from the American Heart Association. Circulation 1994;90:1602–1610.
34. Fletcher GF. How to implement physical activity in primary and secondary prevention: a statement for healthcare professionals from the task force on risk reduction, American Heart Association. Circulation 1997;96:355–357.
35. Wenger NK, Froelicher ES, Smith LK, et al. Cardiac Rehabilitation: Clinical Practice Guideline No.17. AHCPR Publication No. 96-0673. US Dept of Health and Human Services, Public Health Service, Agency for Health Care Policy and Research, Public Health Service, Agency for Health Care Policy and Research, National Heart, Lung, and Blood Institute, Rockville, MD, 1995.
36. American Association of Cardiovascular and Pulmonary Rehabilitation. Guidelines for Cardiac Rehabilitation and Secondary Prevention Programs, 3rd ed. Human Kinetics, Champaign, IL, 1999, p. 281.
37. Shephard RJ, Balady GJ. Exercise as cardiovascular therapy. Circulation 1999;99:963–972.
38. Paffenbarger RS, Hyde RT, Wing AL, et al. The association of changes in physical activity level and other lifestyle characteristics with mortality among men. N Engl J Med 1993;328:538–545.
39. Lee IM, Sesso HD, Paffenbarger RS. Physical activity and coronary heart disease risk in men. Does the duration of exercise episodes predict risk? Circulation 2000;102:981–986.
40. Sesso HD, Paffenbarger RS, Lee IM. Physical activity and coronary heart disease in men. The Harvard Alumni Health Study. Circulation 2000;102:975–980.
41. Hakim AA, Curb JD, Petrovitch H, et al. Effects of walking on coronary heart disease in elderly men. The Honolulu Heart Program. Circulation 1999;100:9–13.
42. Hedblad B, Ogren M, Isacsson SO, et al. Reduced cardiovascular mortality risk in male smokers who are physically active. Arch Intern Med 1997;157:893–899.
43. Hu FB, Stampfer MJ, Solomon C, et al. Physical activity and risk for cardiovascular events in diabetic women. Ann Intern Med 2001;134:96–105.
44. Wannamethee SG, Shaper A, Walker MA. Physical activity and mortality in older men with diagnosed coronary heart disease. Circulation 2000;102:1358–1363.
45. Blumenthal JA, Emery CF, Madden DJ, et al. Effects of exercise training on cardiorespiratory function in men and women >60 years of age. Am J Cardiol 1991;67:633–639.
46. Ades PA, Coello CE. Effects of exercise and cardiac rehabilitation on cardiovascular outcomes. Med Clin North Am 2000;84:251–265.
47. Wei M, Gibbons LW, Mitchell TL, et al. The association between cardiorespiratory fitness and impaired fasting glucose and type 2 diabetes mellitus in men. Ann Intern Med 1999;130:89–96.

48. Dylewicz P, Bienkowska S, Szczesniak L, et al. Beneficial effect of short-term endurance training on glucose metabolism during rehabilitation after coronary bypass surgery. Chest 2000;117:47–54.

49. Koenig W, Ernst E. Exercise and thrombosis. Coronary Artery Dis 2000;11:123–127.

50. Sherman, DL. Exercise and endothelial function. Coronary Artery Dis 2000;11:117–122.

51. Taddei S, Galetta F, Virdis A, et al. Physical activity prevents age-related impairment in nitric oxide availability in elderly athletes. Circulation 2000;101:2896–2901.

52. DeSouza CA, Shapiro LF, Clevenger CM, et al. Regular aerobic exercise prevents and restores age-related declines in endothelium-dependent vasodilation in healthy men. Circulation 2000;102:1351–1357.

53. Tanaka H, Dinnenno FA, Monahan KD, et al. Aging, habitual exercise, and dynamic arterial compliance. Circulation 2000;102:1270–1275.

54. Higashi Y, Sasaki S, Kurisu S, et al. Regular aerobic exercise augments endothelium dependent vascular relaxation in normotensive as well as hypertensive subjects. Circulation 1999;100:1194–1202.

55. Czernin J, Barnard J, Sun KT, et al. Effect of short-term cardiovascular conditioning and low-fat diet on myocardial blood flow and flow reserve. Circulation 1995;92:197–204.

56. Hambrecht R, Wolf A, Gielen S, et al. Effect of exercise on coronary endothelial function in patients with coronary artery disease. N Engl J Med 2000;342:454–460.

57. Coats AJS. Exercise rehabilitation in chronic heart failure. J Am Coll Cardiol 1993;22(Suppl A): 172A–177A.

58. Malfatto G, Facchini M, Bragato R, et al. Short and long term effects of exercise training on the tonic autonomic modulation of heart rate variability after myocardial infarction. Eur Heart J 1996;17: 532–538.

59. Stahle A, Nordlander R, Bergfeldt L. Aerobic group training improves exercise capacity and heart rate variability in elderly patients with a recent coronary event: a randomized controlled study. Eur Heart J 1999;20:1638–1646.

60. Goldsmith RL, Bloomfield DM, Rosenwinkel ET. Exercise and autonomic function. Coronary Artery Dis 2000;11:129–135.

61. Iellamo F, Legramante JM, Maassaro M, et al. Effects of a residential exercise training on baroreflex sensitivity and heart rate variability in patients with coronary artery disease. Circulation 2000;102: 2588–2592.

62. Hambrecht R, Niebasuer J, Marburger C, et al. Various intensities of leisure time physical activity in patients with coronary artery disease: effects on cardiorespiratory fitness and progression of coronary atherosclerotic lesions. J Am Coll Cardiol 1993;22:468–477.

63. Niebauer J, Hambrecht R, Velich T, et al. Attenuated progression of coronary artery disease after 6 years of multifactorial risk intervention. Circulation 1997;96:2534–2541.

64. Niebauer J, Hambrecht R, Schlierf G, et al. Five years of physical exercise and low fat diet: effects on progression of coronary artery disease. J Cardiopulmonary Rehabil 1994;15:47–64.

65. Niebauer J, Hambrecht R, Marburger C, et al. Impact of intensive physical exercise and low-fat diet on collateral vessel formation in stable angina pectoris and angiographically confirmed coronary artery disease. Am J Cardiol 1995;76:771–775.

66. Senti S, Fleisch M, Billinger M, et al. Long-term physical exercise and quantitatively assessed human coronary collateral circulation. J Am Coll Cardiol 1998;32:49–56.

67. Linke A, Schoene N, Gielen S, et al. Endothelial dysfunction in patients with chronic heart failure: systemic effects of lower-limb exercise training. J Am Coll Cardiol 2001;37:392–397.

68. Keteyian S, Brawner CA. Chronic heart failure and cardiac rehabilitation for the elderly: is it beneficial? Am J Geriatr Cardiol 1999;8:80–86.

69. Giannuzzi P, Tavazzi L, Temporelli PL, et al. Long-term physical training and left ventricular remodeling after anterior myocardial infarction: results of exercise in anterior myocardial infarction (EAMI) trial. J Am Coll Cardiol 1993;22:1821–1829.

70. Specchia G, DeServi S, Scire A, et al. Interaction between exercise training and ejection fraction in predicting prognosis after a first myocardial infarction. Circulation 1996;94:978–982.

71. Tyni-Lenne R, Gordon A, Jansson E, et al. Skeletal muscle endurance training improves peripheral oxidative capacity, exercise tolerance, and health-related quality of life in women with chronic congestive heart failure secondary to either ischemic cardiomyopathy or idiopathic dilated cardiomyopathy. Am J Cardiol 1997;80:1025–1029.

72. Guerra-Garcia H, Taffet G, Protas E. Considerations related to disability and exercise in elderly women with congestive heart failure. J Cardiovasc Nurs 1997;11:60–74.

73. Piepoli M. European Heart Failure Training Group. Experience from controlled trials of physical training in chronic heart failure: protocol and patient factors in effectiveness in the improvement in exercise tolerance. Eur Heart J 1998;19:466–475.

74. Tyni-Lenne R, Gordon A, Europe E, et al. Exercise-based rehabilitation improves skeletal muscle capacity, exercise tolerance, and quality of life in both women and men with chronic heart failure. J Cardiac Failure 1998;4:9–17.

75. Wielenga RP, Huisveld IA, Bol E, et al. Safety and effects of physical training in chronic heart failure: results of the Chronic Heart Failure and Graded Exercise study (CHANGE). Eur Heart J 1999;20: 872–879.

76. Gottlieb SS, Fisher ML, Freudenberger R, et al. Effects of exercise training on peak performance and quality of life in congestive heart failure patients. J Cardiac Failure 1999;5:188–194.

77. Lavie CJ, Milani RV. Effects of cardiac rehabilitation and exercise training on exercise capacity, coronary risk factors, behavioral characteristics, and quality of life in women. Am J Cardiol 1995;75: 340–343.

78. Lavie CJ, Milani RV. Effects of cardiac rehabilitation, exercise training, and weight reduction on exercise capacity, coronary risk factors, behavioral characteristics, and quality of life in obese coronary patients. Am J Cardiol 1997;79:397–401.

79. Pollock ML, Franklin BA, Balady GJ, et al. Resistance exercise in individuals with and without cardiovascular disease: benefits, rationale, safety, and prescription. An advisory from the Committee on Exercise, Rehabilitation, and Prevention, Council on Clinical Cardiology, American Heart Association. Circulation 2000;1001:828–833.

80. Feigenbaum M, Gentry RK. Prescription of resistance training for clinical populations. Am J Med Sports 2001;3:146–158.

81. Braith RW, Vincent KR. Resistance exercise in the elderly person with cardiovascular disease. Am J Geriatr Cardiol 1999;8:63–70,79.

82. Borg GAV. Psychophysical bases of perceived exertion. Med Sci Sport Exerc 1982;14:377–381.

83. Belardinelli R, Paolini I, Cianci G. Exercise training intervention after coronary angioplasty: the ETICA trial. J Am Coll Cardiol 2001;37:1891–1900.

84. Brechue WF, Pollock ML. Exercise training for coronary artery disease in the elderly. Clin Geriatr Med 1996;12:207–229.

85. Stewart KJ, McFarland LD, Weinhofer JJ, et al. Safety and efficacy of weight training soon after acute myocardial infarction. J Cardiopulmonary Rehabil 1998;18:37–44.

86. Fragnoli-Munn K, Savage PD, Ades PA. Combined resistive-aerobic training in older patients with coronary artery disease early after myocardial infarction. J Cardiopulmonary Rehabil 1998;18:416–420.

87. Meyer K, Hajric R, Westbrook S, et al. Hemodynamic responses during leg press exercise in patients with chronic congestive heart failure. Am J Cardiol 1999;83:1537–1543.

88. Hare DL, Ryan TM, Selig SE, et al. Resistance exercise training increases muscle strength, endurance, and blood flow in patients with chronic heart failure. Am J Cardiol 1999;83:1674–1677.

89. Aronow WS. Treatment of older persons with hypercholesterolemia with and without cardiovascular disease. J Gerontol 2001;56A:M138–M145.

90. Massing MW, Sueta CA, Chowdhury M, et al. Lipid management among coronary artery disease patients with diabetes mellitus or advanced age. Am J Cardiol 2001;87:646–649.

91. Campeau L, Hunninghake DB, Knatterud GL, et al. Aggressive cholesterol lowering delays saphenous vein graft atherosclerosis in women, the elderly, and patients with associated risk factors: NHLBI post coronary artery bypass graft clinical trial. Circulation 1999;99:3241–3247.

92. Executive summary of the third report of the National Cholesterol Education Program (NCEP) expert panel on detection, evaluation, and treatment of high blood cholesterol in adults (Adult Treatment Panel III). JAMA 2001;285:2486–2497.

93. Gordon NF, Haskell WL. Comprehensive cardiovascular disease risk reduction in a cardiac rehabilitation setting. Am J Cardiol 1997;80:69H–73H.

94. Ornish D. Avoiding revascularization with lifestyle changes: the Multicenter Lifestyle Demonstration project. Am J Cardiol 1998;82:72T–76T.

95. Williams PT. Coronary heart disease risk factors of vigorously active sexagenarians and septuagenarians. J Am Geriatr Soc 1998;46:134–142.

96. Brochu M, Poehlman ET, Savage P, et al. Modest effects of exercise training alone on coronary risk factors and body composition in coronary patients. J Cardiopulmonary Rehabil 2000;20:180–188.

97. Savage PD, Brochu M, Scott P, et al. Low caloric expenditure in cardiac rehabilitation. Am Heart J 2000;140:527–533.

98. Yu CM, Lau CP, Cheung BMY, et al. Clinical predictors of morbidity and mortality in patients with myocardial infarction or revascularization who underwent cardiac rehabilitation, and importance of diabetes mellitus and exercise capacity. Am J Cardiol 2000;85:344–349.

99. Gordon NF, Hoogwerf BJ, Olin JW, et al. Associated medical conditions. In: Pashkow FJ, Dafoe WA, eds. Clinical Cardiac Rehabilitaion: A Cardiologist's Guide, 2nd ed. Williams & Wilkins, Philadelphia, PA, 1999, p. 216.

100. Rosal MC, Ockene IS, Ockene JK. Smoking cessation as a critical element of cardiac rehabilitation. In: Pashkow FJ, Dafoe WA, eds. Clinical Cardiac Rehabilitaion: A Cardiologist's Guide, 2nd ed. Williams & Wilkins, Philadelphia, PA, 1999, p. 368.

101. Rozanski A, Blumenthal JA, Kaplan J. Impact of psychological factors on the pathogenesis of cardiovascular disease and implications for therapy. Circulation 1999;99:2192–2217.

102. Sesso HD, Kawachi I, Vokonas PS, et al. Depression and the risk of coronary heart disease in the normative aging study. Am J Cardiol 1998;82:851–856.

103. Kawachi I, Sparrow D, Spiro A, et al. A prospective study of anger and coronary heart disease. Circulation 1996;94:2090–2095.

104. Kubzansky LD, Kawachi I, Spiro A, et al. Is worrying bad for your heart?: a prospective study of worry and coronary heart disease in the Normative Aging Study. Circulation 1997;95:818–824.

105. Mendes de Leon CF, Krumholz HM, Seeman T, et al. Depression and risk of coronary heart disease in elderly men and women. Arch Intern Med 1998;158:2341–2348.

106. Milani RV, Lavie CJ. Prevalence and effects of cardiac rehabilitation on depression in the elderly with coronary heart disease. Am J Cardiol 1998;81:1233–1236.

107. Sotile WM, Miller HS. Helping older patients to cope with cardiac and pulmonary disease. J Cardiopulmonary Rehabil 1998;18:124–128.

108. Milani RV, Lavie CJ, Cassidy MM. Effects of cardiac rehabilitation and exercise training programs on depression in patients after major coronary events. Am Heart J 1996;132:726–732.

109. Franklin BA, Bonzheim K, Gordon S, et al. Safety of medically supervised outpatient cardiac rehabilitation exercise therapy. Chest 1998;114:902–906.

110. Vongvanich P, Merz CNB. Supervised exercise and electrocardiographic monitoring during cardiac rehabilitation. J Cardiopulmonary Rehabil 1996;16:233–238.

111. Oka RK, DeMarco T, Haskell WL, et al. Impact of a home-based walking and resistance training program on quality of life in patients with heart failure. Am J Cardiol 2000;85:365–369.

112. Brubaker PH, Rejeski WJ, Smith MJ, et al. A home-based maintenance exercise program after center-based cardiac rehabilitation: effects on blood lipids, body composition, and functional capacity. J Cardiopulmonary Rehabil 2000;20:50–56.

113. Carlson JJ, Johnson JA, Franklin BA. Program participation, exercise adherence, cardiovascular outcomes, and program cost of traditional versus modified cardiac rehabilitation. Am J Cardiol 2000;86: 17–23.

114. King PA, Savage P, Ades PA. Home resistance training in an elderly woman with coronary heart disease. J Cardiopulmonary Rehabil 2000;20:126–129.

115. Lavie CJ, Milani RV. Disparate effects of improving aerobic exercise capacity and quality of life after cardiac rehabilitation in young and elderly coronary patients. J Cardiopulmonary Rehabil 2000;20:235–240.

116. Lavie CJ, Milani RV. Effects of cardiac rehabilitation and exercise training programs in patients ≥75 years of age. Am J Cariol. 1996;78:675–677.

117. Kim JR, Oberman A, Fletcher GF, et al. Effect of exercise intensity and frequency on lipid levels in men with coronary heart disease: training level comparison trial. Am J Cardiol 2001;87:942–946.

118. Meyer K, Schwaibold M, Westbrook S, et al. Effects of short-term exercise training and activity restriction on functional capacity in patients with severe chronic congestive heart failure. Am J Cardiol 1996; 78:1017–1022.

119. Kong KH, Kevorkian G, Rossi CD. Functional outcomes of patients on a rehabiitation unit after open heart surgery. J Cardiopulmonary Rehabil 1996;16:413–418.

120. Blumenthal JA, Jiang W, Babyak MA, et al. Stress management and exercise training in cardiac patients with myocardial ischemia. Arch Intern Med 1997;157:2213–2223.

121. van Dixhoorn JJ, Duivenvoorden HJ. Effect of relaxation therapy on cardiac events after myocardial infarction: a 5 year follow-up study. J Cardiopulmonary Rehabil 1999;19:178–185.

122. Zamarra JW, Schneider RH, Besseghini I, et al. Usefulness of the transcendental meditation program in the treatment of patients with coronary artery disease. Am J Cardiol 1996;77:867–870.
123. Lan C, Chen S-Y, Lai J-S, et al. The effect of Tai Chi on cardiorespiratory function in patients with coronary artery bypass surgery. Med Sci Sports Exerc 1999;31:634–638.
124. Newman MF, Croughwell ND, Blumenthal JA, et al. Effect of aging on cerebral autoregulation during cardiopulmonary bypass: association with postoperative cognitive dysfunction. Circulation 1994;90 (Suppl II):II-243-II-249.
125. Tuman KJ, McCarthy RJ, Najafi H, et al. Differential effects of advanced age on neurological and cardiac risk of coronary artery operations. J Thorac Cardiovasc Surg 1997;104:1510–1517.
126. Selnes OA, Goldsborough MA, Borowicz LM, et al. Neurobehavioural sequelae of cardiopulmonary bypass. Lancet 1999;353:1601–1606.
127. Newman MF, Kirchner JL, Phillips-Bute B, et al. Longitudinal assessment of neurocognitive function after coronary artery bypass surgery. N Engl J Med 2001;344:395.

8 Ethical Issues in the Elderly

Kenneth M. Prager, MD

CONTENTS

INTRODUCTION

The field of medical ethics has evolved and grown over the past 30 yr in response to the increasing sophistication and complexity of medical technology. Issues are raised that were unheard of in prior years. The increased number of medical choices facing patients and their doctors, coupled with a rising assertiveness of patients seeking to become more involved in the medical decisions affecting their lives, nurtured the birth and growth of the new discipline of medical ethics.

The purpose of this chapter is not to provide an exhaustive analysis of these ethical dilemmas but merely to point to the issues that frequently confront the physician who deals with geriatric patients. The elderly population is most likely to raise subtle distinctions between treatments that prolong dying rather than prolong life. Often such patients are on ventilators or receive artificial nutrition and hydration.

Medical ethics committees seek to assist physicians, patients, and their families in navigating through the thicket of ethical and legal issues that arise daily in today's practice of medicine. The questions often relate to such end-of-life issues as withholding or withdrawing treatment, interpreting advance directives, and mediating differences of opinion among patients, surrogates, and physicians. There are also questions of medical futility and determining patient capacity.

Elderly patients are particularly likely to pose questions of medical ethics. First, they are more likely to be critically ill, often suffering from progressive and chronic cardiopulmonary, neurologic, or neoplastic illness. Second, they are far more likely than younger patients to lack decisional capacity just when it becomes critical to decide important questions raised by the progression of their illnesses [1]. The combination of very sick patients and

From: *Aging, Heart Disease, and Its Management: Facts and Controversies*
Edited by: N. Edwards, M. Maurer, and R. Wellner © Humana Press Inc., Totowa, NJ

their lack of decisional capacity accounts for a large proportion of the consultations performed by medical ethics commitees.

SOURCES OF MEDICAL ETHICS

Erich Fromm is said to have stated: "There are no medical ethics; there are universal ethics applied to particular circumstances." At first blush, this seems true. However, closer consideration reveals that the discipline of medical ethics in Western society is composed of principles that are both ancient and new, and incorporates societal norms as well as principles that are unique to the medical profession.

A cardinal ethical concept for physicians is the sanctity of human life. This is embedded in Western culture and derives from our Judeo-Christian religious tradition. Some philosophers refer to the existence of a "common" or "universal" morality that also infuses medical ethics *(2)*. Codes of behavior deriving from professional morality provide another source of moral norms for the practice of medicine. The Hippocratic Oath is one of the earliest examples of such a source. Contemporary standards of behavior adopted by various medical organizations contribute up-to-date ethical guidelines. Finally, current societal values as expressed through legal rulings, both statutory and case-based, provide a legal framework within which many of the questions facing physicians must be considered.

Although what is ethical and what is legal may not always be the same, the recommendations of medical ethics consultants inevitably reflect the legal requirements of their particular state. Law and ethics are inextricably bound up in the field of medical ethics, and it is critical for the ethicist to be familiar with relevant laws if for no other reason than to protect the physician and hospital from possible litigation.

Thus, common morality, which is often religion-based, professional medical standards, and civil law are the three major contributors to the corpus of medical ethics.

PRINCIPLES OF MEDICAL ETHICS

The four common accepted principles of medical ethics are the following:

Patient autonomy
Beneficence
Nonmaleficence
Justice

Let us consider each principle in turn and demonstrate aspects of each that uniquely pertain to the elderly patient.

Patient Autonomy

When used in medical ethics, the term *autonomy,* which means self-rule, refers to the right of a patient to accept or reject medical or surgical treatment and the associated right to obtain the necessary information to make an informed decision about one's medical care. Although we take this right for granted today, it must be stressed that from time immemorial, physicians considered it ethical to make medical decisions for their patients, providing them with only as much information as the doctors saw fit.

Although today there are few debates about revealing to patients such unfavorable diagnoses as cancer or terminal illness of any sort, the issue is complicated by cultural differences. Patients from different cultural backgrounds may vary greatly in their desire to know details of their illnesses or to participate in medical decision making. As a young physician patient of mine with incurable cancer once told me: "It's true that patients have a right to know, but they also have a right *not* to know."

Autonomy issues in the elderly are particularly varied and extremely important. Because elderly patients often have cognitive difficulties that limit their ability to assimilate information presented by their physicians, their ability to make informed decisions about their treatment may often be compromised. The high incidence of hearing impairment in the elderly, usually untreated, presents another obstacle to critical communication between physician and patient, and too often prevents truly informed consent. Therefore, it is the obligation of every physician treating elderly patients to take the time to adequately explain the medical issues affecting them and to encourage involvement of relatives or other surrogates who can assist the patient in making decisions. Careful explanation of medical issues is important to the elderly surgical candidate who must understand the risks and benefits of the procedure before giving informed consent.

The elderly need clear and unhurried physician input in order to exercise their autonomy regarding end-of-life issues. As the options for end-of-life care become more complex and varied, it becomes especially important for physicians to try and solicit input from their patients—particularly elderly and infirm ones—concerning their wishes regarding end-of-life care. Would the patient with severe emphysema ever want to be placed on a ventilator? If so, would there be limits to such care? If the patient sustains neurologic damage, as with a devastating stroke or hypoxic brain damage, how much aggressive life-sustaining care would they want? What are their wishes concerning treatment of serious illness in case they become severely demented?

The point must be stressed that physicians have an obligation to their elderly patients to facilitate the expression of their wishes regarding medical and surgical treatment, including end-of-life options. This can only be done if the physician raises these issues with patients in a nonthreatening way, preferably when the patient is medically stable and lucid. There is no substitute for an expenditure of time to explain options, answer questions, and clear up misunderstandings. Unfortunately, the current climate of American medicine, characterized by health maintenance organization (HMO) efficiency militating against an appropriate expenditure of time with patients, presents a major obstacle to realizing this goal. Passage by the US Congress in 1991 of the Federal Patient Self Determination Act underscores the importance of enabling patients to exercise their autonomy in medical decision making. The act mandates all hospitals receiving Medicare funds to supply every patient being admitted with written information concerning their rights as patients as well as explanations of advance directives and health care proxies in order to encourage patients to exercise their medical decision-making autonomy. Unfortunately, passage of this law has not appreciably increased the number of patients who obtain advance directives, in part because patients are not receptive to thinking about these issues when being hospitalized. Unless physicians raise the issue of advance directives in their offices, attainment of full autonomy for the majority of patients will remain an unrealized goal.

Although it is commonly assumed that most patients want the opportunity to express their preferences concerning end-of-life care, it must be stressed that there are significant numbers of patients who do *not* wish to discuss these issues, preferring instead to allow their loved ones, in concert with their trusted physicians, to make these decisions for them. For these patients, insistence by their physicians that they execute living wills would be unethical and inappropriate. A skilled physician must be able to distinguish between patients who want and need to know the facts in order to be able to exercise their autonomy, and patients who do not, for either psychosocial or cultural reasons, wish to discuss these issues.

All states have some formal way of enabling patients to appoint health care proxies who can exercise powers of medical decision making for them if they lack capacity. Every physician must acquaint himself with the laws of his state in order to facilitate the expression of patient autonomy.

A brief description of some of the formal vehicles that allow patients to delineate their wishes about medical care is in order.

ADVANCE DIRECTIVES

An advance directive is a written document—such as a living will, medical power of attorney, or designation of a health care proxy—in which a patient discusses his wishes concerning treatment options in situations where he lacks capacity. Many standardized forms exist that allow patients to check off treatment options (ventilator care, resuscitation, artificial feeding, antibiotics, etc.) in various clinical scenarios. The problem with these forms is that they cannot predict nuanced medical situations that so often face the physician with a patient who lacks capacity. Not infrequently, the inflexibility of the directives contained in these documents force the physician into uncomfortable situations of either violating the letter of the directive or of following medical decisions of dubious medical appropriateness. For this reason, many clinicians involved with end-of-life care prefer a health care proxy, who is familiar with the patient's broad philosophy of life and wishes for care.

HEALTH CARE PROXY

Many states allow designation by a patient of a health care proxy who is invested with legal powers to make decisions concerning virtually all aspects of medical treatment, including termination of life support and nutrition/hydration. The health care proxy has broad powers over decision making and acts in the patient's place. This person can be anyone of the patient's choosing except for his personal physician. It is presumed that when selecting a health care proxy, the patient has discussed personal preferences regarding care in the events that are likely to require intervention by the agent.

SURROGATES

The term "surrogates" refers to the people consulted by physicians when patients lack capacity and have not left written advance directives or designated health care proxies/agents. Surrogates are usually spouses, significant others, close family members, or close friends.

Unfortunately, only 10–15% of patients in the United States have written advance directives or health care proxies. In those situations where advance directives or proxies are lacking, most states permit decision making by surrogates, in consultation with the patients' physician, even if patients had never given clear and convincing evidence of their wishes through prior discussions with family or friends. In many states, the decisions can extend even to such matters as removal of life support and discontinuation of nutrition and hydration. Even though these surrogates often lack legal powers to make decisions, most states have not challenged their decision-making authority when it is done responsibly in concert with physicians.

The accuracy of surrogates in reflecting the incapacitated patient's presumed wishes is very questionable, however, as shown by a number of studies. These studies have documented the inaccuracy of surrogate decision making, except when the patient had prior discussions with the surrogate (3–5).

PROBLEMS THAT IMPEDE ELDERLY PATIENTS FROM EXERCISING THEIR AUTONOMY

Elderly patients are particularly at risk for not being able to make their wishes known concerning end-of-life or critical illness care because of the significant incidence of dementia in this population. They are also more prone to confusion and agitation in the hospital setting, which may place insurmountable obstacles in the way of a physician trying to determine the patient's wishes.

For these reasons, it is particularly important for physicians treating the elderly to raise the issue of advance directives and of designating a health care proxy as early as possible in the physician–patient relationship. Physicians must develop their skills in discussing these issues in a tactful and nonthreatening manner with their patients—in particular, when the latter are not ill—so that the entire matter assumes a more comfortable, matter-of-fact atmosphere.

Ideally, in the near future, a portion of the intake forms every primary care physician uses for evaluating a new patient will contain an entry for advance directives, thereby reminding the physician of his or her obligation to inquire about and discuss their patients' wishes.

Beneficence

The ethical value of beneficence is the core of being a healer. The relationship between beneficence and autonomy may be accurately described in this manner: "...beneficence provides the primary goal and rationale of medicine and health care, whereas respect for autonomy (along with nonmaleficence and justice) sets moral limits on the professional's action in pursuit of this goal" (6). Over 2000 yr ago, Hippocrates in his work *Epidemics* wrote "as to disease, make a habit of two things—to help, or at least to do no harm." Two millennia and the technology of organ transplantation, ventilators, dialysis, and ventricular-assist devices have not changed the importance of this principle one iota. In fact, beneficence remains the core value of medical ethics, although its pure expression may need to be modified by consideration of the values of nonmaleficence, autonomy, and justice.

One major aspect of the principle of beneficence as it pertains to medical ethics in the elderly that deserves careful attention is that of *proportionalism*. In assessing the ultimate benefit of a treatment, one must balance the potential good that may result against the cost in terms of patient suffering—the burden–benefit ratio. This assessment is particularly important and complex in the elderly patient for whom there is a lower likelihood of benefit from a particular treatment and a higher probability of experiencing deleterious side effects (7).

The question of chemotherapy provides a clear example or proportionalism. Whether or not to embark on a course of chemotherapy in an octogenarian with inoperable non-small-cell lung carcinoma is a more complex question than whether or not to use the same protocol in a 50-yr-old patient. Although in both cases the patient must be suitably informed of medication side effects, likelihood of response, and prognosis with and without therapy, the assessment is more complex in the elderly patient.

Even the relatively simple issue of anticoagulation in the elderly patient with atrial fibrillation presents greater difficulty than it would in a younger one. The patient's susceptibility to falls, the problem of coumadin interacting with other medications, the greater likelihood of faulty patient compliance because of confusion or forgetfulness, and the logistical problems posed by the need for frequent visits to a lab for prothrombin time monitoring are some of the issues that make this mode of therapy more problematic in the elderly patient.

Decisions regarding both elective and emergency surgery present an even greater ethical challenge in the elderly patient. If we revisit the example of lung cancer, the question of operating on an octogenarian with a resectable malignancy is more vexing than operating on a younger patient. Comorbid conditions weigh heavily in the decision-making process, and only a skilled, unhurried assessment by a physician can give meaningful and accurate projections of the risks of an operation as well as predicted life expectancy with and without successful surgery. The physician must also become familiar with the patient's social setting, support system, coping mechanisms, and personality lest an inaccurate assessment be made and an operation, despite its technical success, produce a depressed, dependent, and debilitated person who will forever view with regret the day he consented to surgery.

Cardiac surgery in the elderly is another expanding field where the principle of beneficence must be tempered by the realities of the patient's physical and mental condition, as well as his social support system. A Clinical Problem-Solving feature article of *The New England Journal of Medicine* discussed the pros and cons of cardiac bypass and aortic valve replacement surgery in an otherwise healthy 87-yr-old woman. Although the patient survived the operation, transferred to a rehabilitation center 3 wk later, and was able to resume her household duties 5 mo later, the discussant raised important questions of the appropriateness of such surgery in the very elderly and underscored the difficulties in making balanced and objective recommendations to such patients. He noted:

> Even when randomized clinical trials have been performed (which is true for only a small number of clinical problems), they will often not answer the question [whether to operate] specifically for the patient sitting in front of us.... The changing demographic characteristics of our patient population will present us with these difficult decision-making conundrums more often as we have to make therapeutic decisions for older and older patients *(8)*.

In some cases, however, statistical analyses of certain medical and surgical treatments or operations can provide us with important information to assist us in deciding whether or not to proceed with treatment. For example, a recent retrospective review of 24 octogenarians who underwent emergency surgery for acute type A aortic dissection showed that there was an in-hospital mortality of 83% and a 6-mo postoperative mortality of 100%. The intraoperative mortality was 33% *(8)*. If surgeons at other medical centers confirm the accuracy of these figures, it can surely be argued that operating on an octogenarian with acute type A aortic dissection at the present time would be unethical.

Another aspect of the principle of beneficence particularly relevant to the care of the elderly is the potential conflict between what the physician feels is her duty to do for her patient and the exercise by the patient of her autonomous rights. "Whether respect for the autonomy of patients should have priority over professional beneficence directed at those patients is a central problem in biomedical ethics" *(9)*. When a physician, in the interests of his patient, overrides the latter's regard for treatment or nontreatment or does not fully disclose the medical facts at hand, he is said to be paternalistic. In other words, a physician acts paternalistically when he feels that beneficence should override autonomy.

However, the issue is often not as simple as stated and many, if not most, cases of paternalism involve instances where the patient's autonomy is not fully violated or where an incomplete and selective recitation of the medical facts is made by the physician to the patient for her benefit. The reason that issues of paternalism affect the elderly disproportionately is because of the higher incidence of both serious illness and impaired cognition among the elderly, both of which create scenarios in which physicians are more likely to have to make decisions for patients, with or without their full understanding and in the face of an inability to achieve truly informed consent.

Nonmaleficence

The principle of nonmaleficence requires physicians to abstain from any action that causes harm to a patient. The principle of *primum non nocere*, namely "first do no harm," is well known to all physicians. It is immediately apparent to any clinician, however, that medical practice is filled with instances in which inflicting harm on patients is acceptable as long as the harm is compensated for by a more significant good. The pain of surgery and the side effects of many chemotherapeutic agents are but two obvious examples of acceptable harm in the course of daily medical and surgical practice.

There are other areas of medicine, often involving elderly patients, in which the benefit–burden ratio of medical actions is far more subtle than the above examples. Specifically, the ethical issues involved in withholding or withdrawing treatment from patients, including removal of life support or artificial nutrition and hydration, raise the question of whether the physician who orders these actions violates the principle of "first do no harm." Is it harmful or beneficial to a patient who is dying of metastatic cancer with no hope of leaving the hospital alive to remove him from a ventilator that is prolonging the dying process? Does a physician who removes a feeding tube from a severely demented patient in accordance with his previously expressed wishes violate the principle of nonmaleficence? Is there an ethical difference between not placing a patient on a ventilator and removing him from it or between not placing a feeding tube and removing one already in place?

Clearly, the ethical complexity of these questions attests to the fact that what distinguishes unacceptable maleficence from acts that may appear maleficent but which, upon closer reflection, are acceptable and perhaps even laudable are notions of benefit–burden and quality of life that go to the heart of medical ethics. Certainly, the values (often religious) of the patient must be respected in these situations.

Regardless of one's position on these issues, the direction our society has taken since the landmark Quinlan case of 1976 that permitted the parents of a young woman in a persistent vegetative state to remove her from a ventilator (she lived for 10 more years, however, while being fed through a feeding tube) is clear: in appropriate circumstances, patients may be removed from life-sustaining ventilatory support and may even have feeding tubes removed. The legal requirements for these actions vary from state to state, but the principles are similar: they reflect the patient's autonomous wishes as expressed in advance directives or as interpreted by a designated health care proxy. Alternatively, they are warranted by careful consideration of the benefit–burden factors of the case at hand.

The controversy over the ethical propriety of discontinuing artificial nutrition and hydration is more vigorous than the debate over so-called terminal extubation. The debate is over whether artificial nutrition/hydration should be considered a form of treatment, such as antibiotics or dialysis, or basic care, such as cleaning and grooming. In most states, discontinuing artificial nutrition/hydration can be carried out when certain criteria are met. Finally, the ethical distinction between withholding and withdrawing treatment has been rejected in many legal decisions and by the vast majority of medical ethicists.

Justice

The final principle of medical ethics is justice, by which we usually mean fairness and equity in allocation of limited health care resources. It represents the principle that people should receive health care based on need rather than entitlement based on class, wealth, race, age, or other criteria unrelated to medical factors. This principle is different from the others in that it usually relates to issues that are most properly decided in the larger arena of societal health care policies. These choices are usually made by government rather than by individual physicians or hospital committees.

The factors that influence how decisions are made by society regarding allocation of limited health care resources reflect different values. A libertarian approach views the rights of property and personal liberty as paramount and does not regard health care *per se* as a right. It holds individuals responsible for procuring health care insurance. A utilitarian view values the greatest good for the greatest number as the ideal and supports government activism in pursuit of this goal. In fact, most societies fall somewhere between these extremes and enact policies closer or farther from them depending on the country's cultural values, traditions, and politics.

The issue of age is raised in many questions relating to the principle of justice in medical ethics. Should age play a role in the allocation of limited health resources? If so, in what manner and to what extent? The term "agism" was coined to refer pejoratively to policies that discriminate against people solely on the basis of their advanced age. Nevertheless, age often plays a significant positive role in the allocation of resources.

The most obvious example is Medicare, an entitlement program as inviolable as Social Security, which discriminates in favor of the elderly by allocating huge sums of money for the medical care of citizens over the age of 65. No other group in the United States is favored in this manner. Medicaid, which targets the poor, is far less ambitious and less costly.

One might argue that Medicare unjustly favors the elderly at the expense of the young by unfairly allocating health care dollars disproportionately to those who have already lived most of their life-span and away from those who have not. Younger taxpayers, who subsidize Medicare, may not be able to afford health care, which may cause their health to suffer.

On the other hand, one can argue that justice requires both giving to the infirm elderly the care that they are likely to need far more than the healthy young as well as returning the fruits of their labor to them by repaying them with money they contributed to the program during their years of employment.

A stark example of how age can affect the distribution of health care is the difficulty faced by elderly patients in the United Kingdom in obtaining hemodialysis. Clearly, British society views the principle of justice in allocating limited medical resources differently from Americans.

On the other hand, age limits exist in virtually every transplant program, even in the United States. The difference in the American approach to the elderly regarding dialysis and organ transplantation may be summarized by stating that when the limited resource is money—as in the provision of dialysis—our wealthy society is willing to draw on its financial resources as much as necessary to provide a life-sustaining technology. When the limiting factor is the number of available donor organs, however, age issues impact more decisively for two reasons. The first is for strictly medical considerations, namely the often better medical prognosis of younger patients. In addition, a value judgment is made that a younger patient is more entitled to the scarce organ to be able to enjoy those years of life that might be denied him because of illness to a greater extent than his older counterpart.

In the vast majority of questions involving individual doctor–patient relationships, a patient's age should not impact on the question of the just allocation of medical resources. These are questions that need to be addressed by governmental and medical professional bodies considering society as a whole and not by doctors at the bedside. This standard is reinforced in the recently reformulated Principles of Medical Ethics of the American Medical Association. The eighth principle states: "A physician shall, while caring for a patient, regard responsibility to the patient as paramount" *(10)*.

COMMON ETHICAL ISSUES IN THE ELDERLY
Withdrawal of Life Support

Until the landmark 1976 Karen Anne Quinlan Case, it was considered unethical and illegal for physicians to remove patients from life support. The New Jersey Supreme Court Justices ruled that physicians could to remove a young woman in a persistent vegetative state from a ventilator based on her rights to refuse treatment as expressed through her surrogates—her parents. Since then, as physicians and Western society in general have become more "comfortable" with this practice, it has become commonplace for patients meeting certain legal and clinical criteria to be removed from life support.

In general, the criteria involve either written advance directives that relate to the clinical situation at hand, the appointing of a health care proxy/agent who has the legal power to act in the patient's place, or previously expressed verbal statements relating to the current case. Most states allow surrogates to request removal of life support even in the absence of any of the three previous criteria based on the surrogate's estimate of the patient's wishes or on their assessment of what is in the patient's best interests. In general, these criteria differ from state to state, and it behooves physicians to be familiar with the laws in their particular locale regarding this sensitive issue.

The issue is particularly relevant to the elderly who comprise the majority of patients in whom so-called "terminal extubation" is considered. This is because they are prone to the sorts of illnesses and medical catastrophes that give rise to these questions.

The circumstances under which this action is considered is usually one of the following:

1. A patient with severe and irreversible brain damage, often as a result of a hypoxic insult suffered at the time of a cardiac arrest or as a result of a devastating cardiovascular accident.
2. A patient with multiorgan failure and no reasonable chance of survival to hospital discharge, for whom continued ventilator care represents prolongation of the dying process.
3. The ethically challenging patient who can survive to discharge but with permanent disability of a degree that precludes him or her from having an acceptable quality of life, based on prior written or verbal evidence of the patient.

The ethical pitfall to avoid in removing life support from an elderly patient is to inappropriately factor in age, independent of the patient's known or suspected directives. An elderly patient is entitled to as much aggressive care as a younger patient. Age should enter into decisions of terminating life support only insofar as it impacts on the patient's medical prognosis.

Physician-Assisted Suicide

Oregon is the only state in which physician-assisted suicide (PAS) is legal. However, there is clearly significant public interest in PAS. Both the American Medical Association and the American College of Physicians—American Society of Internal Medicine have officially come out against the practice (11). Because the incidence of depression and suicide is higher among the elderly, this group of patients would probably make up a disproportionate percentage of those requesting PAS. In addition, feelings of being a financial and emotional burden on children are prevalent among the elderly and might well serve as further incentives to request physicians' assistance in committing suicide. No built-in safeguards can be so effective as to remove the unintended burden that legalizing PAS might have on the elderly and the disabled. Arguments against PAS have been well articulated many times and need not be repeated here (12,13).

Do Not Resuscitate (DNR)

Because elderly patients are more likely to be suffering from end-stage chronic degenerative or neoplastic illnesses than younger patients, they are more likely than younger patients to have a DNR order in their charts. In theory, these orders have been written after the patient has had a discussion with his physician during which the pros and cons of the decision have been carefully weighed. In practice, DNR orders are often not discussed with elderly patients, who may be either demented or too ill for a meaningful discussion to take place. In part, this is unavoidable, given circumstances surrounding these deliberations. At times, however, physician discomfort about raising these issues hinders the process. Ideally, the issue should be raised by physicians as early as is appropriate and under more relaxed circumstances than those surrounding a desperately ill patient. If the patient lacks capacity, the DNR discussion should be conducted with the patient's proxy or surrogate.

There is nothing more medically inappropriate and ethically questionable than to carry out cardiopulmonary resuscitation on a patient with a terminal illness in whom a "successful" resuscitation will merely prolong the dying and suffering process by days or weeks of ventilator-dependent ICU existence. In general, this misuse of medical technology and gratuitous assault on a dying patient can be avoided if appropriate DNR discussions are held with the patient or the family. Physicians have raised the question as to whether it should even be necessary to obtain patient consent for DNR when resuscitation will almost certainly prolong the dying process (14).

Patients who are DNR are *not* likewise DNT—"do not treat." It is unfortunate that patients and families are sometimes appropriately fearful of the implications of a DNR order in the chart. They have either experienced or been warned by others of examples of patients in whom nonresuscitative care was affected negatively by the DNR order. There is simply no excuse for this. A patient who does not wish to suffer the indignities of an inappropriate resuscitation should not be spared any other forms of treatment unless these are his wishes. For example, there is no reason that a DNR patient should not benefit from the added care of an ICU if it is appropriate. A patient with end-stage Chronic Obstructive Pulmonary Disease (COPD), for instance, who refuses to be placed on a ventilator, should not be denied the benefit of frequent pulmonary toilet, blood gas monitoring, and other features of ICU care that might help him survive an exacerbation of his illness.

Finally, the question of DNR status in the operating room is one that has perplexed anesthesiologists and ethicists for over a decade. Different hospitals have their own policies on this question. Some continue to mandate canceling the DNR order in the operating room (OR), but many hospitals now permit the DNR order to carry through the operation under certain guidelines. If, for example, the patient can be resuscitated quickly and effectively because of a problem specifically related to the operation or the anesthesia, resuscitation is carried out despite the DNR order. If, however, resuscitation is required for an arrest that is more directly related to the patient's underlying disease, it may be withheld. Despite common practice, often the distinction is blurred.

In general, if the DNR is to be carried over to the OR, a detailed discussion with the patient should be held prior to the operation, in which the criteria for withholding or implementing resuscitation are discussed *(15)*.

Evaluation of Decision-Making Capacity

In order for a patient to adequately exercise his right of autonomy, he must possess mental capacity. As a group, the elderly are problematic in this regard because of their far higher incidence of dementia and alterations of mental status resulting from illness and hospitalization, whether or not the patient has the mental capacity to give informed consent for a procedure is a common problem experienced by the clinician treating the elderly. ("Competence" is a similar term, but, strictly speaking, it should be used only after a legal determination has been made, not a clinical one).

Usually, the patient's physician can ascertain capacity without the need for psychiatric or neurologic evaluation. In cases of psychiatric illness, however, a psychiatrist should be consulted.

In determining capacity, a physician should ask the following questions *(16)*:

1. Does the patient understand the nature of his illness?
2. Does the patient understand the various treatment options, their benefits, and their risks?
3. Does the patient understand the probable consequences of refusing medical treatment or surgery?
4. Can the patient manipulate the information rationally and make a choice?

Physicians are often tempted to question an elderly patient's capacity solely because the patient refuses what appears to the physician to be a straightforward decision favoring a proposed course of action. In such cases, the physician must engage the patient in unhurried discussion of the reason for his choice and should consult with the patient's family when appropriate.

Even when a patient is found to lack capacity, the physician must exercise sensitive discretion when considering a course of action that will conflict with the patient's wishes. *Just because a patient lacks capacity does not mean that he thereby loses his rights to refuse or accept proposed treatment.* The impact of a course of unwanted medical or surgical treatment on a patient lacking capacity must be carefully considered in assessing the benefit–burden assessment of a planned course of action. For example, the decision of a patient lacking capacity who refuses a straightforward and life-saving appendectomy should not carry the same weight as a patient refusing cancer surgery when there is only a 50% chance for cure.

Futility

Futility is the "F word" of medical ethics. Clinicians are often admonished against using it because of its imprecision and its tendency to be used without careful and accurate analysis. A recent review of the subject concludes that the medical community has yet to agree on a precise definition of the term and that this is the major reason why courts have not upheld physicians who wish to terminate what they consider futile care against the wishes of patients or their surrogates *(17)*.

Nevertheless, physicians continue to use the term indiscriminantly in medical records, most often when justifying a recommendation to withhold or withdraw further treatment from a desperately ill patient. Therefore, it is important to briefly analyze the concept of futility and offer suggestions as to how best to use this powerful term.

In general, there are three kinds of futility encountered in clinical practice. The first and most narrow definition of the term is "physiologic" futility. A treatment may be considered futile in this sense if it cannot achieve the physiologic goals it aims to achieve. For example, adding further pressors to a moribund patient in profound and irreversible septic shock could be considered physiologically futile and, therefore, unwarranted. Continuing to transfuse a massively bleeding patient with esophageal varices, profound liver failure, and an uncorrectable coagulopathy cannot achieve the intended physiologic aim of hemodynamically stabilizing the patient and restoring a falling hematocrit and is, therefore, physiologically futile and unwarranted. This is the narrowest and least controversial definition of futility, but it is also least often used in this manner.

A second way in which the term is used can loosely be referred to as "quantitative" futility. It refers to a situation in which the "quantity" of the patient's life, usually measured by survivability to discharge, is almost certainly not going to be influenced by the treatment in question, rendering treatment futile. Just how unlikely survival to discharge must be in order to qualify for appropriate usage of the term is debatable. Every clinician, however, can point to instances when the likelihood of a patient getting well enough to be discharged is virtually nil. Continuing certain treatments such as dialysis, pressors, and ventilators in such situations can legitimately be said to merely prolong the dying and suffering process.

The third and most controversial context in which the term is used is that of "qualitative" futility. In this case, a treatment is said to be futile if it cannot restore a patient to the quality of life that the patient considers the *sine qua non* of further existence. Thus, for example, a conscious patient with amyotrophic lateral sclerosis (ALS) might refuse treatment with a ventilator because such life support would be futile in the sense of restoring a quality of life sought by the patient, even though the patient might be stabilized medically and remain mentally alert for months or years in that condition. A diabetic patient might wish to have dialysis stopped because of an insufferably poor quality of life due to renal and cardiac failure, even though he might be kept alive for months with continued treatment.

Instead of rejecting use of the word "futility," we should encourage its *appropriate* use, because it conveys a powerful message but only when the precise sense in which the specified treatment is futile can be clearly defined. Such a definition is not only imperative in clarifying why a treatment is considered futile, but it also forces the physician to step back from the details of daily lab values and writing orders in order to define the goals of his patient's treatment. Articulation of these goals then becomes extremely useful not only to the entire medical and nursing team but also to the patient and his family.

One final point: in those few cases which have gone to court over the issue of physicians refusing a family's or patient's request for treatment because of alleged futility, the courts have, except in one case, ruled in favor of the patient *(18)*. This should give pause to physicians who wish to push confrontations with patients over allegedly futile treatments to their legal limits. Although the American Medical Association Council on Ethical and Judicial

Affairs has stated that it is ethically acceptable to halt futile treatments even against the wishes of patients. It notes, "The legal ramifications of this course of action are uncertain." In fact, when push comes to shove, almost all physicians are unwilling to act against patient or family wishes for fear of potential legal consequences.

At present, only one state has enacted legislation giving physicians the right to withdraw futile care against patient wishes. The Texas Advance Directives Act of 1999 allows futile treatment to be unilaterally withdrawn, but only after a detailed five-part process has been carried out *(19)*. This involves ethics consultation and mediation with the family, attempts at finding other hospitals that would be willing to provide the care in question, and an opportunity for legal appeal by the patient's family.

In practice, in the vast majority of cases where futility is invoked, either the family eventually agrees with the physician's assessment of the situation or, in case of persistent disagreement, the physician reluctantly comes around to the family's position for fear of legal consequences should he disobey their requests. Compromise positions are sometimes reached after suitable deliberations, usually with involvement of the ethics committee.

Medical Ethics Committees

Over the past 20 yr, as the field of medical ethics has evolved, an increasing number of hospitals have created ethics advisory committees to assist clinicians with difficult cases that raise the sorts of ethical issue discussed in this chapter. Several years ago, the Joint Commission on Accreditation of Healcare Organizations (JCAHO) required hospitals to have ethics committees in order to be accredited.

Ethics committees serve three major roles:

1. Consultations are provided when requested by physicians, patients, their surrogates, or any hospital personnel. Ethics committees can help resolve conflicts, and clarify ethical, legal, or procedural issues in complex cases.
2. Ethics committees provide education to physicians, nurses, and hospital employees.
3. Ethics committees assist in drawing up policies and procedures for hospitals to deal with questions posed by the ever-increasing sophistication of medical technology.

The medical ethics committee at the Columbia Presbyterian Center of New York–Presbyterian Hospital is called for consultations approx 180 times annually. Almost all of the requests involve end-of-life issues, cases of medical futility, and questions of patient capacity. A significant majority of these patients are elderly, underscoring the need for internists to familiarize themselves with the medical ethics issues discussed in this chapter.

HOW TO APPROACH A CASE
RAISING QUESTIONS OF MEDICAL ETHICS

When a physician encounters a clinical problem that involves questions of medical ethics, there are a number of steps that should be taken to clarify and organize the issues.

1. What are the precise questions that need to be answered? Is it a matter of interpreting an advance directive, assessing patient capacity, or dealing with family–physician or intrafamilial conflict and misunderstanding? Posing the question clearly is helpful both to the clinician and to the ethics consultant.
2. What are the medical facts of the case? It is surprising how often basic medical issues are overlooked in the confusion that may surround a complex case. A simple review of the

medical facts can often clarify the questions that are asked and point to their answers. It also affords the physician an opportunity to step back and look at the big picture: Where is this patient going medically? Do we need an updated and clarified prognosis from the consulting neurologist, cardiologist, and so forth?

3. In trying to ascertain the patient's wishes, it is obviously most important to make sure that the patient been consulted. When, as is often the case, the patient is too ill or lacks capacity, the family must be asked if there are any advance directives that are lying in a safe or in an attorney's office. Was a health care proxy ever designated? Did the patient ever discuss his wishes concerning end-of-life care? What was his reaction to the illnesses of friends of family? It is surprising how often meaningful written or verbal information can be obtained by simply asking the patient or the family.

4. It is imperative that the physician in charge of the patient's care have a sit-down conference with the patient or, when not possible, with members of the patient's family. There is no substitute for spending time with people to clarify issues and answer their questions. The major service provided by the ethics consultant is often simply to spend the time necessary with families for them to understand the facts and analyze the options in complex cases. What initially appear as insurmountable problems and unbridgeable positions often resolve after skilled and patient counseling of families.

It is not possible to practice clinical medicine responsibly today without knowledge of the basic issues of medical ethics that involve one's specialty. Especially for physicians who deal with the elderly, familiarity with the ethical issues raised by the broad range of questions relating to end-of-life matters is essential if one is to be an effective, skilled, and compassionate physician. Just as it would be inconceivable for a cardiologist to consider himself a good physician without knowing the latest recommendations for the treatment of angina, it would be a similar disservice to his patient to be ignorant of the laws, policies, and procedures of his state and hospital with regard to issues of DNR, capacity, advance directives, and removal of life support.

As medicine becomes ever more sophisticated, these issues will become even more prevalent and important. Future clinical research is sure to modify current practices on such questions as substituted judgment and futility. New ethical questions such as those raised by genetic testing, artificial hearts, and problems of patient confidentiality in the age of the electronic medical record are sure to appear in the next decade. To enable the busy physician to keep up with these questions, many medical journals are devoting more space to articles dealing with medical ethics.

The new field of medical ethics is thus faced with the great challenge of dealing in a balanced and skillful way with the issues raised by a medical technology that is evolving with breathtaking speed. How to balance respect for life, patient autonomy, and a just utilization of limited resources is a vexing and never-ending question. As soon as some answers are proposed, new challenges arise. Far from being a frustrating task, grappling with the questions of medical ethics can only enrich and deepen the satisfaction of what it means to be a doctor.

REFERENCES

1. Hayley DC, Cassel CK. Overview of ethical issues. In: Cassel CK, Cohen HJ, Larson EB, Meier DE, Resnick NM, Rubenstein LZ, Sorenson LB, eds. Geriatric Medicine, 3rd ed. Springer-Verlag, New York, 1997, p. 969.
2. Beauchamp TL, Childress JF. Moral norms. In: Principles of Biomedical Ethics, 5th ed. Oxford University Press, New York, 2001, pp. 2–3.

3. Seckler AB, Meier DE, Mulvihill M, Cammer BE. Substituted judgment: how accurate are proxy predictions? Ann Intern Med 1991;115:92–98.

4. Suhl J, Simons P, Reedy T, Garrick T. Myth of substituted judgment. Arch Intern Med 1994;154:90–96.

5. Sulmasy DP, Terry PB, Weisman CS, Miller DJ, Stallings RY, Vettese MA, et al. The accuracy of substituted judgment in patients with terminal diagnoses. Ann Intern Med 1998;128:621–629.

6. Beauchamp TL, Childress JF. Moral norms. In: Principles of Biomedical Ethics, 5th ed. Oxford University Press, 2001, p. 177.

7. Welch HG, Albertsen PC, Nease RF, Bubolz TA, Wasson JH. Estimating treatment benefits for the elderly: the effect of competing risks. Ann Intern Med 1996;124:577–584.

8. Thibault GE. Clinical problem-solving. Too old for what? N Engl J Med 1993;328:946–950.

9. Neri E, Toscano T, Massetti M, Capannini G, Carone E, Tucci E, et al. Operation for acute type A aortic dissection in octogenarians: is it justified? J Thorac Cardiovasc Surg 2001;121:259–267.

10. Principles of Medical Ethics, Committee on Ethics of the American Medical Association, adopted by AMA's House of Delegates, June 17, 2001.

11. Snyder L, Sulmasy D. Position paper: physician-assisted suicide. Ann Intern Med 2001;135:209–216.

12. The New York State Task Force on Life and the Law. When death is sought: assisted suicide and euthanasia in the medical context. New York State Task Force on Life and the Law. Albany, NY, 1994.

13. Hendin H. Suicide, assisted suicide, and medical illness. J Clin Psychiatry 1999;60(Suppl 2):46–50.

14. Blackhall LJ. Must we always use CPR? N Engl J Med 1987;317:1281–1285.

15. Truog R, Waisal D, Burns J. DNR in the OR, a goal-directed approach. Anesthesiology 1999;90:289–285.

16. Appelbaum PS, Grisso T. Assessing patient's capacities to consent to treatment. N Engl J Med 1988;319:1635–1638.

17. Helft P, Siegler M, Lantos J. The rise and fall of the futility movement. N Engl J Med 2000;343:293–296.

18. Daar JF. Medical futility and implications for physician autonomy. Am J Law Med 1995;21:221–240.

19. Fine RL. Medical futility and the Texas advance directives act of 1999. BUMC Proc 2000;13:144–147.

III   CARDIOVASCULAR CARE FOR THE ELDERLY

9

Cardiovascular Changes with Aging

Mathew S. Maurer, MD
and Myron L. Weisfeldt, MD

CONTENTS

INTRODUCTION

Over the past several decades, a body of literature has accumulated regarding the effects of aging on the structure and function of the cardiovascular system. The purpose of the present summary is to describe these changes and place them in a clinical context. It is clear from these data that aging is a selective process affecting certain portions of the cardiovascular system dramatically, while leaving others unaffected (*see* Table 1). Additionally, age-related changes in cardiovascular structure and function result in a phenotype that can significantly contribute to the development of disorders such as diastolic heart failure and syncope that disproportionately afflict the older individual. The management of cardiovascular disease in aged subjects can and should be undertaken with a basic understanding of the physiologic changes that are characteristic of the aging individual. It is with an understanding of these changes that the clinician can distinguish pathology from normative aging and ultimately provide more effective care for the elderly patient with cardiovascular disease.

There are several important lessons to be learned from previous endeavors of investigations of normative human aging of the cardiovascular system. First, the general problem of separating disease-related changes from age-related changes is a difficult one, and it has plagued research on aging. This is a particularly difficult dilemma in studies of the cardiovascular system in human beings because of the high prevalence of ischemic heart disease and generalized arteriosclerosis *(1)* with a minority of subjects manifesting symptoms. Extensive literature describes how cardiovascular function differs in older versus

From: *Aging, Heart Disease, and Its Management: Facts and Controversies*
Edited by: N. Edwards, M. Maurer, and R. Wellner © Humana Press Inc., Totowa, NJ

Table 1
Age-Related Changes in Cardiovascular Structure and Function

Altered with age	Stable with age
Prolonged contraction	Myocardial contractility
Diminished β-adrenergic responsiveness	Coronary blood flow
Increased myocardial and vascular stiffness	α-Adrenergic mediated vasoconstriction
Altered autonomic nervous system control	Autonomic nervous system control
Decreased arterial baroreflexes	Preserved cardiopulmonary baroreflexes
Increased sympathetic outflow	
Decreased vagal outflow	
Decreased VO_2	

younger individuals, yet confusion often arises in the interpretation of these data because of a failure to acknowledge or control for interactions with age, disease, and lifestyle. Initial studies (2) noted a significant decline in ejection fraction with exercise in the elderly as compared with younger individuals that was attributable to an age-related decrease in contractility. However, when subjects were rigorously screened for the absence of underlying cardiac disease by not only histories and physical examinations but also resting and stress electrocardiographs with supplemental imaging, the age-associated decline in ejection fraction was attenuated and the increase in cardiac output with exercise was found not to be limited with advancing age (3).

Second, although the "perfect study of aging," which controls for both disease and lifestyle, has yet to emerge, the study design can complicate and even limit the interpretations of various measures. In general, cross-sectional studies neither quantify nor control for lifestyle issues (exercise, nutrition, etc.) or birth cohort effects and thus intrinsically provide less insight into effects attributable to "aging" than longitudinal studies do. Longitudinal studies, on the other hand, are fraught with other problems, including confounding from the development of occult disease, changes in lifestyle such as reduction in body weight, smoking, or increase in physical activity over the lifetime of the individual. Also, techniques change over time and standardization of new methods is imperfect. In acknowledgment of these issues regarding the study of aging, scientists have delineated primary aging, that results from part of the genetic program and the influence of the passage of time, thus an inevitable part of the aging process, from secondary aging, which is attributable to the influence of extrinsic factors such as the development of disease or a confounding lifestyle issue. With this in mind, let us review the age-related changes in cardiovascular structure and function.

CARDIOVASCULAR STRUCTURE

Left-Ventricular Hypertrophy

Progressive cellular and overall left-ventricular hypertrophy with age occurs in parallel with the rise in arterial systolic blood pressure. Autopsy data from 7112 human hearts have demonstrated that the mass of the heart increased an average of 1 g/yr in men and 1.5 g/yr in women (4). The ratio of heart weight to body weight also increased. Other smaller autopsy studies *(5)*, which more carefully excluded patients with underlying cardiovascular disease, have demonstrated a reduction in volume of the myocardial mass resulting from myocyte loss. Although there is also reactive hypertrophy of the spared myocytes, which is more prominent in men than in women *(6)*, the loss of myocardial cells with age in men by far exceeds any change in mass. Thus, there is more striking cell hypertrophy than any change in cardiac mass or size *(7,8)*; this corresponds to the age-dependent rise in mean arterial blood pressure.

The effect of age on heart size has been assessed by several techniques, including echocardiography and gated blood pool scans. Most cross-sectional studies of sedentary volunteer subjects without heart disease have demonstrated that end-diastolic and end-systolic left-ventricle (LV) wall thickness and estimates of left-ventricular mass, measured via M-mode echocardiography, increase with age *(9–12)*. Other studies using M-mode echocardiography have found only a minor increase in LV mass with age in healthy women and no change in men *(13)*. It should be noted that M-mode echocardiography samples only a single small area of the left-ventricular posterior wall or ventricular septum and uses geometric assumptions that presuppose a constant left-ventricular shape at all ages. Data utilizing a three-dimensional echocardiographic reconstruction technique that is extremely accurate for measuring left-ventricular mass and volumes *(14)* have shown that left-ventricular mass declined with age, more so in men than in women *(see* Fig. 1). The end-diastolic volume (EDV) indexed to body surface area (BSA) declined from 0.75 for women <40 yr to 0.65 for women ≥60 and did not change in men (0.74 to 0.77). As a result, the ratio of EDV index to LV mass index did not correlate with age for either the entire cohort or among men, but declined in women. Similar data on LV cavity size in the seated position by gated cardiac blood pool scans demonstrated moderate increases in end-diastolic and end-systolic volume with age in healthy, normotensive sedentary men but did not vary in women *(15)*. The differences in left-ventricular structure with age between men and women are corroborated by both pathologic studies in humans, which have delineated that aging does not lead to striking myocyte loss and myocyte reactive hypertrophy in women *(16)*, and cross-sectional studies demonstrating that the cardiac adaptation to chronic pressure overload differs by gender in humans *(17)* and animals *(18)*. Whether or not these gender differences contribute to the pathophysiology of disorders that are observed with increased frequency in elderly women, such as diastolic dysfunction, is not clear.

Myocardial Collagen and Amyloid

Increases in the amount and physical properties of collagen (because of altered cross-linking) may play a role in causing the functional cardiovascular changes of aging *(19)*. Studies in humans have revealed that the cardiac muscle-to-collagen ratio either remains constant or increases in the older heart *(20)*. Measurements of collagen content in myocardial tissue suggest that both perimysial and endomysial collagen Type I fibers increase in number and thickness in the old *(21)*. These histochemical results coincided with the electron microscopic observations, showing an increase in the number of collagen fibrils with large diameter in the old hearts. This may be attributable to alterations in either the expression or activity of matrix metalloproteinases *(22)*.

The age-associated accumulation of amyloid in the human heart is well documented *(23)*. The prevalence and severity of cardiac amyloidosis is significantly related to age and gender, with females demonstrating the higher prevalence. Amyloid protein is found in approx 50% of elderly patients >70 yr of age and is frequently limited to the atrium. Whether

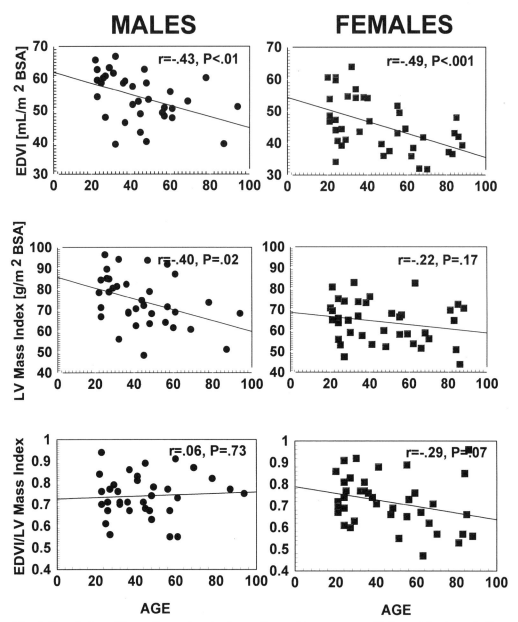

Fig. 1. Correlation of three-dimensional echocardiographic measures of left-ventricular end-diastolic volumes, mass, and volume-to-mass ratio with age in a population of normal subjects. All measures are indexed to body surface area.

or not cardiac amyloid can be considered a part of the normal aging process is debatable. Although cardiac amyloidosis was significantly correlated with the occurrence of both atrial fibrillation and cardiac failure, the histopathologic pattern (i.e., extent and pattern of deposits) is valuable in distinguishing primary amyloidosis from senile cardiac amyloidosis. "Senile" cardiac amyloid is often *(24)* but not exclusively associated with a mutant transthyretin *(25)*.

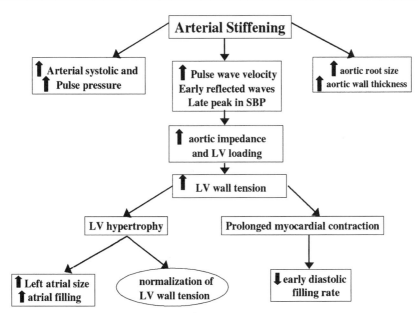

Fig. 2. Impact of age-related increases in central conduit artery stiffness on cardiovascular structure and function. (Adapted from ref. *93*.)

Arterial Stiffness and Pressure

An increase in central conduit artery stiffness with advancing age is a universal phenomenon in every society and contributes to many of the changes in the cardiovascular system with age (*see* Fig. 2). Unlike the vascular intimal changes that are characteristic of arteriosclerosis, the increase in vascular stiffness that accompanies advancing age results from changes in the vascular media.

Changes in arterial stiffness with advancing age are accompanied by an increase in arterial diameter and wall thickness. Up to the age of 60 yr, the buffering capacity of the aorta is not markedly affected by the age-associated increase in arterial stiffness, because the aorta enlarges. Thus, the increasing stiffness is offset by increasing volume *(26)*, and the volume elasticity (change in pressure for a given change in volume) shows no age-associated changes up to approx 60 yr of age, reflecting the increase in aortic volume up to that age *(27)*. After 60, volume elasticity markedly decreases and less diastolic aortic recoil occurs, resulting in a decreased aortic contribution to forward flow. As a result, a larger share of the burden of forward flow is imposed upon the left ventricle during systole *(28)*. Both the reduced distensibility and the increased volume of blood that has to be accelerated during systole increase the impedance to blood flow *(29)*.

Increases in aortic pulse wave velocity with aging are another result of increased aortic stiffness. This causes waves reflected from peripheral sites to the ascending aorta to occur at an earlier time (i.e., during the ventricular ejection period). Thus, the reflected waves merge with the incident (i.e., forward) wave generated by left-ventricular ejection and influence the contour of measured pulse contour (*see* Fig. 3) and systolic left-ventricular load or impedance. Another consequence of arterial stiffening, aside from the augmentation of late systolic pressure as a result of earlier wave reflection, is a reduction in diastolic

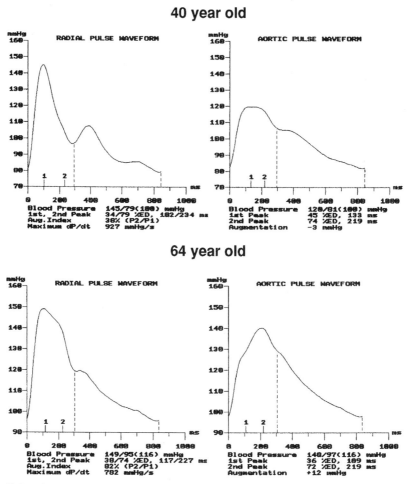

Fig. 3. Radial and central aortic derived waveforms from two subjects with similar cuff pressures but with markedly different central aortic waveforms. The aortic waveform in the older subject is characterized by early wave reflection during left-ventricular ejection, augmenting the central pressure by 12 mm Hg, which is not present in the younger subject.

blood pressure (because the reflected wave normally returns after the aortic valve closes and thus contributes to the diastolic blood pressure) *(30)*. Because coronary perfusion is achieved during diastole, the changes in arterial waveforms can impair coronary perfusion and has been associated with the potential harm of further reducing the diastolic pressure with antihypertensive therapy, especially in patients with coronary heart disease that underlies the controversial "J curve" *(31)*.

The biologic processes that have been implicated in the development of central conduit arterial stiffness with age include loss of elastin and increase in collagen content *(32)*, change in the composition of collagen with a decrease in coiling and twisting of molecular chains resulting in a reduction in effective chain length *(33)*, and an increase in Ca^{2+} content *(34)* and collagen crosslinking *(35)*. The latter process has been the most widely studied *(36)*, and the advent of a new class of therapeutic agents, collagen crosslink breakers, has been recently shown to be effective in treating the primary manifestation of increased central conduit artery stiffness, namely a high pulse pressure *(37)*. In this study, 93 individuals >50 yr of age with a pulse pressure of >60 mm Hg, systolic blood pressure >140 mm Hg, and large artery compliance <1.25 mL/mm Hg were randomized to oral ALT-711 (210 mg, once per day) or placebo for 56 d in a 2:1 fashion. ALT-711 resulted in a greater decline in pulse pressures than placebo (−5.3 vs −0.6 mm Hg), and total arterial compliance rose 15% in ALT-711-treated subjects vs no change with placebo, an effect that did not depend on reduced mean pressure. Therapy with this collagen cross-link breaker improves total arterial compliance in aged humans with vascular stiffening, and it may represent a novel therapeutic approach for this abnormality, which occurs with aging, diabetes, and isolated systolic hypertension. Whether this therapeutic approach is associated with long-term development of aneurysm is a concern.

Venous Stiffness and Capacitance

It is clear that profound peripheral arterial abnormalities are an integral part of the aging process. Changes in structure have been demonstrated in both the arteries and the veins, although the major emphasis of study over the past two decades has been placed on the arterial system. This is because (1) measuring arterial vasoconstriction, changes in afterload, and indices of ejection are much easier than quantifying changes in preload, venoconstriction, and indices of filling and (2) it was recognized that cardiac performance is significantly enhanced by afterload reduction (*see* the section Clinical Implications later in this chapter).

Veins serve an important yet often overlooked variable blood storage function. The large capacity of these vessels permits this low-pressure reservoir to contain as much as 85% of the systemic blood volume based on data from nonhuman species; 70% of this is in the systemic veins and 15% in the heart and lungs *(38)*. The pronounced capacity of this reservoir implies that even small volume changes in the peripheral veins are followed by substantial differences in central blood volume. Thus, reflex alterations in venous vasomotor tone provide a rapidly acting mechanism for compensatory redistribution of the blood volume. For example, venoconstriction acts to partially restore a normal cardiac preload during the assumption of upright posture. Additionally, Guyton *(39)* has shown that intact cardiovascular reflexes mediated through venous vasoconstriction prevent pooling of blood in the peripheral circulation, which is essential to the development of a full cardiac output response to increased metabolism. The research into changes in venous properties with age is limited.

Stress–strain relations of human pulmonary veins have shown an age-related increase in venous stiffness but to a much smaller degree than that observed in the pulmonary arteries *(40)*. The venous compliance of the calf is reduced by 45% with age, with a concomitant reduction in the capacitance response of the calf veins during lower-body negative pressure *(41)*. The pathophysiologic significance of changes in the venous system with age has several clinical implications. This may account for a generalized reduction in baroreceptor reflexes in response to orthostasis, which would be attributable to a decrease in the central blood volume (i.e., deactivation of the baroreceptors) rather than an abnormality in efferent baroreceptor function *(42)*. Additionally, an increase in central blood volume that would result from reduced peripheral venous capacitance may cause an increased preload and provide an explanation for the higher filling pressures, which are characteristic of diastolic heart failure.

Venous characteristics vary markedly from region to region in such a way that the hydrostatic forces associated with upright posture are counteracted *(43)*. In dependent regions of the human body, there is a thickening of the vein walls that tends to oppose some of the hydrostatic pressure encountered during upright posture. In contrast, veins near or above the heart are thin walled and more distensible *(44)*. A majority of the venous volume is stored in the splanchnic bed, which is difficult to study noninvasively. A significant negative correlation has been observed between age and liver blood volume *(45)*, and postprandial changes in blood pressure can exacerbate orthostatic hypotension in elderly subjects *(46)*. In summary, the venous system is not only an understudied and underappreciated regulator of cardiovascular function but also, based on classic physiologic principles, likely plays a significant mechanistic role in the development of disorders that disproportionately afflict the elderly, including diastolic dysfunction and orthostatic hypotension.

FUNCTIONAL PARAMETERS

Coronary Blood Flow

In both experimental animals *(47)* and in man, the maximum capacity of the coronary vascular bed is not altered by aging. When myocardial blood flow was measured in subjects without coronary artery disease at rest and at maximum vasodilatation with dipyridamole and assessed by either coronary sinus flow techniques during cardiac catherization or with positron-emission tomography, no significant correlation was observed with increasing age *(48)*. Myocardial blood flow in response to limitations of oxygen supply is correlated with the age-associated increase in heart weight. Above the age of 60, there is significant increase in basal flow that is associated with an increase in systolic blood pressure *(49)*. Because histologic examination reveals no evidence of structural changes in the coronary vessels, any age-related decrease in coronary flow is likely the result of a failure of the vascular bed to increase in proportion to heart mass. These data suggest that the reduced flow reserve with age is primarily the result of increased cardiac work and blood flow at rest rather than to an abnormal vasodilator capacity *(50)*. The clinical implications of these findings are that manifested coronary ischemia is never a result of normative aging but, rather, reflects the superimposition of arteriosclerosis.

Myocardial Contractility

In vivo measurement of myocardial contractility is difficult in humans. The relationship between heart rate-corrected velocity of fiber shortening and circumferential end-systolic stress is a standard echocardiographic measure of muscle contractility that is relatively load independent *(51,52)*. The rate-corrected velocity of fiber shortening and circumferential end-systolic stress (Vcf–cESS) relationship is plotted in Fig. 4 for younger and older subjects free of cardiovascular disease, with the slope of the regression line representing a measure of inotropic state. Analysis of covariance was employed to compare the slope of the Vcf–cEss relation between cohorts and did not demonstrate a difference in slope or elevation, confirming the lack of an age-related change in contractility.

End-systolic elastance (E_{es}), an index of ventricular chamber contractility, is defined as the slope of the end-systolic pressure–volume relationship (ESPVR) and is normally derived from a series of pressure-volume loops obtained during a vena-caval occlusion and invasive measurement of end-systolic pressure (P_{es}) and volume. This is a load-independent measure of contractility, but the invasive nature of this approach has limited its

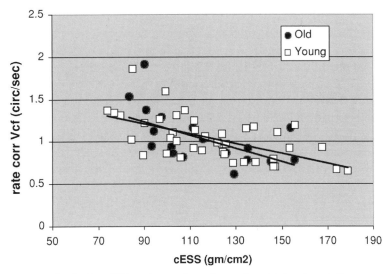

Fig. 4. Rate-corrected velocity of fiber shortening–circumferential end systolic stress relationship in a cohort of healthy young and old subjects. The slope of this relationship does not differ between the two cohorts, indicating preservation of myocardial contractility.

widespread application. We and others *(53)* have employed echocardiographic derived measurements of volume on steady-state beats to derive two related estimates of E_{es} by making two assumptions: (1) that end-systolic pressure is equivalent to either mean arterial pressure (MAP) or systolic aortic blood pressure (SBP) (both assumptions have been made in the literature) and (2) that volume of the ventricle at zero pressure (V_0), the volume–axis intercept of the ESPVR, is 0 mL. Following these assumptions, E_{es} can be estimated as either $E_{es.m} \cong MAP/ESV$ or $E_{es.p} \cong SBP/ESV$, where ESV is the end-systolic volume. These measures have not demonstrated a significant decrease in myocardial contractility with age.

Other more global measures of the left-ventricular function at rest, including ejection fraction, cardiac output, and cardiac index, have all been documented to remain stable with age at least until the seventh decade *(54)*. This is corroborated by animal data that demonstrate that the peak twitch force generated by isolated muscle strips does not alter with age *(55)*. Thus, all of the data support the construct that there is no age-related change in the intrinsic ability of cardiac muscle to develop force or exhibit contractility. Any change in left-ventricular performance is more related to a profound decrease in cardiac β-adrenergic responsiveness with aging *(56)*.

Heart Rate

The majority of cross-sectional studies have demonstrated no difference in supine basal heart rates in young versus older individuals *(57)*. Longitudinal studies of rigorously screened healthy individuals indicate that in the seated position, the heart rate decreases with age in both males and females *(53,58)*. Resting heart rate is modulated by the balance of the two arms of the autonomic nervous system, with parasympathetic innervation dominating. Changes in autonomic control that modulate the heart rate are responsible for the interaction of age and posture on heart rate (*see* the Baroreflex/Autonomic Nervous System Control section).

With exercise, the maximal heart rate response declines significantly in the older individual. The decrease in maximal heart rate achieved during exercise has been defined for decades by the formula 220 − age. This decline in maximal heart rate is not attributable to disease or sedentary lifestyle, because a decline of similar magnitude occurs in healthy sedentary men and women as well as older athletes *(59)*. A recent meta-analysis of 351 studies involving 18,712 subjects determined that maximal heart rate was strongly related to age ($r = -0.90$), using the equation 208 − 0.7 (age). Cross-validation of the new equation in a population of 514 healthy subjects revealed a virtually identical equation to that obtained from the meta-analysis. The regression line was not different between men and women, nor was it influenced by wide variations in habitual physical activity levels *(60)*.

Baroreflex/Autonomic Nervous System Control

The general perception is that baroreflex sensitivity is reduced in older individuals. This assumption is based mainly on observations of an attenuated heart rate slowing during experimental baroreceptor activation *(61)*.

Just as aging exerts a selective effect on the human cardiovascular system, senescence affects autonomic cardiovascular control mechanisms selectively. Attenuation of arterial baroreflex control of heart rate, which manifests clinically as decreased respiratory sinus arrhythmia, has been shown to be impaired with age and is attributable to a decline in parasympathetic control of sinus node function with age *(62)*. However, elevations in basal levels of plasma catecholamines *(63)* and muscle sympathetic nerve activity *(64)* along with preserved response to the cold pressor test *(65)* indicate the selective effect of aging on autonomic control mechanisms.

The data on changes in baroreflex control of sympathetic nervous system activity with age have been inconsistent. Some studies document impairments in baroreflex control, including impaired cardiopulmonary baroreflex control of renal sympathetic nerve activity in animals *(66)* and impaired reflex control of forearm vascular resistance in response to orthostatic stress in humans *(67,68)*. Others have documented preservation *(69)* or even augmentation of forearm vascular resistance to lower-body negative pressure, indicating preservation of the sympathetic component of the baroreflex in healthy elderly individuals at least until the seventh decade of life *(70)*. The apparent inconsistencies between findings of various studies are probably related to several factors. Differences in sites at which the sympathetic activity was sampled (i.e., renal, splanchnic, muscle, etc.) may be explanatory. It is likely that the sympathetic outflow to one vascular bed is not necessarily representative of sympathetic activity in other regions and suggests that the aging process may affect baroreflex regulation of sympathetic outflow to the various regional circulations in a nonuniform manner. Additionally, there is significant redundancy and interaction of various baroreceptor systems, which has been reported to decline with age *(71)*. Selectively studying each system (aortic, carotid, cardiopulmonary) in intact human subjects is not possible. Thus, the differences between reports may be related to differences in techniques used to elicit various baroreceptor responses, some of which invoke reflexes in several receptor systems simultaneously.

The mechanisms involved in the selective loss of baroreceptor function with age are not clear. Defects in the afferent, central nervous system processing, and efferent response in the reflex arc have been postulated, with the evidence favoring the former two mechanisms. With age-related increases in arterial stiffness, the transduction of pulsatile pressure to the baroreceptors is significantly impaired and mechanistically contributes to the age-related decline in cardiovagal baroreflex sensitivity *(72)*. Recent data suggest that both mechanical and neural components are linked to age-related impairments in baroreflex-mediated control of heart rate but that alterations in central nervous system control may be the more important mechanism *(73)*.

Prolonged Contraction/Abnormal Diastolic Filling

Although a complete review of the complexities of diastole is beyond the scope of this review, traditionally, abnormalities of both active relaxation (indexed by increased time constant of pressure fall, τ) and passive diastolic ventricular properties (decreased chamber compliance, which is most accurately measured from end-diastolic pressure-volume relationships, EDPVR) are thought to contribute to the age-associated decrease in diastolic filling *(74)*. Despite the commonly held belief that left-ventricular compliance decreases with aging, the EDPVR has not been measured in healthy humans because of the invasive nature of such a measurement.

The time-course of isovolumic myocardial relaxation (IVRT) is prolonged with aging in both men and women *(75)*. The peak rate at which the left ventricle fills during early diastole is significantly reduced with age, as demonstrated by echo-Doppler and radionuclide techniques *(76,77)*. Factors other than age, including physical activity and loading conditions, affect the left-ventricular filling rate as measured by Doppler techniques *(78)*. However, age appears to be the predominant factor, with peak left-ventricular filling rates being similar between older endurance-trained athletes and age-matched sedentary controls *(79,80)*. These data, along with that of Hajjar et al. demonstrating that diastolic parameters were significantly improved by overexpression of sarcoplasmic reticulum calcium transport pump 2a (SERCA2a), suggest that alterations in diastolic function may be a consequence of altered systolic loading *(81)*. Despite the uncertainties of the mechanism underlying the observed age-associated decline in early left-ventricular filling, atrial augmentation of late left-ventricular filling increases *(82)* and is the basis of a fourth heart sound in most healthy older individuals.

Diminished β-Adrenergic Responsiveness

There is a marked decrease in the response of the cardiovascular system to β-adrenergic stimulation with age. In studies of isolated muscle from rats, the intrinsic inotropic response to catecholamines was diminished *(83)*. Human cardiac muscle shows a very similar pattern of reduction in the response to isoproterenol with age. This occurs by multiple mechanisms, including downregulation and decreased agonist binding of β_1 receptors, uncoupling of β_2 receptors, abnormal G-protein-mediated signal transduction and decreased phosphorylation of regulatory proteins *(84,85)*. Presumably, in an attempt to compensate for the age-related decline in β-adrenergic responsiveness, an augmentation of plasma catecholamines is seen during dynamic exercise in older as compared with younger individuals *(86)*.

As already mentioned, there is a significant decrease in the maximal heart rate with age, which is largely attributable to decreases in β-adrenergic responsiveness. Ejection fraction and cardiac index increase more in younger vs older individuals in response to β-adrenergic stimulation *(87)*. Failure of the β-adrenergic relaxant effect on aortic smooth muscle is partially responsible for the increase in impedance to left-ventricular ejection. Decreases in venous responses to β- but not α-adrenergic stimulation may alter important circulatory responses during exercise *(88)*. These changes with aging are similar to those observed in the β-adrenergic system of patients with heart failure and suggest that age-related differences in exercise cardiovascular performance with advancing age are the result, at least partially, of diminished target-organ responsiveness to adrenergic stimulation (*see* the section Clinical Implications: Cardiovascular Responses to Exercise).

CLINICAL IMPLICATIONS

Cardiovascular Responses to Exercise

Despite the age-related changes delineated thus far, cardiac output during maximal exercise does not decline significantly with age. Because maximal heart rate declines with age, it follows that in order to achieve a maximum cardiac output with exercise similar to a younger individual, the older subject must rely more on the Frank–Starling mechanism *(89)*. Thus, the stroke volume index at maximal exercise increases in older men, because of substantial end-diastolic dilatation, and offsets the heart rate deficit. In women, with normative aging, there is a greater heart rate response to exercise than in men across relative work rates *(90)*.

The age-associated decline in the heart rate response and the increase in left-ventricular volumes at maximal exercise are manifestations of the age-related decline in the efficacy of the sympathetic response during exercise stress. This has been demonstrated rather elegantly in a study in which young male subjects were "made old" through the administration of propanolol to mimic the age-related decline in maximal heart rate response with exercise. In response to β-adrenergic blockade, younger subjects demonstrated many of the age-related changes during maximal exercise testing, including an increase in end-diastolic volume index *(91)*.

Greater Potential Benefit
of Afterload Reduction Especially in Heart Failure

As described previously, an increase in the vascular component of LV afterload with normal aging results in a limitation of the augmentation of stroke volume (SV) elicited by the Frank–Starling mechanism in healthy older persons during exercise because of failure of the LV to empty as completely in older persons as it does in younger ones *(92)*. This results in an age-associated increase in end-systolic volume during exercise. During vigorous exercise, the increased LV vascular afterload and LV preload in older individuals cause the heart to dilate relative to the heart in younger individuals throughout the cardiac cycle *(93)*. This cardiac dilatation increases LV wall stress throughout the cardiac cycle in older vs younger individuals and contributes to the reduction in maximum LV ejection capacity with aging. This particular phenomenon is exacerbated even more under conditions associated with impaired myocardial contractility, such as with systolic heart failure. Indeed, among 25 patients with dilated cardiomyopathy, nitroprusside infusion decreased resistance, increased arterial compliance, and lowered pulse wave velocity in all groups but the effect was greater with advancing age *(94)*. These data demonstrate that in older patients with dilated cardiomyopathy, the left ventricle is coupled to an arterial circulation that has a greater pulsatile load, despite a similar steady load, and that these age-related changes in the arterial system affect the hemodynamic response to pharmacologically induced vasodilatation.

Decreased Response to Stress/Injury

From a physiologic standpoint, aging can be described as the progressive constriction of homeostatic reserve (homeostenosis) of every organ system; the cardiovascular system is no exception. Specifically, in response to physiologic stress or injury, a decreased responsiveness on an organ and cellular level has been observed. For example, the capacity for the left ventricle to hypertrophy to a volume overload stress *(95)* or acute pressure overload *(96)* diminishes with age. This reduced left-ventricular hypertrophic response resulted in persistent elevation of LV end-diastolic pressure and wall stress, potentially being an important mechanism in the observed increase in heart failure with normal systolic function in the elderly. Additionally, angiogenesis, the growth of new vessels from existing microvasculature, is delayed in aged humans *(97)* and may be attributable to changes in the levels of growth factors and proteins in the extracellular matrix *(98)*. This implies that restoration of the favorable mileu with the addition of growth factors can restore normal angiogenic potential. Thus, advanced age does not preclude augmentation of collateral vessel development in response to exogenous angiogenic cytokines *(97)*.

SUMMARY AND CONCLUSIONS

We have attempted to highlight the selective nature of changes in the cardiovascular system with age. Although these age-related alterations have been elucidated through physiologic experiments over the past few decades, the future challenge is for clinicians and physiologists to apply these lessons to the growing population of elderly patients with cardiovascular diseases in the hopes of developing rational and biology-based treatment strategies.

REFERENCES

1. Elveback L, Lie JT. Continued high incidence of coronary artery disease at autopsy in Olmsted County, Minnesota, 1950 to 1979. Circulation 1984;70(3):345–349.
2. Port S, Cobb FR, Coleman RE, Jones RH. Effect of age on the response of the left ventricular ejection fraction to exercise. N Engl J Med 1980;303(20):1133–1137.
3. Rodeheffer RJ, Gerstenblith G, Becker LC, Fleg JL, Weisfeldt ML, Lakatta EG. Exercise cardiac output is maintained with advancing age in healthy human subjects: cardiac dilatation and increased stroke volume compensate for a diminished heart rate. Circulation 1984;69(2):203–213.
4. Linzbach AJ, Akuamoa-Boateng E. Changes in the aging human heart. I. Heart weight in the aged. Klin Wochenschr 1973;51(4):156–163.
5. Melissari M, Balbi T, Gennari M, Olivetti G. The aging of the heart: weight and structural changes in the left ventricle with age. G Ital Cardiol 1991;21(2):119–130.
6. Olivetti G, Giordano G, Corradi D, Melissari M, Lagrasta C, Gambert SR, et al. Gender differences and aging: effects on the human heart. J Am Coll Cardiol 1995;26(4):1068–1079.
7. Unverferth DV, Baker PB, Arn AR, Magorien RD, Fetters J, Leier CV. Aging of the human myocardium: a histologic study based upon endomyocardial biopsy. Gerontology 1986;32(5):241–251.
8. Olivetti G, Melissari M, Balbi T, Quaini F, Cigola E, Sonnenblick EH, et al. Myocyte cellular hypertrophy is responsible for ventricular remodelling in the hypertrophied heart of middle aged individuals in the absence of cardiac failure. Cardiovasc Res 1994;28(8):1199–1208.
9. Gardin JM, Henry WL, Savage DD, Ware JH, Burn C, Borer JS. Echocardiographic measurements in normal subjects: evaluation of an adult population without clinically apparent heart disease. J Clin Ultrasound 1979;7(6):439–447.
10. Henry WL, Gardin JM, Ware JH. Echocardiographic measurements in normal subjects from infancy to old age. Circulation 1980;62(5):1054–1061.
11. Sjogren AL. Left ventricular wall thickness determined by ultrasound in 100 subjects without heart disease. Chest 1971;60(4):341–346.

12. Gerstenblith G, Frederiksen J, Yin FC, Fortuin NJ, Lakatta EG, Weisfeldt ML. Echocardiographic assessment of a normal adult aging population. Circulation 1977;56(2):273–378.

13. Dannenberg AL, Levy D, Garrison RJ. Impact of age on echocardiographic left ventricular mass in a healthy population (the Framingham Study). Am J Cardiol 1989;64(16):1066–1068.

14. Gopal AS, Schnellbaecher MJ, Shen Z, Akinboboye OO, Sapin PM, King DL. Freehand three-dimensional echocardiography for measurement of left ventricular mass: in vivo anatomic validation using explanted human hearts. J Am Coll Cardiol 1997;30(3):802–810.

15. Rodeheffer RJ, Gerstenblith G, Becker LC, Fleg JL, Weisfeldt ML, Lakatta EG. Exercise cardiac output is maintained with advancing age in healthy human subjects: cardiac dilatation and increased stroke volume compensate for a diminished heart rate. Circulation 1984;69(2):203–213.

16. Olivetti G, Giordano G, Corradi D, Melissari M, Lagrasta C, Gambert SR, et al. Gender differences and aging: effects on the human heart. J Am Coll Cardiol 1995;26(4):1068–1079.

17. Douglas PS, Otto CM, Mickel MC, Labovitz A, Reid CL, Davis KB. Gender differences in left ventricle geometry and function in patients undergoing balloon dilatation of the aortic valve for isolated aortic stenosis. NHLBI Balloon Valvuloplasty Registry. Br Heart J 1995;73(6):548–554.

18. Weinberg EO, Thienelt CD, Katz SE, Bartunek J, Tajima M, Rohrbach S, et al. Gender differences in molecular remodeling in pressure overload hypertrophy. J Am Coll Cardiol 1999;34(1):264–273.

19. Gerstenblith G, Lakatta EG, Weisfeldt ML. Age changes in myocardial function and exercise response. Prog Cardiovasc Dis 1976;19(1):1–21.

20. Olivetti G, Melissari M, Capasso JM, Anversa P. Cardiomyopathy of the aging human heart. Myocyte loss and reactive cellular hypertrophy. Circ Res 1991;68(6):1560–1568.

21. Gazoti Debessa CR, Mesiano Maifrino LB, Rodrigues de Souza R. Age related changes of the collagen network of the human heart. Mech Ageing Dev 2001;122(10):1049–1058.

22. Robert V, Besse S, Sabri A, Silvestre JS, Assayag P, Nguyen VT, et al. Differential regulation of matrix metalloproteinases associated with aging and hypertension in the rat heart. Lab Invest 1997;76(5): 729–738.

23. Hodkinson HM, Pomerance A. The clinical significance of senile cardiac amyloidosis: a prospective clinico-pathological study. Q J Med 1977;46(183):381–387.

24. Falk RH, Comenzo RL, Skinner M. The systemic amyloidoses. N Engl J Med 1997;337(13):898–909.

25. Westermark P, Sletten K, Johansson B, Cornwell GG III. Fibril in senile systemic amyloidosis is derived from normal transthyretin. Proc Natl Acad Sci USA 1990;87:2843–2845.

26. Smulyan H, Csermely TJ, Mookherjee S, Warner RA. Effect of age on arterial distensibility in asymptomatic humans. Arteriosclerosis 1983;3(3):199–205.

27. Bader H. Dependence of wall stress in the human thoracic aorta on age and pressure. Circ Res 1967;20(3): 354–361.

28. Gerstenblith G, Lakatta EG, Weisfeldt ML. Age changes in myocardial function and exercise response. Prog Cardiovasc Dis 1976;19(1):1–21.

29. O'Rourke MF. Aging and arterial function. In: Arterial Function and Health Disease (O'Rourke MF, ed.). Churchill Livingstone, New York, 1982, pp. 185–195.

30. Smulyan H, Safar ME. The diastolic blood pressure in systolic hypertension. Ann Intern Med 2000; 132(3):233–237.

31. Smulyan H, Safar ME. The diastolic blood pressure in systolic hypertension. Ann Intern Med 2000; 132(3):233–237.

32. Roach MR, Burton AC. The effect of age on the elasticity of human iliac arteries. Can J Biochem Physiol 1959;37:557–570.

33. Harding SE, Jones SM, O'Gara P, del Monte F, Vescovo G, Poole-Wilson PA. Isolated ventricular myocytes from failing and non-failing human heart: the relation of age and clinical status of patients to isoproterenol response. J Mol Cell Cardiol 1992;24(5):549–564.

34. Lansing AI. Elastic tissue. In: The Arterial Wall: Aging, Structure and Chemistry (Lansing AI, ed.). Williams & Wilkins, Baltimore, MD, 1959, pp. 136–160.

35. Airaksinen KE, Salmela PI, Linnaluoto MK, et al. Diminished arterial elasticity in diabetes: association with fluorescent advanced glycosylation end products in collagen. Cardiovasc Res 1993;27:942–945.

36. Lee AT, Cerami A. Role of glycation in aging. Ann NY Acad Sci 1992;663:63–70.

37. Kass DA, Shapiro EP, Kawaguchi M, Capriotti AR, Scuteri A, deGroof RC, et al. Improved arterial compliance by a novel advanced glycation end-product crosslink breaker. Circulation 2001;104:1464–1470.

38. Rothe CF. Reflex control of the veins in cardiovascular function. Physiologist 1979;22(2):28–35.

39. Banet M, Guyton AC. Effect of body metabolism on cardiac output: role of the central nervous system. Am J Physiol 1971;220:662–666.
40. MacKay EH, Banks J, Sykes B, Lee G de J. Structural bases for the changing physical properties of human pulmonary vessels with age. Thorax 1978;33:335–344.
41. Olsen H, Lanne T. Reduced venous compliance in lower limbs of aging humans and its importance for capacitance function. Am J Physiol 1998;275(3 Pt 2):H878–H886.
42. Olsen H, Vernersson E, Lanne T. Cardiovascular response to acute hypovolemia in relation to age. Implications for orthostasis and hemorrhage. Am J Physiol Heart Circ Physiol 2000;278(1):H222–H232.
43. Rothe C. Venous system: physiology of the capacitance vessels. In: Handbook of Physiology: The Cardiovascular System. Peripheral Circulation and Organ Blood Flow (Shepherd JT and Abboud FM, eds.). American Physiology Society, Bethesda, MD, 1983, Sect. 2, Vol. III, Part 1, pp. 397–452.
44. Rowell L. Hydrostatics and distribution of vascular transmural pressures. In: Human Cardiovascular Control. Oxford University Press, New York, 1993, pp. 1–36.
45. Wynne HA, Cope LH, Mutch E, Rawlins MD, Woodhouse KW, James OF. The effect of age upon liver volume and apparent liver blood flow in healthy man. Hepatology 1989;9(2):297–301.
46. Maurer MS, Karmally W, Rivadeneira H, Parides MK, Bloomfield DM. Upright posture and postprandial hypotension in elderly persons. Ann Intern Med 2000;133(7):533–536.
47. Weisfeldt ML, Wright JR, Shreiner DP, Lakatta E, Shock NW. Coronary flow and oxygen extraction in the perfused heart of senescent male rats. J Appl Physiol 1971;30(1):44–49.
48. Senneff MJ, Geltman EM, Bergmann SR. Noninvasive delineation of the effects of moderate aging on myocardial perfusion. J Nucl Med 1991;32(11):2037–2042.
49. Uren NG, Camici PG, Melin JA, Bol A, de Bruyne B, Radvan J, et al. Effect of aging on myocardial perfusion reserve. J Nucl Med 1995;36(11):2032–2036.
50. Czernin J, Muller P, Chan S, Brunken RC, Porenta G, Krivokapich J, Chen K, Chan A, et al. Influence of age and hemodynamics on myocardial blood flow and flow reserve. Circulation 1993;88(1):62–69.
51. Borow KM, Green LH, Grossman W, Braunwald E. Left ventricular end-systolic stress-shortening and stress-length relations in humans. Normal values and sensitivity to inotropic state. Am J Cardiol 1982; 50:1301–1308.
52. Colan SD, Borow KM, Neumann A. Left ventricular end-systolic wall stress-velocity of fiber shortening relation: a load-independent index of myocardial contractility. J Am Coll Cardiol 1984:4;715–724.
53. Fleg JL, Gerstenblith G, Schulman P, Becker LC, O'Connor FC, Lakatta EG. Gender differences in exercise hemodynamics of older subjects: effects of conditioning status. Circulation 1990;81:III–239.
54. Rodeheffer RJ, Gerstenblith G, Becker LC, Fleg JL, Weisfeldt ML, Lakatta EG. Exercise cardiac output is maintained with advancing age in healthy human subjects: cardiac dilatation and increased stroke volume compensate for a diminished heart rate. Circulation 1984;69(2):203–213.
55. Wei JY, Spurgeon HA, Lakatta EG. Excitation–contraction in rat myocardium: alterations with adult aging. Am J Physiol 1984;246(6 Pt 2):H784–H791.
56. White M, Roden R, Minobe W, Khan MF, Larrabee P, Wollmering M, et al. Age-related changes in beta-adrenergic neuroeffector systems in the human heart. Circulation 1994;90(3):1225–1238.
57. Schwartz JB, Gibb WJ, Tran T. Aging effects on heart rate variation. J Gerontol 1991;46(3):M99–M106.
58. Simpson DM, Wicks R. Spectral analysis of heart rate indicates reduced baroreceptor-related heart rate variability in elderly persons. J Gerontol 1988;43(1):M21–M24.
59. Heath GW, Hagberg JM, Ehsani AA, Holloszy JO. A physiological comparison of young and older endurance athletes. J Appl Physiol 1981;51(3):634–640.
60. Tanaka H, Monahan KD, Seals DR. Age-predicted maximal heart rate revisited. J Am Coll Cardiol 2001;37(1):153–156.
61. Gribbin B, Pickering TG, Sleight P, Peto R. Effect of age and high blood pressure on baroreflex sensitivity in man. Circ Res 1971;29(4):424–431.
62. Pfeifer MA, Weinberg CR, Cook D, Best JD, Reenan A, Halter JB. Differential changes of autonomic nervous system function with age in man. Am J Med 1983;75(2):249–258.
63. Lake CR, Ziegler MG, Coleman MD, Kopin IJ. Age-adjusted plasma norepinephrine levels are similar in normotensive and hypertensive subjects. N Engl J Med 1977;296(4):208–209.
64. Sundlof G, Wallin BG. Human muscle nerve sympathetic activity at rest. Relationship to blood pressure and age. J Physiol 1978;274:621–637.
65. Taylor JA, Hand GA, Johnson DG, Seals DR. Augmented forearm vasoconstriction during dynamic exercise in healthy older men. Circulation 1992;86(6):1789–1799.

66. Hajduczok G, Chapleau MW, Abboud FM. Increase in sympathetic activity with age. II. Role of impairment of cardiopulmonary baroreflexes. Am J Physiol 1991;260(4 Pt 2):H1121–H1127.

67. Cleroux J, Giannattasio C, Grassi G, Seravalle G, Sampieri L, Cuspidi C, et al. Effects of ageing on the cardiopulmonary receptor reflex in normotensive humans. J Hypertens 1998;6(4)(Suppl):S141–S144.

68. Cleroux J, Giannattasio C, Bolla G, Cuspidi C, Grassi G, Mazzola C, et al. Decreased cardiopulmonary reflexes with aging in normotensive humans. Am J Physiol 1989;257(3 Pt 2):H961–H968.

69. Sowers JR, Mohanty PK. Effect of advancing age on cardiopulmonary baroreceptor function in hypertensive men. Hypertension 1987;10(3):274–279.

70. Ebert TJ, Morgan BJ, Barney JA, Denahan T, Smith JJ. Effects of aging on baroreflex regulation of sympathetic activity in humans. Am J Physiol 1992;263(3 Pt 2):H798–H803.

71. Shi X, Gallagher KM, Welch-O'Connor RM, Foresman BH. Arterial and cardiopulmonary baroreflexes in 60- to 69- vs. 18- to 36-yr-old humans. J Appl Physiol 1996;80(6):1903–1910.

72. Monahan KD, Tanaka H, Dinenno FA, Seals DR. Central arterial compliance is associated with age- and habitual exercise-related differences in cardiovagal baroreflex sensitivity. Circulation 2001;104: 1627–1632.

73. Hunt BE, Farquhar WB, Taylor JA. Does reduced vascular stiffening fully explain preserved cardiovagal baroreflex function in older, physically active men? Circulation 2001;103(20):2424–2427.

74. Downes TR, Nomeir AM, Smith KM, Stewart KP, Little WC. Mechanism of altered pattern of left ventricular filling with aging in subjects without cardiac disease. Am J Cardiol 1989;64(8):523–527.

75. Schirmer H, Lunde P, Rasmussen K. Mitral flow derived Doppler indices of left ventricular diastolic function in a general population: the Tromso study. Eur Heart J 2000;21(16):1376–1386.

76. Klein AL, Burstow DJ, Tajik AJ, Zachariah PK, Bailey KR, Seward JB. Effects of age on left ventricular dimensions and filling dynamics in 117 normal persons. Mayo Clin Proc 1994;69(3):212–224.

77. Arora RR, Machac J, Goldman ME, Butler RN, Gorlin R, Horowitz SF. Atrial kinetics and left ventricular diastolic filling in the healthy elderly. J Am Coll Cardiol 1987;9(6):1255–1260.

78. Voutilainen S, Kupari M, Hippelainen M, Karppinen K, Ventila M, Heikkila J. Factors influencing Doppler indexes of left ventricular filling in healthy persons. Am J Cardiol 1991;68(6):653–659.

79. Schulman SP, Lakatta EG, Fleg JL, Lakatta L, Becker LC, Gerstenblith G. Age-related decline in left ventricular filling at rest and exercise. Am J Physiol 1992;263(6 Pt 2):H1932–H1938.

80. Forman DE, Manning WJ, Hauser R, Gervino EV, Evans WJ, Wei JY. Enhanced left ventricular diastolic filling associated with long-term endurance training. J Gerontol 1992;7(2):M56–M58.

81. Schmidt U, del Monte F, Miyamoto MI, Matsui T, Gwathmey JK, Rosenzweig A, et al. Restoration of diastolic function in senescent rat hearts through adenoviral gene transfer of sarcoplasmic reticulum Ca(2+)-ATPase. Circulation 2000;101(7):790–796.

82. Swinne CJ, Shapiro EP, Lima SD, Fleg JL. Age-associated changes in left ventricular diastolic performance during isometric exercise in normal subjects. Am J Cardiol 1992;69(8):823–826.

83. Lakatta EG, Gerstenblith G, Angell CS, Shock NW, Weisfeldt ML. Diminished inotropic response of aged myocardium to catecholamines. Circ Res 1975;36(2):262–269.

84. Jiang MT, Moffat MP, Narayanan N. Age-related alterations in the phosphorylation of sarcoplasmic reticulum and myofibrillar proteins and diminished contractile response to isoproterenol in intact rat ventricle. Circ Res 1993;72(1):102–111.

85. White M, Roden R, Minobe W, Khan MF, Larrabee P, Wollmering M, et al. Age-related changes in beta-adrenergic neuroeffector systems in the human heart. Circulation 1994;90(3):1225–1238.

86. Fleg JL, Tzankoff SP, Lakatta EG. Age-related augmentation of plasma catecholamines during dynamic exercise in healthy males. J Appl Physiol 1985;59(4):1033–1039.

87. Stratton JR, Cerqueira MD, Schwartz RS, Levy WC, Veith RC, Kahn SE, Abrass IB. Differences in cardiovascular responses to isoproterenol in relation to age and exercise training in healthy men. Circulation 1992;86(2):504–512.

88. Pan HY, Hoffman BB, Pershe RA, Blaschke TF. Decline in beta adrenergic receptor-mediated vascular relaxation with aging in man. J Pharmacol Exp Therap 1986;239(3):802–807.

89. Rodeheffer RJ, Gerstenblith G, Becker LC, Fleg JL, Weisfeldt ML, Lakatta EG. Exercise cardiac output is maintained with advancing age in healthy human subjects: cardiac dilatation and increased stroke volume compensate for a diminished heart rate. Circulation 1984;69(2):203–213.

90. Fleg JL, O'Connor F, Gerstenblith G, Becker LC, Clulow J, Schulman SP, et al. Impact of age on the cardiovascular response to dynamic upright exercise in healthy men and women. J Appl Physiol 1995; 78(3):890–900.

91. Fleg JL, Schulman S, O'Connor F, Becker LC, Gerstenblith G, Clulow JF, Renlund DG, et al. Effects of acute beta-adrenergic receptor blockade on age-associated changes in cardiovascular performance during dynamic exercise. Circulation 1994;90(5):2333–2341.

92. Fleg JL, O'Connor F, Gerstenblith G, Becker LC, Clulow J, Schulman SP, et al. Impact of age on the cardiovascular response to dynamic upright exercise in healthy men and women. J Appl Physiol 1995; 78:890–900.

93. Lakatta EG. Cardiovascular regulatory mechanisms in advanced age. Physiol Rev 1993;73:413–467.

94. Carroll JD, Shroff S, Wirth P, Halsted M, Rajfer SI. Arterial mechanical properties in dilated cardiomyopathy. Aging and the response to nitroprusside. J Clin Invest 1991;87(3):1002–1009.

95. Isoyama S, Grossman W, Wei JY. Effect of age on myocardial adaptation to volume overload in the rat. J Clin Invest 1988;81(6):1850–1857.

96. Isoyama S, Wei JY, Izumo S, Fort P, Schoen FJ, Grossman W. Effect of age on the development of cardiac hypertrophy produced by aortic constriction in the rat. Circ Res 1987;61(3):337–345.

97. Rivard A, Fabre JE, Silver M, Chen D, Murohara T, Kearney M, Magner M, et al. Age-dependent impairment of angiogenesis. Circulation 1999;99(1):111–120.

98. Reed MJ, Corsa A, Pendergrass W, Penn P, Sage EH, Abrass IB. Neovascularization in aged mice: delayed angiogenesis is coincident with decreased levels of transforming growth factor beta1 and type I collagen. Am J Pathol 1998;152(1):113–123.

10 Risk Factors and the Prevention of Heart Disease

Nanette K. Wenger, MD

CONTENTS

DIFFERENCES IN THE ELDERLY

Age as a Risk Factor

Cardiovascular disease, and in particular coronary heart disease, is the predominant cause of death and disability worldwide in populations older than 65 yr of age; about half of elderly individuals in industrialized countries have clinical evidence of coronary heart disease. The World Health Organization (WHO) Study Group report on the epidemiology and prevention of cardiovascular diseases in elderly people *(1)* identified coronary heart disease as the major cause of mortality in industrialized nations, where 50% of such deaths occur in the population older than 65 yr of age and 60% at older than age 75. Coronary heart disease is responsible for half of all deaths in the population older than 80 yr of age *(2).* Forty-five percent of octogenarians have clinical evidence of cardiovascular disease, with coronary heart disease being the most common problem. However, the variation in rates of cardiovascular mortality in elderly populations indicates a substantial potential for effective coronary prevention because many risk factors for coronary heart disease are modifiable. The highest risk for development of clinical evidence of coronary heart disease is in the population 65 yr of age and older, double that in the under age 65 population, with the difference more pronounced among women.

Coronary risk factors are highly prevalent at elderly age. Framingham data characterize half of elderly persons as hypertensive, one-third to one-half as hyperlipidemic, 20–30% as obese, 20% as smokers, and 6% as having impaired glucose tolerance. Fourteen percent of male and 11% of female octogenarians have diabetes *(2).* Each decade of older age confers a twofold to threefold increase in cardiovascular mortality at any level of

From: *Aging, Heart Disease, and Its Management: Facts and Controversies*
Edited by: N. Edwards, M. Maurer, and R. Wellner © Humana Press Inc., Totowa, NJ

coronary risk factors. Whether this represents the time-dependent cumulative risk burden over the years remains speculative. The elderly have shared in the dramatic decline in coronary heart disease and stroke rates in the United States during the past three decades, reinforcing the potential for risk reduction and cardiovascular disease prevention at elderly age.

Because of the progressive increase in the world's elderly population, with the greatest acceleration in growth occurring in the subgroup older than 80–85 yr of age, health care and health policy for this population is receiving increasing attention. Life expectancy at age 65 in most industrialized nations is increasing more rapidly than life expectancy at birth, owing to the decline in cardiovascular disease and cardiovascular disease mortality at middle age and older *(1)*. The exponential growth of the elderly population is a social phenomenon without precedent, and a scientific data base is needed to guide both clinical decisions for prevention and management and to shape public policy. Although the prevalence of coronary risk factors and their attributable risks are well-established for younger elderly persons, very limited information is available regarding coronary risk factors in the octogenarian and beyond. Even fewer data are present regarding the efficacy of specific risk interventions at elderly age. This reflects the exclusion of elderly patients in general, and elderly women in specific, from both observational studies and clinical trials *(3)*.

Modifiable cardiovascular risk factors in middle-age are comparable to and continue to remain relevant at elderly age, although the magnitude of the relative risk is lower after age 65. Despite the attenuation of the relative risk of some coronary risk factors with advancing age, the absolute risk tends to increase with age; because morbidity and mortality rates of cardiovascular disease are higher at elderly age and cardiovascular risk factors are more common, the attributable risks of these risk factors are higher at elderly than at middle age *(4)*. This renders risk reduction as cost-effective in elderly populations as at middle-age *(1)*. Global risk assessment best enables identification of the burden of coronary risk factors in the elderly individual and is valuable in targeting appropriate interventions *(5)*. A number of modifiable lifestyle or behavioral factors are associated with the maintenance of good health in older adults; these include physical activity, nonsmoking status, and control of obesity, as well as the control of diabetes, elevated cholesterol levels, and elevated blood pressure *(6)*.

The prevalence of diabetes, hypertension, and electrocardiogram (ECG) evidence of left-ventricular hypertrophy increases with older age, whereas the prevalence of increased body mass index and cigarette smoking declines. Risk factors such as weight and cholesterol levels may be difficult to interpret at an elderly age owing to confounding by associated comorbidities. Nonetheless, hypercholesterolemia, hypertension, diabetes, and obesity appear responsible for much of the coronary heart disease that occurs in elderly populations. During 10 yr of follow-up in the Framingham Heart Study, systolic blood pressure and cigarette smoking in elderly men and women substantially influenced the risk of developing cardiovascular disease *(7)*.

In elderly European men in the FINE (Finland, Italy, Netherlands, Elderly) study, only age, smoking habits, and heart rate were consistently associated with all-cause mortality *(8)*.

In the Cardiovascular Health Study, subclinical evidence of coronary heart disease was a far more powerful predictor of future events at elderly age than were traditional coronary risk factors *(9,10)*. The challenge in the future may be to identify these subclinical attributes (carotid intimal medial thickness, ankle–arm index, major ECG or echocardiographic abnormalities, claudication and Rose questionnaire angina, etc.) as the basis for identifying high-risk elderly populations for aggressive coronary risk intervention. Further tests include electron beam computed tomography (EBCT), helical computed tomography (CT) and magnetic resonance imaging (MRI) *(11)*.

Specifically noted by the Clinical Quality Improvement Network (CQIN) investigators *(12)* was the significantly lesser measurement of risk factors and lesser treatment of risk factors in women and in older patients hospitalized for acute cardiovascular care. This identifies suboptimal risk assessment and risk intervention at elderly age as a confounder of the effect of elderly age *per se*. A recent American Heart Association Advisory addresses secondary prevention of coronary heart disease in the elderly, with emphasis on patients ≥75 yr of age *(13)*.

Evidence for Various Risk Factors in the Elderly

HYPERTENSION

Hypertension is an important modifiable predictor of cardiovascular morbidity and mortality at elderly age, with prominent randomized clinical trial proof available of the efficacy of risk reduction with hypertension control *(4)*. Coronary risk is more closely related to systolic than to diastolic hypertension at elderly age, and hypertension is also an important risk factor for ischemic and hemorrhagic stroke. Isolated systolic hypertension is the most prevalent type of hypertension at elderly age; a wide pulse pressure (≥50 mm Hg) may better predict cerebrovascular disease and heart failure at elderly age *(14)*.

Fewer than 10% of elderly individuals with hypertension do not have other major cardiovascular risk factors *(15)*. Hypertension was present in 40% of elderly men and 50% of elderly women in the Framingham Heart Study *(16)*. African-Americans are more likely to have hypertension than their white counterparts. In NHANES III, hypertension was present in 60% of non-Hispanic whites, 71% of non-Hispanic African-Americans, and 61% of Mexican-Americans older than 60 yr of age *(17)*. The goal of treatment in older patients should be the same as at younger age (<140/90 mm Hg if possible), although an interim goal of systolic blood pressure below 160 mm Hg is reasonable in patients with marked isolated systolic hypertension *(18)*.

At every level of elevated blood pressure, elderly individuals have a greater risk of cardiovascular events. There was a linear relationship between hypertension and cardiovascular mortality in men and women aged 75–94 yr in the Framingham Heart Study *(19)*. At blood pressure levels above 160/95 mm Hg, men aged 65–74 were 2.4 times as likely as normotensive men to incur fatal cardiovascular events, and women 8 times as likely. A comparison of subset analysis of individuals older and younger than 60 yr of age showed a comparable reduction in events with control of hypertension at an elderly age, but a greater absolute reduction in these events in the elderly population. The absolute reduction in coronary events related to hypertension control in older subjects was 2.7 per 1000 person-years, more than twice as great as that seen in younger subjects *(20)*.

Systolic blood pressure, fasting glucose level, and selected subclinical disease measures were important predictors of myocardial infarction in the Cardiovascular Health Study, but uncontrolled hypertension potentially explained one-fourth of all coronary events *(21)*. Systolic blood pressure was the best single predictor of cardiovascular events in the Cardiovascular Health Study *(22)*. Low blood pressure, on the other hand is likely to be a consequence of underlying disease and not a result of antihypertensive therapy

(19). In older persons, elevated systolic blood pressure better predicts coronary and cardiovascular disease, heart failure, stroke, end-stage renal disease, and all-cause mortality than diastolic blood pressure elevation *(18)*. In the Rotterdam Study *(23)*, the relationship between the risk of initial myocardial infarction and increasing levels of both systolic and diastolic blood pressure persisted into older age, without evidence of a J- or U-shaped relationship in the elderly. There was a gradual shift with increasing age from diastolic blood pressure to systolic blood pressure and then to pulse pressure as predictors of coronary risk in the Framingham Heart Study *(24)*; from 60 yr of age and older, pulse pressure was superior even to systolic blood pressure *(25)*. In a Veterans Administration study, pulse pressure predicted cardiovascular death at elderly age better than either systolic blood pressure or diastolic blood pressure alone *(26)*.

Important data regarding nonpharmacologic therapy for hypertension derive from the randomized controlled Trial of Nonpharmacologic Interventions in the Elderly (TONE) *(27)*, which evaluated sodium intake reduction and weight loss in the treatment of hypertension in older persons. A reduction in sodium intake and weight loss were shown to constitute a feasible, effective and safe approach to the nonpharmacologic therapy of hypertension in older persons. Nonpharmacologic interventions appear more effective in older than in younger age populations *(13)*. As well, a meta-analysis of randomized controlled trials suggested that a chronic high sodium chloride diet in patients with essential hypertension was associated with an increase in both systolic and diastolic blood pressures, but that the effect was more pronounced in older patients *(28)*. Lifestyle modifications are the initial therapeutic step, with pharmacologic treatment if the blood pressure remains elevated *(18)*. Included among the recommended lifestyle modifications are weight reduction to ideal body weight, dietary sodium restriction to less than 2 g daily, which may help reduce the dosage and numbers of antihypertensive drugs needed even if it does not normalize arterial pressure, moderation of alcohol consumption to less than 1 oz daily, a regular program of aerobic exercise, and cessation of tobacco use *(29)*.

The Systolic Hypertension in the Elderly Program (SHEP) provided valuable randomized controlled trial data regarding the effectiveness of pharmacologic control of isolated systolic hypertension in this population. Low-dose diuretic-based treatment (with the addition of β-blockade if needed) was an effective low-cost intervention, with the favorable result of preventing stroke, myocardial infarction, and the later occurrence of heart failure; the evidence was most powerful for stroke prevention. Effective treatment of isolated systolic hypertension reduced coronary risk by about 27%. Evaluation of risk factors in this elderly cohort showed a 73% increase in risk associated with cigarette smoking, a 121% increase with diabetes, and a 113% increase associated with the presence of a carotid bruit *(30)*. In this cohort, the low-dose diuretic-based treatment was effective in preventing these major cardiovascular events both in non-insulin-treated diabetic and nondiabetic older patients *(31)*. The chlorthalidone therapy had relatively mild effects on other cardiovascular risk factors *(32)*. In an ancillary study to SHEP, elderly individuals who had both isolated systolic hypertension and peripheral atherosclerosis were at high risk for cardiovascular events; antihypertensive therapy in this group was postulated to result in the prevention of a large number of cardiovascular events *(16)*.

Meta-analysis of a number of clinical trials showed the justification of the treatment of isolated systolic hypertension in older patients with a systolic blood pressure in excess of 160 mm Hg. The absolute benefit was greater in men, in patients aged 70 yr or older, and in those with previous cardiovascular complications or a wider pulse pressure *(33)*.

Meta-analysis of clinical trials of antihypertensive therapy showed a significant reduction in both overall mortality and cardiovascular morbidity and mortality related to pharmacologic treatment in the elderly, with benefits particularly high at ages 60–80 *(34)*. There was also a decrease in cerebrovascular mortality *(2)* and heart failure. Antihypertensive treatment in elderly patients not only prevented major coronary events and stroke and prolonged life, but significant treatment benefits were observed within only 5 yr of therapy *(35)*.

Few patients older than age 80 were included in the large randomized treatment trials of hypertension; the Systolic Hypertension Europe (SYST-EUR) trial and subgroup meta-analyses of other studies demonstrated stroke, heart failure, and cardiovascular event benefit in patients over age 80, although cardiovascular death and total mortality were not reduced *(36,37)*.

Few studies addressed quality of life. In the National Intervention Cooperative Study in Elderly Hypertensives Study Group, nicardipine and trichlomethiazide had nearly equivalent effects on quality-of-life and neither resulted in a deterioration of quality-of-life *(38)*.

Provided that medication is started at low dosage and the dosage is increased slowly, elderly hypertensive patients generally respond well to drug therapy. The increased availability of safer and effective antihypertensive preparations enables the physician to tailor hypertensive treatment to the needs of individual patients and allows for blood pressure control that adds to longevity without compromising the quality-of-life.

Recommendations of the Sixth Report of the Joint National Committee on Prevention, Detection, Evaluation, and Treatment of High Blood Pressure (JNCVI) *(39)* specifically address hypertension in older persons.

Should We Evaluate for Secondary Causes of Hypertension in the Elderly? When?

The initial onset of hypertension after age 60, drug-resistant hypertension *(40)*, sudden onset of hypertension, or previously well-controlled hypertension with new increases in blood pressure warrant investigation for secondary hypertension. Atherosclerotic renal artery stenosis is an important consideration in an elderly patient.

LIPID ABNORMALITIES

Men and women over age 60 have the highest prevalence of hypercholesterolemia. Both total and high-density lipoprotein (HDL) cholesterol levels predict coronary death at elderly age; although the relative risk associated with higher total cholesterol and lower HDL cholesterol levels is lower than at middle age, the attributable risk is greater because of the greater number of coronary events in older persons. Low levels of HDL cholesterol predict coronary disease in older women. The significance of hypertriglycer-idemia as an independent risk factor is controversial. About one-third of elderly men and one-half of elderly women have total cholesterol levels in excess of 240 mg/dL *(2)*.

Forty-six percent of 5201 community dwelling individuals in the Cardiovascular Health Study older than age 65 had an LDL cholesterol level in excess of 160 mg/dL *(41)*. Although hypercholesterolemia is more common in elderly women than elderly men, in the Framingham Heart Study only 11% of men and 21% of women aged 85–94 yr had a total cholesterol in excess of 240 mg/dL; this may represent a survivor effect in that those with the highest levels of cholesterol died at earlier ages *(42)*. Total cholesterol remained an important risk factor for myocardial infarction for both men and women age 70 and older in the population-based Rotterdam Study, whereas HDL at older age was important only in women (43).

The total/HDL cholesterol ratio best predicts coronary heart disease in the elderly, with this prediction valid into the octogenarian age group. Based on Framingham data, although total cholesterol level is not predictive of coronary heart disease in men older than age 70, it continues to predict coronary heart disease in women well into the ninth decade. Total and LDL cholesterol levels in women increase with age, at least to age 80; therefore, lipid levels should be measured at elderly age even for women whose lipid levels were normal at middle age. Importantly, lipid abnormalities at elderly age are not isolated risk attributes but rather cluster with diabetes, hypertension, obesity, and increased fibrinogen. In the Zutphen Elderly Study, a high intake of transfatty acids contributed to coronary risk in this prospective population-based study (44).

In the Finland, Italy, and the Netherlands Elderly (FINE) study, total but not HDL cholesterol was consistently associated with coronary mortality in elderly men (45). Thus, although different studies and different populations identify different components of elevated lipid levels as predictive of coronary heart disease risk, the totality of evidence supports that elevated lipid levels are associated with increased coronary risk in the elderly age population.

The apparent adverse effects associated with low cholesterol levels are likely not a reflection of the low cholesterol levels per se, but rather impute that these low cholesterol levels are secondary to comorbidity and frailty (46).

In the US Health and Nutrition Examination Survey, 40–50% of men and 50–60% of women older than age 65 years were candidates for dietary intervention per the National Cholesterol Education Program Adult Treatment Panel II guidelines (47), with about 5 million individuals older age 65 being candidates for drug treatment (48).

In primary and secondary prevention trials of statin therapy, cholesterol lowering reduced the risk for coronary heart disease comparably in younger and older populations (49). For elderly patients with known coronary heart disease, the composite data from statin therapy given for secondary prevention in randomized controlled trials showed a reduction in the 5-yr risk of coronary heart disease morbidity and mortality up to age 70–75 yr in patients with LDL cholesterol levels in excess of 125 mg/dL. Data are limited for populations older than age 75.

In the secondary prevention Scandinavian Simvastatin Survival Study (4S) 1021 of the 4444 coronary patients were older than 65 yr of age. Five years of therapy with simvastatin was associated with a 34% decline in all cause mortality, in great part the result of a 43% decline in coronary heart disease mortality (50). The relative risk reduction for major coronary events in patients older and younger than age 65 was similar, 42% vs 43%; however, the absolute risk reduction for both coronary and all-cause mortality was twice as great in older patients because the mortality rates increased substantially with age. In the Cholesterol and Recurrent Events (CARE) trial that enrolled patients with prior myocardial infarction and a total cholesterol level under 240 mg/dL, subset analysis of the 1283 patients aged 65-75 years showed that pravastatin decreased major coronary events (coronary death, nonfatal myocardial infarction, coronary angioplasty, or coronary artery bypass surgery) by 32% vs 19% in those below age 65 (51). The decrease in coronary death was 45% and in stroke was 40%. Treatment of 1000 older patients prevented 225 cardiovascular hospitalizations, in contrast to 121 hospitalizations in one thousand younger

patients. Thus, for patients aged 65–75 with myocardial infarction and average cholesterol levels, there was a clinically important decrease in the risk of major coronary events
and stroke. In another secondary prevention statin trial, the Long-Term Intervention with
Pravastatin in Ischemic Disease (LIPID) study *(52)*, 3514 of the 9014 patients enrolled
following myocardial infarction or unstable angina were older than age 65. They had
average or below average cholesterol levels. Pravastatin comparably reduced the risk of
major coronary events, 25%, in patients older and younger than 65 yr of age.

The West of Scotland Coronary Prevention Study (WOSCOPS) primary prevention
trial *(53)* did not include elderly patients. In the AirForce/Texas Coronary Atherosclerosis
Prevention Study (AFCAPS/TexCAPS), a primary prevention trial, 1416 of the 6605 participants were older than 65 yr of age *(54)*. Entry into the trial required an HDL ≤45 mg/
dL for men and ≤47 mg/dL for women. There was a 32% decrease in first acute coronary
events (unstable angina, fatal and nonfatal myocardial infarction or sudden death) in the
below 65-yr age group compared with a 38% decline in the older than 65-yr age group. A
meta-analysis of these statin trials showed that the risk reduction in major coronary events
was similar in elderly (older than age 65) and in younger (under age 65) patients *(55)*.

In the Scandinavian Simvastatin Survival Study (4S), the number of patients needed
to treat for 5 yr to prevent a coronary event was 10 below 60 yr of age and 14 at age 60–
70 *(56)*. In CARE, the numbers were 20 patients below age 60 yr vs 14 patients in the 60–
75 yr age group. In the WOSCOPS primary prevention trial, where the age range was
younger, 38 patients had to be treated under age 55 yr compared with 40 at ages 55–64.

In the Prospective Pravastatin Pooling Project *(57)*, pravastatin reduced coronary events
in patients with both high- and low-risk factor status and across a wide range of pretreat-
ment lipid concentrations. Effects were equal in patients younger and older than 65 yr of
age. In the NHLBI Post-CABG trial *(58)*, aggressive LDL lowering with lovastatin with
or without cholestyramine decreased obstructive changes in the saphenous vein grafts by
31%, with comparable benefit in elderly and younger patients, defined as older and younger
than age 60. The PROSPER (Prospective Study of Pravastatin in the Elderly at Risk) trial
(59) in progress will assess the efficacy and safety of pravastatin in men and women 70–
82 yr of age to determine the effect on major cardiovascular events in this elderly age group.

In the British Heart Protection Study which enrolled over 20,000 patients with coronary disease or at increased risk of coronary death up to age 80, elderly individuals bene-
fited equally to younger persons, including individuals older than 75. Treatment with 40
mg of simvastatin daily reduced by at least one-third the risk of myocardial infarction,
stroke, and myocardial revascularization; the safety data are impressive *(60)*.

A recent report from the Canadian Study of Health and Aging suggested that lipid lowering agent use was associated with a lower risk of dementia, and specifically of Alzheimer
disease, in those younger than age 80 *(61)*. The issue is under study in other cohorts.

Interventions for hypercholesterolemia in high-risk elderly persons remain relatively
cost-effective *(62,63)*. Lipid-lowering drugs, particularly statins, appear to be well-toler-
ated by older as by younger patients. In the Cholesterol Reduction In Seniors Program
(CRISP) pilot study *(64)* which involved patients older than age 65, there was no statistically significant difference in health-related quality-of-life measures or symptoms in men
and women randomized to placebo or lovastatin. Therapy was extremely well tolerated
in older cohort. Despite the equal or enhanced efficacy of lipid-lowering drugs at an elderly
age, there was consistently less use among older patients in a Canadian study *(65)*; therefore, suboptimal pharmacotherapy may contribute to the enhanced risk at an elderly age.

The initial recommended approach is reduction of dietary saturated fat and cholesterol, with associated weight control and regular physical activity. In middle-aged and elderly subjects *(66)* NCEP step 2 diets, both those relatively high and low in fish-derived fatty acids, significantly reduced both total and HDL-cholesterol levels without changing the total/ HDL cholesterol ratio. In a Dutch study, dietary fish intake had coronary protective effects in middle-aged and elderly individuals *(67)*. Although short-term aerobic exercise did not change the lipid profile at elderly age, long-term exercise, particularly when associated with improvements in body fat distribution or weight loss, improved lipid levels in elderly individuals, particularly HDL cholesterol and triglycerides *(68)*.

Specific issues regarding lipid lowering in elderly individuals are addressed in the NCEP ATP III guidelines *(69)*.

OBESITY

Obesity at an elderly age is associated with hypertension and diabetes *(1)*. Whether obesity is an independent risk factor at elderly age remains unclear, but a body mass index of 27 or greater appears to increase coronary risk at an elderly age *(70)*. Data from the Framingham Heart Study identify obesity as a risk factor for recurrent events in older men and women with coronary heart disease *(71)*. There is little information about the effect of dietary or exercise interventions for weight reduction in obese older patients with coronary heart disease *(72)*. Weight reduction may reduce surrogate endpoints for coronary risk, such as hyperglycemia, hyperlipidemia, insulin resistance, and hypertension.

The 2000 Revision of the AHA Dietary Guidelines *(73)* recommends that, with aging, foods be eaten that are dense in nutrients and low in calories.

What is the Role of Body Weight and Adverse Events from Cardiovascular Disease? Is a Higher BMI Protective in the Oldest Old?

As with many other risk factors, a very low BMI may reflect frailty or comorbidity. Higher BMI (beyond desirable levels) has as its associates: hypertension, hypercholesterolemia, hyperglycemia, all adverse attributes. One review suggests that current US guideline standards for ideal weight (BMI 18.7 to <25) may be overly restrictive at elderly age; studies did not support overweight, as opposed to obesity, as conferring an excess mortality risk *(74)*.

TOBACCO USE

Cigarette smoking is less common at elderly age and the relative risks are lower than at middle age. There is substantial evidence for cigarette smoking cessation benefit, predominantly deriving from observational data in younger age populations. However, observational studies suggest benefit for smoking cessation even at an elderly age *(75)*, in individuals both with and without identified coronary heart disease. Within 3–5 yr of smoking cessation, risk decreases to that of nonsmokers. The reduction in relative risk of myocardial infarction and death over age 70 is similar to that in younger individuals *(13)*.

Among elderly patients with coronary heart disease, a 52% reduction in mortality was associated with smoking cessation. In the EPESE (Established Populations for the Epidemiologic Studies of the Elderly) population, within 5 yr of smoking cessation, coronary mortality among elderly former smokers was similar to that of elderly persons who had never smoked *(2)*. Smoking cessation in patients older than 55 yr of age in the Coronary

Artery Surgery Study (CASS), indicated that those who continued smoking postoperatively had a relative risk of dying 1.7 times higher than those who quit; the benefit did not diminish with advanced age *(76)*. In the Norweign Multicenter Group Study, mortality following myocardial infarction decreased by 26% and reinfarction decreased by 45% associated with smoking cessation. Exposure to passive smoke also should be discouraged.

Smoking cessation interventions shown to be effective in younger persons are effective in elderly patients with cardiovascular disease *(77)*. Both nicotine replacement therapy and other pharmacologic agents are safe for elderly persons *(78)*.

DIABETES

The prevalence of diabetes and insulin resistance increases with increasing age, particularly in association with abdominal obesity *(79)*; noninsulin-dependent diabetes is most prominent in elderly populations. Diabetes increases coronary risk twofold to fivefold, with the increase in risk more pronounced for women. Diabetes at an elderly age should be treated according to guidelines for the nonelderly, but with particular care to avoid hypoglycemia and the side effects of antidiabetic agents. Treatment of other risk factors is requisite. Atherosclerotic complications account for 75% of deaths in diabetic patients, who have both higher case fatality rates with coronary heart disease and greater morbidity and mortality from stroke *(1)*.

Exercise improves both insulin resistance and diabetic control in healthy older individuals *(80)*, possibly more related to favorable effects on fat mass or body fat distribution than to fitness *(81)*.

There are few or no data regarding the benefits of precise control of hyperglycemia in elderly patients with type II diabetes, nor is there an organized study that defines the safety of newer hypoglycemic agents or their efficacy in lowering cardiovascular risk at elderly age. With recent myocardial infarction, precise blood glucose control reduced the risk of recurrent events *(82)*. In elderly diabetic patients in the Swedish Trial in Old Patients with hypertension *(83)*, the treatment of hypertension with conventional antihypertensive drugs (diuretics, β blockers or both) was as effective as the treatment with newer drugs (calcium antagonists or angiotensin-converting enzyme [ACE] inhibitors). Emphasis for coronary prevention must also address nonglycemic risk factors. Diabetes is considered a coronary disease risk equivalent in NCEP ATP III *(69)*.

SEDENTARY LIFESTYLE

Despite the prominent inverse association of coronary risk with physical activity at middle age, limited information is available for the elderly population *(84)*; only about 30% of older persons exercise regularly and fewer than 10% routinely exercise vigorously *(2)*. Nonetheless, some observational data suggest a reduction in coronary risk related to physical activity.

Among Harvard alumni, those aged 70–84 who participated in higher level exercise had lower rates of overall mortality, cardiovascular mortality and had increased longevity *(2)*. Framingham data comparably showed pronounced exercise benefit beyond age 80 *(7)*. Leisure-time physical activity in elderly individuals both improved physical function and had a beneficial effect on weight maintenance and lipid measures *(68)*.

In the Cardiovascular Health Study (mean age 73 yr), the intensity of exercise in later life was associated with both more favorable coronary risk factor levels and a reduced prevalence of several markers of subclinical disease *(85)*. In the same study, physical activity level was an independent predictor of 5-yr mortality *(86)*. Based on observational data, even modest increases in the level of habitual activity in older adults appears to limit the decline in functional reserve, to improve functional capacity, to decrease the coronary risk profile and to lessen mortality *(87)*.

Men in the Honolulu Heart Program (mean age 69 yr) who walked regularly had a lower overall mortality rate *(88)*. There was also an inverse association between physical activity and all-cause mortality in women, mean age 62, in the Iowa Women's Health Study *(89)*.

Stronger evidence than was previously available now emerges to support advising older men and women to embark on or maintain a sustained program of walking to prevent cardiovascular events. Walking more than 4 hr weekly appears to reduce the risk of hospitalization for cardiovascular events and may be mediated by the effects of walking on other risk factors *(90)*. In the Harvard Alumni Health Study, physical activity was also associated with decreased coronary risk; shorter sessions of physical activity had comparable benefit to long continuous sessions *(91)*. Coronary risk in elderly men was reduced with the increase in the distance walked *(92)*. In a recent report of a randomized trial, moderate intensive aerobic exercise and light exercise appeared to have similar effects on reducing blood pressure in previously sedentary adults *(93)*. If confirmed, the efficacy of light intensity activity as a means of reducing blood pressure in older adults could have substantial public health benefit. Active exercise may enhance both the quality and quantity of life of elderly persons and potentiate interventions on other risk factors including obesity, hypertension, diabetes, and hyperlipidemia.

Exercise training in elderly patients with coronary heart disease improves functional capacity similar to that at younger age, although absolute levels are less in the elderly *(94, 95)*. In a British study of men with coronary heart disease, light-to-moderate physical activity was associated with decreased all-cause mortality; however the mean age was 63 *(96)*.

Principles of exercise prescription are comparable for younger and older cardiac patients *(97)*, with modifications based on comorbidities such as arthritis and peripheral vascular disease. Strength training can improve muscular strength and endurance *(98)*.

A recent study suggests that ACE inhibitor therapy can decrease the decline in muscle strength in disabled elderly women with hypertension but without heart failure; clearly further study is needed *(99)*.

HORMONE REPLACEMENT THERAPY IN MENOPAUSAL WOMEN

Interest in estrogen for cardioprotection relates to biologically plausible preventive benefits, including improved lipid profiles, lower fibrinogen levels, antioxidant effects and favorable effects on the vascular endothelium and vascular reactivity, among others; as well, meta-analyses of observational studies consistently suggest a 35–50% reduction in coronary risk in current users of estrogen or estrogen/progestin. Selection, compliance, ascertainment, and survivor biases likely overestimate benefit and underestimate risk in these observational data *(100)*.

In prior years, both the American Heart Association and the National Cholesterol Education Program Adult Treatment Panel II *(47)* recommended menopausal hormone replacement therapy (HRT) as an initial approach to lipid lowering for menopausal women. NCEP ATP III no longer recommends HRT as initial management, statins are advised. Based on recent data from randomized controlled trials for the secondary prevention of coronary heart disease *(101)*, as well as other information involving menopausal women up to 80 yr of age, the American Heart Association has made the following recommendations *(102)*:

For women who have cardiovascular disease, hormone replacement therapy should not be initiated for the secondary prevention of cardiovascular disease. The decision to continue or stop hormone replacement therapy in women with cardiovascular disease who have been undergoing such therapy long term should be based on established noncoronary benefits and risks and patient preference. In a woman who develops an acute cardiovascular event, such as a heart attack or stroke, or who is immobilized while receiving hormone replacement therapy, it is prudent to consider discontinuance of such therapy or to consider venous thromboembolism prophylaxis while she is hospitalized to minimize the risk of venous thromboembolism (VTE) associated with immobilization. Reinstitution of hormone replacement therapy should be based on established noncoronary benefits and risks, as well as patient preference.

The Heart and Estrogen/Progestin Replacement Study Follow-up *(102a)* showed no reduction in coronary events over almost 7 yr, with a twofold increase in venous thromboembolism and an almost 50% increase in gallbladder disease requiring surgery. Thus, HRT provides coronary benefit in women with coronary heart disease and may cause harm.

For women who do not have known cardiovascular disease (i.e., treatment for primary prevention) firm clinical recommendations for HRT await the results of ongoing randomized clinical trials. In the interim, there are insufficient data to suggest that HRT should be initiated for the sole purpose of the primary prevention of cardiovascular disease. The initiation and continuation of HRT should be based on established noncoronary benefits and risks, possible coronary benefits and risks, and patient preference *(102)*.

The Women's Health Initiative *(102b)* terminated the estrogen plus progestin randomized trial in healthy menopausal women because the overall health risks exceeded the benefits. Excess risks included coronary events, stroke, venous thromboembolism, and breast cancer; there was benefit for colorectal cancer and hip fracture. The unopposed estrogen component of the randomized hormone trial is continuing.

NEWER RISK FACTORS

Carotid Artery Intima and Media Thickness

In the Cardiovascular Health Study, increases in ultrasound-measured carotid IMT (carotid artery intima and media thickness) were associated an with increased risk of myocardial infarction and stroke in older adults without a history of cardiovascular disease *(103)*. This and other novel risk factors may identify a higher-risk subset of elderly individuals for more intensive risk intervention, a hypothesis that remains to be tested.

Ankle-Arm Index (AAI)

An ankle-arm index (AAI) < 0.9 in the Cardiovascular Health Study was an independent risk factor for incident cardiovascular disease, recurrent cardiovascular disease and mortality in community-dwelling older adults. As is the case with carotid IMT, this subclinical evidence for cardiovascular disease may identify a high risk subset of elderly individuals *(104)*.

Depression

Depressive symptoms in the Cardiovascular Health Study constituted an independent risk factor for the development of coronary heart disease as well as for total mortality in community-dwelling elderly individuals *(105)*. In the Systolic Hypertension in the Elderly (SHEP) study, there was a significant and substantial excess risk of death and stroke or myocardial infarction in elderly patients associated with an increase in depressive symptoms over time *(106)*. Symptomatic depression among older men in the Normative Aging Study was associated with increased coronary risk *(107)*. Although depressive symptoms were not an independent risk factor for coronary outcomes in the elderly population in general in the EPESE (Established Populations for the Epidemiologic Studies of the Elderly) cohort, risk appeared increased among relatively healthy older women *(108)*. This suggests that interventions to ameliorate depressive symptoms warrant evaluation in an elderly population.

Social Status

Whether measured by occupation, income, or education, there is a strong inverse association between social status and cardiovascular morbidity and mortality at elderly age. Whether these are surrogates for access to information or access to care remains uncertain. In developed countries, the level of education bears a strong reverse relationship to the prevalence of major cardiovascular risk factors *(1)*.

Homocysteine

Elevated nonfasting plasma homocysteine levels were independently associated with increased rates of all-cause and cardiovascular mortality in the elderly in the Framingham Heart Study *(109)*. In the Rotterdam Study, *(110)* elevated homocysteine levels were associated with an increased risk of atherosclerosis and cardiovascular disease at ages 55–74; lack of association beyond age 75 may reflect selective mortality.

Although hyperhomocysteinemia is present in between 5–10% of the general population, it may be as high as 30–40% in the elderly. Nonetheless, a Canadian Task Force on Preventive Health Care concluded that at present there was insufficient evidence to recommend screening or management of hyperhomocysteinemia *(111)*.

In the Bronx Aging Study, based on the relationship of vitamin B_{12} and folate blood levels to cardiovascular morbidity and mortality in the old, the investigators concluded that vitamin B_{12} supplementation should not be routinely provided as a management for hyperhomocysteinemia unless a deficiency state was identified *(112)*.

Proteinuria

In older patients with adult-onset diabetes mellitus, both microalbuminuria and gross proteinuria were significantly associated with subsequent mortality from all causes and from cardiovascular, cerebrovascular, and coronary heart disease. This was independent of known cardiovascular risk factors and diabetes-related variables. These measures may help identify a very high-risk subset of elderly diabetic individuals *(113)*.

Chronic Renal Insufficiency

In the Heart and Estrogen/Progestin Replacement Study (HERS) *(114)* both mild and moderate renal insufficiency were independent risk factors for cardiovascular events in menopausal women with known coronary heart disease.

C-Reactive Protein

C-reactive protein (CRP) has been identified as an independent risk factor for coronary heart disease both for men and women. In the Cardiovascular Health Study, CRP was associated with incident events at elderly age, especially in individuals with subclinical cardiovascular disease at baseline *(115)*.

Although CRP was associated with several cardiovascular risk factors in an elderly cohort in the Helsinki Ageing Study, it alone predicted cardiovascular mortality only in the 75 yr old cohort *(116)*.

CRP levels were associated with future cardiovascular risk in other elderly populations as well *(117)*.

STANDARDS OF CARE

Relevance/Applicability of NCEP ATP III Guidelines: Third Report of the National Cholesterol Education Program (NCEP) Expert Panel on Dectection, Evaluation, and Treatment of High Blood Cholesterol in Adults (Adult Treatment Panel III) (69)

There is substantial evidence of undertreatment of hypercholesterolemia at elderly age. In the Cardiovascular Health Study, among community-dwelling individuals older than 65 yr of age, there was little increase in the use of cholesterol-lowering agents between 1989–1990 and 1995–1996. Fewer than 20% of untreated eligible patients at baseline, based on NCEP ATP II guidelines, initiated therapy in the 6 yr of follow-up, even among those with a history of coronary heart disease *(118)*.

Screening is recommended for adults age 20 and older without an upper age limit.

Older adults in the NCEP-ATP III guidelines are defined as men older than 65 and women older than 75 yr. Because most new coronary events and most coronary deaths occur in persons older than 65 yr of age and because high LDL and low HDL cholesterol levels continue to carry predictive power for the development of coronary disease in older persons, intervention is appropriate in this population using the cholesterol levels and the risk category as guidelines for the institution of therapeutic lifestyle changes and for the institution of pharmacologic therapy. For postmenopausal women, there are changes from the NCEP ATP II guidelines in that previously hormone replacement therapy was recommended as their initial intervention for lipid lowering. However, recent secondary and primary prevention trials have cast doubt on the role of hormone replacement therapy in the reduction of coronary risk; by contrast, favorable effects of statin therapy in women in clinical trials make this cholesterol-lowering drug preferable to hormone replacement therapy for coronary risk reduction.

In the estimation of 10-yr risk based on Framingham point scores, older age confers increased risk points both for men and women, with higher point scores accorded for elderly women than elderly men. Secondary prevention trials with statins included a sizeable number of older persons aged 65–75. Because of significant risk reduction with statin therapy, no age-based restrictions were considered necessary when selecting persons with established coronary heart disease for LDL-lowering therapy.

Lifestyle changes are considered the first line of therapy for primary prevention in older persons, although LDL-lowering drugs can be considered in older persons at higher risk because of multiple risk factors or advanced subclinical atherosclerosis. Advanced subclinical atherosclerosis detected by noninvasive testing may help in confirming the presence of higher risk in older persons, as well as the presence of diabetes and clinical evidence of noncoronary cardiovascular disease.

Should Pharmacologic Therapy Be Instituted for Lipid Lowering at an Elderly Age? Should These Agents Be Prescribed to the Oldest Old (i.e., Subjects Over 75–80 yr)?

Based on epidemiologic data, there is a higher attributable risk of hypercholesterolemia at an elderly age, as well as a higher prevalence of established coronary heart disease. Because the pathobiology of atherosclerosis does not appear to change with advancing age, lipid-lowering therapy should not be curtailed based on very elderly age alone. Lipid lowering in the elderly and nonelderly had a similar incidence of adverse drug events and laboratory abnormalities in clinical trials of statin therapy *(60)*. The lowering of LDL in both primary and secondary coronary prevention trials using statins decreased coronary risk and all cause mortality, with a similar risk reduction, about 30%, in middle-aged and elderly patients treated for about 5 yr; data are available to age 75. Extrapolation of data from statin trials suggests that benefit in the old old may be similar to that seen in middle-aged and younger elderly populations. Nonetheless, more information is needed on patients older than 75 yr of age, particularly in the primary prevention setting; and evaluation is requisite of the role of more aggressive lipid lowering at elderly age.

Relevance/Applicability of JNC VI Guidelines: Sixth Report of the Joint National Committee on Prevention, Detection, Evaluation, and Treatment of High Blood Pressure (39)

The JNC VI recommends initial therapy of hypertension with lifestyle modifications, with pharmacologic management if goal blood pressure is not achieved. Older patients respond well to modest reduction in sodium intake and to weight loss; modest intensity exercise may be beneficial. The concept of normotension has changed such that goal blood pressure is defined as <140/90 mm Hg where possible.

Large clinical trials of antihypertensive drug therapy in patients older than 60 yr of age have shown that control of hypertension reduces stroke, coronary heart disease, cardiovascular disease, heart failure and mortality. Thiazide diuretics or β blockers in combination with thiazide diuretics are recommended as initial therapy because of randomized controlled trial evidence in older individuals showing their efficacy in the reduction of morbidity and mortality *(119,120)*. Diuretics (hydrochlorothiazide with amiloride) in one study were superior to the β blocker atenolol *(121)*. Although patients with stage I isolated systolic hypertension have a significant increase in cardiovascular risk, the benefits of pharmacologic therapy for these individuals have not been demonstrated in a randomized controlled trial.

Diuretics are the preferred therapy for isolated systolic hypertension because of the significant reduction in multiple endpoints *(120)*. The calcium blocking drug nitrendipine in a randomized controlled trial *(122)* showed a 42% reduction in fatal and nonfatal stroke over an average of 2 yr, although effect on coronary events and heart failure did not reach statistical significance; thus a long-acting dihydropyridine calcium antagonist may be an appropriate alternative for elderly patients.

Caution is indicated with drugs that exaggerate orthostatic hypotension (peripheral adrenergic blockers, α blockers, and high dose diuretics) or drugs that can cause cognitive dysfunction (central α_2 agonists). Blood pressure should be measured in the standing as well as the seated position to assess for orthostasis.

Recommendations for HRT for Cardioprotection (102)

SECONDARY PREVENTION

* Hormone replacement therapy (HRT) should not be initiated for the secondary prevention of cardiovascular disease (CVD).
* The decision to continue or stop HRT in women with CVD who have been undergoing long-term HRT should be based on established noncoronary benefits and risks and patient preference.
* If a woman develops an acute CVD event or is immobilized while undergoing HRT, it is prudent to consider discontinuance of the HRT or to consider VTE prophylaxis while she is hospitalized to minimized risk of VTE associated with immobilization. Reinstitution of HRT should be based on established noncoronary benefits and risks, as well as patient preference.

PRIMARY PREVENTION

* Firm clinical recommendations for primary prevention await the results of ongoing randomized clinical trials.
* There are insufficient data to suggest that HRT should be initiated for the sole purpose of primary prevention of CVD.
* Initiation and continuation of HRT should be based on established noncoronary benefits and risks, possible coronary benefits and risks, and patient preference.

Recommendations for Risk Factor Management of Elderly Patients at Present

Clinical assessment of elderly patients should include evaluation for subclinical indices of cardiovascular disease, as well as traditional coronary risk factors. A sizeable number of ongoing research studies involve elderly individuals. Until the results of these studies become available, it appears reasonable to extrapolate information from middle-aged individuals to those of younger elderly age, although it remains controversial as to whether extrapolation is appropriate to individuals older than age 80, for whom even less information is available.

SUMMARY

Promotion of cardiovascular health for elderly individuals requires emphasis on adoption of healthy lifestyles and the use of appropriate pharmacotherapy. There is evidence that preventive interventions can be undertaken at elderly age without adversely affecting the quality-of-life. A WHO report *(1)* emphasizes the need to change attitudes and behaviors among elderly individuals in some populations who misperceive themselves as too old to benefit from preventive interventions. The report further emphasizes the principle of equity of care for elderly individuals—in particular, elderly women—in their opportunity for preventive services.

Questionnaire data suggest that an elderly population is concerned about and willing to attempt changes in lifestyle to maintain health *(123)*. Elderly patients were concerned about their cholesterol values, and the majority reported making dietary changes to lower cholesterol levels and prevent heart disease. In a demonstration program of the US Health Care Financing Administration, older rural Americans were shown to use some disease prevention and health promotion services if the costs were covered by Medicare *(124)*; such use was higher among those with more education. The finding that elderly patients were more likely to use preventive services if encouraged to do so by their physicians highlights the need for physician encouragement of preventive services at elderly age. Another study of rural elderly persons identified that follow-up and reinforcement of health promotion interventions played an important role in changing health behavior for elderly patients in rural settings and further highlighted that the family was an important source of support and should be incorporated in health care programs for the elderly *(125)*.

REFERENCES

1. WHO Study Group on Epidemiology and Prevention of Cardiovascular Disease in the Elderly. Epidemiology and Prevention of Cardiovascular Diseases in Elderly People. Report of a World Health Organization Study Group. WHO Technical Report Series No. 853. World Health Organization, Geneva, 1995.
2. Abrams J, Coultas DB, Malhotra D, Vela BS, Samaan SA, Roche RJ. Coronary risk factors and their modification: lipids, smoking, hypertension, estrogen, and the elderly. Curr Prob Cardiol 1995;20:535–610.
3. Lee PY, Alexander KP, Hammill BG, Pasquali SK, Peterson ED. Representation of elderly persons and women in published randomized trials of acute coronary syndromes. JAMA 2001;286:708–713.
4. Kannel WB. Clinical misconceptions dispelled by epidemiological research. Circulation 1995;92: 3350–3360.
5. Kannel WB. Coronary heart disease risk factors in the elderly. Am J Geriatr Cardiol 2002;11:101–107.
6. Burke GL, Arnold AM, Bild DE, et al. Factors associated with healthy aging: the Cardiovascular Health Study. J Am Geriatr Soc 2001;49:254–262.
7. Larson MG. Assessment of cardiovascular risk factors in the elderly: the Framingham Heart Study. Stat Med 1995;14:1745–1756.
8. Menotti A, Mulder I, Nissinen A, et al. Cardiovascular risk factors and 10-year all-cause mortality in elderly European male populations. The FINE study. Eur Heart J 2001;22:573–579.
9. Kuller L, Borhani N, Furberg C, et al. Prevalence of subclinical atherosclerosis and cardiovascular disease and association with risk factors in the Cardiovascular Health Study. Am J Epidemiol 1994;139: 1164–1179.
10. Kuller LH, Shemanski L, Psaty BM, et al. Subclinical disease as an independent risk factor for cardiovascular disease. Circulation 1996;92:720–726.
11. Maroo A, O'Connell CJ. CME Paper. Current practice and future promise for clinical noninvasive measurements of subclinical atherosclerotic disease in the elderly. Am J Geriatr Cardiol 2002;11:108–116.
12. The Clinical Quality Improvement Network (CQIN) Investigators. Low incidence of assessment and modification of risk factors in acute care patients at high risk for cardiovascular events, particularly among females and the elderly. Am J Cardiol 1995;76:570–573.
13. Williams MA, Fleg JL, Ades PA, et al. Secondary prevention of coronary heart disease in the elderly (with emphasis on patients ≥75 years of age): An American Heart Association Scientific Statement from the Council on Clinical Cardiology Subcommittee on Exercise Testing, Cardiac Rehabilitation, and Prevention. Circulation 2002;105:1735–1743.
14. Glynn RJ, Chae CU, Guralnik JM, et al. Pulse pressure and mortality in old people. Arch Intern Med 2000;160:2765–2772.
15. O'Donnell CJ, Kannel WB. Epidemiologic appraisal of hypertension as a coronary risk factor in the elderly. Am J Geriatr Cardiol 2002;11:86–92.
16. Sutton-Tyrrell K, Alcorn HG, Herzog H, Kelsey SF, Kuller LH. Morbidity, mortality, and hypertensive treatment effects by extent of atherosclerosis in older adults with isolated systolic hypertension. Stroke 1995;26:1319–1324.
17 Burt VL, Whelton P, Roccella EJ, et al. Prevalence of hypertension in the US adult population: results from the third National Health and Nutrition Examination Survey, 1988–1991. Hypertension 1995;25: 305–313.
18. National High Blood Pressure Education Program Working Group. National High Blood Pressure Education Program Working Group report on hypertension in the elderly. Hypertension 1994;23:275–285.
19. Kannel WB, D'Agostino RB, Silberschatz H. Blood pressure and cardiovascular morbidity and mortality rates in the elderly. Am Heart J 1997;134:758–763.

20. 27th Bethesda Conference. Matching the intensity of risk factor management with the hazard for coronary disease events. J Am Coll Cardiol 1996;27:957–1047.

21. Psaty BM, Furberg CD, Kuller LH, et al. Traditional risk factors and subclinical disease measures as predictors of first myocardial infarction in older adults: the Cardiovascular Health Study. Arch Intern Med 1999;159:1339–1347.

22. Psaty BM, Furberg CD, Kuller LH, et al. Association between blood pressure level and the risk of myocardial infarction, stroke, and total mortality: the Cardiovascular Health Study. Arch Intern Med 2001; 161:1183–1192.

23. van den Hoogen PC, van Popele NM, Feskens EJ, et al. Blood pressure and risk of myocardial infarction in elderly men and women: the Rotterdam Study. J Hypertension 1999;17:1373–1378.

24. Franklin SS, Larson MG, Khan SA, et al. Does the relation of blood pressure to coronary heart disease risk change with aging? The Framingham Heart Study. Circulation 2001;103:1245–1249.

25. Madhavan S, Ooi WL, Cohen H, Alderman MH. Relation of pulse pressure and blood pressure reduction to the incidence of myocardial infarction. Hypertension 1994;23:395–401.

26. Lee ML, Rosner BA, Weiss ST. Relationship of blood pressure to cardiovascular death: the effects of pulse pressure in the elderly. Ann Epidemiol 1999;9:101–107.

27. Whelton PK, Appel LJ, Espeland MA, et al. Sodium reduction and weight loss in the treatment of hypertension in older persons: a randomized controlled trial of nonpharmacologic interventions in the elderly (TONE). TONE Collaborative Research Group. JAMA 1998;279:839–846.

28. Alam S, Johnson AG. A meta-analysis of randomised controlled trials (RCT) among healthy normotensive and essential hypertensive elderly patients to determine the effect of high salt (NaC1) diet on blood pressure. J Hum Hypertens 1999;13:367–374.

29. Sowers JR, Farrow AL. Treatment of elderly hypertensive patients with diabetes, renal disease, and coronary heart disease. Am J Geriatr Cardiol 1996;5:57–70.

30. Frost PH, Davis BR, Burlando AJ, et al. Coronary heart disease risk factors in men and women aged 60 years and older: findings from the Systolic Hypertension in the Elderly Program. Circulation 1996; 94:26–34.

31. Curb JD, Pressel SL, Cutler JA, et al. Effect of diuretic-based antihypertensive treatment on cardiovascular disease risk in older diabetic patients with isolated systolic hypertension. Systolic Hypertension in the Elderly Program Cooperative Research Group. JAMA 1996;276:1886–1892.

32. Savage PJ, Pressel SL, Curb JD, et al. Influence of long-term, low-dose, diuretic-based, antihypertensive therapy on glucose, lipid, uric acid, and potassium levels in older men and women with isolated systolic hypertension: The Systolic Hypertension in the Elderly Program. SHEP Cooperative Research Group. Arch Intern Med 1998;158:741–751.

33. Staessen JA, Gasowski J, Wang JE, et al. Risks of untreated and treated isolated systolic hypertension in the elderly: meta-analysis of outcome trials. Lancet 2000;355:865–872.

34. MacMahon S, Rodger A. The effects of blood pressure reduction in older patients: an overview of five randomized controlled trials in elderly hypertensives. J Clin Exp Hypertension 1993;15:967–978.

35. Pearce KA, Furberg CD, Rushing J. Does antihypertensive treatment of the elderly prevent cardiovascular events or prolong life? A meta-analysis of hypertension treatment trials. Arch Fam Med 1995;4: 943–949.

36. Staessen JA, Fagard R, Thijs L, et al. Randomised double-blind comparison of placebo and active treatment for older patients with isolated systolic hypertension. The Systolic Hypertension in Europe (Syst-Eur) Trial Investigators. Lancet 1997;350:757–764.

37. Gueyffier F, Bulpitt C, Boissel J-P, et al. Antihypertensive drugs in very old people: a subgroup meta-analysis of randomised controlled trials. Lancet 1999;353:793–796.

38. Ogihara T, Kuramoto K. Effect of long-term treatment with antihypertensive drugs on quality of life of elderly patients with hypertension: a double-blind comparative study between a calcium antagonist and a diuretic. NICS-EH Study Group. National Intervention Cooperative Study in Elderly Hypertensives. Hypertension Res 2000;23:33–37.

39. The Sixth Report of the Joint National Committee on Prevention, Detection, Evaluation, and Treatment of High Blood Pressure. Arch Intern Med 1997;157:2413–2446.

40. Setaro JF, Black HR. Refractory hypertension. N Engl J Med 1992;327:543–547.

41. Ettinger WH, Wahl PW, Kuller LH, et al., for the CHS Collaborative Research Group. Lipoprotein lipids in older people. Results from the Cardiovascular Health Study. Circulation 1992;86:858–869.

42. Kannel WB. Range of serum cholesterol values in the population developing coronary artery disease. Am J Cardiol 1995;76:69C–77C.

43. Houterman S, Verschuren WM, Hofman A, Witteman JC. Serum cholesterol is a risk factor for myocardial infarction in elderly men and women: the Rotterdam Study. J Intern Med 1999;246:25–33.

44. Oomen CM, Ocke MC, Feskens EJ, van Erp-Baart MA, Kok FJ, Kromhout D. Association between trans fatty acid intake and 10-year risk of coronary heart disease in the Zutphen Elderly Study: a prospective population-based study. Lancet 2001;357:746–751.

45. Houterman S, Verschuren WM, Giampaoli S, et al. Total but not high-density lipoprotein cholesterol is consistently associated with coronary heart disease mortality in elderly men in Finland, Italy, and The Netherlands. Epidemiology 2000;11:327–332.

46. Corti MC, Guralnik JM, Salive ME, et al. Clarifying the direct relation between total cholesterol levels and death from coronary heart disease in older persons. Ann Intern Med 1997;126:753–760.

47. Expert Panel on Detection, Evaluation, and Treatment of High Blood Cholesterol in Adults: Summary of the second report of the National Cholesterol Education Program (NCEP) Expert Panel on Detection, Evaluation, and Treatment of High Blood Cholesterol in Adults (Adult Treatment Panel II). JAMA 1993;269:3015–3023.

48. Sempos CT, Cleeman JI, Carroll MD, et al. Prevalence of high blood cholesterol among U.S. adults: an update based on guidelines from the Second Report of the National Cholesterol Education Program Adult Treatment Panel. JAMA 1993;269:3009–3014.

49. Grundy SM, Cleeman JI, Rifkind BM, Kuller LH. Cholesterol lowering in the elderly population. Coordinating Committee of the National Cholesterol Education Program. Arch Intern Med 1999;159:1670–1678.

50. Miettinen TA, Pyorala K, Olsson AG, et al., for the Scandinavian Simvastatin Study Group. Cholesterol-lowering therapy in women and elderly patients with myocardial infarction or angina pectoris. Findings from the Scandinavian Simvastatin Survival Study (4S). Circulation 1997;96:4211–4218.

51. Lewis SJ, Moye LA, Sacks FM, et al., for the CARE Investigators. Effect of pravastatin on cardiovascular events in older patients with myocardial infarction and cholesterol levels in the average range. Results of the Cholesterol and Recurrent Events (CARE) Trial. Ann Intern Med 1998;129:681–689.

52. The Long-Term Intervention with Pravastatin in Ischemic Disease (LIPID) Study Group. Prevention of cardiovascular events and death with pravastatin in patients with coronary heart disease and a broad range of initial cholesterol levels. N Engl J Med 1998;339:1349–1357.

53. West of Scotland Coronary Prevention Study Group. Influence of pravastatin and plasma lipids on clinical events in the West of Scotland Coronary Prevention Study (WOSCOPS). Circulation 1998;97:1440–1445.

54. Downs JR, Clearfield M, Weis S, et al., for the AFCAPS/TexCAPS Research Group. Primary prevention of acute coronary events with lovastatin in men and women with average cholesterol levels. Results of AFCAPS/TexCAPS. JAMA 1998;279:1615–1622.

55. LaRosa JC, He J, Vupputuri S. Effect of statins on risk of coronary disease. A meta-analysis of randomized controlled trials. JAMA 1999;282:2340–2346.

56. Lilly LS. Drug therapy of lipid disorders: benefits and limitations in elderly patients. Am J Geriatr Cardiol 1996;5:15–16, 21–26.

57. Sacks FM, Tonkin AM, Shepherd J, et al. Effect of pravastatin on coronary disease events in subgroups defined by coronary risk factors: the Prospective Pravastatin Pooling Project. Circulation 2000;102:1893–1900.

58. Campeau L, Hunninghake DB, Knatterud GL, et al., and Post CABG Trial Investigators. Aggressive cholesterol lowering delays saphenous vein graft atherosclerosis in women, the elderly, and patients with associated risk factors. NHLBI Post Coronary Artery Bypass Graft Clinical Trial. Circulation 1999;99:3241–3247.

59. Shepherd J, Blauw GJ, Murphy MB, et al. The design of a prospective study of Pravastatin in the Elderly at Risk (PROSPER). PROSPER Study Group. Prospective Study of Pravastatin in the Elderly at Risk. Am J Cardiol 1999;84:1192–1197.

60. Heart Protection Study Collaborative Group. MRC/BHF Heart Protection study of cholesterol lowering with simvastatin in 20,536 high-risk individuals: a randomised placebo-controlled trial. Lancet 2000;360:7–22.

61. Rockwood K, Kirkland S, Hogan DB, et al. Use of lipid-lowering agents, indication bias, and the risk of dementia in community-dwelling elderly people. Arch Neurol 2002;59:223–227.

62. Hamilton VH, Racicot F-E, Zowall MA, Coupal L, Grover SA. The cost-effectiveness of HMG-CoA reductase inhibitors to prevent coronary heart disease: estimating the benefits of increasing HDL-C. JAMA 1995;273:1032–1038.

63. Ganz DA, Kuntz KM, Jacobson GA, et al. Cost-effectiveness of 3-hydroxy-3-methylglutaryl coenzyme A reductase inhibitor therapy in older patients with myocardial infarction. Ann Intern Med 2000; 132:780–787.

64. Santanello N, Barber BL, Applegate WB, et al., for the CRISP Collaborative Study Group. Effect of pharmacologic lipid lowering on health-related quality of life in older persons: results form the Cholesterol Reduction in Seniors Program (CRISP) Pilot Study. J Am Geriatr Soc 1997;45:8–14.

65. McAlister FA, Taylor L, Teo KK, et al. The treatment and prevention of coronary heart disease in Canada: do older patients receive efficacious therapies? The Clinical Quality Improvement Network (CQIN) Investigators. J Am Geriatr Soc 1999;47:811–818.

66. Shaefer EJ, Lichtenstein AH, Lamon-Fava S, et al. Effects of National Cholesterol Education Program Step 2 diets relatively high or relatively low in fish-derived fatty acids on plasma lipoproteins in middle-aged and elderly subjects. Am J Clin Nutr 1996;63:234–241.

67. Kromhout D, Feskens EJM, Bowles CH. The protective effect of a small amount of fish on coronary heart disease mortality in an elderly population. Int J Epidemiol 1995;24:340–345.

68. Ades PA, Poehlman ET. The effects of exercise training on serum lipids in the elderly. J Am Geriatr Cardiol 1996;5:27–31.

69. Expert Panel on Detection, Evaluation, and Treatment of High Blood Cholesterol in Adults. Executive Summary of the Third Report of the National Cholesterol Education Program (NCEP) Expert Panel on Detection, Evaluation, and Treatment of High Blood Cholesterol in Adults (Adult Treatment Panel III). JAMA 2001;285:2486–2497.

70. Harris TB, Launer LJ, Madans J, Feldman JJ. Cohort study of effect of being overweight and change in weight of coronary heart disease in old age. Br Med J 1997;314:1791–1794.

71. Vokonas PS, Kannel WB. Epidemiology of coronary heart disease in the elderly. In: Tresch DD, Aronow WS, eds., *Cardiovascular Disease in the Elderly Patient.* Marcel Dekker, New York, 1994, pp. 91–123.

72. Harvey-Berino J. Weight loss in the clinical setting: applications for cardiac rehabilitation. Coronary Artery Dis 1998;9:795–798.

73. Krauss RM, Eckel RH, Howard B, et al. AHA Dietary Guidelines. Revision 2000: A Statement for Healthcare Professionals from the Nutrition Committee of the American Heart Association. Circulation 2000;102:2284–2299.

74. Heiat A, Vaccarino V, Krumholz HM. An evidence-based assessment of federal guidelines for overweight and obesity as they apply to elderly persons. Arch Intern Med 2001;161:1194–1203.

75. LaCroix AZ, Lang J, Scherr P, et al. Smoking and mortality among older men and women in three communities. N Engl J Med 1991;324:1619–1625.

76. Hermanson B, Omenn GS, Kronmal RA, Gersh BJ, and participants in the Coronary Artery Surgery Study. Beneficial six-year outcome of smoking cessation in older men and women with coronary artery disease. Results from the CASS Registry. N Engl J Med 1988;319:1365–1369.

77. Morgan GD, Noll EL, Orleans BK, et al. Reaching midlife and older smokers: tailored interventions for routine medical care. Prev Med 1996;25:346–354.

78. Fiore MC, Bailey WC, Cohen SJ, et al. *Treating Tobacco Use and Dependence.* Clinical Practice Guideline. Rockville, MD. US Department of Health and Human Services. Public Health Service. June, 2000.

79. Kohrt WM, Kirwan JP, Staten MA, et al. Insulin resistance in aging is related to abdominal obesity. Diabetes 1993;42:273–281.

80. Kirwan JP, Lohrt WM, Wojta DM, et al. Endurance exercise training reduces glucose-stimulated insulin levels in 60- to 70-year-old men and women. J Gerontol 1993;48:M84–M90.

81. Brochu M, Poehlman EP, Savage PD, et al. Coronary risk profiles in male coronary patients: effects of body composition, fat distribution, age and fitness. Coronary Artery Dis 2000;1:137–144.

82. Diabetes and the heart. Lancet 1997;350(Suppl I):1–32.

83. Lindholm LH, Hansson L, Ekbom T, et al. Comparison of antihypertensive treatments in preventing cardiovascular events in elderly diabetic patients: results from the Swedish Trial in Old Patients with Hypertension-2. STOP Hypertension-2 Study Group. J Hypertens 2000;18:1671–1675.

84. Wannamethee SG, Shaper AG, Walker M. changes in physical activity, mortality, and incidence of coronary heart disease in older men. Lancet 1998;351:1603–1608.

85. Siscovick DS, Fried L, Mittelmark M, Rutan G, Bild D, O'Leary DH. Exercise intensity and subclinical cardiovascular disease in the elderly. The Cardiovascular Health Study. Am J Epidemiol 1997;145:977–986.

86. Fried LP, Kronmal RA, Newman AB, et al. Risk factors for 5-year mortality in older adults. JAMA 1998;279:585–592.

87. Wenger NK. Physical inactivity and coronary heart disease in elderly patients. Clin Geriatr Med 1996; 12:79–88.

88. Hakim AA, Petrovitch H, Burchfiel CM, et al. Effects of walking on mortality among nonsmoking retired men. N Engl J Med 1998;338:94–99.

89. Kushi LH, Fee RM, Folsom AR, et al. Physical activity and mortality in postmenopausal women. JAMA 1997;277:1287–1292.

90. LaCroix AZ, Leveille SG, Hecht JA, Grothaus LC, Wagner EH. Does walking decrease the risk of cardiovascular disease hospitalizations and death in older adults? J Am Geriatr Soc 1996;44:113–120.

91. Lee IM, Sesso HD, Paffenbarger RS Jr. Physical activity and coronary heart disease risk in men: does the duration of exercise episodes predict risk? Circulation 2000;102:981–986.

92. Hakim AA, Curb JD, Petrovitch H, et al. Effects of walking on coronary heart disease in elderly men: the Honolulu Heart Program. Circulation 1999;100:9–13.

93. Young DR, Appel LJ, Jee S, Miller ER III. The effects of aerobic exercise and T'ai Chi on elderly men: blood pressure in older people: results of a randomized trial. J Am Geriatr Soc 1999;47:277–284.

94. Williams MA, Maresh CM, Esterbrooks DJ, et al. Early exercise training in patients older than age 65 years compared with that in younger patients after acute myocardial infarction or coronary artery bypass grafting. Am J Cardiol 1985;55:263–266.

95. Lavie CJ, Milani RV, Littman AB. Benefits of cardiac rehabilitation and exercise training in secondary coronary prevention in the elderly. J Am Coll Cardiol 1993;22:678–683.

96. Wannamethee SG, Shaper AG, Walker M. Physical activity and mortality in older men with diagnosed heart disease. Circulation 2000;102:1358–1363.

97. Williams MA. Exercise testing in cardiac rehabilitation: exercise prescription and beyond. Cardiology Clinics 2001;19:415–431.

98. Pollock ML, Franklin BA, Balady GJ, et al. Resistance exercise in individuals with and without cardiovascular disease: benefits, rationale, safety, and prescription. Circulation 2000;101:828–833.

99. Onder G, Penninx BWJH, Balkrishnan R, et al. Relation between use of angiotensin-converting enzyme inhibitors and muscle strength and physical function in older women: an observational study. Lancet 2002;359:926–930.

100. Wenger NK. A cardiologist's view of hormone replacement therapy and alternatives for cardioprotection. Women's Health Gender-Based Med 2001;10:257–260.

101. Hulley S, Grady D, Bush T, et al. Randomized trial of estrogen plus progestin for secondary prevention of coronary heart disease in postmenopausal women. Heart and Estrogen/progestin Replacement Study (HERS) Research Group. JAMA 1998;280:605–613.

102. Mosca L, Collins P, Herrington DM, et al. Hormone replacement therapy and cardiovascular disease. A statement for healthcare professionals from the American Heart Association. Circulation 2001;104: 499–503.

102a. Grady D, Herrington D, Bittner V, et al. Cardiovascular disease outcomes during 6.8 years of hormone therapy. Heart and Estrogen/progestin Replacement Study follow-up (HERS II). JAMA 2002;288: 49–57.

102b. Writing Group for the Women's Health Initiative Investigators. Risks and benefits of estrogen plus progestin in healthy postmenopausal women: principal results from the Women's Health Initiative randomized controlled trial. JAMA 2002;288:321–333.

103. O'Leary DH, Polak JF, Kronmal RA, et al. Carotid-artery intima and media thickness as a risk factor for myocardial infarction and stroke in older adults. Cardiovascular Health Study Collaborative Research Group. N Engl J Med 1999;340:14–22.

104. Newman AB, Shemanski L, Manolio TA, et al. Ankle-arm index as a predictor of cardiovascular disease and mortality in the Cardiovascular Health Study. The Cardiovascular Health Study Group. Arterioscler Thromb Vasc Biology 1999;19:538–545.

105. Ariyo AA, Haan M, Tangen CM, et al. Depressive symptoms and risks of coronary heart disease and mortality in elderly Americans. Cardiovascular Health Study Collaborative Research Group. Circulation 2000;102:1773–1779.

106. Wassertheil-Smoller S, Applegate WB, Berge K, et al. Change in depression as a precursor of cardiovascular events. SHEP Cooperative Research Group (Systolic Hypertension in the Elderly). Arch Intern Med 1996;156:553–561.

107. Sesso HD, Kawachi I, Vokonas PS, Sparrow D. Depression and the risk of coronary heart disease in the Normative Aging Study. Am J Cardiol 1998;82:851–856.

108. Mendes de Leon CF, Krumholz HM, Seeman TS, et al. Depression and risk of coronary heart disease in elderly men and women: New Haven EPESE, 1982–1991. Established Populations for the Epidemiologic Studies of the Elderly. Arch Intern Med 1998;158:2341–2348.
109. Bostom AG, Silbershatz H, Rosenberg IH, et al. Nonfasting plasma total homocysteine levels and all-cause and cardiovascular disease mortality in elderly Framingham men and women. Arch Intern Med 1999;159:1077–1080.
110. Bots ML, Launer LJ, Lindemans J, Hofman A, Grobbee DE. Homocysteine, atherosclerosis and prevalent cardiovascular disease in the elderly: The Rotterdam Study. J Intern Med 1997;242:339–347.
111. Booth GL, Wang EE. Preventive health care, 2000 update: screening and management of hyperhomocysteinemia for the prevention of coronary artery disease events. The Canadian Task Force on Preventive Health Care. Canadian Medical Association Journal 2000;163:21–29.
112. Zeitlin A, Frishman WH, Chang CJ. The association of vitamin B_{12} and folate blood levels with mortality and cardiovascular morbidity incidence in the old old: the Bronx Aging Study. Am J Therap 1997;4: 275–281.
113. Valmadrid CT, Klein R, Moss SE, Klein BE. The risk of cardiovascular disease mortality associated with microalbuminuria and gross proteinuria in persons with older-onset diabetes mellitus. Arch Intern Med 2000;160:1093–1100.
114. Shlipak MG, Simon JA, Grady D, Lin F, Wenger NK, Furberg CD, for the Heart and Estrogen/progestin Replacement Study (HERS) Investigators. Renal insufficiency and cardiovascular events in postmenopausal women with coronary heart disease. J Am Coll Cardiol 2001;38:705–711.
115. Tracy RP, Lemaitre RN, Psaty BM, et al. Relationship of C-reactive protein to risk of cardiovascular disease in the elderly. Results from the Cardiovascular Health Study and the Rural Health Promotion Project. Arterioscler Thromb Vasc Biol 1997;17:1121–1127.
116. Strandberg TE, Tilvis RS. C-reactive protein, cardiovascular risk factors, and mortality in a prospective study in the elderly. Arterioscler Thromb Vasc Biol 2000;20:1057–1060.
117. Tracy RP. Hemostatic and inflammatory markers as risk factors for coronary disease in the elderly. Am J Geriatr Cardiol 2002;11:93–100, 107.
118. Lemaitre RN, Furberg CD, Newman AB, et al. Time trends in the use of cholesterol-lowering agents in older adults. The Cardiovascular Health Study. Arch Intern Med 1998;158:1761–1768.
119. MacMahon S, Rodgers A. The effects of blood pressure reduction in older patients: an overview of five randomized controlled trials in elderly hypertensives. Clin Exp Hypertens 1993;15:967–978.
120. SHEP Cooperative Research Group. Prevention of stroke by antihypertensive drug treatment in older persons with isolated systolic hypertension: final results of the Systolic Hypertension in the Elderly Program (SHEP). JAMA 1991;265:3255–3264.
121. MRC Working Party. Medical Research Council trial of treatment of hypertension in older adults: principal results. Br Med J 1992;304:405–412.
122. Staessen JA, Fagard R, Thijs L, et al., for the Systolic Hypertension – Europe (Syst-Eur) Trial Investigators. Morbidity and mortality in the placebo-controlled European Trial on Isolated Systolic Hypertension in the Elderly. Lancet 1997;260:757–764.
123. Soons KR, Little DN, Harvey J. Cholesterol screening in the elderly: changing attitudes. Gerontol 1995; 41:57–62.
124. Lave JR, Ives DG. Participation in health promotion programs by the rural elderly. Am J Prev Med 1995; 11:46–53.
125. Dellasega C, Brown R, White A. Cholesterol-related health behaviors in rural elderly persons. J Gerontol Nurs 1995;21:6–12.

11 Arrhythmias in the Elderly
With an Emphasis on Atrial Fibrillation

James A. Reiffel, MD

CONTENTS

INTRODUCTION
STANDARDS OF CARE
ARRHYTHMIA CONTROVERSIES: REAL AND PERCEIVED
REFERENCES

INTRODUCTION

Cardiac arrhythmias know no age restrictions; they occur *in utero*, in youth, in middle age, and in the elderly. However, an age-related predilection or altered incidence does exist for specific arrhythmias *(1)* (Table 1). Automatic junctional tachycardias are substantially more frequent in youth than in later life. Atrioventricular re-entrant tachycardias (AVRTs) utilizing accessory pathways often present in childhood, the teenage years, or young adulthood. AV nodal re-entrant tachycardias (AVNRT) most frequently first occurs between the fourth and sixth decades of life, whereas the risk of developing atrial fibrillation (AF) increases with age *(1–5)*. In observational studies such as those performed in Framingham *(6)*, less than 5% of the male 60-yr old population had AF, whereas the incidence approximates 10% by age 70 and >15% by age 75–80. Similarly, ventricular premature depolarizations (VPDs) increase with age, presenting in approximately two-thirds of subjects by age 50 on routine Holter monitoring *(7,8)*. In contrast, vagal-mediated dysrhythmias, such as marked nocturnal sinus bradycardia (sleeping rates <40 bpm) or nocturnal AV Wenckebach, are more common in the autonomically innervated young heart and less frequent in healthy elderly subjects, where autonomic sensitivity is routinely diminished *(9–14)*. When the same bradyarrhythmias are seen in the elderly, disease-mediated, drug-mediated, or degenerative nodal dysfunction rather than a vagotonic mechanism must be suspected.

Arrhythmias occur in the setting of organic heart disease—unrelated to either the loss of myocytes or the increase in fibrosis that occurs with aging. Many of the common cardiovascular diseases, other than the congenital, also increase with age. Most striking among these are coronary artery disease, hypertension, and congestive heart failure, which are

From: *Aging, Heart Disease, and Its Management: Facts and Controversies*
Edited by: N. Edwards, M. Maurer, and R. Wellner © Humana Press Inc., Totowa, NJ

Table 1
Arrhythmias vs Age

Common age of onset
  Youth: AVRT
  Middle age: AVNRT, VPDs
  Older age: AF
Age-related therapy modifiers
Choice of anticoagulation for AF
Age-related structural disorders
  Autonomic sensitivity
  Primary therapy for SCD

Abbreviations: AVRT = atrioventricular reentrant tachycardia; AVNRT = atrioventricular nodal reentrant tachycardia; AF = atrial fibrillation; VPDs = ventricular premature depolarization; SCD = sudden cardiac death.

more prevalent with age, and are associated with an increase in the frequency of AF, ventricular ectopy, ventricular tachycardia (ventricular tachycardia), and sudden cardiac death (SCD).

Accordingly, similar symptom presentations or clinical syndromes will commonly represent different pathophysiologic mechanisms or dysrhythmic states in young versus geriatric patients. For example, a new onset, rapid, narrow QRS tachycardia at a rate of 150 bpm is likely to be atrioventricular re-entrant tachycardias in a teenager, AV nodal re-entrant tachycardias in a 50-yr old, and atrial flutter with a 2:1 ventricular response in the elderly. Similarly, unexplained syncope in a healthy young adult is commonly neurocardiogenic in its mechanism and more likely to be diagnosed with a tilt-table test than with Holter monitoring (HM) or an electrophysiologic study (EPS). In contrast, in the elderly, dysrhythmic syncope is more likely to represent ventricular tachycardia; a rapid supraventricular tachyarrhythmia in a diseased heart; organic sinus node, or conduction disease than an autonomically mediated mechanism (aside from orthostatic hypotension) and is more likely to be elucidated with HM or EPS than with a tilt test (aside from orthostatic hypotension) (15–21). Consequently, recognition of the impact of age and its alterations on the presence and frequency of specific arrhythmias and clinical syndromes is important in evaluating patients with suspected cardiac dysrhythmias.

Interacting with the above are several other age-related phenomena that can modify both arrhythmogenesis and antiarrhythmic therapy. Because the autonomic influence on the sinus node, AV node, and cardiovascular reflexes declines as we go from youth to our geriatric years (9–14), the effectiveness of therapeutic modalities changes. Additionally, because both renal function and muscle mass decline with age, the excretory rate and volume of distribution of many drugs will also decline, resulting in a need to use lower doses of many agents in elderly subjects in order to avoid toxicity and risk. Dofetilide and sotalol, both renally excreted agents, are important examples of drugs with doses that must be exquisitely matched to renal function as judged by creatinine clearance rates and, hence, must usually be reduced in geriatric subjects.

Finally, the clinical presentation of and therapeutic options for arrhythmogenic disorders may also be altered by age. Hyperthyroidism (22), e.g., may present as AF without its other typical, often hyperadrenergic-like signs (so-called apathetic hyperthyroidism) in geriatric patients such that otherwise common clinical clues may be absent. Structural heart disorders (SHDs), which occur more commonly in the elderly, may adversely interact with antiarrhythmic drugs, increasing pro-arrhythmic risk. Class IC anti-arrhythmics as determined from placebo-controlled clinical trials (23–25) should be avoided in patients with ischemic heart disease or ventricular failure, limiting their use in elderly patients. This is probably true for other class I anti-arrhythmics (24,25). Accordingly, because of such phenomena and concerns, the standard of care for several arrhythmias differs in the elderly as compared to the young. This may be true for AF or for ventricular tachycardia/sudden cardiac death, where drug suppression or device therapy is usually either the initial or the only approach to therapy; this is in contrast to curative ablation that may be feasible in only the minority of older patients with structural heart disorders but in a substantial fraction of young, otherwise healthy patients, with atrioventricular re-entrant tachycardias, AV nodal re-entrant tachycardias, idiopathic ventricular tachycardia, and some AF.

STANDARDS OF CARE

Atrial Fibrillation

Most patients with AF encountered by clinicians, particularly those with structural heart disease, will be 60 yr of age or older. Although treatment approaches for this arrhythmia are generally similar, regardless of age, attention to differences is critical (Table 1). All patients with AF require that any underlying disorder be identified and treated, heart rate controlled, and anticoagulation considered. Age- or disease-associated changes in atrial electrophysiology and size, however, are more likely to be present in older individuals.

Age may play a role in the management of lone AF. In patients older than 60–65 yr, for example, warfarin is the standard recommendation, rather than aspirin, and should be used in the absence of a contraindication (26–30). This is true for paroxysmal and persistent AF in all nontransitory settings, including following cardiac surgery. Patients of all ages with AF who have other risk markers for enhanced embolic rates also require warfarin rather than aspirin (see more below) (31–37).

Digoxin can play a role in ventricular rate control for older patients, especially those with congestive heart failure (CHF), whereas the effectiveness of this drug is usually suboptimal in younger, active patients. Digoxin's effect predominantly occurs through indirect vagomimmetic actions (38) and secondarily via direct effects. Vagal withdrawal during activity in young, autonomically innervated patients allows exercise rates to increase significantly, simultaneously reducing the rate-slowing potential of digitalis. In contrast, in elderly less active patients, particularly when disease or age has altered AV nodal function, digoxin may be more effective for ventricular rate control in AF than it is in the young. Digoxin's positive inotropic effects in the failing ventricle, which may reduce reflex sympathetic activation, may also serve to help control the ventricular response in such patients. There may be a reduced role for the calcium channel blockers (CCBs), particularly verapamil, because of its constipating effects in geriatric patients. Reduced autonomic influence on the cardiac conduction system in later life may reduce the rate-slowing potential of β-receptor inhibition. Because β-blocker or CCB drugs are often used for the management of concomitant disorders in the elderly, they frequently are used as first-line agents for rate control in many older subjects; digoxin is only added later if necessary (39). Notably, some elderly patients do not require therapy for control of the ventricular rate during AF, because they have intrinsic AV nodal disease. Nodal disease may also contribute to AF in the elderly because sinus node dysfunction, which is most common in older patients, may enhance the genesis of AF (the "brady-tachy syndrome") *(40)*. Accordingly, pacemaker implantation to support drug therapy and reduce bradycardia-related paroxysms of AF *(41–44)* is also more common in this age group.

Choice of Phamacologic Treatment for AF

The use of pharmacologic agents to produce cardioversion or to maintain sinus rhythm (antiarrhythmic drugs, AAD) is similar in both elderly and younger patients. In recent years, several algorithms for AF management have been published *(45–49)*; these guidelines have become the norm in management decisions. Aside from anticoagulation, none have used age as a discriminator for therapy. However, age-related differences in the presence and nature of underlying structural heart disease and in metabolic and excretory function often reduces either the choice of agents or the doses that can be used in older patients. Class IC drugs are useful as single-dose therapy to produce cardioversion of recent-onset AF *(50,51)*, but they are less useful in older than in younger patients for the maintenance of sinus rhythm. Multiple clinical trials and analyses *(23–25)* have taught us that drugs in this class are either absolutely or relatively contraindicated in the presence of structural heart disease. Prior to initiating therapy with class I drugs, structural heart disease must be ruled out. Normal baseline electrocardiogram (ECG), echocardiogram, and exercise test are prerequisites for the use of a class I drug in this age group. Such trials have included Cardiac Arrhythmic Suppression Trial (CAST) as well as other post-MI (myocardial infarction) analyses of antiarrhythmic drug safety and risk *(23,24)*, which have shown a mortality risk vs placebo, and CASH *(52)*, CASCADE *(53)*, and ESVEM *(54,55)*, which have shown a mortality risk of class I drugs versus class III antiarrhythmic drugs. During the course of AFFIRM *(50–57)*, class I anti-arrhythmic drugs for AF were withdrawn.

In contrast, dofetilide, sotalol, and amiodarone are the antiarrhythmics of choice in patients with structural heart disease, per all the published algorithms *(45–48)*, and thus in most elderly subjects with AF. In placebo-controlled trials in patients with structural heart disease, including DIAMOND, EMIAT, CAMIAT, and the Julian study *(58–62)*, dofetilide, sotalol, and amiodarone have been found not to have a mortality risk versus placebo in post-MI or heart failure patients. Because both sotalol and dofetilide are renally excreted, the drug dose must be adjusted accordingly and the QT interval monitored. Extra caution is also required with dofetilide and amiodarone because of their numerous drug interactions with the polypharmacy commonly used in the older patient.

Particular concern is also needed when using dofetilide or sotalol if the patient is concomitantly taking a diuretic, because hypokalemia or hypomagnesia will increase the risk of ventricular proarrhythmia with these agents. Fortunately, many elderly patients with structural heart disease will often be on an angiotension-converting enzyme (ACE) inhibitor that reduces hypokalemia or hypomagnesemia.

Choice of Pharmacologic Therapy for Other Arrhythmias

For ventricular arrhythmias, pharmacologic therapy is not determined so much by age as it is by arrhythmia mechanism and setting. In younger patients without structural heart disease, ventricular tachycardia is frequently the result of triggered or re-entrant foci in the right ventricular (RV) outflow tract and/or left-ventricular postero-septal fascicular tissues. The former is often responsive to β-blockers, antiarrhythmic drugs, ablation, and sometimes, to calcium channel blockers. The latter is usually ablatable, sensitive to anti-arrhythmic drugs, and sometimes to calcium channel blockers, which are contraindicated in most other ventricular tachycardias because of inefficacy and high risk for hypotension. In older subjects, when structural heart disease such as cardiomyopathy or coronary artery disease (e.g., post-MI) is frequent, these idiopathic ventricular tachycardias are much less common. In this setting, β-blockers as monotherapy are rarely effective [although they are useful to augment the efficacy of other antiarrhythmic drugs (63–64)], CCBs are contraindicated, class IA drugs are relatively ineffective, and sotalol and amiodarone have proven superior in comparative efficacy studies such as ESVEM, CASH, and CASCADE (52–55). However, even more effective in reducing SCD is the implantable cardioverter-defibrillator (ICD), which has now become the treatment of first choice for SCD prevention in most ventricular tachycardia/ventricular fibrillation patients with structural heart disease. Even less influenced by age are the decisions to treat bradyarrhythmias. Guidelines for treatment of sinus node/AV node dysfunction indicate pacemaker implantation for symptoms of marked bradycardia, without age-specific differences (65,66). Similarly, advanced His–Purkinje block, such as Mobitz II or complete heart block, requires pacing independent of age.

ARRHYTHMIA CONTROVERSIES: REAL AND PERCEIVED

Anticoagulation for AF, Which Type and for Whom?

There should be no controversy over whether or not to anticoagulate a patient with AF. The guidelines are well established and quite clear (26–30). A simple summary would be that aspirin (325 mg) may be reasonable for lone AF in patients without known risk factors, including the presence of structural heart disease, age ≥ 60 yr, hypertension, diabetes mellitus, prior emboli, CHF, rheumatic heart disease, and/or echocardiographically defined markers (26–30). Warfarin is more effective at reduction of emboli, and therefore clearly preferred, in patients of greater age. The guidelines are the same for all forms of AF: permanent, persistent, and paroxysmal, and for atrial flutter. Controversial questions include the following:

1. *Is anticoagulation required for very brief and infrequent episodes?*
   There is neither a clear answer nor a formal set of guidelines. Anticoagulation prior to cardioversion is not customary for new-onset AF of <24–48 h duration. Therefore, it may not be needed for infrequent recurrent AF of similar duration. In general, such patients were not enrolled in the major anticoagulation trials, and therefore comparative data are lacking. Physicians will have to use their best judgment, but extrapolation from anticoagulation guidelines would make it more advisable in older patients with these types of presentations than in younger ones.

2. *How long to anticoagulate if NSR is restored and maintained?*
   An increasing number of experts are now advising lifelong anticoagulation in patients placed on warfarin, because it is rare for AADs to prevent all recurrences and because many AF recurrences have been found to be asymptomatic and thus unrecognized by the patient (particularly if rate-control drugs are continued). The incidence of stroke in asymptomatic and symptomatic AF is similar. Nonetheless, it may be reasonable to consider discontinuation of warfarin in patients who have maintained NSR for several months if (1) rate-control agents can also be stopped, thereby increasing the likelihood of early detection of recurrent AF and (2) the patient can be taught to check his/her pulse daily so as to recognize

any recurrent AF on the first day it occurs. Because in the elderly, particularly those with structural heart disease, hemodynamic symptoms with recurrent AF may be more severe (e.g., pulmonary edema, syncope) and discontinuation of rate-control agents may be hazardous due to the presentation of recurrent AF, therefore, discontinuation of warfarin may be more difficult in the more elderly patient with AF than in a younger subject.

3. *Is there a role for nonwarfarin anticoagulants, such as heparin or low-molecular-weight heparinoids (LMWH)?*

   In addition to aspirin therapy for lone AF, there are neither trial data nor formal guidelines to support nonwarfarin anticoagulation *(67)*. Thus, although heparin or LMWH is often used during warfarin loading or for precardioversion management with new onset AF, blinded, placebo-controlled, and/or dose-ranging data upon which to formulate guidelines do not exist.

Rate vs Rhythm Control for AF: Which Is the Best Management Strategy?

This is a topic of endless debate and the subject of several recent trials. Clearly, anticoagulation and rate control can substantially reduce the major morbidity/mortality risks of AF, namely emboli and tachycardic induced cardiomyopathy. However, whether or not survival is better with maintenance of NSR than with rate-control plus anticoagulation is unproven and uncertain. Given this uncertainty, the only mandatory reason for the pursuit of sinus rhythm at present is to improve quality-of-life (i.e., to reduce symptoms that persist despite rate control). Although NSR may, in theory, enhance survival and reduce embolic risk better than leaving the patient in rate-controlled, anticoagulated AF, it is possible that the adverse effects of antiarrhythmic strategies and/or incomplete resolution of atrial enlargement or mechanical dysfunction may offset or minimize any benefit. Thus, the need for clinical trials in this arena. The largest and most important trial is AFFIRM *(56,57)*, which is comparing, in a randomized trial, the outcome of patients maintained in AF with rate control plus anticoagulation to the outcome in patients whose treatment strategy is pursuit of sinus rhythm, with an intention-to-treat analysis. The population, however, is somewhat atypical in that patients have to be able to tolerate assignment to the rate-control arm and have been chosen from a population with a relatively high likelihood of morbid events. Moreover, because of a high incidence of structural heart disease and other factors, the use of class I AAD was discontinued early in the trial. Thus, there will undoubtedly be questions as to how widely the results of AFFIRM can be extrapolated.

Initial results of AFFIRM presented at the March 2002 American College of Cardiology Annual Scientific Sessions and in press but not yet published, showed no mortality reduction with rhythm control as compared to rate control. In fact, there was a small trend toward harm. This is in keeping with the two small, already published trials PIAF *(68)* and STAF *(69)*. Neither showed a particular major advantage to one arm vs the other. Both were too small to be powered to detect a mortality difference. In both, failure to maintain NSR in the rhythm control arm was common. Thus, despite the debate, reality may indicate that most patients will ultimately have a management strategy of rate control plus anticoagulation.

Post-CABG AF: Is There a Difference in Management?

Atrial fibrillation is common after coronary artery bypass grafting (CABG), occurring in approximately one-third of patients. It is the most common cause of prolonged hospital stay. Its onset is usually in the first few days; it may be paroxysmal or persistent, and in patients without prior AF, sinus rhythm usually returns by 2 mo postoperatively. Older age, heart failure, long pump times, prior AF, and other markers can identify patients with a greater propensity for developing post-CABG AF *(70–72)*.

In general, management strategies for postoperative AF are the same as for AF in other settings *(45–49)*, except that *(73–78)* (1) the duration of management may be measured in weeks to months so that long-term adverse events attributable to antiarrhythmic drugs concerns are reduced. Thus, procainamide has been used frequently in this setting, as has amiodarone. (2) In this setting, β-blockers have consistently been found to decrease the incidence of AF, particularly if patients were taking them preoperatively, as well as to control rate, and are considered by many to be the agents of first choice. In patients who have AF despite β-blockers, adding another antiarrhythmic drug or changing to sotalol usually reduces AF further. (3) Atrial fibrillation may occur in the first few hours postoperatively, while the patient is still intubated or on pressor support, requiring an intravenous antiarrhythmic drug. Procainamide has been used in this setting for years, as has amiodarone more recently. Amiodarone will usually afford rate control, even in these high catecholamine states (generally with the first 400 mg), which affords it an advantage *(75–78)*. Long loading times, multiple-drug interactions, including those with warfarin and digoxin, the possibility of hypotension, and high cost, however, can limit its attractiveness.

In high-risk patients (i.e., those clearly prone to postoperative AF), preoperative drug loading (e.g., β-blockers, sotalol, amiodarone) may be useful. Because few postoperative comparative trials have been performed, aside from sotalol vs standard β-blockers, with sotalol usually proving superior, comparative efficacy among antiarrhythmic drugs in this setting has not been directly examined. However, indirect comparisons of data from various sources and a few small amiodarone vs class I trials probably indicate that sotalol and amiodarone are more effective than class IA antiarrhythmic drugs, digitalis, and CCBs *(73–78)*. Recent studies also appear to indicate that atrial pacing—particularly perhaps, biatrial—may further reduce postoperative AF during the in-hospital phase where temporary pacing is practical.

Anticoagulation guidelines for postoperative AF are no different than for AF in other circumstances. But because patients are generally on aspirin following CABG and often have normal LV function and expectation for short AF duration, some would advocate using aspirin (325 mg) and not warfarin.

Other Arrhythmias

For non-AF arrhythmias, perhaps the major controversy related to age is whether intracardiac devices (ICDs) should be used in the very elderly. In part, the controversy arises from concerns about impaired wound healing and the risk of infection in older, frailer, and more wasted subjects. In part, it relates to the greater probability of comorbid diseases with reduced life expectancy as a result of other illnesses, rendering the relative cost of an intracardiac device excessive. In AVID *(79–82)*, for example, which compared ICD therapy to antiarrhythmic drugs therapy (essentially amiodarone) in survivors of ventricular tachycardia/ventricular fibrillation, life expectancy was greater in ICD-treated patients than in drug-treated patients by about 30% (relative efficacy) and 7% per year (absolute efficacy), for each of the 3 yr of follow-up, but the average extension of life was small (months) and the cost per life-year high (>$100,000). Clearly, the ICDs should be most cost-effective for younger patients without comorbid diseases and only moderately impaired LV function, where a reduction of arrhythmic mortality should strongly equate with a reduction of total mortality as compared to older, sicker patients with multiple modes of death.

Additionally, the alternative strategies of drug therapy may appear more attractive in older patients than in younger ones, particularly with amiodarone. Many of amiodarone's toxic manifestations are progressive over time, such as pulmonary fibrosis, which probably occurs at a rate of 1.5–2%/yr with low-dose therapy. Thus, concern for toxic risk is greater in younger patients with otherwise longer life expectancy than it is in geriatric patients. This is commonly one of the decision points in choosing between drug treatment and ICD therapy in the older aged patient. In light of these issues, I find it more difficult to be as dogmatic about making an ICD uniformly the first-line therapy for ventricular tachycardia/ventricular fibrillation for the geriatric patient as would be the case for younger patients.

REFERENCES

1. Kadish A, Passman R. Mechanisms and management of paroxysmal supraventricular tachycardias. Cardiol Rev 1999;2:254–264.
2. Okane P, Jackson G. Cardiovascular disease in the elderly. Practitioner 1999;243:574–580.
3. Falk RH. Atrial fibrillation. N Engl J Med 2001;344:1067–1078.
4. Chugh SS, Blackshear JL, Shen WK, Hammill SC, Gersh BJ. Epidemiology and natural history of atrial fibrillation: clinical implications. J Am Coll Cardiol 2001;37:371–378.
5. Sra J, Dhala A, Blenck Z, Dashpande S, Couley R, Akhtar M. Atrial fibrillation: epidemiology, mechanisms, and management. Curr Probl Cardiol 2000;25:405–524.
6. Benjamin EJ, Wolf PA, Kannel WB. The epidemiology of atrial fibrillation. In: Falk RH, Podrid PJ, eds. Atrial Fibrillation Mechanisms and Management, 2nd ed. Lippincott Williams & Williams, Philadelphia, PA, 1997, pp. 1–22.
7. Bigger JT Jr, Reiffel JA, Coromilas J. Ambulatory electrocardiography. In: Platia E, ed. Nonpharmacologic Management of Cardiac Arrhythmias. JB Lippincott, Philadelphia, PA, 1986, pp. 36–61.
8. Hinkle LE Jr, Carver ST, Stevens M. The frequency of asymptomatic disturbances of cardiac rhythm and conduction in middle aged men. Am J Cardiol 1969;24:629–650.
9. Reiffel JA. Clinical Electrophysiology of the sinus node. In: Mazagalev T, Dreifus LS, Micholson EL, eds. Electrophysiology of the Sinoatrial and Atrioventricular Nodes: Integrative Physiologic, Morphologic, Autonomic, and Pharmacologic Aspects. Alan R Liss, New York, 1988, pp. 239–257.
10. Lakatta EG. Cardiovascular aging in health. Clin Geriatr Med 2000;10:419–444.
11. Rutenberg HL, Spann JF Jr. Alterations in cardiac sympathetic neurotransmitter activity in congestive heart failure. Am J Cardiol 1973;32:472–480.
12. Ruoke GA. Autonomic and cardiovascular function in the geriatric patient. Anesthesiol Clin North Am 2000;18:31–46.
13. Opthof J. The normal range and determinants of the intrinsic heart rate in man. Cardiovasc Res 2000;45:177–184.
14. Brodde OE, Michel ML. Adrenergic and muscarinic receptors in the human heart. Pharmacol Rev 1999;51:651–690.
15. Reiffel JA, Wang P, Basner R, Bigger JT Jr, Livelli FD Jr, Glicklich JI. Electrophysiological testing in patients with recurrent syncope: are results predicted by prior ambulatory monitoring. Am Heart J 1985;110:1146–1153.
16. Reiffel JA. Role of invasive electrophysiological testing in the evaluation and management of bradyarrhythmias/sinus node dysfunction. Clin Electrophysiol Rev 1997;4:414–416.
17. Dickey JQ Jr, Calkins H. Diagnostic evaluation and management of syncope. Curr Opin Cardiol 1991;6:56–59.
18. Grubb BP, Kosinski DJ. Syncope resulting from autonomic insufficiency syndromes associated with orthostatic intolerance. Med Clin North Am 2001;85:457–472.
19. Luria DM, Shen WK. Syncope in the elderly: new trends in diagnostic approaches and nonpharmacologic management. Am J Geriatr Cardiol 2001;10:41–46.
20. Meyer MD, Handler J. Evaluation of the patient with syncope: an evidence based approach. Emerg Med Clin North Am 1999;17:187–201.

21. Schnipper JL, Kapoor WN. Diagnostic evaluation and management of patients with syncope. Med Clin North Am 2001;85:423–456.
22. Tuft AD, Boon NA. Thyroid disease and the heart. Heart 2000;84:455–460.
23. The Cardiac Arrhythmia Suppression Trial (CAST) Investigators. Preliminary report: effect of encainide and flecainide on mortality in a randomized trial of arrhythmia suppression after myocardial infarction. N Engl J Med 1989;321:406–412.
24. Teo KK, Yusuf S, Furberg CD. Effects of prophylactic antiarrhythmic drug therapy in acute myocardial infarction. An overview of results from randomized controlled trials. JAMA 1993;270:1589–1595.
25. Reiffel JA. Date driven decisions: the importance of clinical trials in arrhythmia management. J Cardiovasc Pharmacol Therap 1996;1:79–88.
26. Anonymous. Guidelines for medical treatment for stroke prevention. American College of Physicians. Ann Intern Med 1994;121(1):54–55.
27. Kottlamp H, Hinkricks G, Breithardt G. Role of anticoagulant therapy in atrial fibrillation. J Cardiovasc Electrophysiol 1998;9(Suppl):S86–S96.
28. Singer DE, Go AS. Antithrombotic therapy in atrial fibrillation. Clin Geriatr Med 2001;17:131–147.
29. Bungard TJ, Shuaib A, Tsuyuki RT. Stroke prevention in non-valvular atrial fibrillation. Curr Opin Neurol 2001;14:59–65.
30. Prystowsky EN, Benson DW Jr, Fuster V, Hart RG, Kay GN, Myerberg RJ, et al. Management of patients with atrial fibrillation: a statement for health care professionals. From the Subcommittee on Electrocardiography and Electrophysiology, American Heart Association. Circulation 1996;93:1162–1177.
31. The Stroke Prevention in Atrial Fibrillation Investigators. Predictors of thromboembolism in atrial fibrillation: 1. Clinical features of patients at risk. Ann Intern Med 1992;116(1):1–5.
32. The Stroke Prevention in Atrial Fibrillation Investigators. Predictors of thromboembolism in atrial fibrillation: II. Echocardiographic features of patients at risk. Ann Intern Med 1992;116(1):6–12.
33. Cairns JA, Connolly SJ. Nonrheumatic atrial fibrillation. Risk of stroke and role of antithrombotic therapy. Circulation 1991;84:469–481.
34. Hart RG, Halperin JL. Atrial fibrillation and stroke: concepts and controversies. Stroke 2000;32:803–808.
35. Thalmilarasan M, Klein AL. Transesophageal echocardiography (TEE) in atrial fibrillation. Cardiol Clin 2000;18:819–831.
36. Hart RG, Halperin JL. Atrial fibrillation and thromboembolism: a decade of progress in stroke prevention. Ann Intern Med 1999;131(9):688–695.
37. Hart RG, Benavente O, McBride R, Pearce LA. Antithrombotic therapy to prevent stroke in patients with atrial fibrillation: a meta-analysis. Ann Intern Med 1999;131:492–501.
38. Reiffel JA, Bigger JT, Cramer M. Effects of digoxin on sinus nodal function before and after vagal blockade in patients in sinus nodal dysfunction. Am J Cardiol 1979;43:983–989.
39. Blitzer M, Costeas C, Kassotis J, Reiffel J. Rhythm management in atrial fibrillation with a primary emphasis on pharmacologic therapy—Part 1. Pacing Clin Electrophysiol 1998;21:590–602.
40. Reiffel JA. Sinus node dysfunction: sinus bradyarrhythmias and the bradytachy syndrome. In: Horowitz LN, ed. Current Management of Arrhythmias. BG Decker, Philadelphia, PA, 1991, pp. 235–237.
41. Saksena S. Pacing therapy for atrial fibrillation. Thorac Cardiovasc Surg 1999;47(Suppl 3):339–341.
42. Glikson M, Espinosa RE, Hayes DL. Expanding indications for permanent pacemakers. Ann Intern Med 1995;123:443–451.
43. Barold SS. Prevention of atrial fibrillation by mulitsite atrial pacing. J Electrocardiol 2001;34:49–52.
44. Kassotis J, Costeas C, Blitzer M, Reiffel JA. Rhythm management in atrial fibrillation with a primary emphasis on pharmacologic therapy—Part 3. Pacing Clin Electrophysiol 1998;21:1133–1145.
45. Reiffel JA. Selecting an antiarrhythmic agent for atrial fibrillation should be a patient-specific data-driven decision. Am J Cardiol 1998;82:72N–81N.
46. Reiffel JA. Drug choices in the treatment of atrial fibrillation. Am J Cardiol 2000;85:12D–19D.
47. Reiffel JA, Camm AJ, Haffajee CJ, Kowey PR, Luderitz B, Naccarelli GV, et al. International consensus roundtable on atrial fibrillation. Cardiol Rev 2000;12(Suppl):1–19.
48. Prystowsky EN. Management of atrial fibrillation: therapeutic options and clinical decisions. Am J Cardiol 2000;85:3D–11D.
49. Aronow WS. Management of the older person with atrial fibrillation. J Am Geriatr Soc 1999;47: 740–748.
50. Boriani G, Biffi M, Capucci A, Botto G, Broffoni T, Ongari M, et al. Conversion of recent-onset atrial fibrillation to sinus rhythm: effects of different drug protocols. Pacing Clin Electrophysiol 1998;21: 2470–2474.

51. Costeas C, Kassotis J, Blitzer M, Reiffel J. Rhythm management in atrial fibrillation with a primary emphasis on pharmacologic therapy—Part 2. Pacing Clin Electrophysiol 1998;21:742–752.

52. Kuck KH, Cappato R, Siebels J, Ruppel R. Randomized comparison of antiarrhythmic drug therapy with implantable defibrillators in patients resuscitated from cardiac arrest: the Cardiac Arrest Study Hamburg (CASH). Circulation 2000;102:748–754.

53. Greene HL and the CASCADE Investigators. The CASCADE Study: randomized antiarrhythmic drug therapy in survivors of cardiac arrest in Seattle. Am J Cardiol 1993;72:70F–74F.

54. Mason JW, for the ESVEM Investigators. A comparison of seven antiarrhythmic drugs in patients with ventricular tachyarrhythmias. N Engl J Med 1993;329:452–458.

55. Mason JW, Marcus FI, Bigger JT Jr, Lazzara R, Reiffel JA, Reiter MJ, et al. A summary and assessment of the findings and conclusions of the ESVEM trial. Prog Cardiovasc Dis 1996;38:347–358.

56. The Planning and Steering Committees of the AFFIRM Study for the NHLBI AFFIRM Investigators. Atrial fibrillation follow-up investigation of rhythm management—the AFFIRM Study Design. Am J Cardiol 1997;79:1198–1202.

57. Wyse DG. The AFFIRM trial: main trial and substudies—what can we expect. J Intervent Cardiac Electrophysiol 2000;I:171–176.

58. Kober L, Bloch Thomsen PE, Moller M, Torp-Pedersen C, Carlsen J, Sandoe E, et al. Danish Investigations of Arrhythmia and Mortality on Dofetilide (DIAMOND) Study Group. Effect of dofetilide in patients with recent myocardial infarction and left-ventricular dysfunction: a randomized trial. Lancet 2000;356:2052–2058.

59. Boutitie F, Boissel JP, Connolly SJ, Camm AJ, Cairns JA, Julian DG, et al. Amiodarone interaction with beta-blockers: analysis of the merged EMIAT (European Myocardial Infarct Amiodarone Trial) and CAMIAT (Canadian Amiodarone Myocardial Infarction Trial) databases. Circulation 1999;99:2268–2275.

60. Cairns JA, Connolly SJ, Roberts R, Gent M. Randomized trial of outcome after myocardial infarction in patients with frequent or repetitive ventricular premature depolarizations: CAMIAT. Lancet 1997;349:675–682.

61. Jafri SM, Borzak S, Goldberger J, Gheorghiade M. Role of antiarrhythmic agents after myocardial infarction with special reference to the EMIAT and CAMIAT trials of amiodarone. Prog Cardiovasc Dis 1998;41:65–70.

62. Julian DG, Prescott RJ, Jackson FS, Szekely P. Controlled trial of sotalol for one year after myocardial infarction. Lancet 1982;1:1142–1147.

63. Reiffel JA, Hahn E, Hartz V, Reiter MJ, and the ESVEM Investigators. Sotalol for ventricular tachyarrhythmias: beta-blocking and class III contributions, and relative efficacy versus class I drugs after prior drug failure. Am J Cardiol 1997;79:1048–1053.

64. Reiter MJ, Reiffel JA. Importance of beta blockade in the therapy of serious ventricular arrhythmias. Am J Cardiol 1998;82:9I–19I.

65. Dreifus LS, Fisch C, Griffin JC, Gillette PC, Mason JW, Parsonnet V. Guidelines for implantation of cardiac pacemakers and antiarrhythmia devices. A report of the American College of Cardiology/American Heart Association Task Force on Assessment of Diagnostic and Therapeutic Cardiovascular Procedures. J Am Coll Cardiol 1991;18:1–13.

66. Gregoratos G. Permanent pacemakers in older persons. J Am Geriatrics Soc 1999;47:1125–1135.

67. Schulman RI. Assessment of low molecular weight heparin trials in cardiology. Pharmacol Therapeut 2000;87:1–9.

68. Hohnloser SH, Kuck KH, Lilienthal J. Rhythm or rate control in atrial fibrillation—Pharmacological Intervention in Atrial Fibrillation (PIAF): a randomized trial. Lancet 2000;356:1789–1794.

69. Carlson J, Tebbe U. Rhythm control versus rate control in atrial fibrillation: results from the STAF Pilot Study. Pacing Clin Electrophysiol 2001;24:II–561.

70. Hogue CW, Hyder ML. Atrial fibrillation after cardiac operation: risks, mechanisms, and treatment. Ann Thorac Surg 2000;69:300–306.

71. Bharucha DB, Kowey PR. Management and prevention of atrial fibrillation after cardiovascular surgery. Am J Cardiol 2000;85:20D–24D.

72. Cox JL. A perspective on postoperative atrial fibrillation. Semin Thorac Cardiovasc Surg 1999;11:299–302.

73. Solomon AJ. Treatment of postoperative atrial fibrillation: a non-surgical perspective. Semin Thorac Cardiovasc Surg 1999;11:320–324.

74. Borzok S, Silverman NA. Treatment of postoperative atrial fibrillation. Semin Thorac Cardiovasc Surg 1999;11:314–319.

75. Pinter A, Doran P. Intravenous antiarrhythmic agents. Curr Opin Cardiol 2001;16:17–22.
76. Reiffel JA. Intravenous amiodarone in the management of atrial fibrillation. J Cardiovasc Pharmacol Therap 1999;4:199–204.
77. Connolly SJ. Evidence-based analysis of amiodarone efficacy and safety. Circulation 1999;100:2025–2034.
78. Kowey PR, Reiffel JA. Section on Pharmacokinetics, antiarrhythmic drugs, proarrhythmia. In: Electrophysiology Self-assessment Program (EPSAP). American College of Cardiology, Bethesda, MD, 2000.
79. The Antiarrhythmics Versus Implantable Defibrillator (AVID) Investigators. A comparison of antiarrhythmic drug therapy with implantable defibrillators in patients resuscitated from near-fatal ventricular arrhythmias. N Engl J Med 1997;337:1576–1583.
80. Reiffel JA, Reiter MJ, Blitzer M. Antiarrhythmic drugs and devices for the management of ventricular tachyarrhythmias in ischemic heart disease. Am J Cardiol 1998;82:31I–40I.
81. Hallstrom P, Anderson JL, Cobb L, Friedman PL, Herre JM, Klein RC, et al., for the AVID Investigators. Advantages and disadvantages of trial designs: a review of analysis methods for ICD studies. Pacing Clin Electrophysiol 2000;23:1029–1038.
82. Reiffel JA. Prolonging survival by reducing sudden death: pharmacological therapy of ventricular tachycardia and fibrillation. Am J Cardiol 1997;80:45G–55G.

12 Syncope in the Elderly

Daniel M. Bloomfield, MD, FACC
and Chandra Kunavarapu, MD

CONTENTS

SIGNIFICANCE OF THE PROBLEM

Epidemiology: Incidence, Recurrence Rates, Morbidity, Mortality

Syncope is a symptom defined as a transient, self-limited loss of consciousness, often leading to a fall with loss of muscle tone. Syncope in elderly individuals is common, recurrent, and can often be disabling, and it may be associated with a risk of sudden death, but its etiology is often elusive. Consequently, syncope often leads to hospital admission, multiple consultations, and the performance of many diagnostic tests. Syncope is not a disease but, rather, represents a clinical manifestation of one or more disease processes, which results in cerebral hypoperfusion. Although syncope is common in all ages, complex physiologic and pathophysiologic changes that occur with aging combined with frequently occurring comorbid conditions and an increased susceptibility to the adverse effects of polypharmacy predispose elderly patients to recurrent syncope *(1,2)*.

Syncope accounts for 1–6% of all hospital admissions and 3% of all emergency room visits (80% of which are over 65 yr of age) *(3)*. Little is known about the epidemiology of syncope in elderly persons. Accurate historical data are difficult to ascertain, because episodes are often unwitnessed and patients frequently fail to recall the event. A retrospective analysis of syncope in very old (mean age 87 yr) institutionalized patients revealed a 10 yr prevalence of 23% and a yearly incidence of 6% with a recurrence rate of 30% *(4)*. The finding of a cardiovascular cause is common in 34% of the elderly and a strong predictor of mortality, which is as high as 30% at the end of 2 yr *(5–7)*. Cumulative mortality at the end of 2 yr was 26% in the elderly as compared with 8% in the young, and the 2 yr incidence of sudden death in elderly subjects with syncope was 10.5% *(6)*. Even if the cause

From: *Aging, Heart Disease, and Its Management: Facts and Controversies*
Edited by: N. Edwards, M. Maurer, and R. Wellner © Humana Press Inc., Totowa, NJ

of syncope is benign, the consequences of the resultant fall may not be. Injuries from syncope occur frequently in elderly patients *(8,9)*.

Multivariate analysis from several studies has demonstrated a number of risk factors for syncope. In institutionalized elderly patients, the risk factors include a history of coronary artery disease, functional impairment, postural blood pressure reduction, aortic stenosis, abnormal electrocardiogram (ECG), history of ventricular arrhythmia, and congestive heart failure *(4)*. In the Framingham heart disease study, predictors for syncope in a community sample were history of transient ischemic attack, use of cardiac medications, diabetes, and high blood pressure *(10)*.

Data from the early 1980s showed that in nearly 40–50% of patients, the cause of syncope was not determined after initial, often extensive, investigations *(11)*. More recently, the use of head-up tilt-table testing, carotid sinus massage, memory loop monitors, and electrophysiologic studies with a better guided history, physical exam, and diagnostic algorithm has reduced the proportion of undiagnosed cases to 10% from 26% *(12)*.

Syncope vs Falls

The traditional definitions of falls (transient loss of postural tone without loss of consciousness) and syncope (transient loss of postural tone and loss of consciousness) consider these entities to be two separate diagnoses with separate etiologies. However, distinguishing falls from syncope relies upon obtaining either an accurate history of the event or an eyewitness account. This is unlikely in up to one-third of older patients, who have retrograde amnesia regarding the episode *(13,14)*. Cummings et al. *(13)* found that 32% of cognitively normal patients with documented falls could not remember falling 3 mo after the event. Other investigators have found that 21–32% of subjects with witnessed syncope during carotid sinus massage had amnesia for the loss of consciousness *(15,16)*. Furthermore, a witness account is usually unavailable in many cases of falls brought to medical attention *(8,14,17)*.

The epidemiologic importance of falls in the elderly is astounding. Unintentional injury ranks as the fifth leading cause of death among people over 65, and falls represent the single most common cause of accidental mortality, accounting for 70% *(18)*. Close to one-third of those 65 and older living at home suffer a fall each year; 18% fall once and 12% two or more times *(19,20)*. Also, 5–30% of falls in the community result in injury. Most of the injuries are mild and superficial, but up to 5% result in fracture and 1% results in hip fracture. About 1 in 40 community-dwelling elders who fall will be hospitalized, and only about half of the elderly patients hospitalized as a result of a fall will be alive 1 yr later *(21)*. Incidence rates for falls increase with advancing age and frailty. Recent data have shown that the incidence of falls has increased by 31% since 1992, primarily as a result of the aging of the population *(22)*. Each year, about 1800 fatal falls occur in nursing homes. Nursing home residents demonstrate a disproportionately high incidence of hip fractures and have been shown to experience higher mortality rates after hip fractures than community-dwelling elderly persons do *(23)*.

Many patients with falls or syncope, after a comprehensive evaluation, are found to have similar diagnoses *(8,15,24,25)*. Moreover, as further proof of this concept, treating patients with unexplained falls (not syncope) and documented bradycardia from carotid sinus hypersensitivity with a pacemaker prevents falls in follow-up *(26)*. In our practice, we consider unexplained falls and unexplained syncope to be an equivalent presentation and evaluate each in a similar fashion.

DIFFERENCES IN THE ELDERLY

Pathophysiology

Multiple factors predispose elderly patients to syncope. These include physiologic processes associated with normal aging, age-associated diseases, and increased use of medications, often with concomitant polypharmacy. In many cases, syncope results not simply from one pathological process but from the combination of multiple processes that "synergistically" result in a patient's syncopal episode.

Physiologic Processes Associated with Normative Aging That Predispose the Elderly Patient to Syncope

In the vast majority of patients, syncope results from a transient reduction in cerebral blood flow (the exception to this would be seizures, hypoglycemia, or psychogenic syncope). Aging has been associated with a reduction in cerebral blood flow *(27)*. Other diseases, such as hypertension, which may impair cerebral autoregulation, often compound this reduction in cerebral blood flow. Anemia or chronic obstructive pulmonary disease may further impair oxygen-carrying capacity. When cerebral blood flow is sufficiently impaired, challenge by even small hemodynamic stresses may result in syncope.

A number of age-related physiologic changes result in an impairment of blood pressure regulation that increases the likelihood of developing transient hypotension and syncope. The integrity and function of the baroreflexes is impaired in elderly subjects, which may result in attenuated compensatory responses to decreases in blood pressure *(28)*. Renal salt and water conservation is impaired in elderly subjects *(29)*. This is likely the result of a combination of factors, including reductions in renin and aldosterone levels *(30)*, which impair salt retention and elevate atrial natriuretic peptide *(31)*, which results in salt loss. In addition, elderly subjects may not develop thirst, which potentially further compromises intravascular volume *(32)*.

Impairment in diastolic filling (diastolic dysfunction) also occurs with aging, further compromising the maintenance of blood pressure in certain settings *(33)*. Patients with diastolic dysfunction are more dependent on preload than with normal diastolic filling. Conditions that compromise preload such as volume depletion, tachycardia, upright posture (from lower extremity venous pooling), and meal ingestion (from splanchnic pooling), as well as medications that reduce preolad, such as nitrates, may result in hypotension in an elderly subject with diastolic dysfunction.

Age-Associated Diseases That May Increase the Risk of Developing Syncope

A number of diseases that are common in the elderly exacerbate and compound the physiologic changes that occur in normal aging, further impairing the regulation of blood pressure. Hypertension is extremely common in elderly subjects, such that nearly one-third of elderly subjects older than 70 yr have a systolic blood pressure >170 mm Hg. Hypertension impairs cerebral autoregulation and baroreflex responsiveness and increases myocardial stiffness, resulting in greater diastolic dysfunction. These effects of hypertension further diminish an individual's ability to regulate blood pressure and may increase an individual's risk of developing syncope. Hypertension can also cause conduction system disease that may cause syncope if it becomes severe. Diabetes is also common among elderly subjects and is associated with autonomic dysfunction that impairs the regulation of blood pressure. In addition, both diabetes and hypertension increase the risk of having coronary artery disease and myocardial infarction, which increases an individual's risk of developing ventricular arrhythmias. Finally, a number of other conditions that are associated with autonomic dysfunction are more common in elderly subjects, including Parkinson's disease, multisystem atrophy, and pure autonomic failure.

Situational Syncope in the Elderly: Common Situational Stresses Compound Age and Disease-Associated Changes, Resulting in Syncope

In a prospective study by Lipsitz et al., the cause of syncope in one-third of institutionalized elderly patients with syncope was related to a common stress, such as eating a meal, defecating, urinating, or changing posture *(2)*. These common stresses challenge the homeostatic system that regulates blood pressure. When blood pressure regulation is impaired in elderly subjects, even these simple stresses can result in significant transient hypotension and syncope.

One clear example of this phenomenon is postprandial hypotension. Although postprandial hypotension is cited as a potential cause of falls and syncope, most studies have measured postprandial declines in blood pressure either in the supine or sitting position *(34,35)*. These studies did not demonstrate that postprandial hypotension, by itself, is an important risk factor for falls or syncope *(36)*. Because falls in the elderly are often the result of the interaction of multiple coexistent clinical abnormalities, we hypothesized that postprandial and orthostatic hypotension would be additive, resulting in symptomatic hypotension in a subset of elderly subjects. We found that meal ingestion was associated with an 8 mm Hg decline in systolic blood pressure that was additive to the orthostatic response. Although this average additional decline in blood pressure is small, the number of elderly subjects with symptomatic hypotension during head-up tilt after meal ingestion increased from 12% to 22% of subjects. In addition, symptomatic hypotension tended to occur earlier after meal ingestion rather than before meal ingestion for the same subjects. These data indicate that the combination of a meal and upright posture is associated with symptomatic hypotension in a significant number of functionally independent elderly subjects. In the evaluation of an elderly patient with falls, syncope, or dizziness, attention to the relationship of these symptoms to a meal or postural change may be useful in identifying the potential etiology. An example of the clinical significance of post-prandial hypotension in an elderly subject with recurrent syncope is illustrated in Fig. 1.

Common Etiologies of Syncope in the Elderly

BRADYARRHYTHMIAS

Compared to younger patients, bradyarrhythmias are a much more common etiology of syncope in the elderly. It is important to recognize the distinction between intrinsic bradyarrhythmias from diseases of the conduction system and extrinsic or reflex bradyarrhythmias that result from transient increases in vagal tone. Reflex bradyarrhythmias are common in both young and elderly subjects with syncope. Pauses associated with carotid hypersensitivity are much more common in the elderly and are rare in younger patients. In many cases, however, bradyarrhythmias causing syncope may be the result of both intrinsic conduction system disease and a transient increase in vagal tone.

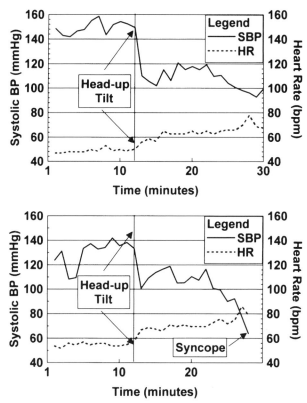

Fig. 1. Demonstration of the clinical significance of the interaction between upright posture and post-prandial hypotension in an elderly patient with recurrent syncope following meals. Tilt-table testing was done before (top panel) and after (bottom panel) a standardized liquid meal. Prior to the meal, there was an asymptomatic 35 mm Hg fall in blood pressure immediately after being tilted head-up, but she was able to complete 20 min of tilt. Following the meal, her supine blood pressure dropped from 145 mm Hg (before the meal) to approx 135 mm Hg. Immediately after being tilted, her blood pressure once again fell 35 mm Hg, this time to 100 mm Hg. Over the next 15 min, however, her blood pressure gradually but progressively fell to a low value of 66 mm Hg, which was associated with syncope.

The distinction between intrinsic and extrinsic causes of bradycardia has important ramifications with respect to both the decision to implant a permanent pacemaker and determining the type of pacemaker best suited for a given patient. The decision to implant a standard pacemaker with rate-responsive pacing, if chronotropic incompetence is present, for patients with intrinsic causes of bradycardia is straightforward. However, patients with bradycardia resulting from extrinsic causes (vasovagal syncope or carotid sinus hypersentitivity) may also exhibit a vasodepressor component to their syndrome. These patients will vasodilate and become hypotensive at the same time as they are becoming bradycardic. Standard single chamber (VVI) or dual chamber (DDD) pacing is often ineffective for these patients *(37)*. More advanced sensing and pacing algorithms are available in certain pacemakers, which have been shown to be beneficial in ameliorating hypotension during these episodes by pacing at a more rapid rate *(38–40)*.

SICK SINUS SYNDROME

Sick sinus syndrome is identified as the cause of syncope in 3–10% of patients *(2,6,8)*. Sick sinus syndrome is a condition characterized by abnormal sinus node function in which there is episodic failure in sinus node output with consequent failure of the normal conduction system to depolarize. The resulting sinus pause leads to cardiac stand-still until either sinus rhythm is restored or a subsidiary pacemaker assumes control of cardiac rhythm. Sinus node dysfunction is a common entity in the elderly and has significant clinical implications. The prevalence of sick sinus syndrome was found to be 3 in 5000 in patients greater than 50 yr of age *(41)* and accounts for more than 50% of new pacemaker implantations *(42)*. Most commonly, adults develop sick sinus syndrome in the sixth and seventh decades of life *(43)*.

Sick sinus syndrome can result from a number of processes. In many cases, no etiology is identified, but many patients with sick sinus syndrome have structural heart disease. Sick sinus syndrome is common after certain types of cardiac surgery, especially after correction of congenital heart disease and heart transplantation. Less commonly, sick sinus syndrome may be a manifestation of atrial amyloidosis or of diffuse fibrosis associated with either collagen vascular disease or some other disease process.

The diagnosis of sick sinus syndrome is usually made either during electrophysiologic (EP) testing *(44–47)* or during some type of ECG monitoring. Recently, investigators have suggested that it can be diagnosed by examining the sinus node response to an adenosine challenge *(48,49)*, although definitive studies of this diagnostic approach have not been done. The diagnostic yield of electrophysiologic testing for sick sinus syndrome remains unknown, although it is thought to be low. Fujimura et al. evaluated eight patients with spontaneous sinus pauses documented during ambulatory ECG recordings, and only three had evidence of sinus node dysfunction during electrophysiologic testing (EPS) (sensitivity of 37.5%) *(46)*. This assumes, however, that all eight patients had sinus node dysfunction as the cause of their spontaneous pause. Notably, two of the patients had pauses in response to carotid sinus massage, suggesting that the cause of their spontaneous pause was carotid sinus hypersensitivity rather than sick sinus syndrome. Unfortunately, because neither carotid sinus massage nor tilt-table testing were performed on all patients, it is not clear whether these patients all had sick sinus syndrome and, thus, the estimate of the sensitivity of EP testing in this study is unreliable.

This issue was addressed by Brignole et al. in a subsequent article that evaluated 25 patients with documented sinus arrest or transient atrioventricular (AV) block during ambulatory ECG recordings *(47)*. In this study tilt table testing and carotid sinus massage were performed in all patients in addition to EPS. Unfortunately, nearly all of the patients with documented sinus arrest had either carotid sinus hypersensitivity or vasovagal syncope with a pause during tilt-table testing; therefore, it is impossible to determine the diagnostic accuracy of EPS for sick sinus syndrome. These data could suggest that sick sinus syndrome in and of itself is an unusual cause of syncope.

TRANSIENT AV BLOCK

Transient or persistent complete heart block is thought to account for 6–10% of patients with syncope. A number of processes can affect the conduction system, the most common of which are fibrosis and sclerosis. Lenegre disease is a sclerodegenerative disease of the conduction system. Lev disease is caused by fibrosis or calcification extending from any of the adjacent fibrous structures into the conduction system.

Syncope caused by transient AV block may be infrequent and unpredictable and is most often diagnosed by ECG monitoring. The sensitivity of EP testing for the diagnosis of AV block is low. Fujimura et al. *(46)* described the results of EP testing in 13 patients with documented AV block from ambulatory ECG monitoring. Only four of these patients had a prolonged His–Ventricular (HV) interval (≥70 ms) during EPS. Brignole et al. *(47)* described 12 patients with documented AV block from ambulatory ECG monitoring, of which 5 had a prolonged HV interval. No patient demonstrated infra-Hissian block in the drug-free state during EP testing, although two patients developed complete AV block during the infusion of a Type Ia antiarrhythmic drug used to stress His–Purkinje conduction. Notably, 9 of these 12 patients also had either carotid sinus hypersensitivity or vasovagal syncope during tilt-table testing, suggesting that reflex increases in vagal tone may be required to trigger AV block.

The ability of EP testing to predict the subsequent development of complete AV block in patients with bundle branch block was evaluated by Scheinman et al. *(50)*. Patients with an HV interval ≥70 ms had a greater incidence of progression to high-degree AV block (12%) compared to patients with an HV <70 ms (3%). Of the patients with an HV interval >100 ms, 24% developed high-degree AV block.

The limitation of using EP testing to identify patients with AV block as the cause of syncope was demonstrated by Brignole et al., who evaluated 52 patients with syncope and bundle branch block, all of whom had a negative EP study, including measurement of the HV during pharmacologic stress with a class Ia antiarrhythmic drug *(51)*. These patients all had implantable loop recorders placed and were followed for 2 yr. Syncope recurred in 42% of patients after a median of 48 d, and the majority of these demonstrated AV block with an asystolic pause. This study demonstrates that patients with syncope and bundle branch block with a negative EP study remain at high risk for recurrent syncope, which is most likely caused by AV block. The implantable loop recorder was an effective method of making the diagnosis in these patients. (*See* Chapter 17 for a discussion of cardiac pacing/defibrillators.)

Disorders in Blood Pressure Regulation

Disorders in blood pressure regulation represent the most common causes of syncope in both the young and the elderly patients. These disorders primarily include orthostatic hypotension and vasovagal syncope (the vasodepressor form of carotid sinus hypersensitivity is discussed separately below). One confusing feature of these disorders in elderly patients is the lack of specific symptoms reported by many elderly subjects, despite demonstrable hypotension. In younger subjects, when systolic blood pressure falls below approx 90 mm Hg, symptoms of lightheadedness nearly always occurs. However, it is not uncommon for elderly subjects to present with syncope and no prodrome. During tilt-table testing, they remain asymptomatic despite a drop in systolic blood pressure to values as low as 70 mm Hg before developing abrupt syncope.

ORTHOSTATIC HYPOTENSION

Orthostatic hypotension is defined as a fall in blood pressure with standing (>20 mm Hg fall in systolic or >10 mm Hg fall in diastolic blood pressure). Patients with the most obvious form of orthostatic hypotension demonstrate a significant fall in blood pressure within 1–3 min of standing up. When systolic blood pressure falls to values <90 mm Hg and is associated with symptoms of lightheadedness, it is extremely likely that orthostatic

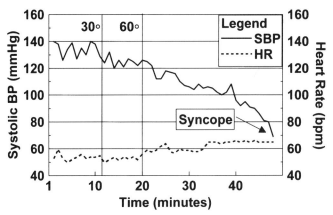

Fig. 2. Tilt study with progressive orthostatic intolerance in an elderly patient with recurrent syncope. The patient is tilted initially to 30° and then to 60°. The blood pressure fell from approx 135 mm Hg supine to ~115 mm Hg over the first 5 min of tilt. Over the next 25 min, however, her blood pressure gradually but progressively fell to a low value of 68 mm Hg. During this time, she remained asymptomatic, even when her blood pressure was <80 mm Hg. When her blood pressure dropped below 70 mm Hg, she abruptly lost consciousness. This is an example of why elderly patients may present without a prodrome even if the cause of syncope was related to a disorder in blood pressure regulation.

hypotension is the cause of syncope. However, many elderly patients demonstrate an asymptomatic 30–40 mm Hg fall in systolic blood pressure to a value of 110–120 mm Hg. In these cases, it is unclear whether or not orthostatic hypotension is the cause of syncope or an unrelated finding. In addition, some of these patients will demonstrate only a mild to moderate fall in blood pressure immediately upon standing, but their blood pressures will progressively fall while they are upright for prolonged periods of time. This can be easily demonstrated during tilt-table testing and has been described as a dysautonomic response to upright posture (*see* Fig. 2).

The pathophysiology of orthostatic hypotension in elderly subjects is often multifactorial, as described earlier. Ultimately, orthostatic hypotension results from inadequate vasoconstriction in the setting of a reduction in circulatory volume caused by pooling of blood in the lower extremities. In elderly subjects, attenuation of baroreflex function, diastolic dysfunction, and a propensity to become hypovolemic, contribute to this pathophysiology. Splanchnic vasodilation following a meal further exacerbates this problem, leading to postprandial hypotension. In addition, diseases that directly cause autonomic dysfunction are more common in the elderly, including Parkinson's disease, diabetes mellitus, multisystem atrophy, and pure autonomic failure.

The treatment of orthostatic hypotension begins with the discontinuation of drugs that may exacerbate the problem. Patients with Parkinson's disease, however, should not have their anti-parkinsonian drugs stopped, given their established benefits to quality of life. Rather, these patients should have their blood pressure supported with other agents to allow them to continue taking their anti-parkinsonian treatments. The mainstay of therapy for patients with symptomatic orthostatic hypotension is the α-agonist midodrine, which has been shown to improve blood pressure when standing *(52)*. Many physicians use fludrocortisone as the first line of therapy, although this approach is rarely effective if the orthostatic hypotension is severe. In addition, fludrocortisone is not well tolerated by elderly

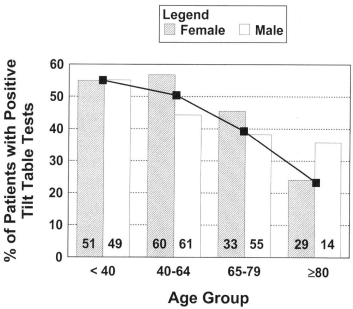

Fig. 3. Percentage of positive tilt-table tests by age and gender. Numbers at the bottom of each bar represent the total number of subjects tested. Although there is a statistically significant decline in positive tilt-table tests with age ($p < 0.05$), a significant proportion of patients age ≥65 had a positive tilt-table test. Reproduced with permission from ref. *56.*

subjects; nearly half of elderly patients stop the drug within a year because of unpleasant side effects (primarily edema) *(53).* A number of other treatments are available, although their efficacy has not been clearly established *(54).*

VASOVAGAL SYNCOPE

It is traditional teaching that vasovagal syncope is common in young women and rare in the elderly *(3,55).* Specifically, Lipsitz et al. found that vasovagal syncope accounted for only 1–5% of episodes in the elderly *(4),* but tilt-table testing was not employed in the diagnostic evaluation. Kapoor et al., in a study of 210 elderly subjects and 190 younger patients evaluated for syncope, found that 3 (1.4%) of the elderly and 29 (15.3%) of the young were identified as having vasovagal syncope *(5).* However, once again, tilt-table testing was not utilized in the evaluation. These studies utilized clinical criteria such as pallor, nausea, sweating associated with a precipitating event such as fear, severe pain, or instrumentation to diagnose patients with vasovagal syncope. In our experience, many elderly patients have syncope without a prodrome and without a clear precipitating event, thereby making a diagnosis on clinical grounds difficult.

We examined the results of tilt-table testing in 352 subjects with unexplained syncope including 133 patients >65 yr of age and 43 patients >80 yr of age *(56).* The average age was 54 ± 20.8 yr (range 11–99 yr), 51% were male, and 164 subjects (46.6%) had a positive tilt-table test (defined by symptomatic hypotension with a systolic blood pressure <80 mm Hg). As expected, there was an age-related decline in positive tilt-table testing. However, a surprisingly high proportion of elderly patients with unexplained syncope had a positive tilt-table test (37% of patients age 65 and older, and 23% patients age 80 and older) *(see* Fig. 3). These data demonstrate that a large proportion of elderly patients with syncope may have neurally mediated syncope that may be difficult to diagnose based on clinical grounds alone.

A recent study contributes further evidence that vasovagal syncope may be more common than previously believed and suggests that tilt-table testing may not be that sensitive for diagnosing neurally mediated syncope in older patients (mean age 64 yr) *(57)*. In this study, 111 patients who underwent tilt-table testing for the evaluation of unexplained syncope all had implantable loop recorders placed regardless of the outcome of their tilt-table tests. Interestingly, comparing patients with positive (29/111) and negative (82/111) tilt-table tests, the rate of recurrent syncope was similar (8/24 [28%] vs 24/82 [27%]). In addition, the majority of the syncopal episodes in both groups demonstrated progressive sinus bradycardia followed by an asystolic pause (mean pause approx 15 s) that was interpreted as a pattern consistent with vasovagal syncope. These data suggest that the patients with negative tilt-table studies were as likely as the patients with positive tilt-table studies to have vasovagal syncope. It would be wrong to interpret these data as suggesting that tilt-table testing is not useful. More correctly, it would be fair to say that even though the sensitivity of tilt-table testing is suboptimal (it only identified 8/32 patients with vasovagal syncope), its yield is still extremely high compared to other tests used to evaluate unexplained syncope. In addition, given that the test is simple and easy to perform, it is certainly worth performing prior to implantation of a loop recorder.

Considerable uncertainty remains in our understanding of the mechanism of vasovagal syncope *(58)*. The triggering mechanism in vasovagal syncope is thought to be a relative central hypovolemia (reduced ventricular preload) that occurs because of venous pooling. The afferent end of this reflex is mediated by left-ventricular mechanoreceptors that are activated during vigorous contraction around an underfilled chamber—a situation similar to severe hemorrhage *(59)*. Information from these mechanoreceptors travels along vagal C fibers to the brainstem, which mediates an abrupt and characteristic efferent response consisting primarily of withdrawal of sympathetic vasomotor tone and often (but not always) a vagally mediated bradycardia. This characteristic efferent response is often referred to as a Bezold–Jarisch reflex and most likely represents a hypersensitive response to an otherwise normal stimulus.

The characteristic efferent "vasovagal-like" response that results in hypotension and a paradoxical relative bradycardia can also occur in other settings, some of which may involve mechanoreceptor activation from other sources, such as the bladder in micturition syncope and the rectum in defecation syncope. This characteristic efferent response is also observed in carotid sinus hypersensitivity *(60)* and during what appears to be vasovagal syncope while undergoing phlebotomy. Vasovagal syncope during blood-injury phobia highlights the possibility of a central nervous system mechanism directly initiating the vasovagal efferent response.

This proposed pathophysiology has been called into question by the observation of vasovagal-like syncopal episodes in patients who have undergone cardiac transplantation (and thus have a denervated heart) *(61–63)*. These observations implicate either the potential importance of other vascular mechanoreceptors or an alternative afferent mechanism. In addition, the role of increased sympathetic activity in the pathogenesis of vasovagal syncope has been called into question by a study that demonstrated that clonidine worsened and yohimbine improved orthostatic tolerance in patients with vasovagal syncope *(64)*. These data and others suggest that the peripheral arteriolar vasoconstriction may not function normally in patients with vasovagal syncope *(65)*.

It is important to recognize the differences in the pathophysiology of vasovagal syncope and the dysautonomic response (or progressive orthostatic hypotensive response) to upright posture *(54,66–68)*. These two disorders can be distinguished from one another based on the cardiovascular and autonomic response to upright posture. In both disorders, the provocative stimulus is an orthostatic challenge caused by either venous pooling in the lower extremities or in the splanchnic vasculature. In vasovagal syncope, the initial cardiovascular response to upright posture appears to be relatively normal. Syncope occurs after an abrupt fall in blood pressure, sometimes accompanied by a fall in heart rate (suggesting a "hypersensitive response") after a delayed period of standing or head-up tilt. In a few large series of patients undergoing tilt-table testing, the mean time to syncope was approx 25 min with a standard deviation of 10 min *(56,69)*. The dysautonomic response results when the autonomic nervous system appears to be failing. These patients are unable to compensate for the drop in venous return that occurs acutely with upright posture. When this failure to compensate becomes severe, frank orthostatic hypotension occurs. However, in many patients, frank orthostatic hypotension may not develop immediately after assuming an upright posture. Patients with a failing autonomic nervous system may demonstrate a progressive type of orthostatic hypotension after prolonged periods of head-up tilt: As blood continues to pool in the lower extremities with prolonged periods of upright posture, blood pressure continues to fall. This has been described as delayed or progressive orthostatic intolerance *(70)* or a dysautonomic response to upright posture *(54)*.

This distinction between a hypersensitive and a failing autonomic response to upright posture is particularly important in understanding differences in this condition between younger and older patients. Younger patients almost exclusively suffer from the classic hypersensitive, vasovagal response; a dysautonomic response is extremely rare in otherwise healthy younger patients. In contrast, elderly patients commonly suffer from an inadequate or failing autonomic response to upright posture, which may result in progressive orthostatic hypotension or a Bezold–Jarisch reflex and vasovagal syncope. This distinction in the mechanism of vasovagal syncope and the dysautonomic response to upright posture has important ramifications in the choice of the treatment for syncope.

Many patients with vasovagal syncope can be effectively treated with education, reassurance, and a simple increase in dietary salt. In others treatment involves removal or avoidance of agents that predispose to hypotension or dehydration, including alcohol, vasodilating antihypertensive medications (such as α-antagonists), and diuretics. However, when these measures fail to prevent the recurrence of symptoms, pharmacologic therapy is usually recommended. Although many pharmacologic agents have been proposed and/or demonstrated to be effective based on nonrandomized clinical trials, there is a remarkable absence of data from large prospective clinical trials *(71,72)*. In fact, no clinical trial on the treatment of vasovagal syncope has involved more than 100 subjects and no study has included a large number of elderly patients. There are data from small randomized placebo controlled studies supporting the efficacy of β-blockers, midodrine, serotonin reuptake inhibitors, and angiotensin-converting enzyme (ACE) inhibitors. In addition to these agents, there is also considerable clinical experience and a consensus suggesting that fludrocortisone is also effective, although it is often not well tolerated by elderly subjects because of the development of edema *(73)*.

With regard to the treatment of elderly patients with vasovagal syncope, many elderly patients have hypertension, which is a contraindication to a number of treatments used for vasovagal syncope (salt, fludrocortisone, and midodrine). In elderly subjects, selective serotonin reuptake inhibitors (SSRIs) may be effective at preventing vasovagal syncope in highly symptomatic patients. Although there is no specific data on SSRIs in older patients, the use of SSRIs for the treatment of vasovagal syncope is appealing for a number of reasons. First, if an older patient has vasovagal syncope in the setting of a dysautonomic response to upright posture, then β-blockers, which further attenuate the autonomic response, may not be effective. Second, there is anecdotal evidence that SSRIs may be effective in treating refractory neurogenic orthostatic hypotension (74), suggesting that treatment with SSRIs augment rather than attenuate the autonomic response to upright posture. If pharmacologic therapy is either not tolerated or ineffective, implantation of a pacemaker with a specialized sensing and pacing algorithm may be an effective alternative treatment (40).

Carotid Sinus Hypersensitivity

Several studies have demonstrated that carotid sinus hypersensitivity is a common etiology for syncope and falls in the elderly (8,25,75). A study of patients evaluated in a "syncope" clinic demonstrated that 44% had documented carotid sinus hypersensitivity (8). Of those with carotid sinus hypersensitivity (CSH), 39% had presented with falls or dizziness, denying syncope. Kenny and Traynor found that among 130 elderly subjects who attended a geriatric outpatient clinic, 33 (25%) had CSH (16). Dey and Kenny evaluated 35 patients with drop attacks and found that 18 (51%) had CSH and symptoms directly attributable to carotid sinus hypersensitivity (76). Once again, the original studies of syncope in the 1980s likely underestimated the prevalence of carotid sinus hypersensitivity, because carotid sinus massage was not performed routinely (1).

The initial study documenting an association between carotid sinus hypersensitivity and falls involved 100 nursing home residents, 14 of whom were found to have carotid sinus hypersensitivity (77). In this study, only electrocardiographic monitoring was used for diagnosis; thus, the prevalence may have been underestimated. Over a follow-up of 33 mo, the incidence of falls complicated by fractures or lacerations were significantly more common among patients with carotid sinus hypersensitivity. In a larger epidemiologic study of 598 patients >50 yr of age presenting to an emergency room with an unexplained fall, Richardson et al. (25) performed carotid sinus massage (CSM) on 279 subjects, 34% of whom had CSH. More recent data have demonstrated a high prevalence of CSH among elderly subjects with femoral fractures (78). The most convincing evidence linking CSH to unexplained falls is from a study in which 175 patients with nonaccidental falls and cardioinhibitory CSH were randomized either to a permanent pacemaker implantation or to a control group (26). Treatment with a pacemaker resulted in a 66% reduction in falls in 1 yr of follow-up.

Carotid sinus massage has been employed as a provocative maneuver to elicit CSH. Carotid sinus massage is performed by applying digital pressure at the bifurcation of the internal and external carotid arteries below the angle of the jaw at the level of the cricothyroid cartilage for no more than 5 s on only one side. Because some patients may be exquisitely sensitive, carotid massage should be initiated with very gentle pressure, which should be applied with a longitudinal or rotatory movement. Care should be taken to avoid carotid occlusion, as this will reduce rather than increase carotid sinus nerve traffic and might increase the risk of neurologic complications in subjects with disease in the contralateral artery.

Carotid sinus hypersensitivity is classified according to its predominant hemodynamic manifestation—either prolonged sinus pauses (>3 s; cardioinhibitory) or marked falls in

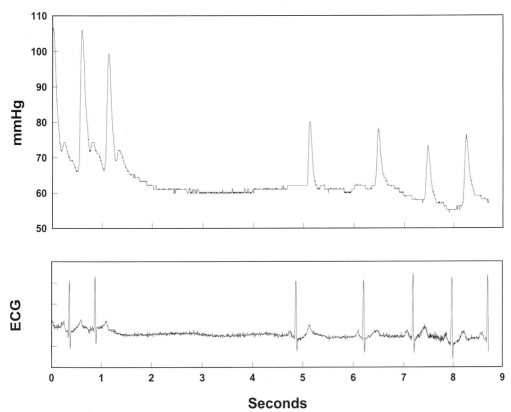

Fig. 4. Mixed CSH in an elderly patient with recurrent syncope. Following carotid sinus massage (at time 0), there is a 4.5-s pause. Despite the return of sinus rhythm, the blood pressure is 70–80 mm Hg, demonstrating that the vasodilation has occurred.

systolic blood pressure (>50 mm Hg, vasodepressor), or both (mixed CSH). These diagnostic criteria have been reaffirmed as appropriate after a study documented responses to CSM among 25 asymptomatic elderly subjects who demonstrated mean maximal cardioinhibitory responses of 1038 ± 195 ms and mean maximal vasodepressor responses of 21 ± 14 mm Hg *(79)*. Although CSM is typically performed during continuous electrocardiographic monitoring, the realization that a large percentage of subjects with CSH have a predominantly vasodepressor component argues for performance of the procedure with continuous blood pressure as well as heart rate monitoring. The former is easily obtained with noninvasive devices that utilize plethysmography or applanation tonometry to record beat-to-beat arterial waveforms accurately (*see* Fig. 4). Carotid sinus massage should be performed initially in the supine position. However, performing carotid sinus massage during erect posture enhances its sensitivity in identifying subjects with CSH *(80)*.

Physicians occasionally hesitate to perform CSM for fear of complications. The contraindications to CSM include the presence of carotid bruits, a history of ventricular tachycardia, recent myocardial infarction, and cerebral infarction. In the absence of these contraindications, CSM has a low incidence of complications, and the potential benefit of diagnosing CSH outweighs this small risk. Recent data confirmed an extremely low incidence of neurologic complications (11 in 16,000; an incidence of <0.1%) when appropriate screening criteria are utilized *(81)*. Notably, almost all of the neurologic events in this extremely large series were without long-term sequelae. In addition, there were no episodes of ventricular tachyarrhythmias in this large series of patients.

The pathophysiology of CSH is not well understood and is beyond the scope of this chapter and has been reviewed elsewhere *(75)*. Abnormalities have been proposed in each portion of the reflex arc: the afferent limb (i.e., baroreceptor itself or vessel wall), and central processing or efferent limb (i.e., sinus node dysfunction). The predominance of the evidence implicates a theory of "underuse hypersensitivity," in which an impairment of afferent limb stimulation either secondary to age-related arterial stiffening or abnormalities of proprioceptive input result in abnormal central nervous system processing and a hypersensitive efferent response *(82,83)*.

The use of pacemakers for the treatment of CSH is straightforward in patients with the predominantly cardioinhibitory form. Randomized prospective data performed in two studies have documented the significant benefit of pacing, with recurrence rates for syncope of 57% and 47% of the nonpacing group and in 0% and 9% of the pacing group *(84, 85)*. Moreover, 65% in the nonpacing group needed a pacemaker implanted because of the ongoing severity of symptoms. Pacing has been ineffective in treating subjects with pure vasodepressor responses or mixed responses with a significant vasodepressor component. However, the use of specialized sensing and pacing algorithms (rate-drop pacing or rate hysteresis) has led to improved outcomes in patients with mixed CSH. These algorithms sense a sudden drop in heart rate and pace at a rapid rate (approx 100 bpm) for a few minutes in an attempt to overcome the drop in blood pressure with rapid pacing *(38,39,86)*.

Few data demonstrating beneficial treatments for the pure vasodepressor form of CSH exist. Case reports have suggested the benefit of SSRIs *(87,88)*. Others have suggested the use of carotid sinus denervation as a treatment for these patients *(75,89,90)*.

Ventricular Arrhythmias

Ventricular tachyarrhythmias are an important and life-threatening cause of syncope in both young and elderly patients. Given the increasing prevalence of diabetes, hypertension, hypercholesterolemia, and coronary artery disease with age, elderly patients are more likely to have reduced left-ventricular function, whether from prior myocardial infarction or from cardiomyopathy and are, therefore, at increased risk for developing ventricular tachycardia as the cause of their syncope. In addition, patients with significant left-ventricular hypertrophy or aortic stenosis are also at increased risk for developing ventricular tachyarrhythmias. Finally, given that elderly patients are often faced with polypharmacy, syncope from torsades de pointes may result from a drug that may prolong the QT interval, especially when taken in combination with diuretics or in the setting of any illness that may cause hypokalemia.

The gold standard for evaluating the syncope patient with an increased risk of having ventricular arrhythmias has been EP testing. When monomorphic ventricular tachycardia is induced during EP testing, the patient is clearly at increased risk for having ventricular arrhythmias as the cause of his or her syncope and requires treatment aimed at preventing (antiarrhythmic drugs) or treating (implantable cardiac defibrillators) these arrhythmias. However, the sensitivity of EP testing is suboptimal, especially in patients with a nonischemic cardiomyopathy *(91)*. Patients with a nonischemic cardiomyopathy and syncope are at high risk for developing ventricular arrhythmias and require definitive treatment, regardless of the outcome of an EP study *(92)*. The sensitivity of EP testing in patients with an ischemic cardiomyopathy has been recently called into question by the relatively high rate (approx

12% over 2 yr) of arrhythmic events in the "registry" arm (i.e., negative EP study) of the MUSTT study *(93)*.

An alternative strategy for identifying patients at high risk for developing ventricular arrhythmias has emerged over the past few years with the advent of microvolt T-wave alternans testing. Microvolt T-wave alternans is strongly associated mechanistically with the genesis of ventricular arrhythmias *(94)* and patients with T-wave alternans have been shown to be at markedly increased risk of developing ventricular arrhythmias *(95)*. In patients with syncope, microvolt T-wave alternans is a better predictor of spontaneous ventricular arrhythmia during 1 yr of follow-up than an EP study *(96)*. In addition, the association between microvolt T-wave alternans and ventricular arrhythmias is equally strong in patients with ischemic and nonischemic heart disease *(97)*. Microvolt T-wave alternans can be measured during a standard exercise stress test with specialized electrodes and computer processing that is now commercially available (Cambridge Heart Inc., Bedford, MA).

The signal-averaged ECG is another noninvasive test that identifies patients at increased risk of having ventricular arrhythmias as the cause of syncope *(98)*. In a head-to-head comparison, however, T-wave alternans appeared to be a more powerful marker of arrhythmia risk than the signal-averaged ECG *(95)*. The two tests may be complementary; T-wave alternans cannot be measured in patients in atrial fibrillation but can have a signal-averaged ECG measured. Alternatively, the signal-averaged ECG is not reliable in patients with bundle branch block, but these patients can have T-wave alternans measured.

Other Causes of Syncope in the Elderly

It is beyond the scope of this chapter to review in detail all of the causes of syncope in the elderly. A few points deserve mention regarding other causes of syncope in order to point out how elderly patients may differ from their younger counterparts.

Aortic stenosis is a well-known cause of syncope in elderly patients. In patients with critical aortic stenosis, syncope may result from a number of pathophysiologic processes. Syncope during exercise or exertion may be the result of exercised-induced hypotension. Although this is often thought to result from an inability to increase cardiac output in the face of a fixed obstruction, there is evidence that hypotension may be caused by vasodilation from a Bezold–Jarisch reflex caused by elevated left-ventricular systolic pressures during exertion *(99)*. Syncope in patients with aortic stenosis may also result from ventricular tachyarrhythmias or from bradyarrhythmias, the latter caused by the combination of left-ventricular hypertrophy and fibrosis as well as extension of valvular calcification into the conduction system. In patients with critical aortic stenosis, syncope is an ominous sign.

Supraventricular tachycardias uncommonly cause syncope in younger subjects but are more likely to cause syncope in elderly patients. Rapid heart rates during a supraventricular tachycardia in the setting of diastolic dysfunction and even mild hypovolemia may result in hypotension in elderly subjects. This is often difficult to prove unless the supraventricular tachycardia is documented on an ECG from a monitor or telemetry during an episode of syncope. It is uncommon to provoke syncope in the electrophysiology laboratory when a supraventricular tachycardia is induced, because the patient is supine. In addition, elderly patients with supraventricular tachycardias may develop syncope from a pause following the tachycardia (tachy-brady syndrome).

Neurologic causes of syncope are relatively uncommon in the absence of neurologic findings from the history or the physical examination (unilateral weakness or paresthesias, dysarthria, etc.). When syncope is the result of a cerebrovascular accident or transient ischemic attack, these findings are almost always present. Seizure disorder can present as unexplained syncope, although this type of presentation is uncommon. Seizures tend to present with tonic–clonic movements and with a prolonged period of disorientation following the event. The prolonged period of disorientation is relatively specific for seizure disorder; the majority of patients with syncope have a clear sensorium within a minute or two of regaining consciousness. Tonic–clonic movements, however, are not specific for seizure disorder. Patients with syncope and a prolonged period of hypotension, often from a long asystolic pause, can develop myoclonic jerking movements that can be confused with seizure. In a study of 70 patients carrying the diagnosis of epilepsy who did not have clear EEG evidence of seizure disorder, nearly half were found to have a cardiovascular cause of syncope, such as a long asystolic pause (either from vasovagal syncope, carotid sinus hypersensitivity, or from sick sinus syndrome) *(100)*.

STANDARD OF CARE

Evaluation of Elderly Patient with Unexplained Syncope

In many patients who present with syncope, the diagnosis can either be made or is strongly suggested by the history, physical examination, basic laboratory values, and an ECG. This initial workup should be able to identify patients with complete heart block, severe orthostatic hypotension, supraventricular or ventricular tachycardia, and critical aortic stenosis. The evaluation of the elderly patient with unexplained syncope after an initial workup should follow a diagnostic algorithm that first utilizes noninvasive, high-yield diagnostic tests (*see* Fig. 5).

The first step in the algorithm is to determine whether or not there is evidence (by history or on physical examination) of a neurologic cause for syncope. In the majority of patients, there is no such evidence and there is no need for neurologic testing. Numerous studies have demonstrated that imaging studies of the brain and electroencephalograms (EEGs) have an extremely low diagnostic yield in patients with unexplained syncope *(101–103)*. Some patients may require a computed tomography (CT) scan of the head to exclude a subdural hematoma in the setting of syncope with a traumatic fall. However, CT scans of the head are vastly overutilized in the evaluation of the patient with unexplained syncope *(103,104)*.

The second step in the algorithm is to determine if the patient has structural heart disease and to assess the possibility of ventricular arrhythmias as the cause of syncope. Echocardiography or some other assessment of left-ventricular function is often done to determine whether or not structural heart disease is present and, if so, to estimate its extent. Patients with a prior myocardial infarction or with left-ventricular dysfunction from any cause require an assessment of their risk of having ventricular arrhythmias. Patients without any evidence of structural heart disease are at low risk for having ventricular arrhythmias and may not require further risk stratification. Patients with left-ventricular hypertrophy, a history of coronary artery disease without a prior myocardial infarction, or patients with valvular heart disease with normal left-ventricular function probably have an intermediate risk for having ventricular arrhythmias and may require further risk stratification.

As discussed earlier, microvolt T-wave alternans testing or the signal-averaged ECG are useful noninvasive diagnostic tests that may be used to risk-stratify patients with syncope and structural heart disease. Both of these tests have an excellent negative predictive accuracy, suggesting that they can be used to identify patients at low risk for having ventricular arrhythmias, thus directing their workup toward other causes of syncope (brady-

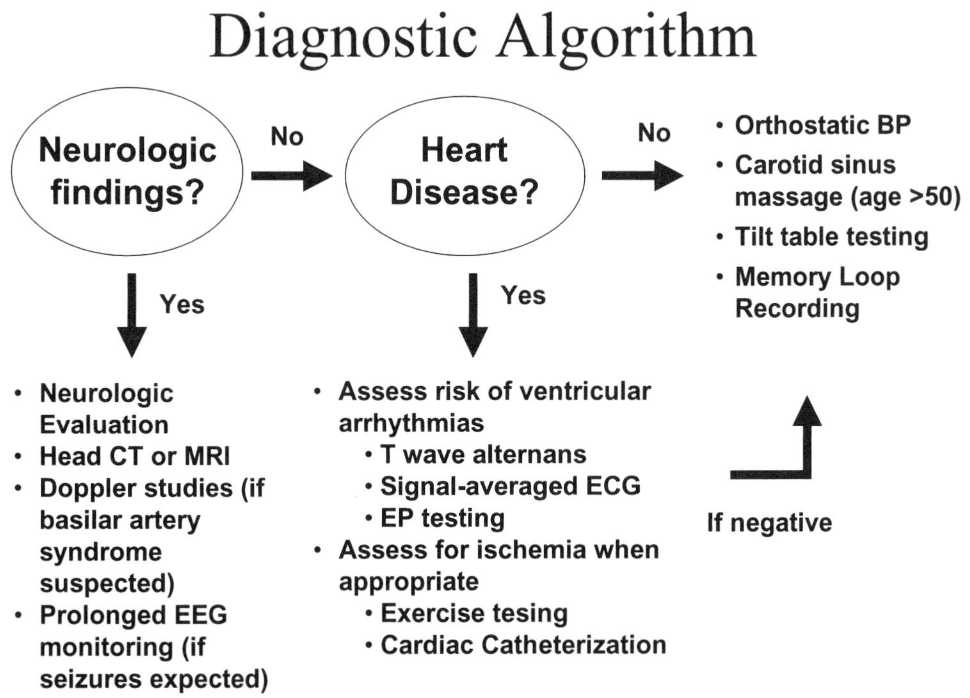

Diagnostic Algorithm

Neurologic findings? — No → Heart Disease? — No →
- Orthostatic BP
- Carotid sinus massage (age >50)
- Tilt table testing
- Memory Loop Recording

Neurologic findings? ↓ Yes
- Neurologic Evaluation
- Head CT or MRI
- Doppler studies (if basilar artery syndrome suspected)
- Prolonged EEG monitoring (if seizures expected)

Heart Disease? ↓ Yes
- Assess risk of ventricular arrhythmias
  - T wave alternans
  - Signal-averaged ECG
  - EP testing
- Assess for ischemia when appropriate
  - Exercise tesing
  - Cardiac Catheterization

↑ If negative

Fig. 5. Diagnostic algorithm for the patient with unexplained syncope. This simple algorithm is meant to direct the evaluation of the patient with unexplained syncope (after an initial history, physical examination, and ECG) toward tests with the highest yield. The diagnostic evaluation of an individual patient must be tailored based on the history and physical examination.

arrhythmias or disorders in blood pressure regulation). Patients who have positive tests may go on to have EP studies or, in some cases (patients with a nonischemic cardiomyopathy and syncope), may be treated directly.

The majority of elderly patients with syncope will have neither neurologic findings nor will be at high risk for having ventricular arrhythmias as the cause of their syncopal episode(s). In most elderly patients, the cause of syncope will either be a bradyarrhythmia or a transient hypotensive episode from one of the disorders of blood pressure regulation. For these patients, the two diagnostic tests with the highest yield are carotid sinus massage and tilt-table testing. Both of these tests are noninvasive, simple to perform, and safe. Unfortunately, these tests are vastly underutilized, leaving many elderly patients with no explanation for their syncope *(104)*.

In patients with a normal response to carotid sinus massage and a nondiagnostic tilt-table test, memory loop recorders may be useful in identifying the cause of syncope. These small and unobtrusive recorders are worn by patients for approx 30 d and provide continuous ECG recording over a 5 min "loop." When they have a recurrent syncopal episode, they activate the device upon regaining consciousness, which triggers the device to store the previous few minutes of ECG on the loop, hopefully capturing the ECG at the time of the syncopal episode. The overall concept of documenting the ECG during an episode of syncope, providing so-called "symptom rhythm correlation," is powerful. Unfortunately, these external loop recorders are problematic for a number of reasons. First, it is difficult to determine whether or not patients activated the device within the 3 to 4 min window following the event. This lack of certainty is problematic if the ECG demonstrates sinus rhythm without an arrhythmia: was the rhythm normal, implicating a transient hypotensive event as the cause of syncope, or did the patient fail to activate the device quickly enough? Second, recurrent syncope is often infrequent and is not captured with only 1 mo of monitoring. These external loop recorders are cumbersome to wear for more than 1 mo, often leaving patients without a diagnosis after 1 mo of monitoring.

The recent development of implantable loop recorders (Reveal Plus™; Medtronic, Minneapolis, MN) has improved our ability to accomplish "symptom–rhythm correlation" (105,106). Implantable monitors have 14 mo of battery life, can store up to 42 min of ECG rhythm, and can be programmed to store one or more episodes. For patients who may have trouble activating the device within a few minutes of a syncopal episode, the device can be set to store 41 min of ECG data prior to the time of activation. In addition, this device can now be activated automatically when the heart rate is outside of a programmable range (e.g., <30 bpm or >150 bpm). This automatic activation allows the device to capture potentially asymptomatic arrhythmias, in addition to guaranteeing that symptomatic arrhythmias will be captured, even if the patient forgot to activate the device. In two studies of patients with unexplained syncope, the diagnostic yield of the implantable loop monitor was 64%, of which 23% of patients had a documented arrhythmic event at the time of syncope, the vast majority of which were bradyarrhythmias (107,108). Ten percent had either a normal rhythm or sinus bradycardia along with symptoms suggesting vasovagal syncope. Another 31% had documentation of a normal rhythm during a syncopal event, which effectively excludes the diagnosis of a dysrhythmia and strongly suggests an alternative diagnosis such as a transient hypotensive episode or a psychogenic cause of syncope.

Another study randomized 60 patients with unexplained syncope either to a conventional evaluation (with an external loop recorder and tilt and electrophysiologic testing) or to prolonged monitoring with an implantable loop recorder with 1 yr of monitoring. A diagnosis was obtained in 14 of 27 patients randomized to prolonged monitoring compared with 6 of 30 patients undergoing conventional testing (52% vs 20%, $p < 0.05$). Bradyarrhythmias were much more likely to be identified as the cause of syncope in patients randomized to the implantable monitor (40% vs 8%) (see Fig. 6). Overall, the diagnostic yield of implantable monitors is extremely high. Further studies are underway to better define how an implantable monitor should be used in the evaluation of the patient with unexplained syncope.

Issues with Treating Elderly Patients

The decision to treat elderly patients with syncope depends on a number of factors, including the patients' risk of developing recurrent syncope and the risk of having trauma related to another syncopal event (patients without a prodrome are at much greater risk for a traumatic fall than patients with a predictable prodrome that allows them to sit down when symptoms occur). The decision to treat is also based in part on the intrinsic risk of the cause of syncope; life-threatening causes of syncope, such as ventricular tachycardia or aortic stenosis, require urgent treatment, whereas vasovagal syncope with a long prodrome may not require any specific treatment. Finally, the decision to treat is based in part on one's confidence in the diagnosis. It is not a difficult decision to treat an elderly patient with a 10 s pause during carotid sinus massage. On the other hand, the decision to treat an asymptomatic 2.5 s pause is more difficult.

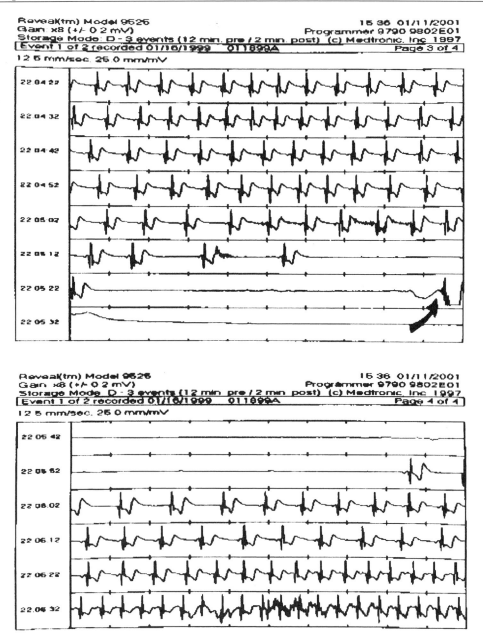

Fig. 6. Electrocardiogram documentation of asystole from an implantable loop recorder. Down-loaded rhythm strip from 55-yr old patient with 11 previous episodes of syncope over 7 yr before enrollment. Conventional testing did not yield a diagnosis. Patient was crossed over to monitoring strategy. Seven months after implantation of loop recorder, patient had recurrent syncope and captured a 43 s pause with a single QRS complex after 4 s. There is an impact artifact (arrow) at the point at which the patient fell to the floor. The device was removed, and a pacemaker was implanted. Reproduced with permission from ref. *106*.

Many physicians opt to treat patients empirically without a clear diagnosis. Unfortunately, many of these patients have had neither carotid sinus massage nor tilt-table testing performed; thus, the decision to treat empirically was made prior to a complete workup.

Pacemakers are often used as empiric treatment for syncope in elderly subjects, especially when any bradycardia has been documented (even asymptomatic sinus bradycardia or asymptomatic short pauses <3 s). This approach is problematic, because hypotensive disorders are common in elderly subjects and are often ineffectively treated by the implantation of a simple pacemaker. In a study of 206 patients with unexplained syncope who underwent long-term monitoring with an implantable loop recorder, the clinical characteristics of patients ultimately diagnosed with a bradyarrhythmia as the cause of syncope were not sufficiently distinct from those of patients who had syncope unrelated to a bradyarrhythmia (107). These data suggest that it would be difficult to target a group of patients prospectively that are likely to benefit from a pacemaker. A better option would be to use an implantable loop monitor and wait for one additional syncopal episode to document the rhythm prior to implanting a pacemaker.

Long-term monitoring with an implantable loop recorder is effective in establishing a diagnosis in any patient who has evidence of nondiagnostic, nonspecific, asymptomatic, nonsustained arrhythmias. For example, prior to treating patients with short runs of supraventricular tachycardia documented on a Holter recorder in a patient with syncope, it would be better to document the supraventricular tachycardia during an episode of syncope. Occasionally, these patients are empirically treated with β-blockers, rate-slowing calcium channel blockers, or even amiodarone and continue to have recurrent syncope from bradyarrhythmias that were exacerbated by the empiric treatment. The same type of situation exists for patients with nonsustained ventricular tachycardia, with either a negative EP study, signal-averaged ECG, or microvolt T-wave alternans test. Treating these patients with amiodarone or sotalol may exacerbate undetected bradyarrhythmias causing syncope.

Another issue that commonly arises in elderly patients with unexplained syncope is the treatment of asymptomatic orthostatic hypotension. Many patients with asymptomatic orthostatic hypotension on physical examination will demonstrate a gradual and progressive drop in blood pressure to the point of syncope during tilt-table testing. However, in those patients in whom tilt-table testing is not diagnostic, it remains unclear if the asymptomatic fall in blood pressure is the cause of syncope or is an unrelated finding. Once again, the use of an implantable loop recorder would be helpful in these patients by potentially excluding dysrhythmias as the cause of syncope, thereby offering additional evidence that transient hypotension is the most likely cause of syncope.

CONTROVERSIES

Role of Tilt-Table Testing in Elderly Subjects

Tilt-table testing is a simple, noninvasive technique that identifies abnormalities in the regulation of blood pressure that may be the cause of syncope. Tilt-table testing has a high diagnostic yield in both young and elderly patients (56). In addition, two international expert consensus panels recommend the use of tilt-table testing in the evaluation of patients with unexplained syncope (12,109). Despite these recommendations, tilt-table testing is a vastly underutilized diagnostic test for patients with unexplained syncope (104). There are a number of potential explanations for the under use of tilt-table testing.

First, tilt-table testing requires specialized equipment that is not available in some hospitals. In addition, the reimbursement for tilt-table testing is extremely low (Medicare reimburses approx $250 (global: technical and professional), providing a disincentive for investing in this equipment and the time involved in testing. On the other hand, the cost of this equipment ($10,000 to $25,000) is relatively low, given its potential usefulness. Furthermore, the tilt-table can be used in rehabilitation medicine for patients with spinal cord injury and other debilitated patients following prolonged bedrest, enhancing the value of the investment.

Second, physicians question the uncertain link between what happens during a tilt-table test and what happens during a spontaneous episode of syncope. This uncertainty is present with most diagnoses identified as the cause of unexplained syncope. For example, there is an uncertain link between a 4 s asymptomatic pause on telemetry and the actual cause of unexplained syncope. However, most physicians would not hesitate to implant a pacemaker for this 4 s pause. The plausibility of linking the response of tilt-table testing to the cause of spontaneous episodes of syncope was recently made clear by a study in which patients (mean age 64 yr) had implantable loop monitors placed following their tilt-table test (57). In this study in patients with positive tilt-table tests, the ECG rhythm documented during a spontaneous episode of syncope (progressive sinus bradycardia with a variable asystolic pause) was similar to the patient's response during the tilt test.

Third, physicians question the specificity of tilt-table testing. This line of thinking derives from the proportion of positive tilt-table tests in healthy volunteers. A meta-analysis of more than 400 tilt-table tests on healthy volunteers suggests that approx 13% will have a positive tilt-table test without drug provocation (110). Although the use of isoproterenol is known to reduce the specificity of tilt-table testing (111,112), recent studies using nitroglycerin as a provocative agent have demonstrated that its specificity is excellent (113,114). Ultimately, the question of specificity should be viewed in the context of Bayes' theorem. For those patients with syncope who have had other potential diagnoses excluded, the pretest likelihood of a disorder in blood pressure regulation is high. Thus, an abnormal tilt-table test in these patients is likely to be a true positive rather than a false-positive test result. In addition, the response to tilt-table testing may directly influence the choice of therapy based on whether the response is vasovagal or orthostatic.

Ultimately, tilt-table testing is extremely useful for a large number of patients with unexplained syncope. Most patients with normal left-ventricular function who have a normal response to carotid sinus massage are left at the end of their workup with a limited differential diagnosis for the cause of their syncope—usually either bradycardic syncope or syncope from one of the disorders of blood pressure regulation. Tilt-table testing may help differentiate these disorders and allow the initiation of treatment. The performance of upright carotid sinus massage as part of the tilt-table test will increase the yield of carotid sinus massage (115). In those patients in whom the tilt-table test is normal, implantable loop recorders is the likely next step in the workup.

Role of Implantable Loop Recorders

The implantable loop recorder (Reveal, Medtronic, Minneapolis, MN) is a new technology supported by a growing body of literature demonstrating its efficacy (see Fig. 6). The role of loop recorders in the evaluation of the patient with unexplained syncope is based on the large number of patients without an etiology for their syncope despite an extensive evaluation. If the patient is likely to have recurrent syncope despite an extensive but unrevealing workup, then one has the option of doing nothing and waiting for the next episode to occur or to implant a loop recorder, so that the ECG rhythm is documented during the next syncopal episode. In our opinion, the decision to use an implantable loop recorder in these patients is clear. If the choice is made not to utilize the implantable loop recorder, then it is likely that when the patient returns with recurrent syncope a month or a year later, nothing new would have been learned, and the cause of syncope will remain elusive. At that point, the extensive workup is often repeated, but it is still unlikely to demonstrate a cause of syncope. Once again, the patient is sent home, exposed to the risks of another syncopal episode without a diagnosis.

When the implantable loop recorders are used, the diagnostic yield is high *(106–108)*. Approximately 20% of patients will have a bradycardic event documented at the time of their next syncopal episode. Another 10% of patients will have sinus bradycardia documented along with symptoms that strongly suggest the diagnosis of vasovagal syncope, and another 30% will have sinus rhythm documented at the time of syncope. Although one could debate whether these latter two findings are "diagnostic" or "nondiagnostic," the absence of a bradyarrhythmia or tachyarrhythmia at the time of syncope remains an important and valuable finding and focuses our attention on other causes of syncope, usually either a transient hypotensive event, a seizure disorder, or a psychogenic cause of syncope.

The most obvious limitation of the implantable loop recorder is its lack of ability to measure blood pressure. When the recorder documents bradyarrhythmias, it may be difficult to determine if these are intrinsic (e.g., sinus node dysfunction) or extrinsic (e.g., part of a vasovagal episode). The assumption is often that the bradyarrhythmia is intrinsic, prompting placement of a permanent pacemaker, although some of these bradyarrhythmias may respond to pharmacotherapy directed at vasovagal syncope. It is important to note that, to date, there have not been any studies showing the benefits of therapeutic intervention after documented bradyarrhythmias from an implantable loop recorder. Finally, use of an implantable loop recorder, by definition, accepts the risk of at least one subsequent syncopal episode. Although this leaves the patient exposed to all of the risks inherent to traumatic fall, this risk is offset by the knowledge gained from another syncopal episode. Importantly, if an appropriate and extensive evaluation has been done, this risk is present whether an implantable loop recorder is used or whether patients are sent home without a recorder. The only alternative is empiric treatment, which has not been proven effective and is not recommended for these patients.

Although still controversial, we believe that the implantable loop recorder should be placed in patients who have had an unrevealing evaluation that has included, at a minimum, an echocardiogram, a tilt-table test, and carotid sinus massage. In some patients, it may be appropriate to perform an electrophysiology study prior to use of an implantable loop recorder. The relative benefit of an electrophysiology study and an implantable loop recorder is currently being investigated in a large multicenter study.

Role of CSM

Carotid sinus massage should be performed in all elderly subjects with unexplained syncope unless they have one of the contraindications to carotid sinus massage, which include the presence of carotid bruits, a history of ventricular tachycardia, recent myocardial infarction or cerebral infarction. Unfortunately, carotid sinus massage remains a vastly underutilized diagnostic test *(104)*.

The underutilization of this high-yield diagnostic test is likely the result of two misunderstandings. First, there is a perception that CSH is a relatively rare cause of syncope. A recent review suggested that CSH only accounts for 1% of syncopal episode *(116)*, although this is based on studies in which carotid sinus massage was not routinely performed *(6)*.

When carotid sinus massage is routinely performed in the evaluation of the patient with syncope or unexplained falls, the diagnostic yield may be as high as 45% *(8,25,115)*.

Second, in the absence of contraindications, carotid sinus massage has a low incidence of complications (<0.1%), and the potential benefit of diagnosing carotid sinus hypersensitivity outweighs this small risk *(81)*. Importantly, nearly all of the neurologic events that have been reported during carotid sinus massage largely resolved and were without long-term sequelae.

There should be no controversy surrounding the use of carotid sinus massage. It should be done in all patients with unexplained syncope unless contraindicated. In addition, it should be performed both supine and upright because of the increased yield when it is done upright *(115)*. In addition, blood pressure must be measured during carotid sinus massage in order to detect the vasodepressor type and the mixed type, which together account for the vast majority of cases of carotid sinus hypersensitivity. It is difficult to document the transient hypotension that occurs following carotid sinus massage with a manual blood pressure cuff. Ideally, blood pressure should be measured using a noninvasive blood pressure monitor. At least one such monitor is commercially available (Colin Medical Instruments, San Antonio, TX).

Hypertension and Orthostatic Hypotension

A significant number of patients with hypertension will develop orthostatic hypotension, although most of these patients are asymptomatic. The prevalence of orthostatic hypotension is related to the severity of the hypertension (nearly 30% of patients with a systolic blood pressure >160 mm Hg whether they are on medications for hypertension or not) *(117)*. Patients with the combination of hypertension and symptomatic orthostatic hypotension are extremely difficult to treat. Unfortunately, there has been a paucity of literature guiding the treatment of these difficult patients. It is important to document that symptoms are related to hypotension, which is best done with tilt-table testing. Lightheadedness is a nonspecific symptom that can also be caused by hypertension, as well as vestibular problems, central nervous system disorders such as Parkinson's disease, or normal pressure hydrocephalus.

It may be useful to distinguish among three types of patient that demonstrate both orthostatic hypotension and hypertension. First, there are patients with hypertension who have a >20 mm Hg fall in blood pressure that is asymptomatic. To be truly asymptomatic, these patients must not have any history of syncope or significant lightheadedness. Although these patients do have a demonstrable drop in blood pressure when they are upright, their standing blood pressures are often >120 mm Hg. There is no specific treatment necessary for the patient with long-standing hypertension who develops mild, asymptomatic, orthostatic hypotension. It may be possible to ameliorate some of the orthostatic hypotension by changing a patient's antihypertensive medication. For example, α-antagonists are notorious for causing or exacerbating orthostatic hypotension. Organic nitrates can also exacerbate orthostatic hypotension and can be stopped in many patients. In one study of patients who presented to the emergency room with drug-related syncope, organic nitrates were the most common class of drug implicated as the cause of syncope *(118)*.

Second, there are patients with hypertension who have an asymptomatic >20 mm Hg fall in blood pressure when standing, but they also have either vasovagal syncope or a documented progressive fall in blood pressure during a tilt-table test. These patients may also benefit from trying alternative antihypertensive treatment in an attempt to limit the orthostatic hypotension. Unfortunately, this is often not sufficient to prevent recurrent symptoms of syncope or near-syncope. The treatment of their symptoms, either from vasovagal syncope or a delayed and progressive fall in blood pressure is difficult, as many of the commonly used treatments are contraindicated, because they also cause an increase in blood pressure (salt supplementation, fludrocortisone, or midodrine). One class of drugs that may be useful are the selective serotonin reuptake inhibitors (SSRIs). Paroxetine has been shown to prevent vasovagal syncope in a randomized double-blind placebo-controlled trial, although this trial did not include elderly patients with either hypertension or orthostatic hypotension *(119)*. There is also a case report of patients with severe orthostatic hypotension who improved after treatment with fluoxetine *(74)*.

Third, there are patients with hypertension who also have severe and symptomatic orthostatic hypotension who stand up and develop lightheadedness within 3 min with a documented fall in systolic blood pressure to less than 100 mm Hg. Many of these patients do not have a long history of hypertension but rather have one of the causes of severe orthostatic hypotension (multisystem atrophy or pure autonomic failure) and subsequently developed hypertension, which is part of the natural history of severe orthostatic hypotension. It is important to recognize that these patients have developed hypertension as a complication of long-term orthostatic hypotension. These patients often present with recurrent syncope or near-syncope and have severe orthostatic hypotension (supine systolic blood pressures often >160 mm Hg and standing systolic blood pressures often <90 mm Hg). In general, their hypertension should not be treated, because it will exacerbate their orthostatic hypotension. It is important to recognize that during the day, when these patients are either seated or standing, they are usually not hypertensive, because their blood pressure has dropped into the normal range when they have changed from supine to the sitting position. Some investigators have suggested the use of short-acting antihypertensive drugs in the evening. This may be problematic if the patient gets up during the night to go to the bathroom and may become syncopal. An alternative would be to elevate the head of the bed, which is often sufficient to decrease the supine hypertension.

REFERENCES

1. Kapoor WN, Karpf M, Wieand S, Peterson JR, Levey GS. A prospective evaluation and follow-up of patients with syncope. N Engl J Med 1983;309:197–204.
2. Lipsitz LA, Pluchino FC, Wei JY, Rowe JW. Syncope in institutionalized elderly: the impact of multiple pathological conditions and situational stress. J Chronic Dis 1986;39:619–630.
3. Day SC, Cook EF, Funkenstein H, Goldman L. Evaluation and outcome of emergency room patients with transient loss of consciousness. Am J Med 1982;73:15–23.
4. Lipsitz LA, Wei JY, Rowe JW. Syncope in an elderly, institutionalised population: prevalence, incidence, and associated risk. Q J Med 1985;55:45–54.
5. Kapoor W, Snustad D, Peterson J, Wieand HS, Cha R, Karpf M. Syncope in the elderly. Am J Med 1986;80:419–428.
6. Kapoor WN, Karpf M, Wieand S, Peterson JR, Levey GS. A prospective evaluation and follow-up of patients with syncope. N Engl J Med 1983;309:197–204.
7. Lipsitz LA. What's Different About Syncope in the Aged? Am J Geriatr Cardiol 1993;2:37–41.
8. McIntosh S, Da Costa D, Kenny RA. Outcome of an integrated approach to the investigation of dizziness, falls and syncope in elderly patients referred to a "syncope" clinic. Age Ageing 1993;22:53–58.
9. Hori S. Diagnosis of patients with syncope in emergency medicine. Keio J Med 1994;43:185–191.
10. Chen L, Chen MH, Larson MG, Evans J, Benjamin EJ, Levy D. Risk factors for syncope in a community-based sample (the Framingham Heart Study). Am J Cardiol 2000;85:1189–1193.

11. Kapoor WN, Karpf M, Maher Y, Miller RA, Levey GS. Syncope of unknown origin. The need for a more cost-effective approach to its diagnosis evaluation. JAMA 1982;247:2687–2691.
12. Brignole M, Alboni P, Benditt D, Bergfeldt L, Blanc JJ, Bloch TP, et al. Task force on syncope, European Society of Cardiology. Part 1. The initial evaluation of patients with syncope. Europace 2001; 3:253–260.
13. Cummings SR, Nevitt MC, Kidd S. Forgetting falls. The limited accuracy of recall of falls in the elderly. J Am Geriatr Soc 1988;36:613–616.
14. McIntosh SJ, Lawson J, Kenny RA. Clinical characteristics of vasodepressor, cardioinhibitory, and mixed carotid sinus syndrome in the elderly. Am J Med 1993;95:203–208.
15. Shaw FE, Kenny RA. The overlap between syncope and falls in the elderly. Postgrad Med J 1997;73: 635–639.
16. Kenny RA, Traynor G. Carotid sinus syndrome—clinical characteristics in elderly patients. Age Ageing 1991;20:449–454.
17. Dimant J. Accidents in the skilled nursing facility. NY State J Med 1985;85:202–205.
18. Sattin RW. Falls among older persons: a public health perspective. Ann Rev Public Health 1992;13: 489–508.
19. Tinetti ME, Speechley M. Prevention of falls among the elderly. N Engl J Med 1989;320:1055–1059.
20. O'Loughlin JL, Robitaille Y, Boivin JF, Suissa S. Incidence of and risk factors for falls and injurious falls among the community-dwelling elderly. Am J Epidemiol 1993;137:342–354.
21. Kane R, Ouslander J, Abrass I. Essentials of Clinical Geriatrics. McGraw Hill, New York, 1989.
22. Wald ML. Accidental deaths on the rise as the population ages fast. New York Times 26, April 2000, p. A19.
23. Rhymes J, Jaeger R. Falls. Prevention and management in the institutional setting. Clin Geriatr Med 1988;4:613–622.
24. Dey AB, Stout NR, Kenny RA. Cardiovascular syncope is the most common cause of drop attacks in the elderly. Pacing Clin Electrophysiol 1997;20:818–819.
25. Richardson DA, Bexton RS, Shaw FE, Kenny RA. Prevalence of cardioinhibitory carotid sinus hypersensitivity in patients 50 years or over presenting to the accident and emergency department with "unexplained" or "recurrent" falls. Pacing Clin Electrophysiol 1997;20:820–823.
26. Kenny RA, Richardson DA, Steen N, Bexton RS, Shaw FE, Bond J. Carotid sinus syndrome: a modifiable risk factor for nonaccidental falls in older adults (SAFE PACE). J Am Coll Cardiol 2001;38: 1491–1496.
27. Scheinberg P, Blackburn I, Rich M. Effects of aging on cerebral circulation and metabolis. Arch Neurol Psychol 1953;70:70–85.
28. Shimada K, Kitazumi T, Ogura H, Sadakane N, Ozawa T. Differences in age-independent effects of blood pressure on baroreflex sensitivity between normal and hypertensive subjects. Clin Sci (Colch) 1986;70:489–494.
29. Epstein M, Hollenberg NK. Age as a determinant of renal sodium conservation in normal man. J Lab Clin Med 1976;87:411–417.
30. Crane MG, Harris JJ. Effect of aging on renin activity and aldosterone excretion. J Lab Clin Med 1976; 87:947–959.
31. Haller BG, Zust H, Shaw S, Gnadinger MP, Uehlinger DE, Weidmann P. Effects of posture and ageing on circulating atrial natriuretic peptide levels in man. J Hypertens 1987;5:551–556.
32. Phillips PA, Rolls BJ, Ledingham JG, Forsling ML, Morton JJ, Crowe MJ, et al. Reduced thirst after water deprivation in healthy elderly men. N Engl J Med 1984;311:753–759.
33. Schulman SP, Lakatta EG, Fleg JL, Lakatta L, Becker LC, Gerstenblith G. Age-related decline in left ventricular filling at rest and exercise. Am J Physiol 1992;263:H1932–H1938.
34. Lipsitz LA, Fullerton KJ. Post-prandial blood pressure reduction in healthy elderly. J Am Geriatr Soc 1986;34:267–270.
35. Vaitkevicius PV, Esserwein DM, Maynard AK, O'Connor FC, Fleg JL. Frequency and importance of post-prandial blood pressure reduction in elderly nursing-home patients. Ann Intern Med 1991;115: 865–870.
36. Lipsitz LA, Nyquist RP, Wei JY, Rowe JW. Post-prandial reduction in blood pressure in the elderly. N Engl J Med 1983;309:81–83.
37. Almquist A, Gornick C, Benson WJ, Dunnigan A, Benditt DG. Carotid sinus hypersensitivity: evaluation of the vasodepressor component. Circulation 1985;71:927–936.

38. Benditt DG, Sutton R, Gammage MD, Markowitz T, Gorski J, Nygaard GA, et al. Clinical experience with Thera DR rate-drop response pacing algorithm in carotid sinus syndrome and vasovagal syncope. The International Rate-Drop Investigators Group. Pacing Clin Electrophysiol 1997;20:832–839.

39. Crilley JG, Herd B, Khurana CS, Appleby CA, de Belder MA, Davies A, et al. Permanent cardiac pacing in elderly patients with recurrent falls, dizziness and syncope, and a hypersensitive cardioinhibitory reflex. Postgrad Med J 1997;73:415–418.

40. Connolly SJ, Sheldon R, Roberts RS, Gent M. The North American Vasovagal Pacemaker Study (VPS). A randomized trial of permanent cardiac pacing for the prevention of vasovagal syncope. J Am Coll Cardiol 1999;33:16–20.

41. Kulbertus HE, De Leval-Rutten F, Demoulin JC. Sino-atrial disease: a report on 13 cases. J Electrocardiol 1973;6:303–312.

42. Radford DJ, Julian DG. Sick sinus syndrome: experience of a cardiac pacemaker clinic. Br Med J 1974; 3:504–507.

43. Rubenstein JJ, Schulman CL, Yurchak PM, DeSanctis RW. Clinical spectrum of the sick sinus syndrome. Circulation 1972;46:5–13.

44. Benditt DG, Gornick CC, Dunbar D, Almquist A, Pool-Schneider S. Indications for electrophysiologic testing in the diagnosis and assessment of sinus node dysfunction. Circulation 1987;75:III93–III102.

45. Reiffel JA, Ferrick K, Zimmerman J, Bigger JTJ. Electrophysiologic studies of the sinus node and atria. Cardiovasc Clin 1985;16:37–59.

46. Fujimura O, Yee R, Klein GJ, Sharma AD, Boahene KA. The diagnostic sensitivity of electrophysiologic testing in patients with syncope caused by transient bradycardia. N Engl J Med 1989;321:1703–1707.

47. Brignole M, Menozzi C, Bottoni N, Gianfranchi L, Lolli G, Oddone D, et al. Mechanisms of syncope caused by transient bradycardia and the diagnostic value of electrophysiologic testing and cardiovascular reflexivity maneuvers. Am J Cardiol 1995;76:273–278.

48. Burnett D, Abi-Samra F, Vacek JL. Use of intravenous adenosine as a noninvasive diagnostic test for sick sinus syndrome. Am Heart J 1999;137:435–438.

49. Brignole M, Menozzi C, Alboni P, Oddone D, Gianfranchi L, Gaggioli G, et al. The effect of exogenous adenosine in patients with neurally-mediated syncope and sick sinus syndrome. Pacing Clin Electrophysiol 1994;17:2211–2216.

50. Scheinman MM, Peters RW, Suave MJ, Desai J, Abbott JA, Cogan J, et al. Value of the H-Q interval in patients with bundle branch block and the role of prophylactic permanent pacing. Am J Cardiol 1982; 50:1316–1322.

51. Brignole M, Menozzi C, Moya A, Garcia-Civera R, Mont L, Alvarez M, et al. Mechanism of syncope in patients with bundle branch block and negative electrophysiologic test. Circulation 2001;104:2045–2050.

52. Low PA, Gilden JL, Freeman R, Sheng KN, McElligott MA. Efficacy of midodrine vs placebo in neurogenic orthostatic hypotension. A randomized, double-blind multicenter study. Midodrine Study Group. JAMA 1997;277:1046–1051.

53. Hussain RM, McIntosh SJ, Lawson J, Kenny RA. Fludrocortisone in the treatment of hypotensive disorders in the elderly. Heart 1996;76:507–509.

54. Grubb BP, Karas B. Clinical disorders of the autonomic nervous system associated with orthostatic intolerance: an overview of classification, clinical evaluation, and management. Pacing Clin Electrophysiol 1999;22:798–810.

55. Engel GL. Psychologic stress, vasodepressor (vasovagal) syncope, and sudden death. Ann Intern Med 1978;89:403–412.

56. Bloomfield D, Maurer M, Bigger JTJ. Effects of age on outcome of tilt-table testing. Am J Cardiol 1999; 83:1055–1058.

57. Moya A, Brignole M, Menozzi C, Garcia-Civera R, Tognarini S, Mont L, et al. Mechanism of syncope in patients with isolated syncope and in patients with tilt-positive syncope. Circulation 2001;104: 1261–1267.

58. Mosqueda-Garcia R, Furlan R, Tank J, Fernandez-Violante R. The elusive pathophysiology of neurally mediated syncope. Circulation 2000;102:2898–2906.

59. Oberg B, Thoren PN. Increased activity in left ventricular receptors during hemorrhage or occlusion of caval veins in the cat—a possible cause of the vaso-vagal reaction. Acta Physiol Scand 1972;85: 164–173.

60. Sutton R, Petersen ME. The clinical spectrum of neurocardiogenic syncope. J Cardiovasc Electrophysiol 1995;6:569–576.

61. Fitzpatrick AP, Banner NB, Cheng A, Yacoub M, Sutton R. Vasovagal reactions may occur after orthotopic heart transplantation. J Am Coll Cardiol 1993;21:1132–1137.

62. Morgan-Hughes NJ, Dark JH, McComb JM, Kenny RA. Vasovagal reactions after heart transplantation. J Am Coll Cardiol 1993;22:2058.

63. Rudas L, Pflugfelder PW, Kostuk WJ. Vasodepressor syncope in a cardiac transplant recipient: a case of vagal re-innervation. Can J Cardiol 1992;8:403–405.

64. Mosqueda-Garcia R, Fernandez-Violante R, Tank J, Snell M, Cunningham G, Furlan R. Yohimbine in neurally mediated syncope. Pathophysiologic implications. J Clin Invest 1998;102:1824–1830.

65. Manyari DE, Rose S, Tyberg JV, Sheldon RS. Abnormal reflex venous function in patients with neuromediated syncope. J Am Coll Cardiol 1996;27:1730–1735.

66. Grubb BP. Pathophysiology and differential diagnosis of neurocardiogenic syncope. Am J Cardiol 1999; 84:3Q–9Q.

67. Benditt DG. Neurally mediated syncopal syndromes: pathophysiologic concepts and clinical evaluation. Pacing Clin Electrophysiol 1997;20:572–584.

68. Sutton R, Petersen ME. The economics of treating vasovagal syncope. Pacing Clin Electrophysiol 1997; 20:849–850.

69. Fitzpatrick AP, Theodorakis G, Vardas P, Sutton R. Methodology of head-up tilt testing in patients with unexplained syncope. J Am Coll Cardiol 1991;17:125–130.

70. Streeten DHP, Anderson GH. Delayed orthostatic intolerance. Arch Intern Med 1992;152:1066–1072.

71. Calkins H. Pharmacologic approaches to therapy for vasovagal syncope. Am J Cardiol 1999;84:20Q–25Q.

72. Bloomfield DM. Strategy for the management of vasovagal syncope. Drugs Aging 2002;19:179–202.

73. Hussain RM, McIntosh SJ, Lawson J, Kenny RA. Fludrocortisone in the treatment of hypotensive disorders in the elderly. Heart 1996;76:507–509.

74. Grubb BP, Samoil D, Kosinski D, Wolfe D, Lorton M, Madu E. Fluoxetine hydrochloride for the treatment of severe refractory orthostatic hypotension. Am J Med 1994;97:366–368.

75. Maurer MS, Alabre M, Stetson P, Bloomfield DM. Carotid sinus hypersensitivity and falls in the elderly: a renewed interest in an "old" disease. CVR&R 2000;21:669–678.

76. Dey AB, Kenny RA. Drop attacks in the elderly revisited. Q J Med 1997;90:1–3.

77. Murphy AL, Rowbotham BJ, Boyle RS, Thew CM, Fardoulys JA, Wilson K. Carotid sinus hypersensitivity in elderly nursing home patients. Aust NZ J Med 1986;16:24–27.

78. Ward CR, McIntosh S, Kenny RA. Carotid sinus hypersensitivity—a modifiable risk factor for fractured neck of femur. Age Ageing 1999;28:127–133.

79. McIntosh SJ, Lawson J, Kenny RA. Heart rate and blood pressure responses to carotid sinus massage in healthy elderly subjects. Age Ageing 1994;23:57–61.

80. Morillo CA, Camacho ME, Wood MA, Gilligan DM, Ellenbogen KA. Diagnostic utility of mechanical, pharmacological and orthostatic stimulation of the carotid sinus in patients with unexplained syncope. J Am Coll Cardiol 1999;34:1587–1594.

81. Davies AJ, Kenny RA. Frequency of neurologic complications following carotid sinus massage. Am J Cardiol 1998;81:1256–1257.

82. Schweitzer P, Teichholz LE. Carotid sinus massage. Its diagnostic and therapeutic value in arrhythmias. Am J Med 1985;78:645–654.

83. O'Mahony D. Pathophysiology of carotid sinus hypersensitivity in elderly patients. Lancet 1995;346: 950–952.

84. Brignole M, Menozzi C, Lolli G, Bottoni N, Gaggioli G. Long-term outcome of paced and nonpaced patients with severe carotid sinus syndrome. Am J Cardiol 1992;69:1039–1043.

85. Brignole M, Menozzi C, Lolli G, Sartore B, Barra M. Natural and unnatural history of patients with severe carotid sinus hypersensitivity: a preliminary study. Pacing Clin Electrophysiol 1988;11:1628–1635.

86. Bexton RS, Davies A, Kenny RA. The rate-drop response in carotid sinus syndrome: the Newcastle experience. Pacing Clin Electrophysiol 1997;20:840.

87. Grubb BP, Samoil D, Kosinski D, Temesy-Armos P, Akpunonu B. The use of serotonin reuptake inhibitors for the treatment of recurrent syncope due to carotid sinus hypersensitivity unresponsive to dual chamber cardiac pacing. Pacing Clin Electrophysiol 1994;17:1434–1436.

88. Dan D, Grubb BP, Mouhaffel AH, Kosinski DJ. Use of serotonin re-uptake inhibitors as primary therapy for carotid sinus hypersensitivity. Pacing Clin Electrophysiol 1997;20:1633–1635.

89. Schellack J, Fulenwider JT, Olson RA, Smith RB, Mansour K. The carotid sinus syndrome: a frequently overlooked cause of syncope in the elderly. J Vasc Surg 1986;4:376–383.

90. Fachinetti P, Bellocchi S, Dorizzi A, Forgione FN. Carotid sinus syndrome: a review of the literature and our experience using carotid sinus denervation. J Neurosurg Sci 1998;42:189–193.

91. Anderson KP, Mason JW. Clinical value of cardiac electrophyiology studies. In: Zipes DP, Jalife J, eds. Cardiac Electrophysiology: From Cell to Bedside, 2nd ed. WB Saunders, Philadelphia, PA, 1995, pp. 1133–1150.

92. Knight BP, Goyal R, Pelosi F, Flemming M, Horwood L, Morady F, et al. Outcome of patients with nonischemic dilated cardiomyopathy and unexplained syncope treated with an implantable defibrillator. J Am Coll Cardiol 1999;33:1964–1970.

93. Buxton AE, Lee KL, Fisher JD, Josephson ME, Prystowsky EN, Hafley G. A randomized study of the prevention of sudden death in patients with coronary artery disease. N Engl J Med 1999;341:1882–1890.

94. Pastore JM, Girouard SD, Laurita KR, Akar FG, Rosenbaum DS. Mechanism linking T-wave alternans to the genesis of cardiac fibrillation. Circulation 1999;99:1385–1394.

95. Gold MR, Bloomfield DM, Anderson KP, El-Sherif NE, Wilber DJ, Groh WJ, et al. A comparison of T-wave alternans, signal averaged electrocardiography and programmed ventricular stimulation for arrhythmia risk stratification. J Am Coll Cardiol 2000;36:2247–2253.

96. Bloomfield DM, Gold MR, Anderson KP, Wilber DJ, El-Sherif N, Estes NA, et al. T Wave alternans predicts events in patients with syncope undergoing electrophysiology testing. Circulation 1999;100: I-508 (abstract).

97. Bloomfield DM, Gold MR, Anderson KP, Wilber DJ, El-Sherif N, Estes NA, et al. T Wave alternans predicts events independent of ejection fraction and etiology of heart disease in patients undergoing electrophysiologic testing for known or suspected ventricular arrhythmias. PACE 2000;23:593 (abstract).

98. Steinberg JS, Prystowsky E, Freedman RA, Moreno F, Katz R, Kron J, et al. Use of the signal-averaged electrocardiogram for predicting inducible ventricular tachycardia in patients with unexplained syncope: relation to clinical variables in a multivariate analysis. J Am Coll Cardiol 1994;23:99–106.

99. Mark AL, Kioschos JM, Abboud FM, Heistad DD, Schmid PG. Abnormal vascular responses to exercise in patients with aortic stenosis. J Clin Invest 1973;52:1138–1146.

100. Zaidi A, Clough P, Cooper P, Scheepers B, Fitzpatrick AP. Misdiagnosis of epilepsy: many seizure-like attacks have a cardiovascular cause. J Am Coll Cardiol 2000;36(1):181–184.

101. Davis TL, Freemon FR. Electroencephalography should not be routine in the evaluation of syncope in adults. Arch Intern Med 1990;150:2027–2029.

102. Linzer M, Yang EH, Estes NA, Wang P, Vorperian VR, Kapoor WN. Diagnosing syncope. Part 2: Unexplained syncope. Clinical Efficacy Assessment Project of the American College of Physicians. Ann Intern Med 1997;127:76–86.

103. Pires LA, Ganji JR, Jarandila R, Steele R. Diagnostic patterns and temporal trends in the evaluation of adult patients hospitalized with syncope. Arch Intern Med 2001;161:1889–1895.

104. Stetson P, Maurer M, Green R, Quint E, Bloomfield DM. Current diagnostic testing patterns in syncope. PACE 1999;22:782 (abstract).

105. Kenny RA, Krahn AD. Implantable loop recorder: evaluation of unexplained syncope. Heart 1999;81: 431–433.

106. Krahn AD, Klein GJ, Yee R, Skanes AC. Randomized assessment of syncope trial: conventional diagnostic testing versus a prolonged monitoring strategy. Circulation 2001;104:46–51.

107. Krahn AD, Klein GJ, Fitzpatrick AP, Zaidi A, Skanes A, Yee R, et al. Predicting the outcome of patients with unexplained syncope undergoing prolonged monitoring. Pacing Clin Electrophysiol 2002;25: 37–41.

108. Krahn AD, Klein GJ, Yee R, Norris C. Final results from a pilot study with an implantable loop recorder to determine the etiology of syncope in patients with negative noninvasive and invasive testing. Am J Cardiol 1998;82:117–119.

109. Benditt DG, Ferguson DW, Grubb BP, Kapoor WN, Kugler J, Lerman BB, et al. Tilt table testing for assessing syncope. American College of Cardiology. J Am Coll Cardiol 1996;28:263–275.

110. Petersen ME, Williams TR, Gordon C, Chamberlain-Webber R, Sutton R. The normal response to prolonged passive head-up tilt testing. Heart 2000;84:509–514.

111. Kapoor WN, Brant N. Evaluation of syncope by upright tilt testing with isoproterenol: a non-specific test. Ann Intern Med 1992;116:358–363.

112. Natale A, Akhtar M, Jazayeri MR, Dhala A, Blanck Z, Deshpande S, et al. Provocation of hypotension during head-up tilt testing in subjects with no history of syncope or presyncope. Circulation 1995;92: 54–58.

113. Mussi C, Tolve I, Foroni M, Valli A, Ascari S, Salvioli G. Specificity and total positive rate of head-up tilt testing potentiated with sublingual nitroglycerin in older patients with unexplained syncope. Aging (Milano) 2001;13:105–111.

114. Natale A, Sra J, Akhtar M, Kusmirek L, Tomassoni G, Leonelli F, et al. Use of sublingual nitroglycerin during head-up tilt-table testing in patients >60 years of age. Am J Cardiol 1998;82:1210–1213.

115. Parry SW, Richardson DA, O'Shea D, Sen B, Kenny RA. Diagnosis of carotid sinus hypersensitivity in older adults: carotid sinus massage in the upright position is essential. Heart 2000;83:22–23.

116. Kapoor WN. Syncope. N Engl J Med 2000;343:1856–1862.

117. Harris T, Kleinman J, Lipsitz LA, Cornoni-Huntley J, Garrison R. Is age or level of systolic blood pressure related to positional blood pressure change? Gerontologist 1986;26:59A.

118. Davidson E, Fuchs J, Rotenberg Z, Weinberger I, Agmon J. Drug-related syncope. Clin Cardiol 1989; 12:577–580.

119. Di Girolamo E, Di Iorio C, Sabatini P, Leonzio L, Barbone C, Barsotti A. Effects of paroxetine hydrochloride, a selective serotonin reuptake inhibitor, on refractory vasovagal syncope: a randomized, double-blind, placebo-controlled study. J Am Coll Cardiol 1999;33:1227–1230.

13   Ischemic Heart Disease

Susan J. Zieman, MD, Steven P. Schulman, MD, and Jerome L. Fleg, MD

CHARACTERISTICS OF ISCHEMIC HEART DISEASE IN THE ELDERLY

Of all of the known risk factors for coronary artery disease, age remains the most potent. Yet, the specific processes that accompany increasing age and that render it such an important risk factor for cardiovascular disease are not clearly elucidated. Age-associated changes in cardiovascular structure and physiologic function alter the substrate on which disease is superimposed. (*See* Chapter 9 for a discussion on age-related cardiovascular changes) These alterations include increased central arterial stiffness, decreased responsiveness to β-adrenergic stimulation, delayed early left-ventricular diastolic filling, and endothelial dysfunction *(1–3)*. Such changes impact the presentation, diagnosis, clinical manifestations, therapeutic management, and prognosis of cardiovascular disease. Although it is thought that these changes occur universally, the rate at which they change is highly variable. The resultant heterogeneity of the aging process adds further challenge to the clinical care of older patients because no clear markers exist to discern biologic from chronologic age.

In addition to the increased morbidity and mortality of ischemic heart disease (IHD) in the elderly, both the prevalence and the incidence of cardiovascular disease increase with age *(4–6)*. Autopsy studies have demonstrated an increase in the prevalence of obstructive IHD from approx 10–20% in the fourth decade to 50–70% in the eighth decade and beyond *(7,8)*. Nearly half of all deaths in Americans older than 65 yr are the result of IHD. Recent estimates demonstrate approx 500,000 coronary artery bypass graft (CABG) operations are performed annually in North America, more than 30% of which involve patients older than 70 yr old *(9)*. Better understanding and promotion of coronary risk-factor reduction as well as improvements in diagnosis and treatment of acute coronary events in younger

From: *Aging, Heart Disease, and Its Management: Facts and Controversies*
Edited by: N. Edwards, M. Maurer, and R. Wellner © Humana Press Inc., Totowa, NJ

Table 1
Percentage of Initial Uncomplicated MI Patients
with Various Cardiac Risk Factors Stratified by Age Group

	Age (yr)			
	≤49 (n = 14,753)	50–59 (n = 16,799)	60–69 (n = 15,379)	≥70 (n = 14,301)
Gender (male)	83.6	77.8	68.7	53.7
Diabetes mellitus	11.7	16.9	20.5	20.4
Systemic hypertension	32.1	39.5	46.0	50.8
Cigarette smoking	68.1	54.8	35.3	15.9
Hypercholesterolemia	31.5	32.3	30.5	22.2
Family history of myocardial infarction	49.5	43.1	35.4	24.6

Source: Data from the Second National Registry of Myocardial Infarction (adapted from ref. 13).

patients contribute to the increasing prevalence of ischemic heart disease in the older population.

In addition to the increased prevalence of IHD with age noted earlier, the severity of IHD also increases in the elderly. The Duke University Data Bank and Coronary Artery Surgery Study (CASS) Registry demonstrated that triple-vessel and left main IHD more than doubled in prevalence between ages 40 and 80 yr in both sexes (10,11). Older CASS patients also had greater left-ventricular end-diastolic pressures and more prevalent wall-motion abnormalities and congestive heart failure signs. This greater severity of IHD in the elderly probably accounts in large part for their greater morbidity and mortality from acute coronary syndromes. Furthermore, the higher IHD prevalence and severity in the elderly influences the interpretation of most diagnostic modalities, because more extensive disease is easier to detect. For example, the sensitivity of >1 mm ischemic ST-segment depression during treadmill exercise in detecting IHD rose from 56% in patients younger than 40 yr to 84% in those >60 yr old (12). Conversely, a modest reduction in the specificity of the exercise ECG from 84% to 70% was observed between these ages.

The coronary-risk-factor profile changes strikingly with age. The risk-factor profile of 61,232 patients suffering an uncomplicated initial acute myocardial infarction (AMI) is shown as a function of age in Table 1 (13). Compared to the subset ≤49 yr old, the subset ≥70 yr demonstrated nearly three times as many women and nearly double the prevalence of diabetes and hypertension but only one-quarter as many smokers, half as many with a positive family history for IHD, and two-thirds as many with hypercholesterolemia as the younger group. Nevertheless, the existing data suggest similar benefit from treating the modifiable IHD risk factors in older and younger patients. Moreover, newly recognized variables in older individuals can serve as unique markers for cardiovascular disease, including pulse pressure, serum homocysteine levels, and atrial fibrillation (14–18).

DIAGNOSTIC CONSIDERATIONS IN THE ELDERLY
Angina Pectoris

Whereas the diagnosis of angina pectoris and AMI is typically straightforward in younger patients, the elderly often present multiple diagnostic hurdles. For example, the low level of physical activity engaged in by many older patients because of arthritic or other noncardiac conditions may be insufficient to precipitate exertional angina. Similarly, a decrease in activity as a result of an arthritic flare or respiratory disorder may cause anginal symptoms to disappear. Problems with recall in the elderly present another diagnostic challenge. In a longitudinal survey of 252 older adults, nearly half of those who reported positive anginal histories on the initial survey denied such symptoms on a second survey 5 yr later; none who gave positive responses for infarction on the first survey did so 5 yr later *(19)*. An age-associated reduction in general pain sensitivity may further contribute to a lesser reporting of chest pain during myocardial ischemia or infarction in the elderly. However, support for this concept is limited; in several large series of IHD patients, the mean age of those with only silent episodes of ischemia was similar to that in patients experiencing angina pectoris.

Several noncardiac and non-IHD cardiac disorders can confound the diagnosis of IHD induced chest pain in the elderly. Esophageal and musculoskeletal disorders are common in this age group. Esophageal reflux and motility disturbances may mimic angina. Exacerbation by supine posture and relief with antacids are helpful distinguishing features. Calcific aortic valvular stenosis, seen almost exclusively in older adults, often presents as angina pectoris. Because IHD often co-exists with aortic stenosis, coronary angiography is often necessary to determine the source of anginal pain. Angina may be observed in aortic regurgitation, even in the absence of significant valvular stenosis. Patients with hypertrophic cardiomyopathy frequently experience exertional chest pain.

It is often stated that dyspnea as an anginal equivalent is more common in older than younger IHD patients. The age-associated increase in left-ventricular diastolic dysfunction provides a theoretical basis for such a finding. Higher end-diastolic pressures, as found in older IHD patients in the CASS Registry *(11)*, could manifest as dyspnea when transmitted retrograde to the pulmonary capillaries. This mechanism probably accounts for the higher incidence of dyspnea as the presenting symptom in older vs younger patients with AMI.

Acute Myocardial Infarction

The clinical features and prognosis associated with AMI in the elderly warrant special consideration. In several series of elderly patients, the prevalence of chest pain as the dominant symptom during AMI was particularly low *(20–22)*. For example, Pathy reported chest pain in only 19% of patients aged >65 yr, whereas dyspnea was the cardinal manifestation in 20% and neurological symptoms in 33% *(20)*. Such frequent atypical presentations may account, in part, for the longer prehospital delay in older AMI patients *(23)*.

Acute MI in the elderly is more likely to be non-Q-wave, in contrast to younger patients *(6,23,24)*. Although such non-Q-wave AMIs are generally smaller and less likely to result in major complications or death than are Q-wave infarctions, the overall morbidity and mortality from AMI in the elderly markedly exceed those in younger patients. For example, in a large German registry, mortality for patients who received reperfusion therapy increased from 6% in those younger than 65 yr to 29.4% in those ≥85 yr. Corresponding numbers in patients not receiving reperfusion interventions were 9.7% and 38.5%, respectively *(25)*.

Despite having smaller infarct sizes than younger patients *(26)*, the elderly have higher frequency of congestive heart failure, atrial fibrillation, conduction disturbances, stroke, and mechanical complications such as septal or free-wall rupture *(25–27)*. Similar findings have been reported for non-Q-wave AMI *(28)*. Furthermore, the subsequent mortality in the 1–4 yr postinfarction is also strikingly higher in the elderly than in the younger individuals after both Q- and non-Q-wave infarction *(26,28)*. In addition to increased late mortality in older patients, increased age is also a significant risk factor for re-infarction *(29)*. Such findings increase the importance of risk stratification in older infarct patients. Therefore, it is paradoxical that the utilization of several therapeutic interventions proven to reduce morbidity and mortality post-AMI, including converting enzyme inhibitors, β-blockers, and antiplatelet drugs, is lower in elderly than younger patients *(30)*. Rates of cardiac catheterization and coronary revascularization procedures are also inversely related to patient age *(13)*. The risk–benefit ratio of these important medical and invasive strategies must be carefully weighed.

MANAGEMENT CONSIDERATIONS OF IHD IN THE ELDERLY

Many unique aspects of older individuals add further challenges to the management of ischemic heart disease in the elderly. In addition to age-associated changes in the cardiovascular substrate, the presentation, diagnosis, and management is often affected by comorbidities. Both disease processes and age-related changes in other organ systems may influence therapeutic choices. Clinical decision making must also reflect an understanding of the altered drug metabolism of older individuals and the potential for pharmacological interactions *(31)*. Many of the therapeutic options do come with an increased risk of complications in the elderly. Finally, those issues that may be paramount to older patients, such as independence, functional and caregiver status, cognitive function, and financial concerns, are often overlooked in the therapeutic decision-making process.

STANDARDS OF CARE

The heterogeneity of the aging process is the Achilles' heel of inclusion of older subjects in large-scale clinical trials. These studies seek a relatively homogeneous population in order to reduce confounding factors and, therefore, commonly exclude potential subjects with comorbidities (disease-related or impaired renal/hepatic/ hematological function) and those on a multitude of drugs. Moreover, the elderly are often not invited to participate in therapeutic or interventional clinical trials because of a concern over the ability to make follow-up visits, to comply with protocols, or to provide informed consent. The result is a paucity of evidence-based data upon which to support clinical decisions in this important segment of the population. Ethical considerations may also limit future prospective trials in the elderly on cardiovascular drugs that are currently considered the "standard of care" based on findings in younger populations. Thus, most clinical decisions in the elderly are based on anecdotal evidence, extrapolations from trials involving younger subjects, or observational and Medicare beneficiary databases, all of which have limitations. The following subsections review evidence-based support of specific recommendations for older individuals with ischemic heart disease. These recommendations are based on clinical trials and observational databases, where applicable; areas where future research is sought are highlighted.

Efficacy of Drug Treatment in the Elderly

ASPIRIN

Evidence for the benefit of aspirin in older patients during and after acute myocardial infarction was demonstrated in ISIS-2, a prospective trial that reported a 22.3% reduction in 5 wk mortality in 3411 myocardial infarction patients over 70 yr old *(32)*. In this trial,

Table 2
Clinical Trials Evaluating the Use of β-Adrenergic Receptor Blockers After AMI by Age Group

Trial	β-Blocker	Age (yr)	Patients (n)	% Mortality reduction	p-Value	Ref.
BHAT	Propanolol	<60	2589	19	NS[a]	44
		60–69	1248	33	0.01	
Göteburg	Metoprolol	<64	917	21	NS	38
		64–74	478	45	0.03	
Norwegian (33 mo)	Timolol	<65	732	31	0.01	42
		65–74	1152	43	0.05	
Norwegian (72 mo)		65–74	1634 (total)	13	NS	43
				19	0.02	
ISIS-1	Atenolol	<65	10,805	4	NS	39
		≥65	5222	23	0.001	

[a]NS, not significant.

the aspirin dose of 160 mg/d was not associated with an increase in cerebrovascular bleeding in older patients. Further support for the use of aspirin in the elderly as secondary prevention for future cardiovascular events is primarily based on meta-analyses of prospective trials and observational studies, as the number of older subjects enrolled in many large randomized prospective clinical trials is limited. The Antiplatelet Trialists' Collaboration reported a 25% reduction in the odds ratio of recurrent myocardial infarction, stroke, or cardiovascular death in older patients who experienced a myocardial infarction (70%) or unstable angina pectoris (30%) (33).

In the Cooperative Cardiovascular Project, which reviewed the care of over 10,000 myocardial infarction patients over age 65 yr, aspirin use was associated with a 22% reduction in 30 d mortality (34). Despite the evidence that aspirin is associated with a significant reduction in mortality and future myocardial events, Krumholz and colleagues found that only 64–76% of Medicare beneficiaries with no contraindication to its use were prescribed aspirin after an AMI (35,36). Reluctance to prescribe aspirin in older patients may be because of the fear of aspirin-associated gastritis. However, Moore et al. reported that age was not associated with an increased incidence of gastritis with aspirin use (37).

β-Blockers

Among the recommendations of therapies for older patients following myocardial infarction, perhaps the strongest level of evidence exists for the use of β-blockers in this population (see Table 2). In the acute setting of a myocardial infarction, a 23–45% reduction in mortality was associated with the use of intravenous β-blockade in patients over 65 yr (38,39). A significant reduction in mortality and future cardiovascular events is also seen with long-term use of β-blockers in older patients in several large-scale randomized clinical trials (38,40–43). In fact, in the β-Blocker Heart Attack Trial and the Göteborg Metoprolol Trial, the significance of the mortality reduction after a myocardial infarction was driven exclusively by the mortality benefit of those over age 60 and 65 yr, respectively (44). Despite the consistent nature of the findings that β-blocker use reduces mortality and secondary cardiovascular events in the elderly, a startlingly low percentage of older patients without contraindications are prescribed this important medicine following a cardiac event. In one study of over 200,000 Medicare beneficiaries in the Cooperative Cardiovascular Project, only 34% of patients were prescribed β-blockers on hospital discharge following a heart attack *(45)*. In this observational database analysis, a 40% reduction in overall 2 yr mortality was associated with β-blocker use; the same magnitude of mortality benefit was also seen in those older patients following non-Q-wave myocardial infarction and in those with chronic obstructive pulmonary disease (COPD). In another observational study of New Jersey Medicare patients, β-blocker use following myocardial infarction (although only prescribed to 21% of eligible patients) was associated with a 43% reduction in mortality in all age strata (65–74, 75–84, and ≥85 yr) as well as a 22% reduction in hospital readmission *(46)*. Interestingly, in this review, physicians were three times more likely to prescribe a calcium channel blocker than a β-blocker following a heart attack, although the former was associated with a twofold risk of death compared with β-blocker use.

Reluctance to prescribe β-blockers in the elderly is likely multifaceted. Because of their proclivity to cause bronchospasm, β-blockers are often withheld cardiac patients with COPD or asthma. Chen and colleagues report a similar survival benefit of β-blocker use following myocardial infarction in those elderly patients with mild COPD/asthma not requiring β-agonists as those without pulmonary disease *(47)*. Another deterrent to β-blocker use in the elderly is their potential cognitive effects. However, the concern over cognitive and mood changes with β-blockers in older patients has not been substantiated in prospective trials or registry-type database analyses *(48–50)*. Regardless of these concerns, β-blockers have been shown to reduce morbidity and mortality and to be cost-effective in the elderly *(51)*.

ACE INHIBITORS

The decision to use angiotensin converting-enzyme-inhibitors (ACEi) in elderly populations following myocardial infarction is stratified based on the degree of left-ventricular function. Similar to the mortality benefit seen with β-blockers after myocardial infarction, the reduction in mortality associated with the postinfarction use of ACEi has been demonstrated in older patients in several large-scale clinical trials (*see* Table 3). In the Survival and Ventricular Enlargement (SAVE) Trial, which examined the benefit of captopril (50 mg tid) initiated on d 3–16 following a heart attack in those patients with a left-ventricular ejection fraction of less that 40%, a significant reduction in mortality, congestive heart failure, and re-infarction were associated with ACEi use *(52)*. Interestingly, in this trial, captopril was associated with a 23% reduction in death in patients over 65 yr, but only a 9% mortality reduction in those younger than 65 yr. Compared with placebo, a long-term mortality reduction was also seen in elderly myocardial infarction patients with left-ventricular dysfunction taking the ACEi trandolapril *(53)*. Specifically, trandolapril was associated with a 17% risk reduction of death in patients over age 65. Similarly, in the Acute Infarction Ramipril Efficacy study, which compared ramipril to placebo in postinfarction patients with congestive heart failure, a 26% reduction in 15 mo mortality was shown; the survival benefit was larger in those over 65 yr compared with younger patients *(54)*. This degree of mortality reduction with ACEi was also seen in a retrospective observational study of Medicare beneficiaries who had experienced a heart attack and who had reduced left-ventricular function *(35)*. More recently, a meta-analysis of 100,000 postinfarction patients in four placebo-controlled clinical trials evaluating the efficacy of ACEi in reducing mortality demonstrated an 11% mortality reduction in patients aged 65–74 yr (30% of subjects). No significant reduction in 30 d death rates was seen in postinfarction patients over 75 yr taking ACEi. This meta-analysis did demonstrate a small but statistically significant interaction between age and

Table 3
Clinical Trials Evaluating the Use of ACEi
After AMI with Reduced Left-Ventricular Function by Age Group

Trial	ACEi	Age (yr)	Patients (n)	% Mortality reduction	p-Value	Ref.
SAVE	Captopril	<65	1448	9	NS[a]	52
		≥65	783	23	0.02	
AIRE	Ramipril	<65		2	NS	54
		≥65		39	<0.05	
TRACE	Trandolapril	<65	627	17	<0.05	53
		≥65	1122	38	<0.01	
ISIS-IV	Captopril	<60	23,405	17	NS	55
		60–69	18,607	14	<0.05	
		≥70	16,000	0	NS	

[a]NS, not significant.

hypotension and age and renal dysfunction with intravenous ACEi use. In elderly post-infarction patients with reduced left-ventricular function (ejection fraction less than 40%), the use of an ACEi and a β-blocker may have an additive effect of reducing mortality (56).

More recent clinical trials suggest the potential benefit of ACEi after myocardial infarction in patients with normal left-ventricular function (57,58). Although not statistically significant, a greater reduction in the composite end point of myocardial infarction, stroke, and death was associated with the ACEi ramipril in patients over 65 compared to younger patients. However, given the increased risk of hypotension and renal dysfunction of these agents in older patients and the lack of support of significant morbidity and mortality benefit in postinfarction patients with preserved left-ventricular function, their routine use in this clinical scenario is not yet supported by the American College of Cardiology (ACC)/American Heart Association (AHA). Therefore, the recommendation of ACEi use for elderly patients after myocardial infarction is limited to those who have congestive heart failure or reduced left-ventricular ejection fraction. Yet, despite the ACC/AHA guidelines for ACEi use following myocardial infarction in patients with a left-ventricular ejection fraction of under 40% (59), only 58% of Medicare recipients without contraindications to ACEi use were prescribed this medication at hospital discharge (35).

MAGNESIUM

Controversy has surrounded the use of magnesium in the management of AMI for years; the recommendation for its use in older heart attack patients is equally unclear. Following the publication of ISIS-4 (55), a randomized, factorial design, clinical trial investigating the efficacy of early intravenous magnesium use in AMI, the ACC/AHA refined their recommendation of magnesium use to those acute infarction patients with documented hypomagnesemia or with ventricular tachycardia, specifically torsades de pointes (59). A recently published review of the Second National Registry of Myocardial Infarction confirmed that magnesium was only used in 5.1% of AMI patients; its use was associated with younger age, percutaneous interventions, heart failure, ventricular arrhythmias, and thrombolytic therapy (60). Although magnesium use in this retrospective study was associated with a 25% increase in mortality, a cause–effect relationship could not be established. Interestingly, there was no increase in mortality associated with magnesium use in those patients receiving thrombolytics. In a recent randomized placebo-controlled clinical trial of coronary angioplasty after AMI, magnesium was not associated with reductions in infarct size, ventricular arrhythmias, heart failure, or mortality *(61)*. Although suppression of ventricular arrhythmias has been the target of intravenous magnesium therapy in AMI, recent data demonstrating that magnesium is associated with improved endothelial function and the inhibition of platelet-dependent thrombosis suggest alternate mechanisms of benefit of this agent in ischemic heart disease *(62–64)*. A randomized trial of acute intravenous magnesium use early after myocardial infarction is ongoing *(65)*.

NITRATES

The role of nitrate therapy in the treatment of AMI is also controversial. In ISIS-4, a randomized, factorial-designed, study, isosorbide-5-mononitrate (60 mg qd) did not reduce overall mortality compared with placebo *(55)*. In this trial, nitrate use was associated with reduced chest pain, but its association with headache and hypotension often led to the discontinuation of the agent. When combined with ACEi therapy, as in GISSI-3, nitrates were associated with a 17% early mortality reduction *(66)*. A similar decrease in mortality with nitrates and ACEi was also demonstrated in elderly patients, a prespecified end-point. The GISSI-3 investigators were unable to demonstrate a mortality benefit of nitrates, independent of their combined effect with ACEi.

In contrast to their equivocal benefit in AMI, the utility of sublingual and long-acting nitrate therapy in angina pectoris is well established. Although no mortality benefit has ever been associated with the use of nitrates in patients with chronic IHD *(67)*, significant reductions in anginal pain, immobility, psychological distress, and improvements in overall quality of life in all age groups are associated with their use *(68)*. The maximal benefit from nitrates is derived when they are used intermittently, so as to avoid tachyphylaxis *(67)*. Thus, nitrates have an important role in the treatment of elderly patients with severe angina, which limits activity and quality-of-life, and for whom revacularization options are limited. Use of nitrates prior to physical exertion in such patients can be highly effective. However, some caution should be exercised with the use of nitrate therapy in the elderly. Because there is an age-associated shift of the ventricular pressure–volume relationship with age, these preload and afterload reducing agents may cause hypotension and falls more readily in older patients compared with younger ones *(69)*. It is also important to recognize the potential for severe hypotension resulting from the interaction of nitrates and the oral phosphodiesterase inhibitor, sildenafil citrate, which is commonly prescribed for erectile dysfunction in older patients.

CALCIUM CHANNELS BLOCKERS

The use of calcium channel blockers after myocardial infarction is generally not advised. Evidence from randomized placebo-controlled clinical trials as well as retrospective studies and meta-analyses suggest that the short-acting dihydropyridine nifedipine is associated with increased mortality when used after heart attacks *(70,71)*. Moreover, the Multicenter Diltiazem Postinfarction Trial (MDPIT), the second Danish Verapamil Infarction Trial (DAVIT-II), and the Calcium Antagonist Reinfarction Italian Study (CRIS), all randomized placebo-controlled trials investigating the effect of nondihydropyridine calcium antagonists after myocardial infarction, failed to show a morbidity or mortality benefit with these agents after myocardial infarction *(72–74)*. Interestingly, a post hoc analysis of only those patients enrolled in MDPIT and DAVIT-II with non-Q-wave myocardial infarctions and no pulmonary congestion did demonstrate a 42% risk reduction in mortality in this subpopulation taking calcium channel blockers compared with placebo *(75)*. Whether or not elderly patients, who experience an increased incidence of non-Q-wave myocardial infarction, may benefit from nondihydropyridine calcium antagonists after myocardial infarction is uncertain *(76,77)*. To date, there is no clear indication for their use in postinfarction patients of any age. Despite this fact, calcium channel blockers are still widely prescribed to elderly infarct patients upon hospital discharge *(76)*. When calcium channel blockers are prescribed for older individuals, care should be taken to monitor for side effects such as peripheral edema, constipation, atrioventricular conduction abnormalities, and urinary retention *(31)*. The newer second-generation calcium channel blockers, such as amlodipine, may play a role in ischemic heart disease in the elderly. In general, these agents are easily tolerated and are associated with improvement in anginal symptoms, exercise tolerance, and left-ventricular relaxation in patients with stable angina pectoris *(78,79)*.

Glycoprotein IIb/IIIa Inhibitors

Intravenous platelet glycoprotein IIb/IIIa receptor antagonists may have a particularly beneficial role in elderly patients with acute coronary syndromes. Because older patients more commonly present with unstable angina and/or non-ST-elevation myocardial infarction and have a higher morbidity and mortality from these events than younger individuals, these agents provide greater relative and absolute benefit in this population *(80)*. Two of these agents, tirofiban and eptifibatide, are associated with a significant reduction in the composite end-point of death, myocardial infarction and recurrent ischemia compared to placebo or heparin *(81–84)* in unstable angina or non-ST-elevation infarction. In the PRISM and PRISM-PLUS studies, both of which investigated the benefit of tirofiban in unstable angina and non-Q-wave myocardial infarction, the most significant reduction in the composite end-point was seen in those patients over age 65 yr *(81,82)*.

In patients with acute coronary syndromes undergoing percutaneous interventions, abciximab and eptifibatide are associated with reduced short- and long-term morbidity and mortality. This association was demonstrated in patients over 65 yr by subgroup analysis *(85–87)*. The benefit of abciximab over placebo in patients over 70 yr with acute coronary syndromes undergoing percutaneous coronary interventions is also supported by a significant reduction of 30 d death or myocardial infarction (odd ratio [OR] = 0.56, 95% confidence interval [CI] = 0.37–0.83) in 7860 patients over age 70 yr pooled from trials investigating the effects of abciximab vs placebo *(88)*. The benefit of this glycoprotein IIb/IIIa inhibitor was not accompanied by an increase in major bleeding events in older patients.

Thrombolytics

The treatment of ST elevation, or new left bundle branch block, AMI with thrombolytic therapy in the elderly has been a topic of heated debate. Many of the first randomized clinical trials, which established the efficacy of these agents, either excluded older patients or did not enroll a sufficient number of elderly patients to draw conclusions about this segment of the population. Therefore, the Fibrinolytic Therapy Trialists' (FTT) Collaborative Group performed a meta-analysis of data pooled from 9 trials (58,600 patients), which demonstrated a significant mortality benefit of thrombolytics (mainly streptokinase in these trials) in patients ages 65–75 yr *(89)*. However, only a 1% absolute 35 d mortality benefit was seen in those over 75 yr with thrombolytics. In fact, the GISSI-2 investigators report a sharp rise in in-hospital mortality with age; 1.9% in those 40 yr old and younger to 31.9% in those over age 80 yr *(90)*. It is important to consider that the FTT meta-analysis was performed on trials that predated the use of tissue plasminogen activator and included patients who presented over 24 h after onset of their initial symptoms. Despite these caveats, the lack of benefit from thrombolytics in patients over 75 yr was recently reproduced using a retrospective analysis of data from the Cardiovascular Cooperative Project *(91)*. In this analysis, Theimann et al. reported a reduction in 30 d mortality with thrombolytic therapy (hazard ratio [HR] = 0.88; 95% CI = 0.69–1.12) in patients aged 65–75 yr. Conversely, but consistent with prior data, a significant increase in 30 d mortality was associated with thrombolytic use in patients aged 76–86 yr (HR = 1.38, $p = 0.003$). The current ACC/AHA Guidelines for the use of thrombolytics for AMI now includes age criteria: class I indication for those under 75 yr and Class IIa indication for those over age 75 yr without other exclusions *(92)*.

Despite the recommendations for the use of thrombolytics in this population based on evidence that they reduce mortality in older patients with AMI, these agents are often avoided in the elderly. Several factors contribute to the lower usage of thrombolytics in the elderly; many are not eligible because of hypertension, history of cerebrovascular accident, bleeding or recent surgery, presentation to medical care longer than 12 h after the onset of symptoms, and a higher incidence of non-ST-elevation myocardial infarctions *(93,94)*. Another legitimate concern that impacts the use of thrombolytics is the increased risk of hemorrhage in older patients. In the GUSTO-1 trial comparing various thrombolytic regimens, tissue plasminogen activator (tPA), when used with aspirin and heparin, was associated with a significantly greater risk of intracranial hemorrhage in patients over 75 yr compared with those younger than 75 (2.1% vs 0.5%, respectively). It is important to note that a standard rather than a weight-based dose of heparin was used in this trial and was associated with an average activated partial prothrombin time (APTT) of 20 s longer in the older compared with younger patients *(95)*. Weight-based heparin dosing nomograms may reduce rate of hemorrhagic complications in the elderly given thrombolytics *(96)*. There was no interaction of age and intracranial hemorrhage in those patients receiving streptokinase in GUSTO-1. Newer thrombolytic agents, which are more specifically targeted to fibrin, such as TNK–tPA, may have a slightly better safety profile in older patients compared with tPA. In the TIMI 10b trial, a head-to-head comparison between TNK–tPA and tPA, a nonsignificant reduction in mortality was seen in those over 75 yr treated with TNK–tPA versus tPA, but not in younger patients *(97)*. This mortality reduction was not seen in the ASSENT 2 trial, but TNK–tPA was associated with a lower rate of intracranial hemorrhage in patients over 75 yr compared with tPA *(98)*.

Anticoagulants

Heparin has been shown to play an important role in the therapy of acute coronary syndromes alone and in combination with thrombolytics and glycoprotein IIb/IIIa inhibitors. In older patients, the dosing of unfractionated heparin is important, both to maximize efficacy and to avoid bleeding complications. Rather than administering a standard dose, a weight-based bolus and infusion is recommended *(96)*. Use of such weight-based nomograms in the elderly may reduce the previously reported increase in intracranial bleeding in the older patients who were given standard heparin doses with thrombolytics *(91)*.

Low-molecular-weight heparins are emerging as an important option in the treatment of acute coronary syndromes. In the Efficacy and Safety of Subcutaneous Enoxaparin in

Non-Q-Wave Coronary Events (ESSENCE) study, the combination of enoxaparin and aspirin was associated with a significant reduction of the composite end-point of death, myocardial infarction, and recurrent angina, as well as the need for revascularization at 30 d compared with unfractionated heparin and aspirin *(99)*. Whereas the risk of major bleeding events was lower in the enoxaparin arm (p = NS), minor bleeding events were significantly higher in those patients treated with low-molecular-weight heparin compared with unfractionated heparin. Similar results favoring the use of enoxaparin over unfractionated heparin in unstable angina/non-Q-wave myocardial infarction were observed in TIMI 11B with no increase in bleeding events associated with low-molecular-weight heparin use *(100)*. The mean age of both of these studies is 64–65 yr.

LIPID LOWERING

Putting an end to a long-standing debate over the association between elevated serum cholesterol and coronary events in the elderly, evidence from both the Framingham Heart Study and the Established Populations for Epidemiologic Studies in the Elderly supports this relationship *(101,102)*. These reports, combined with recent evidence that cholesterol-lowering drugs reduce the incidence of recurrent cardiac events and death in elderly patients with known coronary artery disease, emphasize the importance of treating hypercholesterolemia in older cardiac patients *(103)*. Several large-scale clinical trials support the use of lipid-lowering agents in older individuals with coronary artery disease as secondary prevention. The Scandinavian Simvastatin Survival Study reported a significant reduction in coronary events (34%), coronary deaths (42%) and overall mortality (30%) in patients taking simvastatin compared with placebo *(104)*. The magnitude and the significance of these reductions were also seen in patients over 65 yr. In the CARE study, which was designed to investigate the effects of pravastatin in patients following myocardial infarction with a total cholesterol under 240 mg/dL and a serum low-density lipoprotein (LDL) cholesterol greater than 115 mg/dL, a 27% reduction in major coronary events was seen in patients 60–75 yr compared with a 20% reduction in patients under 60 yr *(105)*. Although there is now evidence that older postinfarction patients benefit from lipid-lowering therapy, the rate of prescriptions in the elderly is far lower that in younger patients *(106,107)*. This decreased rate may be the result of the fear of increased side effects; however, the safety and efficacy profiles for HMG-CoA reductase inhibitors are similar in older and younger patients *(108–111)*.

The use of lipid-lowering agents for the primary prevention of coronary artery disease in the elderly is less clear. Although the Air Force/Texas Coronary Atherosclerosis Prevention Study demonstrated a 29% reduction in risk of a first coronary event in persons over age 65 treated with lovastatin compared with placebo, this subanalysis of 1387 people did not reach statistical significance *(112)*. The other major primary prevention trial that examined the effect of pravastatin in lowering the risk of a first cardiac event, the West of Scotland Coronary Prevention Study Group, did show a 27% risk reduction in subjects older than 55 yr, but no individuals over age 64 yr were included in this study *(113)*.

Percutaneous Coronary Interventions in the Elderly

Angioplasty outcomes have improved in the elderly over the last 10 yr with increased operator experience, new tools, and the introduction of stents and glycoprotein IIb/IIIa inhibitors. In spite of increasing age and greater comorbidites, the procedural success rate of percutaneous coronary interventions (PCIs) in the elderly has significantly improved with reduction in complications, need for emergent CABG, and decreased length of stay *(114–116)*. Attempts have been made to quantitate the procedural risk and success in octogenarians through several retrospective analyses *(117–121)*. Ang and colleagues performed a retrospective analysis comparing those age 70–79 yr ($n = 524$) with those over 80 yr ($n = 64$): No difference in the procedural success rate was demonstrated (94% vs 96%, p = NS, respectively) *(119)*. In this study, patients over age 80 yr demonstrated complicated anatomy, including more three-vessel disease as well as more calcified and longer lesions than their younger counterparts. Although the rates of complications were similar in the two age groups, the mean length of stay was longer in those over 80 yr old compared with patients aged 70–79 yr (4.1 ± 5.7 vs 2.0 ± 3.5 d, respectively). Another retrospective analysis comparing 7472 octogenarians with 102,236 patients younger than 80 yr undergoing percutaneous coronary interventions reported a slightly lower procedural success rate in the older cohort (84% vs 89%, $p = 0.001$) *(118)*. Octogenarians, compared with younger patients, experienced a twofold to fourfold increase in in-hospital procedural complications including death (3.8% vs 1.1%), Q-wave infarction (1.9% vs 1.3%), stroke (0.58% vs 0.23%), renal failure (3.2% vs 1.0%), and vascular complications (6.7% vs 3.3%) ($p < 0.001$ for all comparisons). Interestingly, over the time-course of the analyses, complication rates significantly decreased in older patients, presumably the result of technological and medical advancements. This study cited several significant predictors associated with increased procedural mortality in octogenarians, including shock, AMI, left-ventricular dysfunction (ejection fraction <0.35), renal insufficiency, first PCI, diabetes mellitus, and age over 85 yr. It is important to note that overall procedural mortality varies widely in older patients and may be related to comorbidities.

Although several trials have randomized patients with stable coronary artery disease to PCI vs CABG, the elderly have generally been excluded. A recent randomized trial included 454 high-risk veterans with medically refractory angina who were randomized to PCI with or without stents or to CABG *(122)*. High-risk criteria included age >70 yr, prior CABG, left-ventricular ejection fraction <35%, recent myocardial infarction, or need for intra-aortic balloon pump. Survival at 30 d was excellent in both groups (95% vs 97% for CABG and PCI, respectively). Survival up to 3 yr remained similar in the two groups. These data suggest that high-risk patients with medically refractory angina, including the elderly, can undergo revascularization with PCI or CABG with excellent survival and relief of angina.

The fear of increased hemorrhagic events associated with PCI in the elderly is further complicated by reports that adjuvant therapies such as the glycoprotein IIb/IIIa receptor antagonists have been associated with increased minor bleeding as well as vascular complications with increasing age *(123)*. Further prospective studies are needed to determine the additional risk posed by these agents in older adults as well as dosing information.

Health-related quality of life has been shown to increase significantly in older patients undergoing PCI and to a similar extent as in younger patients *(124)*. Thus, PCI may have an important role in providing symptomatic relief and preserve independence in older patients with ischemic heart disease who are not candidates for more invasive procedures.

Efficacy of Primary Percutaneous Coronary Interventions and Stents

Given the increased incidence of bleeding complications with thrombolytics in the elderly, primary PCI has a favorable role in elderly patients with AMI. Because of the rapid changes in technology and adjuvant therapies, such as stents and glycoprotein IIb/IIIa inhibitors, evidence regarding PCI lags current experience. Primary PCI and PCIs with stent placement compares favorably to thrombolytic therapy in the management of acute ST-segment elevation MI in the elderly (125). Nevertheless, patients ≥75 yr of age with AMI who are treated aggressively with direct PCI continue to experience a relatively high morbidity and mortality compared to younger patients with ST-segment elevation MI (121). In a series of 3032 patients with acute ST-segment elevation MI treated with direct PCI, of whom 452 were ≥75 yr of age, in-hospital mortality was 10.2% in the elderly vs 1.8% in the younger patients. Older patients had lower PCI success rates, higher frequency of three-vessel coronary disease, and lower left-ventricular ejection fraction compared to younger subjects. Advanced age was a powerful predictor of in-hospital mortality.

Coronary stenting improves outcomes in patients with stable coronary artery disease with less restenosis compared to PCI (126). In the elderly, observational data from the Medicare database also suggests that PCI with stenting results in improved outcomes compared to PCI alone. In a large cohort of elderly who underwent PCI in 1994 and 1996 for stable coronary artery disease, including 74,836 cases with stent placement, stent placement resulted in a large reduction in need for urgent CABG and mortality (127). Outcomes were best at high-volume PCI institutions. Although PCI with coronary stenting does not reduce mortality compared to PCI in patients with AMI, coronary stenting results in a reduced risk of infarct vessel revascularization over 6 mo follow-up (128).

Rescue PCI/Stents

Although age is a powerful predictor of mortality in large thrombolytic trials (90,129), this is not the result of the lower frequency of infarct vessel reperfusion seen in older patients (95). In patients who fail to reperfuse with thrombolytic therapy, rescue PCI is often recommended. Although earlier studies with rescue PCI suggested a high complication rate (130), more recent data with the use of glycoprotein IIb/IIIa inhibitors and stents suggest better outcomes (131). The only randomized trial with rescue PCI conducted enrolled 150 patients with an occluded left anterior descending coronary artery following thrombolytic therapy (132). Six-month survival free of congestive heart failure was improved in patients randomized to left anterior descending rescue PCI as compared to conservative therapy. The largest cohort of rescue PCI patients comes from the GUSTO-1 angiographic substudy (133). One hundred ninety-eight patients who had an occluded vessel on a 90 min angiogram following thrombolytic therapy had rescue angioplasty, as determined by their primary physician. Rescue PCI restored normal infarct vessel flow (Thrombolysis in Myocardial Infarction grade III) in 68% of patients. Only severe heart failure predicted failure of rescue with PCI. Follow-up left-ventricular function was superior in patients with successful rescue PCI compared to patients with an occluded vessel managed conservatively following failed thrombolytics. Survival was best in patients with successful thrombolysis at 90 min, followed by those patients with successful rescue PCI, followed by those in whom no rescue was attempted. Patients with failed rescue attempts had the highest death rate (30.4%), the majority of whom were in cardiogenic shock at the time of the procedure. Age had no influence on the success or failure of rescue PCI. These data suggest that age itself should not influence the decision to proceed with rescue PCI. Although randomized data are limited, older patients with a large infarction, particularly anterior, or with hemodynamic compromise are likely to benefit from rescue PCI following failed thrombolysis.

Intra-Aortic Balloon Pump

By virtue of augmenting coronary perfusion pressure while decreasing afterload without increasing myocardial oxygen consumption, the use of intra-aortic balloon pump (IABP) counterpulsation appears beneficial for temporary clinical and hemodynamic stabilization despite the lack of large randomized trials *(134)*. Two frequent uses for IABP in the elderly are for high-risk CABG and cardiogenic shock. Many elderly CABG patients are designated high risk by virtue of poor left-ventricular function, redo CABG, and extensive coronary artery disease. In this setting, preoperative IABP may improve outcomes *(135)*. One small trial of 52 high-risk CABG patients (defined by the presence of two of the following: low ejection fraction, left main coronary disease, unstable angina or redo CABG) randomized patients to preoperative IABP or not. The IABP group had lower perioperative mortality *(136)*. Although randomized trials are lacking, off-pump CABG may particularly benefit the elderly. In this setting, particularly in elderly patients with critical coronary artery disease, a strategy of prophylactic IABP may also improve outcomes *(137)* *(see* Chapter 15).

Age is a powerful predictor of cardiogenic shock in AMI *(138)*. In the setting of cardiogenic shock, IABP placement is frequently used to interrupt the spiral of worsening ischemia and reduced cardiac output. In a large registry of AMI, 23,180 patients developed cardiogenic shock with a mean age of 72 yr *(139)*. Thirty-one percent of patients in shock received an IABP; this group was younger (67 vs 74 yr) and more likely received reperfusion therapy than the larger subset of cardiogenic shock patients who did not receive an IABP. The overall in-hospital mortality in this large cohort with cardiogenic shock was 70%. There was an important interaction of IABP on survival in those patients treated with thrombolytic therapy. IABP use was associated with a reduction in mortality in patients treated with thrombolytic therapy (OR = 0.82; 95% CI = 0.72–0.93). IABP use was not associated with a reduction in mortality in patients treated with primary PCI. These data support prior thrombolytic trials that show no survival advantage with thrombolytic therapy in the setting of cardiogenic shock *(32)*; angiography studies demonstrate a poor reperfusion rate with thrombolytics when coronary perfusion pressures are low *(140)*. IABP counterpulsation can enhance reperfusion with thrombolytics by increasing coronary perfusion pressure *(141)*. This strategy of IABP support with thrombolytics may be particularly beneficial in the community setting *(142)*.

In the setting of primary PCI in high-risk MI patients, IABP counterpulsation does not appear as useful. Four-hundred and thirty-seven patients with AMI who were treated with direct PCI and felt to be at high risk for complications based on age >70 yr, three-vessel coronary artery disease, left-ventricular ejection fraction ≤45%, saphenous vein graft occlusion, malignant ventricular arrhythmias, or a suboptimal PCI result were randomized to prophylactic IABP for 36–48 h or not following the PCI *(143)*. There was no difference in the primary end-point; in-hospital death, reinfarction, infarct-related artery reocclusion, stroke, new heart failure, or sustained hypotension in patients treated with an IABP versus conservative treatment. These data suggest that in the setting of cardiogenic shock, IABP support is likely helpful if thrombolytic therapy is used as a stabilizing measure prior to emergent cardiac catheterization. IABP support does not prevent morbidity and mortality in high-risk patients who have stabilized following PCI.

Elderly patients with severe coronary disease may develop medically refractory angina pectoris. IABP support is very useful to reduce ischemia in the elderly patient with refractory angina as a bridge to emergent PCI or CABG. IABP support is also indicated in the setting of AMI when devastating mechanical complications, such as a ventricular septal defect or papillary muscle rupture with acute mitral regurgitation, occur. The IABP can be lifesaving as a bridge to emergent cardiac surgery.

Hemodynamic Monitoring

Congestive heart failure is a frequent complication of AMI in the elderly, and hemodynamic monitoring is an important management tool in this setting *(90)*. In older patients with severe or progressive congestive heart failure, cardiogenic shock, or mechanical complications of myocardial infarction, such as ventricular septal defect, hemodynamic monitoring with a balloon floatation right-heart catheter helps guide therapy *(59)*. In the low-cardiac-output setting, precise measurements of filling pressures help to determine the need for volume expansion and inotropic support. These patients should also receive intra-arterial pressure monitoring.

Whether or not pulmonary artery catheterization assists in the management of patients with advanced heart failure (not in the setting of AMI) is controversial. The Evaluation Study of Congestive Heart Failure and Pulmonary Artery Cathterization Effectiveness (ESCAPE) trial is an ongoing randomized trial to test the safety and efficacy of treatment guided by pulmonary artery catheterization plus clinical assessment vs clinical assessment alone in hospitalized patients with severe heart failure *(144)*. Until these prospective, randomized data are available, individual patient assessment as to the utility of pulmonary artery catheterization is recommended.

Efficacy of Surgical Therapy

Use of CABG has increased substantially in the very elderly over the last 10–15 yr *(145)*. (*See* Chapter 15 for a discussion on surgical treatment of ischemic heart disease.) Thirty-day mortality in a large cohort aged 80 yr and older averaged 11.5%, and 1 yr mortality averaged 19.2%, a figure approx 2.5-fold greater than the corresponding mortalities in 65 to 70 yr olds. Independent predictors of mortality include increasing age, female sex, and admission with AMI, congestive heart failure, cerebral or peripheral vascular disease, and chronic renal disease. Older age is also a powerful predictor of perioperative stroke, which occurs in about 8% of the very elderly during CABG *(146)*. Other important predictors of stroke include aortic atherosclerosis, history of neurological disease, use of an IABP, diabetes mellitus, history of hypertension, history of pulmonary disease, and history of unstable angina. In addition to stroke risk, many patients following CABG experience cognitive decline on formal neurocognitive testing compared to baseline. In one study, 53% of 261 CABG patients at discharge and 42% of patients at 5 yr showed evidence of neurocognitive decline *(147)*. Increased age was a powerful predictor of neurocognitive decline in this study. Importantly, however, significant improvement in the quality-of-life with relief of medically refractory angina is achieved in many elderly patients who undergo CABG *(148)*. Therefore, age alone should not be a contraindication for CABG. Careful assessments of the risks (particularly neurologic) and benefits (improved quality-of-life) of bypass surgery should be performed, including consideration of comorbid conditions that increase perioperative morbidity and mortality.

An important addition to the treatment of the elderly patient with critical coronary artery disease is off-pump CABG. Preliminary studies suggest that off-pump CABG (no aortic cross-clamping or cardiopulmonary bypass) may have specific advantages in the elderly, who are at higher risk for neurologic complications with routine CABG. One randomized trial of 40 patients showed that, compared to standard CABG, off-pump CABG resulted in significantly fewer transcranial Doppler ultrasound embolic signals and less postoperative cognitive impairment *(149)*. Larger randomized trials are ongoing to determine whether this new procedure will benefit the elderly.

CONTROVERSIES

Which Test for the Evaluation of IHD in the Elderly?

The performance of an exercise ECG stress test poses several challenges for the elderly. Maximal aerobic capacity declines with age *(150)*. Other noncardiac conditions may also limit the exercise response in the elderly, including an age-associated increase in neurologic and musculoskeletal disorders, associated lung and peripheral vascular disease, and psychological factors *(151)*. Therefore, the best test to evaluate ischemic heart disease in the elderly will depend on these factors (e.g., a bicycle exercise test in a patient with gait difficulties, or a more gradual treadmill protocol in a debilitated elderly patient).

Interpretation of an exercise treadmill test in the elderly may be more difficult than in younger subjects because of a higher incidence of baseline ST-segment abnormalities. The sensitivity (number of true positive tests in those with coronary artery disease) of the exercise ECG is greater in the elderly, increasing from 56% in those younger than 40 yr to 84% in those older 60 yr *(12)*. The specificity (number of true negative tests over those without coronary disease) is lower, decreasing from 84% to 70% in those under 40 yr and over 60 yr of age, respectively *(12)*.

The increased sensitivity is because the frequency and severity of coronary disease increases with age in men and women *(152)*. Lower specificity (more false-positives) in older patients may result from more baseline ST changes, left-ventricular hypertrophy, and conduction disease *(153)*. In an elderly patient able to exercise, a treadmill ECG stress test provides prognostic information about exercise tolerance, blood pressure response, exercise-induced arrhythmias, and heart rate recovery following cessation of exercise, all parameters that add to the ST-segment in predicting prognosis *(154)*.

In elderly patients with baseline ST-segment changes that make the exercise ECG uninterpretable and in patients with prior revascularization procedures, the addition of a radioisotope enhances the diagnostic and prognostic accuracy of the exercise ECG *(155, 156)*. Recent data in a large cohort of elderly patients, who underwent exercise echocardiography, suggest that echocardiographic findings add to the stress ECG and clinical variables in predicting cardiac events and cardiac death over 3 yr of follow-up *(157)*. In older patients with left bundle branch block or a ventricular-paced rhythm, an adenosine/persantine thallium test is the evaluation of choice for diagnostic assessment of coronary artery disease *(153)*. Finally, in older patients unable to walk, stress echocardiography with dobutamine has a high sensitivity and specificity and is well tolerated, and a test positive for ischemia predicts future cardiac events *(158)*.

Is CABG Indicated in the Very Old?

Previous randomized trials of medical vs revascularization therapy in patients with stable coronary artery disease have excluded the elderly. An important recent trial of prospectively randomized patients aged 75 yr and older (mean 80 yr) with moderate angina despite at least two anti-anginal drugs to either coronary angiography and revascularization or optimal medical therapy *(159)*. The primary end point of this trial was quality-of-life scores at 6 mo. Seventy-four percent of patients randomized to the invasive arm had anatomy appropriate for either percutaneous intervention (54%) or CABG (20%). Although the quality-of-life improved in both groups by 6 mo, the group randomized to invasive therapy had a significantly better quality-of-life compared to medically treated patients. Secondary end-points of 6-mo mortality, myocardial infarction, or hospitalization for unstable angina was lower in those elderly patients randomized to invasive therapy (19%) vs medical therapy (49%). Furthermore, one-third of patients in the medical arm crossed over to revascularization because of refractory symptoms. This important study suggests that age alone is not a contraindication to proceed with an interventional approach to the treatment of moderate to severe angina.

Primary PCI vs Thrombolytic for the Elderly

One of the established therapies for acute ST-segment elevation myocardial infarction is thrombolytic therapy. The large FTT meta-analysis *(89)*, did not demonstrate a significant benefit for fibrinolytic therapy compared to control in patients 75 yr of age and older. An observational study from the Medicare database suggested that 30 d mortality was higher in patients >75 yr of age receiving fibrinolytic therapy for acute ST-segment-elevation myocardial infarction compared to eligible patients who did not receive such therapy *(91)*. These data suggest that alternative therapies should be considered in the elderly presenting with ST-segment-elevation myocardial infarction.

In experienced hands, primary PCI in acute ST-segment elevation myocardial infarction results in Thrombolysis in Myocardial Infarction (TIMI) III flow in 75–90% of patients *(160,161)*. With the use of a GPIIb/IIIa inhibitor added to coronary stenting, TIMI III flow and short-term outcomes are also improved *(162)*. Several randomized controlled trials comparing thrombolytic therapy with emergent PCI suggest that the latter therapy results in a decrease in infarct size and short-term mortality, re-infarction rate, and stroke risk *(125,163)*. Long-term survival free of recurrent myocardial infarction is also significantly lowered with PCI compared to fibrinolytic therapy *(164)*. Important caveats include the fact that these randomized studies were performed by experienced interventionists and that the time interval from arrival in the emergency department to the catheterization laboratory arrival was impressively short *(165)*. Patients over 70 yr appeared to have the greatest benefit from PCI as compared to fibrinolytics. Therefore, given the controversies of fibrinolytic therapy in patients 75 yr of age and older, consideration should be made for emergent PCI in patients hospitalized by an experienced interventionalist at high-volume angioplasty centers. In the community hospitals, where the availability of PCI may be limited, considerations for treating the older patients with acute ST-segment elevation myocardial infarction with fibrinolytic therapy versus transfer to a tertiary-care facility must be made on an individual basis. Important factors include the time to reperfusion, size of the infarction, hemodynamic stability, and other patient comorbidities, including cerebral vascular disease, hypertension, and body weight.

Conservative vs Aggressive
Approach to AMI Complicated by Cardiogenic Shock

The incidence of cardiogenic shock has not changed over the last two decades, averaging 7.1% of patients with AMI *(166)*. Patients with AMI who develop shock are substantially older than those who do not, and age is a powerful independent predictor of outcome of this life-threatening condition, the incidence of which rises 47% for every 10 yr age increase *(167,168)*. Although an invasive strategy for the treatment of cardiogenic shock showed a benefit in observational studies in AMI *(169)*, the results of these studies are affected by patient selection bias. The SHOCK trial randomized 302 patients who developed clinical or hemorrhagic cardiogenic shock secondary to left-ventricular dysfunction within 36 h of the infarction *(170)*. Randomization was within 12 h following the diagnosis of shock. Patients were randomized to early revascularization (PCI or CABG) with IABP recommended (86%) or intensive medical therapy that included thrombolytics (63%) and IABP (86%). Delayed revascularization after 54 h from randomization was recommended only if clinically indicated (25%). Thirty-day mortality was 46.7% in patients randomized to early invasive therapy and 56% in patients assigned to intensive medical stabilization ($p = 0.11$). In patients randomized to invasive therapy, 6 and 12 mo mortality were significantly lower *(171)*. Importantly, in subgroup analyses there was an important interaction of age with treatment at 30 d, 6 mo, and 12 mo. In patients <75 yr of age, 30-d, 6-mo, and 12-month mortality was significantly lower in patients randomized to early invasive therapy (41.4%, 44.9%, and 48.4%, respectively) compared to intensive medical therapy (56.8%, 65%, and 65.7%, respectively). In contrast, in patients over 75 yr of age, there was a trend toward greater mortality at 30 d, 6 mo, and 12 mo with early invasive therapy (75%, 79.2%, and 79.2%, respectively) compared to intensive medical therapy (53.1%, 56.3%, and 65.6%, respectively). Small sample size (56 patients) may account for this apparent lack of benefit of an early invasive strategy for cardiogenic shock in older individuals, conflicting with observational data in the elderly *(172)*. Nevertheless, emergent cardiac catheterization with revascularization is recommended in patients <75 yr of age with cardiogenic shock, although routine application of this strategy cannot be recommended in those >75 yr of age. In this situation, careful determination of other comorbidities and functional status must be assessed, with the decision to utilize an invasive approach made only on a case-by-case basis.

REFERENCES

1. Lakatta EG. Cardiovascular regulatory mechanisms in advanced age. Physiol Rev 1993;73:413–467.
2. Lakatta EG, Gerstenblith G, Angell CS, Shock NW, Weisfeldt ML. Diminished inotropic response of aged myocardium to catecholamines. Circ Res 1975;36:262–269.
3. Schulman SP, Lakatta EG, Fleg JL, Lakatta L, Becker LC, Gerstenblith G. Age-related decline in left ventricular filling at rest and exercise. Am J Physiol 1992;263:H1932–H1938.
4. Shirani J, Alaeddini J, Roberts WC. Comparison of modes of death and cardiac necropsy findings in fatal acute myocardial infarction in men and women >75 years of age. Am J Cardiol 2000;86(9): 1010–1012.
5. Foot DK, Lewis RP, Pearson TA, Beller GA. Demography and cardiology, 1950–2050. J Am Coll Cardiol 2000;35(4):1067–1081.
6. Dauerman HL, Lessard D, Yarzebski J, Furman MI, Gore JM, Goldberg RJ. Ten-year trends in the incidence, treatment, and outcome of Q-wave myocardial infarction. Am J Cardiol 2000;86:730–735.
7. Elveback L, Lie JT. Continued high evidence of coronary artery disease at autopsy in Olmstead County, Minnesota 1950 to 1979. Circulation 1984;70:345–349.
8. Roberts WC, Shirani J. Comparison of cardiac findings at necropsy in octogenarians, nonagenarians, and centenarians. Am J Cardiol 1998;82:627–631.
9. Society of Cardiovascular Surgeons Database 2000.
10. Cobb FR, Higginbotham MB, Mark D. Diagnosis of coronary disease in the elderly. In: Wenger N, Furberg C, Pitt E, eds. Coronary Heart Disease in the Elderly. Elsevier, New York, 1986, pp. 303–325.
11. Gersh BJ, Kronmal RA, Frye RL. Coronary arteriography and coronary artery bypass surgery; morbidity and mortality in patients aged 65 years or older: a report from the Coronary Artery Surgery Study. Circulation 1983;67:483–491.

12. Hlatky M, Pryor DB, Harrell FE. Factors affecting sensitivity and specificity of exercise electrocardiography: multivariate analysis. Am J Med 1984;77:64–71.

13. Spencer FA, Goldberg RJ, Frederick PD, Malmgren J, Becker RC, Gore JM. Age and the utilization of cardiac catherrization following uncomplicated first acute myocardial infarction treated with thrombolytic therapy (the Second National Registry of Myocardial Infarction [NRMI-2]). Am J Cardiol 2001;88:107–111.

14. Aronow WS, Ahn C. Increased plasma homocysteine is an independent predictor of new coronary events in older persons. Am J Cardiol 2000;86:346–347.

15. Kopecky SL, Gersh BJ, McGoon MD, Chu C-P, Ilstrup DM, Chesebro JH, et al. Lone atrial fibrillation in elderly persons. A marker for cardiovascular risk. Arch Intern Med 1999;159:1118–1122.

16. Benetos A, Safar M, Rudnichi A, Smulyan H, Richard J-L, Ducimetière P, et al. Pulse pressure: a predictor of long-term cardiovascular mortality in a french male population. Hypertension 1997;30(6): 1410–1415.

17. Franklin SS, Khan SA, Wong ND, Larson MG, Levy D. Is pulse pressure useful in predicting risk for coronary heart disease? The Framingham Heart Study. Circulation 1999;100:354–360.

18. Franklin SS, Larson MG, Khan SA, Wong ND, Leip FP, Kannel WB, et al. Does the relation of blood pressure to coronary heart disease risk change with aging? The Framingham Heart Study. Circulation 2001;103:1245–1249.

19. Kitchen AH, Milne JS. Longitudinal survey of ischemic heart disease in a randomly selected sample of an older population. Br Heart J 1977;39:889–893.

20. Pathy MS. Clinical presentation of myocardial infarction in the elderly. Br Heart J 1967;29:190–198.

21. Wroblewski M, Mikulowski P, Steen B. Symptoms of myocardial infarction in old age: clinical case, retrospective, and prospective studies. Age Ageing 1986;15:99–104.

22. Aronow WS. Prevalence of presenting symptoms of recognized myocardial infarction and of unrecognized healed myocardial infarction in elderly patients. Am J Cardiol 1987;60:1182

23. Tresch DD, Brady WJ, Aufderheide TP. Comparison of elderly and younger patients with out-of-hospital chest pain. Arch Intern Med 1996;156:1089–1093.

24. Nicol P, Gilpin E, Dittrich H. Short and long-term clinical outcome after Q wave and non-Q-wave myocardial infarction in a large patient population. Circulation 1989;79:528–536.

25. Rich MW, Bosner MS, Chung MMK. Is age an independent predictor of early and late mortality in patients with acute myocardial infarction? Am J Med 1992;92:7–13.

26. Tofler GH, Muller JE, Stone PH. Factors leading to shorter survival after acute myocardial infarction in patients 65 to 75 years. Am J Cardiol 1988;62:860–867.

27. Wienberg H, Schiele R, Gitt AK, Schneider S, Heer T, Gottwik M, et al. Incidence, risk factors, and clinical outcome of stroke after acute myocardial infarction in clinical practice. Am J Cardiol 2000;87: 782–785.

28. Chung MMK, Bosner MS, McKenzie JP. Prognosis of patients ≥70 years of age with non-Q-wave acute myocardial infarction compared with younger patients with similar infarcts and with patients ≥70 years of age with Q wave acute myocardial infarction. Am J Cardiol 1995;75:18–22.

29. Schiele R, Gitt AK, Weinbergen H, Schneider S, Zahn R, Grube R, et al. Incidence, determinants, and clinical course of reinfarction in-hospital after index acute myocardial infarction (results from the pooled data of the Maximal Individual Therapy in Acute Myocardial Infarction [MITRA], and the Myocardial Infarction Registry [MIR]). Am J Cardiol 2001;87:1039–1044.

30. Aronow WS. Managment of older persons after myocardial infarction. J Am Geriatr Soc 1998;46: 1459–1468.

31. Leipzig RM. Avoiding adverse drug effects in elderly patients. Clev Clin J Med 1998;65(9):470–478.

32. ISIS-2. Randomised trial of intravenous streptokinase, oral aspirin, both or neither among 17,187 cases of suspected acute myocardial infarction. Lancet 1988;2:349–360.

33. Antiplatelet Trialists' Collaboration. Collaborative overview of randomised trials of antiplatelet therapy-I: prevention of death, myocardial infarction and stroke by prolonged antiplatelet therapy in various categories of patients. Br Med J 1994;308:81–106.

34. Krumholz HM, Radford MJ, Ellerbeck EF, Hennen J, Meehan TP, Petrillo M. Aspirin in the treatment of acute myocardial infarction in elderly Medicare beneficiaries: patterns of use and outcomes. Circulation 1995;92:2841–2847.

35. Krumholz HM, Chen Y-T, Wang Y, Radford MJ. Aspirin and angiotensin-converting enzyme inhibitors among elderly survivors of hospitalization for an acute myocardial infarction. Arch Intern Med 2001; 161:538–544.

36. Krumholz HM, Radford MJ, Ellerbeck EF, Hennen J, Meehan TP, Petrillo M, et al. Aspirin for secondary prevention after acute myocardial infarction in the elderly: prescribed use and outcomes. Ann Intern Med 1996;124:292–298.
37. Moore JG, Bjorkman DJ, Mitchell MD, Avots-Avotins, A. Age does not influence acute aspirin-induced gastric mucosal damage. Gastroenterology 1991;100:1626–1629.
38. Hjalmarson A, Elmfeldt D, Herlitz J. Effect of mortality of metoprolol in acute myocardial infarction: a double-blind randomised trial. Lancet 1981;2:823–827.
39. First International Study of Infarct Survival Collaborative Group. Randomised trial of intravenous atenolol among 16,027 cases of suspected acute myocardial infarction. Lancet 1986;2:57–66.
40. β-Blocker Heart Attack Trial Research Group. A randomized clinical trial of propranolol in patients with acute myocardial infarction, II: morbidity results. JAMA 1983;250:2814–2819.
41. β-Blocker Heart Attack Trial Research Group. A randomized clinical trial of propranolol in patients with acute myocardial infarction, I: mortality results. JAMA 1982;247:1707–1714.
42. Gundersen T, Abrahamsen AM, Kjekshus J, Ronnevik PK. Timolol-related reduction in mortality and reinfarction in patients ages 65-75 years surviving acute myocardial infarction. Circulation 1982;66:1179–1182.
43. Pederson TR. Six-year follow-up of the Norwegian Multicenter Study on timolol after myocardial infarction. N Engl J Med 1985;313:1055–1058.
44. Hawkins CM, Richardson DW, Vokonas PS. Effect of propranolol in reducing mortality in old myocardial infarction patients: the Beta-Blocker Heart Attack Trial Experience. Circulation 1983;67(Suppl I):194–197.
45. Gottlieb SS, McCarter RJ, Vogel RA. Effect of beta-blockade on mortality among high-risk and low-risk patients after myocardial infarction. N Engl J Med 1993;339:489.
46. Soumerai SB, McLaughlin TJ, Speigelman D, Hertzmark E, Thibault G, Goldman L. Adverse outcomes of underuse of β-blockers in elderly survivors of acute myocardial infarction. JAMA 1997;277(2):115–121.
47. Chen J, Radford MJ, Wang Y, Marciniak TA, Krumholz HM. Effectiveness of beta-blocker therapy after acute myocardial infarction in elderly patients with chronic obstructive pulmonary disease or asthma. J Am Coll Cardiol 2001;37(7):1950–1956.
48. Croog SH, Elias MF, Colton T, Baume RM, Leiblum SR, Jenkins CD, et al. Effects of antihypertensive medications on quality of life in elderly hypertensive women. Am J Hypertens 1994;7(4 Pt 1):329–339.
49. Prince MJ, Bird AS, Blizard RA, Mann AH. Is the cognitive function of older patients affected by antihypertensive treatment? Results from 54 months o the Medical Research Council's treatment trial of hypertension in older adults. Br Med J 1996;312:801–805.
50. Skinner MH, Futterman A, Morrissette D, Thompson LW, Hoffman BB, et al. Atenolol compared with nifedipine: effect on cognitive function and mood in elderly hypertensive patients. Ann Intern Med 1992;116(8):615–623.
51. Phillips KA, Shipak MG, Coxson P, Heidenreich PA, Hunink MGM, Goldman PA, et al. Health and economic benefits of increased β-blocker use following myocardial infarction. JAMA 2000;284(21):2748–2754.
52. Pfeffer MA, Braunwald E, Moye LA. Effect of captopril on mortality and morbidity in patients with left ventricular dysfunction after myocardial infarction—results of the Survival and Ventricular Enlargement Trial. N Engl J Med 1992;327:669–677.
53. Kober L, Torp-Pedersen C, Carlsen JE. A clinical trial of the angiotensin-converting enzyme inhibitor trandolapril in patients with left ventricular dysfunction after myocardial infarction. N Engl J Med 1995;333:1670–1676.
54. Acute Infarction Ramipril Efficacy (AIRE) Study Investigators. Effect of ramapril on mortality and morbidity of survivors of acute myocardial infarction with clinical evidence of heart failure. Lancet 1993;342:821–828.
55. ISIS-4 Collaborative Group. ISIS-4: a randomized factorial trial assessing early oral captopril, oral mononitrate, and intravenous magnesium sulfate in 58,050 patients with suspected acute myocardial infarction. Lancet 1995;345:669–685.
56. Shlipak MG, Browner WS, Noguchi H, Massie B, Frances CD, McClellan M. Comparison of the effects of angiotensin converting-enzyme inhibitors and beta blockers on survival in elderly patients with reduced left ventricular function after myocardial infarction. Am J Med 2001;110:425–433.

57. The Heart Outcomes Prevention Evaluation Study Investigators. Effects of an angiotensin-converting enzyme inhibitor, ramipril, on cardiovascular events in high-risk patients. N Engl J Med 2000;342(3): 145–153.
58. Dagenais GR, Yusef S, Bourassa MG, Yi Q, Bosch J, Kouz S, et al. Effects of ramipril on coronary events in high-risk persons. Results of the Heart Outcomes Prevention Evaluation Study. Circulation 2001; 104:522–526.
59. ACC/AHA guidelines for the managment of patients with acute myocardial infarction. J Am Coll Cardiol 1996;28(5):1328–1428.
60. Ziegelstein RC, Hilbe JM, French WJ, Antman EM, Chandra-Strobos N. Magnesium use in the treatment of acute myocardial infarction in the United States (observations from the Second National Registry of Myocardial Infarction). Am J Cardiol 2001;87:7–10.
61. Santoro GM, Antoniucci D, Bolognese L, Valenti R, Buonamici P, Trapani M, et al. A randomized study of intravenous magnesium in acute myocardial infarction treated with direct coronary angioplasty. Am Heart J 2000;140(6):891–897.
62. Shechter M, Merz CN, Paul-Labrador M, Meisel SR, Rude RK, Molloy MD, et al. Beneficial antithrombotic effects of the association of pharmacological oral magnesium therapy with aspirin in coronary heart disease patients. Magnesium Res 2000;13(4):275–284.
63. Shechter M, Sharir M, Paul-Labrador M, Forrester J, Silver B, Bairey-Merz N. Oral magnesium therapy improves endothelial function in patients with coronary artery disease. Circulation 2000;102:2353–2358.
64. Teragawa H, Kato M, Yamagata T, Matsuura H, Kajiyama G. The preventive effect of magnesium on coronary spasm in patients with vasospastic angina. Chest 2000;118:1690–1695.
65. The MAGIC Steering Committee. Rationale and design of the magnesium in coronaries (MAGIC) study: a clinical trial to reevaluate the efficacy of early administration of magnesium in acute myocardial infarction. Am Heart J 2000;139:10–14.
66. GISSI-3: effects of lisinopril and transdermal glyceryl trinitrate singly and together on 6-week mortality and ventricular function after acute myocardial infarction. Gruppo Italiano per lo Studio della Sopravvivenza nell'infarcto Miocardico. Lancet 1994;343(8906):1115–1122.
67. Ishikawa K, Yamamoto T, Hayashi T, Takenaka T, Kimura A, Miyataka M, et al. Intermittent nitrate therapy for prior myocardial infarction does not induce rebound angina nor reduce cardiac events. Intern Med 2000;39(12):1020–1026.
68. Niemeyer JR, Zwinderman AH. Independent determinants of the efficacy of nitrate therapy. Int J Clin Pharmacol Ther 2000;38(12):563–567.
69. Leipzig RM, Cumming RG, Tinetti ME. Drugs and falls in older people: a systematic revies and meta-analysis: II. cardiac and analgesic drugs. J Am Geriatr Soc 1999;47(1):40–50.
70. Goldbourt U, Behar S, Reicher-Reiss H, Zion M, Mandelzweig L, Kaplinsky E. Early administration of nifedipine in suspected acute myocardial infarction: the Secondary Prevention Reinfarction Israel Nifedipine Trial 2 Study. Arch Intern Med 1993;153:345–353.
71. Furberg CD, Psaty BM, Meyer JV. Nifedipine: dose-related increase in mortality in patients with coronary heart disease. Circulation 1995;92:1326–1331.
72. The Multicenter Diltiazem PostInfarction Trial (MDPIT) Research Group. The effect of diltiazem on mortality and reinfarction after myocardial infarction. N Engl J Med 1988;319:385–392.
73. The Danish Study Group on Verapamil in Myocardial Infarction. Effect of verapamil on mortality and major events after myocardial infarction (The Danish Verapamil Infarction Trial II—DAVIT-II). Am J Cardiol 1990;66:779–785.
74. Rengo F, Carbonin P, Pahor M. A controlled trial of verapamil in pateints after acute myocardial infarction: results of the Calcium Antagonist Reinfarction Italian Study (CRIS). Am J Cardiol 1996;77: 365–369.
75. Gibson RS, Hansen JF, Messerli F, Schechtman KB, Boden WE. Long-term effects of diltiazem and verapmil on mortality and cardiac events in non-Q-wave acute myocardial infarction without pulmonary congestion: post-hoc subset analysis of the Multicenter Diltiazem PostInfarction Trial and the Second Danish Verapamil Infarction Trial studies. Am J Cardiol 2000;86:275–279.
76. Jollis JG, Simpson RJ, Chowdhury MK, Cascio WE, Crouse JR, Massing MW, et al. Calcium channel blockers and mortality in elderly patients with myocardial infarction. Arch Intern Med 1999;159:2341–2348.
77. Gillman MW, Ross-Degnan D, McLaughlin TJ, Gao X, Spiegelman D, Hertzmark E, et al. Effects of long-acting versus short-acting calcium channel blockers among older survivors of acute myocardial infarction. J Am Geriatr Soc 1999;47(5):512–517.

78. Meluzin J, Stejfa M, Novak M, Zeman K, Spinarova L, Julinek J, et al. Amlodipine in patients with stable angina pectoris treated with nitrates and beta-blockers. The influence on exercise tolerance, systolic and diastolic functions of the left ventricle. Int J Cardiol 1992;(1):101–109.

79. Langdon C. Treatment of hypertension in patients > or = 65 years of age: experience with amlodipine. Clin Ther 2000;(12):1473–1482.

80. Cannon CP. Elderly patients with acute coronary syndromes: higher risk and greater benefit from antithrombotic and interventional therapies. Am J Geriatr Cardiol 2000;5:265–270.

81. The PRISM-PLUS Investigators. Inhibition of the platelet glycoprotein IIb/IIIa receptor with tirofiban in unstable angina and non-Q-wave myocardial infarction. N Engl J Med 1998;338:1488–1497.

82. The PRISM Investigators. A comparison of aspirin plus tirofiban with aspirin plus heparin of unstable angina. N Engl J Med 1998;338:1498–1505.

83. PURSUIT Trial Investigators. Inhibition of platelet glycoprotein IIb/IIIa with eptifibatide in patients with acute coronary syndromes. N Engl J Med 1998;339:436–443.

84. Simoons ML, GUSTO IV–ACS Investigators. Effect of glycoprotein IIb/IIIa receptor blocker abciximab on outcome in patients with acute coronary syndromes withour early coronary revascualrization: the GUSTO IV–ACS randomised trial. Lancet 2001;357(9272):1915–1924.

85. Anderson KM, Califf RM, Stone GW, Neumann F-J, Montalescot G, Miller DP, et al. Long-term mortality benefit with abciximab in patients undergoing percutnaeous interventions. J Am Coll Cardiol 2001;37(8):2059–2065.

86. Montalescot G, Barragan P, Wittenberg O, et al. Platelet glycoprotein IIb/IIIa inhibition with coronary stenting for acute mayocardial infarction. N Engl J Med 2001;344:1895–1903.

87. O'Shea JC, Hafley GE, Greenberg S, Hasselblad V, Lorenz TJ, Kitt MM, et al. Platelet glycoprotein IIb/IIIa integrin blockade with eptifibatide in coronary stent intervention. The ESPRIT Trial: a randomized controlled trial. JAMA 2001;285:2468–2473.

88. Mak KH, Effron MB, Moliterno DJ. Platelet glycoprotein IIb/IIIa receptor antagonists and their use in elderly patients. Drugs Aging 2000;3:179–187.

89. Fibrinolytic Therapy Trialists Collaborative Group. Indications for fibrinolytic therapy in suspected acute myocardial infarction: collaborative overview of early mortality and major morbidity results from all randomised trials of more that 1000 patients. Lancet 1994;343:311–322.

90. Maggioni AP, Maseri A, Fresco C. Age-related increase in mortality among patients with first myocardial infarction treated with thrombolysis. N Engl J Med 1993;329:1442–1448.

91. Thiemann DR, Coresh J, Schulman SP, Gerstenblith G, Oetgen WR, Powe NR. Lack of benefit of for intravenous thrombolysis in patients with myocardial infarction who are older than 75 years. Circulation 2000;101:2239–2246.

92. Ryan TJ, Antman EM, Brooks NH, et al. ACC/AHA 1999 update: ACC/AHA guidelines for the management of patients with acute myocardial infarction. J Am Coll Cardiol 1999;34(3):890–911.

93. Gurwitz JH, McLaughlin TJ, Willison DJ, Guadagnoli E, Hauptman PJ, Gao X, et al. Delayed hospital presentation in patients who have had acute myocardial infarction. Ann Intern Med 1997;126(8): 593–599.

94. Krumholz HM, Friesinger GC, Cook EF. Relationship of age with eligibility for thrombolytic therapy and mortality among patients with suspected acute myocardial infarction. J Am Geriatr Soc 1994;42: 127–131.

95. White HD, Barbbash GI, Califf RM. Age and outcome with contemporary thrombolytic therapy: results from the GUSTO-1 trial. Circulation 1996;94:1826–1833.

96. Menon V, Berkowitz SD, Antman EM, Fuchs RM, Hochman JS. New heparin dosing recommendations for patients with acute coronary syndromes. Am J Med 2001;110(8):641–650.

97. Cannon CP, Gibson CM, McCabe CH. TNK-Tissue plasminogen activator compared with frontloaded alteplase in acute myocardial infarction: results of the TIMI 10b trial. Circulation 1998;98: 2805–2814.

98. ASSENT Investigators. Single-bolus tenecteplase compared with front-loaded alteplase in acute myocardial infarction. The ASSENT-2 double-blind randomised trial. Lancet 1999;354:716–722.

99. Cohen M, Demers C, Gurfinkel EP, Turpie AG, Fromell GJ, Goodman S, et al. A comparison of lowmolecular-weight heparin with unfractionated heparin for unstable coronary artery disease. N Engl J Med 1997;337(7):447–452.

100. Antman EM, McCabe CH, Gurfinkel EP, Turpie AG, Bernink PJ, Salein D, et al. Enoxaparin prevents death and cardiac ischemic events in unstable angina/non-Q-wave myocardial infarction. Results of the Thrombolysis in Myocardial Infarction (TIMI) 11B Trial. Circulation 1999;100:1593–1601.

101. Harris T, Cook EF, Kannel WB, Goldman L. Proportional hazards analysis of risk factors for coronary heart disease in individuals aged 65 or older: the Framingham Heart Study. J Am Geriatr Soc 1988;36: 1023–1028.

102. Corti MC, Guralnik JM, Salive ME. Clarifying the direct relation between total cholesterol levels and death from coronary heart disease in older persons. Ann Intern Med 1997;126:753–760.

103. Carlsson CM, Carnes M, McBride PE, Stein JH. Managing dyslipidemia in older adults. J Am Geriatr Soc 1999;47:1458–1465.

104. Scandanavian Simvastatin Survival Study. Randomised trial of cholesterol lowering in 4444 patients with coronary heart disease: the Scandinavian Simvastatin Survival Study (4S). Lancet 1994;344: 1383–1389.

105. Sacks FM, Pfeffer MA, Moye LA, Rouleau J-L, Rutherford JD, Cole TG, et al. The effect of pravastatin on coronary events after myocardial infarction in patients with average cholesterol levels. N Engl J Med 1996;335(14):1001–1009.

106. Fonarow GC, French WJ, Parsons LS, Sun H, Malmgren JA. Use of lipid-lowering medications at discharge in patients with acute myocardial infarction. Data from the National Registry of Myocardial Infarction 3. Circulation 2001;103:38–44.

107. Rich SE, Shah J, Rich DS, Shah R, Rich MW. Effects of age, sex, race, diagnosis-related group, and hospital setting on lipid managment in patients with coronary artery disease. Am J Cardiol 2000;86: 328–330.

108. Santinga JT, Rosman HS, Rubenfire M. Efficacy and safety of pravastatin in the long-term treatment of elderly patients with hypercholesterolemia. Am J Med 1994;96:509–515.

109. LaRosa JC, Applegate W, Crouse JR. Cholesterol lowering in the elderly: results of the Cholesterol Reduction in Seniors Program (CRISP) Pilot Study. Arch Intern Med 1994;154:529–539.

110. Miettinen TA, Pyörälä K, Alsson AG. Cholesterol-lowering therapy in women and elderly patients with myocardial infarction or angina pectoris: findings from the Scandanavian Simvastatin Survival Study (4S). Circulation 1997;96:4211–4218.

111. Black DM, Bakker-Arkema RG, Nawrocki JW. An overview of the clinical safety profile of atorvastatin (Lipitor), a new HMG-CoA reductase inhibitor. Arch Intern Med 158, 577–584.

112. Whitney E, Downs JR, Clearfield M. Air Force/Texas Coronary Atherosclerosis Prevention Study: extending the benefit of primary prevention to healthy elderly men and women. Circulation 1998;98:I–46.

113. Shepherd J, Cobbe SM, Ford I, Isles CG, Lorimer AR, MacFarlane PW, et al. Prevention of coronary heart disease with pravastatin in men with hypercholesterolemia. West of Scotland Coronary Prevention Study Group. N Engl J Med 1995;333(20):1301–1307.

114. Weintraub WS, Mahoney E, Ghazzal Z. Trends in outcome and costs of coronary intervention in the 1990's. Am J Cardiol 2001;88:497–503.

115. Thompson RC, Holmes DR Jr, Grill DE, Mock MB, Bailey KR. Changing outcomes of angioplasty in the elderly. J Am Coll Cardiol 1996;27:8–14.

116. Abenhaim HA, Eisenberg MJ, Schechter D. Comparison of six-month outcomes of percutaneous transluminal coronary angioplasty in patients ≥75 with those <75 years of age (The ROSETTA Registry). Am J Cardiol 2001;87:1392–1395.

117. Antoniucci D, Valenti R, Santoro GM, Bolognese L, Moschi G, Trapani M, et al. Systematic primary angioplasty in octogenarian and older patients. Am Heart J 1999;138(4):670–674.

118. Batchelor WB, Anstrom KJ, Muhlbaier LH, Grosswald R, Weintraub WS, O'Neill WW, et al. Contemporary outcome trends in the elderly undergoing percutaneous coronary interventions: results in 7,472 octogenarians. J Am Coll Cardiol 2000;36(3):723–730.

119. Ang PC, Farouque HM, Harper RW, Meredith IT. Percutaneous coronary intervention in the elderly: a comparison of procedural and clinical outcomes between the eighth and ninth decades. J Invasive Cardiol 2000;12(10):488–494.

120. Gravina Taddei CF, Weintraub WS, Douglas JS, Ghazzal Z, Mahoney E, Thompson T, et al. Influence of age on outcome after percutaneous transluminal coronary angioplasty. Am J Cardiol 1999;84:245–251.

121. DeGeare VS, Stone GW, Grines L, Brodie BR, Cox DA, Garcia E, et al. Angiographic and clinical characteristics associated with increased in-hospital mortality in elderly patients with acute myocardial infarction undergoing percutaneous intervention (a pooled analysis of the primary angioplasty in myocardial infarction trials). Am J Cardiol 2000;86:30–34.

122. Morrison DA, Sethi G, Sacks J. Percutaneous coronary intervention versus coronary artery bypass graft surgery for patients with medically refractory myocardial ischemia and risk factors for adverse outcomes with bypass: a multicenter, randomized trial. J Am Coll Cardiol 2001;38:143–149.

123. Cote AV, Berger PB, Holmes DR Jr, Scott CG, Bell MR. Hemmorhagic and vascular complications after percutaneous coronary intervention with adjunctive abciximab. Mayo Clin Proc 2001;76:890–896.

124. Seto TB, Taira DA, Berezin R, Chauhan MS, Cutlip DE, Ho KK, et al. Percutaneous coronary revascularization in elderly patients: impact on functional status and quality of life. Ann Intern Med 2000;132: 955–958.

125. Weaver WD, Simes RJ, Betriu A. Comparison of primary angioplasty and intravenous thrombolytic therapy for acute myocardial infarction. JAMA 1997;278:2093–2098.

126. Fishman DL, Leon MB, Baim DS. A randomized comparison of coronary-stent placement and balloon angioplasty in the treatment of coronary artery disease. N Engl J Med 1994;331:496–501.

127. Ritchie JL, Maynard C, Every NR, Chapko MK. Coronary artery stent outcomes in a Medicare population: less emergency bypass surgery and lower mortality rates in patients with stents. Am Heart J 1999; 138(3):437–440.

128. Zhu MM, Feit A, Chadow H, Alam M, Kwan T, Clark LT. Primary stent implantation compared with primary balloon angioplasty for acute myocardial infarction: a meta-analysis of randomized clinical trials. Am J Cardiol 2001;88:297–301.

129. GUSTO Investigators. An international randomized trial comparing four thrombolytic strategies for acute myocardial infarction. N Engl J Med 1993;329:673–682.

130. The TIMI Research Group. Immediate vs. delayed catheterization and angioplasty following thrombolytic therapy for acute myocardial infarction: TIMI IIA results. JAMA 1988;260:2849–2858.

131. Gimelli G, Kalra A, Sabatine MS, Jang IK. Primary versus rescue percutaneous coronary intervention in patients with acute myocardial infarction. Acta Cardiol 2000;55:187–192.

132. Ellis SG, da Silva ER, Heyndricks G. Randomized comparison of rescue angioplasty with conservative management of patients with early failure of thrombolysis for acute anterior myocardial infarction. Circulation 1994;90:2280–2284.

133. Ross AM, Lundergan CF, Rohrbeck SC, Boyle DH, van den Brand M, Buller CH, et al. Rescue angioplasty after failed thrombolysis: technical and clinical outcomes in a large thrombolysis trial. GUSTO-1 Angiographic Investigators. Global Utilization of Streptokinase and Tissue Plasminogen Activator for Occluded Coronary Arteries. J Am Coll Cardiol 1998;7:1511–1517.

134. Califf RM, Bengston JR. Cardiogenic shock. N Engl J Med 1994;330:1724–1730.

135. Kang N, Edwards M, Larbalestier R. Preoperative intraaortic balloon pumps in high-risk patients undergoing open heart surgery. Ann Thorac Surg 2001;72:54–57.

136. Christenson JT, Simonet F, Badel P, Schmuziger M. Evaluation of preoperative intraaortic balloon pump support in high risk coronary patients. Eur J Cardio-thorac Surg 1997;11:1097–1103.

137. Craver JM, Murrah CP. Elective intraaortic balloon counterpulsation for high-risk off-pump coronary bypass operations. Ann Thorac Surg 2001;71:1220–1223.

138. Hasdai D, Topol EJ, Califf RM, Berger PB, Holmes DR Jr. Cardiogenic shock complicating acute coronary syndromes. Lancet 2000;356:749–756.

139. Barron HV, Every NR, Parsons LS, Angeja B, Goldberg RJ, Gore JM, et al. The use of intra-aortic balloon counterpulsation in patients with cardiogenic shock complicating acute myocardial infarction: data from the National Registry of Myocardial Infarction 2. Am Heart J 2001;141:933–939.

140. Prewitt RM, Gu S, Garber PJ, Ducas J. Marked systemic hypotension depresses coronary thrombolysis induced by intracoronary adminstration of recombinant tissue-type plasminogen activator. J Am Coll Cardiol 1992;20:1626–1633.

141. Prewitt RM, Gu S, Schick U, Ducas J. Intraaortic balloon counterpulsation enhances coronary thrombolysis induced by intravenous administration of a thrombolytic agent. J Am Coll Cardiol 1994;23:794–798.

142. Kovack PJ, Rasak MA, Bates ER, Ohman EM, Stomel RJ. Thrombolysis plus aortic counterpulsation: improved survival in patients who present to community hospitals with cardiogenic shock. J Am Coll Cardiol 1997;29:1454–1458.

143. Stone GW, Marsalese D, Brodie BR. A prospective, randomized evaluation of prophylactic intraaortic balloon counterpulsation in high risk patients with acute myocardial infarction treated with angioplasty. J Am Coll Cardiol 1997;29:1459–1467.

144. Shah MR, O'Connor CM, Sopko G, Hasselblad V, Califf RM, Stevenson LW. Evaluation Study of Congestive Heart Failure and Pulmonary Artery Catherization Effectiveness (ESCAPE): design and rationale. Am Heart J 2001;141:528–535.

145. Peterson ED, Cowper PA, Jollis JG. Outcomes of coronary artery bypass graft surgery in 24461 patients aged 80 years or older. Circulation 1995;92(Suppl II):II-85–II-95.

146. Roach GW, Kanchuger M, Mangano CM. Adverse cerebral outcomes after coronary bypass surgery. N Engl J Med 1996;335:1857–1863.

147. Newman MF, Kirchner JL, Phillips-Bute B. Longitudinal assessment of neurocognitive function after coronary-artery bypass surgery. N Engl J Med 2001;344:395–402.

148. Glower DD, Christopher TD, Milano CA. Performance status and outcome after coronary artery bypass grafting in persons 80 to 93 years. Am J Cardiol 1992;70:567–571.

149. Diegeler A, Hirsch R, Schneider F. Neuromonitoring and neurocognitive outcome in off-pump versus conventional coronary bypass operation. Ann Thorac Surg 2000;69:1162–1166.

150. Stratton JR, Levy WC, Cerqueira MD. Cardiovascular responses to exercise: effects of aging and exercise training in healthy men. Circulation 1994;89:1648–1655.

151. Schulman SP, Fleg JL. Stress testing for coronary artery disease in the elderly. Clin Geriatr Med 1996; 12:101–119.

152. Chaitman BR, Bourassa MG, Davis K. Angiographic prevalence of high-risk coronary artery disease in patient subsets (CASS). Circulation 1981;64:360–368.

153. Ritchie JL, Gibbon RJ, Cheitlin MD. ACC/AHA guidelines for exercise testing. J Am Coll Cardiol 1997; 30:260–315.

154. Cole CR, Blackstone EH, Pashkow FJ, Snader CE, Lauer MS. Heart-rate recovery immediately after exercise as a predictor of mortality. N Engl J Med 1999;341:1351–1357.

155. Fleg JL, Gerstenblith G, Zonderman AB, Becker LC, Weisfeldt ML, Costa PT Jr, et al. Prevalence and prognostic significance of exercise-induced silent myocardial ischemia detected by thallium scintigraphy and electrocardiography in asymptomatic volunteers. Circulation 1990;81:428–436.

156. Iskandrian AS, Heo J, Decoskey D. Use of exercise thallium-201 imaging for risk stratification of elderly patients with coronary artery disease. Am J Cardiol 1988;61:269–275.

157. Arruda AM, Das MK, Roger VL, Klarich KW, Mahoney DW, Pellikka PA. Prognostic value of exercise echocardiography in 2,632 patients ≥65 years of age. J Am Coll Cardiol 2001;37:1036–1041.

158. Anthopoulos LP, Bonou MS, Kardaras FG. Stress echocardiography in elderly patients with coronary artery disease. J Am Coll Cardiol 1996;28:52–59.

159. The TIME Investigators. Trial of invasive versus medical therapy in elderly patients with chronic symptomatic coronary artery disease (TIME): a randomised trial. Lancet 2001;358:951–957.

160. Grines CL, Browne KF, Marco J. A comparison of immediate angioplasty with thrombolytic therapy for acute myocardial infarction. N Engl J Med 1993;328:673–679.

161. GUSTO IIb Angioplasty Substudy Investigators. A clinical trial comparing primary coronary angioplasty with tissue plasminogen activator for acute myocardial infarction. N Engl J Med 1997;336(23): 1621–1628.

162. Montalescot G, Barragan P, Wittenberg O. Platelet glycoprotein IIb/IIIa inhibition with coronary stenting for acute myocardial infarction. N Engl J Med 2001;344:1895–1903.

163. Schomig A, Kastrati A, Dirschinger J. Coronary stenting plus platelet glycoprotein IIb/IIIa blockade compared with tissue plasminogen activator in acute myocardial infarction. N Engl J Med 2000;343: 385–391.

164. Zijlstra F, Hoorntje JCA, de Boer M-J. Long-term benefit of primary angioplasty as compared with thrombolytic therapy for acute myocardial infarction. N Engl J Med 1999;341:1413–1419.

165. Berger PB, Ellis SG, Holmes DR Jr. Relationship between delay in preforming direct coronary angioplasty and early clinical outcome in patients with acute myocardial infarction. Circulation 2001;100:14–20.

166. Goldberg RJ, Samad NA, Yarzebski J, Gurwitz JH, Bigelow C, Gore JM. Temporal trends in cardiogenic shock complicating acute myocardial infarction. N Engl J Med 1999;340:1162–1168.

167. Holmes DR Jr, Berger PB, Hochman JS. Cardiogenic shock in patients with acute ischemic syndromes with and without ST-segment elevation. Circulation 1999;100:2067–2073.

168. Hasdai D, Califf RM, Thompson TD. Predictors of cardiogenic shock after thrombolytic therapy for acute myocardial infarction. J Am Coll Cardiol 2000;35:136–143.

169. Berger PB, Holmes DR Jr, Stebbins AL, Bates ER, Califf RM, Topol EJ. Impact of an aggressive invasive catheterization and revascularization strategy on mortality in patients with cardiogenic shock in the Global Utilization of Streptokinase and Tissue Plasminogen Activator for Occluded Coronary Arteries (GUSTO-I) Trial. Circulation 1997;96:122–127.

170. Hochman JS, Sleeper LA, Webb JG. Early revascularization in acute myocardial infarction complicated by cardiogenic shock. N Engl J Med 1999;341:625–634.

171. Hochman JS, Sleeper LA, White HD. One-year survival following early revascularization for cardiogenic shock. JAMA 2001;285:190–192.

172. Hochman JS, Buller CE, Sleeper LA. Cardiogenic shock complicating acute myocardial infarction—etiologies, management and outcome; overall findings of the SHOCK Trial Registry. J Am Coll Cardiol 2000;36:1063–1070.

14 Heart Failure

With an Emphasis on Diastolic Heart Failure

Dalane W. Kitzman, MD

INTRODUCTION

Until recently, there were almost no data regarding the etiology, pathophysiology, diagnosis, prognosis, and management of older patients with heart failure. Uncertainty as a result of the large gaps in our knowledge, coupled with recognition of the marked public health implications of heart failure among the elderly, lays the foundation for a number of controversies in this area. In order to address these controversies, this chapter will focus on those aspects of heart failure that are particular to the older patient.

EPIDEMIOLOGY AND RISKS FACTORS

The prevalence and incidence of heart failure (HF) increase dramatically with age. In the Framingham Heart Study, the incidence of congestive heart failure (CHF) was observed to increase approximately fivefold from age 40 to 70 *(1)*. In contrast to the decline in overall cardiovascular disease over the past two decades, rates of CHF in the United States are increasing dramatically, as a result of the aging of the population *(2)*.

Even within the older group, CHF prevalence increases substantially with age, in both men and women. In the Cardiovascular Health Study, a population-based observational study of cardiovascular risk conducted exclusively in the elderly, CHF prevalence increased

From: *Aging, Heart Disease, and Its Management: Facts and Controversies*
Edited by: N. Edwards, M. Maurer, and R. Wellner © Humana Press Inc., Totowa, NJ

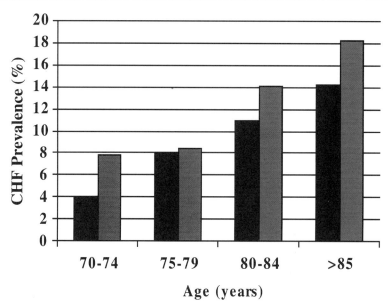

Fig. 1. Prevalence of congestive heart failure versus age in elderly men (solid bars) and women (hatched bars) in the Cardiovascular Health Study. Even in an older cohort such as this, CHF prevalence increased with age. Adapted from ref. *3*.

in women from 4.1% at age 70 to 14.3% at age 85 (*see* Fig. 1) *(3)*. CHF prevalence was higher in men but with a similar age trend (7.8% increasing to 18.4%) *(3)*. During 6 yr of follow-up in the Cardiovascular Health Study, the incidence of CHF was 10.6/1000 person-years at age 65 and 42.5/1000 person-years at age ≥80 *(4)*. Other population-based studies have shown similar results *(2,5)*. In the Cardiovascular Health Study, the prevalence and incidence of CHF were similar in African-Americans and in whites *(3,4)*.

Risk factors for the development of CHF in the elderly were recently reported in the Cardiovascular Health Study (CHS) and in another study *(4,5)*. The strongest risk factors were age, male gender, ischemic heart disease, systolic hypertension, and diabetes. Using a standardized battery of tests, CHS found that additional independent predictors of heart failure in the elderly included reduced force expiratory vital capacity, renal dysfunction, stroke, increased C-reactive protein, reduced ankle–brachial index, atrial fibrillation, and left-ventricular (LV) hypertrophy *(4)*. In the East Boston Senior Health Project, increased pulse pressure, a measure of arterial stiffness, was also an independent risk factor for CHF *(6)*. Systolic hypertension may be one of the most important risk factors for CHF, particularly in older women, and is modifiable *(7–9)*.

Older patients often develop CHF in the presence of preserved left-ventricular systolic function, in contrast to younger patients, in whom systolic dysfunction predominates. This syndrome, presumptively termed diastolic heart failure (DHF), was first described by Luchi et al. in 1982 in a consecutive series of hospitalized elderly men with acute CHF *(10)*. More recently, in the population-based Olmsted Community project, records were reviewed from all patients during a 1 yr period in whom an assessment of LV ejection fraction (EF) was obtained within 3 wk of newly diagnosed CHF *(11)*. The average patient age was 71 yr. A normal EF was found in 43% of patients, and this phenomenon increased with age. This was the form of heart failure seen in all patients age ≥100 yr, whereas it was

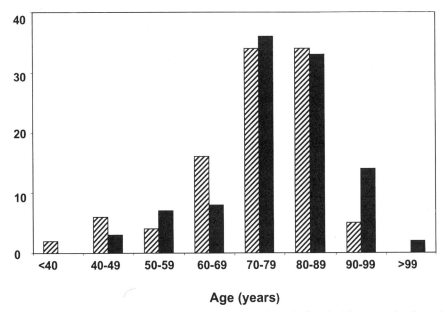

Fig. 2. Numbers of patients in Olmsted County, Minnesota hospitalized with congestive heart failure in 1991 versus age with normal (solid bars) and reduced (hatched bars) ejection fraction. Note that CHF with a normal ejection fraction is absent in the youngest group (age <40 yr) in contrast to the oldest group (age >99), where it comprises essentially all patients. Adapted from ref. *11*.

not seen in those <40 yr old (*see* Fig. 2) *(11)*. Population-based reports are also available from the Framingham Study *(12)*, the Cardiovascular Health Study *(3,13)*, and the Strong Heart Study of American Indians *(14)*. All of these population-based databases suggest that 50% or more of elderly patients with CHF have normal LV ejection fractions.

There is a strong female preponderance in DHF. In the Cardiovascular Health Study, 67% of elderly women and 42% of men with CHF had normal ejection fractions *(3)*. During a 6 yr follow-up in the Cardiovascular Health Study, over 90% of women who developed heart failure had normal systolic function *(4)*. Because women significantly outnumber men in the older population, the population attributable risk of reduced systolic function was relatively small *(4)*. Thus, the typical person with heart failure living in the community is an older woman with normal left-ventricular systolic function and systolic hypertension. This contrasts significantly with the typical patient seen in referral heart failure clinics, who is a middle-aged man with severely reduced systolic function and ischemic heart disease (*see* Table 1) *(15)*.

PATHOPHYSIOLOGY

Relatively little data are available comparing young and old heart failure patients. However, available data suggesting that the pathophysiology of heart failure may differ substantially in older patients because of differences resulting from "normal" aging changes, etiology, comorbidity, and increased heterogeneity. A number of "normal" age-related changes in cardiovascular structure and function are relevant, including increased arterial and myocardial stiffness, decreased diastolic myocardial relaxation, increased LV mass, decreased peak

Table 1
Heart Failure in Older vs Middle-Aged Patients

Characteristic	Elderly	Middle-aged
Prevalence	6–18%	<1%
Gender	Predominantly women	Predominantly men
Etiology	Hypertension	Coronary artery disease
Left-ventricular systolic function	Normal	Impaired
Comorbidities	Multiple	Few

Source: Adapted from ref. *16*.

contractility, reduced myocardial and vascular responsiveness to β-adrenergic stimulation, decreased coronary flow reserve, and decreased mitochondrial response to increased demand for adenosine triphosphate (ATP) production *(16)*. The net effect of these changes is decreased cardiovascular reserve; this can be measured as an approximately 1% per year decline in maximal exercise oxygen consumption *(17)*. Consequently, insults from acute myocardial ischemia or infarction, poorly controlled hypertension, atrial fibrillation, iatrogenic volume overload, and pneumonia, which would be tolerated in younger patients, can cause acute CHF in older persons *(16)*.

Older patients also have normal underlying age-related changes in other organ systems that can impair their ability to compensate for heart failure *(16)*. These include a gradual decline in creatinine clearance, impaired fluid and electrolyte homeostasis, reduced ventilatory capacity and increased ventilation/perfusion (V/Q) mismatching and pulmonary vascular resistance, reduced central nervous system autoregulatory capacity, skeletal muscle sarcopenia, as well as altered pharmacodynamics and pharmacokinetics. Although each of these has been documented in studies of normal aging, their role in altering the compensatory response to HF in older patients is controversial, as there is almost no information on how these affect the older HF patients.

Older HF patients also experience many more comorbidities than those that are younger; these have specific implications (*see* Table 2) *(18)*. Concomitant renal dysfunction or pulmonary disease are particularly problematic in the management of the older HF patient. The combination of comorbidities and age-related changes in cardiovascular function and in other organ systems lowers the threshold for HF, exacerbates symptoms and prognosis, and complicates management.

The pathophysiology of systolic heart failure (SHF) has been examined intensively, but these studies have almost uniformly excluded older patients *(18)*. Given the above discussion, older patients would be expected to differ substantially. Furthermore, older patients with SHF more frequently have an ischemic etiology and more severe exercise intolerance, the mechanisms of which are uncertain even in young SHF patients, who have been intensively studied for years *(18)*. Thus, much of the literature on SHF may not necessarily apply to older patients. One notable exception to the exclusion of older patients was a study by Cody et al. *(19)*, who performed detailed hemodynamic, renal, and hormonal assessments in 128 young vs old HF patients, focusing specifically on age-related differences. The older group had higher systemic vascular resistance, norepinephrine, serum urea, serum creatinine, and lower glomerular filtration rate compared to younger patients *(19)*.

Table 2
Comorbidities in Older Heart Failure Patients

Condition	Implications
Renal dysfunction	Exacerbates symptoms, prognosis; exacerbated by diuretics, ACE[a] inhibitors
Chronic lung disease	Exacerbates symptoms, prognosis; contributes to uncertainty about diagnosis/volume status
Cognitive dysfunction	Interferes with dietary, medication, activity compliance
Depression, social isolation	Exacerbates prognosis, interferes with compliance
Postural hypotension, falls	Exacerbated by vasodilators, diuretics, β-blockers
Urinary incontinence	Aggravated by diuretics, ACE inhibitors (cough)
Sensory deprivation	Interferes with compliance
Nutritional disorders	Exacerbated by dietary restrictions
Polypharmacy	Compliance issues, drug interactions
Frailty	Exacerbates symptoms and quality of life; exacerbated by hospitalization; increased fall risk

[a]ACE: angiotensin-converting enzyme.
Source: Adapted from ref. *16.*

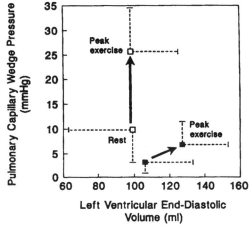

Fig. 3. Left-ventricular diastolic function assessed by invasive cardiopulmonary exercise testing in patients with heart failure and normal systolic function (open boxes) and age-matched normals (filled boxes). The pressure–volume relation was shifted upward and leftward at rest. In the patients with exercise, LV diastolic volume did not increase despite marked increase in diastolic (pulmonary wedge) pressure. Because of diastolic dysfunction, failure of the Frank–Starling mechanism resulted in severe exercise intolerance. From ref. *20* with permission.

The situation is compounded by the fact that the majority of elderly HF patients have preserved systolic function (presumably DHF) and there is very little information regarding the pathophysiology of this disorder. Using invasive cardiopulmonary exercise testing, it was demonstrated that patients with this syndrome have severe exercise intolerance. This is the result of an inability to increase stroke volume via the Frank–Starling mechanism despite increased LV filling pressure, indicative of diastolic dysfunction (*see* Fig. 3) *(20).* This results in severely reduced exercise cardiac output and early lactate formation that appears responsible for the reduced exercise capacity.

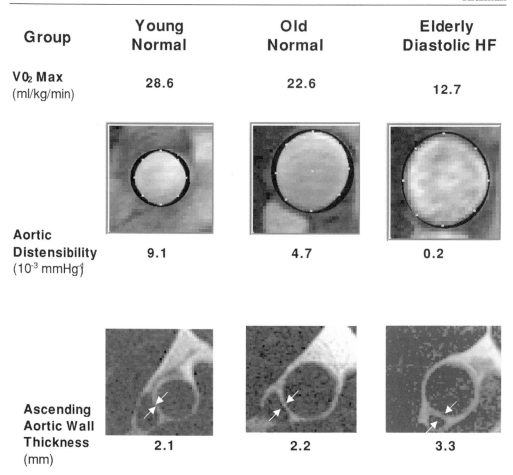

Group	Young Normal	Old Normal	Elderly Diastolic HF
VO$_2$ Max (ml/kg/min)	28.6	22.6	12.7
Aortic Distensibility (10^{-3} mmHg)	9.1	4.7	0.2
Ascending Aortic Wall Thickness (mm)	2.1	2.2	3.3

Fig. 4. Data and images from representative subjects from healthy young, healthy elderly, and elderly patients with diastolic heart failure. Maximal exercise oxygen consumption (VO$_2$max), aortic distensibility at rest, and left-ventricular mass:volume ratio. Patients with diastolic heart failure have severely reduced exercise tolerance (VO$_2$max) and aortic distensibility and increased aortic wall thickness. Adapted from ref. *21* with permission.

Exercise intolerance, manifest as exertional dyspnea and fatigue, is the primary symptom in chronic HF with either a reduced or a normal ejection fraction. A recent study indicates that decreased aortic distensibility, perhaps the result of the combined effects of aging- and hypertension-induced thickening and remodeling of the thoracic aortic wall, may be an important contributor to exercise intolerance in chronic DHF. Magnetic resonance imaging (MRI) and maximal exercise testing with expired gas analysis were performed in a group of elderly patients with isolated DHF and in age-matched healthy subjects. The patients with DHF had increased pulse pressure and thoracic aortic wall thickness and markedly decreased aortic distensibility, which correlated closely with their severely decreased exercise capacity (*see* Figs. 4 and 5) *(21)*.

Several lines of evidence suggest that systemic hypertension plays an important role in the genesis of DHF. In animal models, diastolic dysfunction develops early with systemic hypertension, and LV diastolic relaxation is very sensitive to increased afterload *(22–27)*.

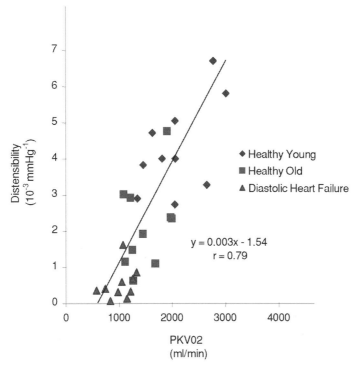

Fig. 5. A close relationship between peak VO$_2$ (horizontal axis) and proximal aortic distensibility (vertical axis) in a group of 30 subjects (10 healthy young, 10 healthy old, and 10 elderly DHF patients). Each symbol represents the data from one participant. From ref. *21* with permission.

Increased afterload may impair relaxation, leading to increased LV filling pressures, decreased stroke volume, symptoms of dyspnea, and congestion *(27)*. Nearly all (88%) DHF patients have a history of chronic systemic hypertension *(3,28)*. In addition, severe systolic hypertension is usually present during acute exacerbations (pulmonary edema) *(9,29)*.

The role of ischemia in DHF is uncertain. It would seem likely that it is a significant contributor in many cases. It has been hypothesized that patients found to have a normal ejection fraction following an episode of CHF may have had transiently reduced systolic function and ischemia at the time of the acute exacerbation. If so, then the term "diastolic heart failure" would be an inappropriate label for this disorder and all therapeutic efforts would be aimed at treatment of ischemia and reversible systolic dysfunction.

A recent study addressed this issue *(29)*. An echocardiogram was performed at the time of presentation in 38 consecutive patients with acute hypertensive pulmonary edema and was repeated again about 3 d later, after resolution of pulmonary edema and control of hypertension. The left-ventricular ejection fraction and wall-motion score index at follow-up were similar to that found during the acute echocardiogram. Furthermore, of those who had LV ejection fraction ≥50% at follow-up (*n* = 18), all but 2 had LV ejection fraction ≥50% acutely, and in those 2 cases, the LV ejection fraction was >40%, above the level that would be expected to cause acute heart failure on the basis of primary systolic dysfunction (*see* Fig. 6). These data suggest that marked transient systolic dysfunction and overt ischemia do not play a primary role in most patients who present with DHF in

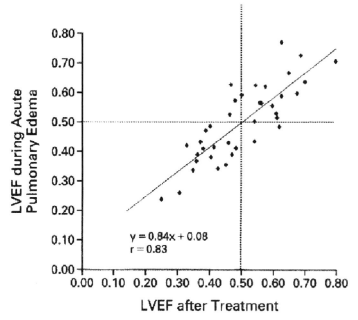

Fig. 6. Left-ventricular ejection fraction (LVEF) measured during acute pulmonary edema and at follow-up, 1–3 d after treatment. Nearly all patients found to have normal EF (>50%) at follow-up also had normal EF during acute pulmonary edema. Adapted from ref. *29*.

the presence of severe systolic hypertension. Furthermore, they support the concept that acute pulmonary edema in these patients is most likely the result of an exacerbation of diastolic dysfunction caused by severe systolic hypertension. The data also suggest that the ejection fraction measurement from an echocardiogram performed in follow-up accurately reflects that during an episode of acute pulmonary edema.

In a related study, 3 yr follow-up was performed in 46 patients who initially presented with acute hypertensive pulmonary edema *(8)*. The majority had a normal ejection fraction. Of those who were referred clinically for coronary angiography ($n = 38$), 33 had obstructive epicardial coronary artery disease and 19 underwent revascularization. However, by 6 mo follow-up, 9 of these 19 had been hospitalized with recurrent pulmonary edema and 1 had died. Severe systolic hypertension was nearly uniformly present at the time of recurrent pulmonary edema *(8)*. These two studies suggest that severe systolic hypertension plays a pivotal role in the pathogenesis of acute exacerbations of DHF.

Neurohormonal activation may play an important role in the pathophysiology of DHF, as it does in patients with SHF. In a group of patients with primary DHF, Clarkson et al. showed that atrial natriuretic peptide and brain natriuretic peptide were substantially increased, and there was an exaggerated response during exercise *(30)*, a pattern similar to that described in patients with SHF. Furthermore, atrial natriuretic peptide levels in older subjects are predictive of the subsequent development of CHF *(31)*.

The role of genetic predisposition in the genesis of DHF in the elderly is unknown. Diastolic LV relaxation is significantly modulated by β-adrenergic stimulation via phospholamban and, to a lesser extent, cardiac troponin-I, both of which are substantially under genetic control. Furthermore, data from the HyperGen study have shown significant herita-

Table 3
Alternate Explanations for Signs/Symptoms Suggestive of CHF in Elderly Patients

Dyspnea and rales
- Chronic pulmonary disease
- Pneumonia

Pedal edema
- Benign idiopathic edema
- Primary venous insufficiency
- Renal or hepatic disease
- Medications

Fatigue
- Anemia
- Hypothyroidism
- Extreme obesity
- Severe deconditioning

Aortic or mitral stenosis/regurgitation
Constrictive pericarditis
Ischemic heart disease

Cautions
- Elderly often have multiple confounding conditions
- Normal aging alone does cause of exertional fatigue, and dyspnea

bility of hypertension *(32)*, LV mass *(33)*, and Doppler diastolic filling *(34)*, all factors that likely play a role in DHF in the elderly. The genetic basis for familial hypertrophic cardiomyopathy, which has substantial phenotypic similarities to isolated DHF in the elderly, has been described *(35,36)*. It is noteworthy that in this disorder, the phenotype may not express itself for 30 to 50 yr. It has been hypothesized that relatively modest point mutations that would not lead to detectable phenotypes in skeletal muscle do so in the heart after several decades because of the constant demands on the heart muscle. This model has important implications for isolated DHF in the elderly and it would not be surprising if genetic studies were to reveal genetic links to this disorder.

DIAGNOSIS AND CLINICAL FEATURES

The clinical diagnosis of HF is complicated by the fact that it is based on a constellation of signs and symptoms, the exclusion of alternative diagnoses, none of the signs and symptoms is specific for CHF, and there is no confirmatory laboratory test. This has led to substantial controversy, as demonstrated by the many competing case definitions used in different studies *(37,38)*. Unfortunately, the diagnostic process is even more challenging in the elderly. First, older patients are much more likely to have comorbid conditions that produce signs and symptoms consistent with heart failure (*see* Table 3). Except for those noted in Table 3, physical signs of CHF are similar in the elderly and in the young. In older persons, a fourth heart sound (S_4 gallop), particularly if soft, can be normal; however, a third heart sound (S_3 or early diastolic gallop) is usually pathologic. Second, a reliable history may be more difficult to obtain because of cognitive or sensory impairment. Third, atypical presentations are more common in elderly patients; CHF may present as somnolence, confusion, disorientation, weakness, fatigue, and failure to thrive. Fourth, patients often fail to perceive substantial declines in exercise tolerance that occur incrementally, or they attribute them to old age. In these cases, it is helpful to encourage patients to recall tasks that have become difficult or are now avoided altogether. Older patients are often voluntarily sedentary, and when impairment develops, they merely decrease their activity level further, thus avoiding symptoms. Fifth, as discussed earlier, elderly heart failure patients often have a normal ejection fraction. Although reduced ejection fraction measurement is not part of the clinical diagnosis of heart failure, its presence is a reassuring confirmation of the presence of one LV substrate known to predispose to CHF.

The distinction between HF resulting from systolic dysfunction versus diastolic dysfunction usually *cannot* be made reliably at the bedside (39), and evaluation of new onset HF in an elderly patient should include an imaging test, usually an echocardiogram. This will not only assess systolic function but also exclude unexpected but important diagnoses, such as aortic stenosis, severe valvular regurgitation, large pericardial effusion, hypertrophic obstructive cardiomyopathy, and cardiac amyloidosis.

Unfortunately, a definitive noninvasive measure is not available for diastolic dysfunction. Doppler left-ventricular diastolic filling indexes and, particularly, the newer tissue Doppler techniques (40) can provide helpful supplementary information, but their role in the clinical diagnosis of the DHF syndrome is unclear and their independent discriminatory power in unselected populations is not known.

The diagnostic criteria from the European Study Group on Diastolic Heart Failure (41) include signs and symptoms of congestive heart failure, a normal or at most mildly reduced LVEF, and evidence of abnormal diastolic function. The modifications of these criteria by Vasan and Levy (38) and those that follow from the findings of Gandhi et al. discussed earlier (29), suggest that DHF diagnosis can usually be made without the mandate for measurement of ejection fraction at the time of the acute event. Invasive measures of diastolic function are impractical and not feasible in most circumstances. The necessity of these abnormal filling parameters for the diagnosis of DHF, required by the European Study Group criteria, has been obviated by a recent report indicating that nearly all patients who meet the other criteria for DHF will have diastolic dysfunction if invasive measurements were made (42). Care must always be taken to consider other causes for the signs and symptoms suggesting heart failure, as displayed in Table 3. Because active myocardial ischemia can present as HF, particularly in the elderly, and has independent prognostic and therapeutic implications, a stress test is often indicated; in the case of concomitant severe or unstable angina, coronary angiography is recommended. Patients with HF, a normal ejection fraction, and no other explanation for their symptoms carry a diagnosis of *isolated* DHF. In the Cardiovascular Health Study, this subgroup comprised 42% of the patients with CHF and a normal ejection fraction (3). Typical patients with isolated DHF often have high normal or super normal ejection fraction (70% or more), normal or small left-ventricular chamber size, thick walls with concentric hypertrophy, and no segmental wall-motion abnormalities.

Recent studies suggest that rapid brain natriuretic peptide (BNP) assays could aid in the diagnosis of HF, particularly in the emergency setting, and may help in judging disease severity (18). Recently, rapid-assay kits have become commercially available and have been heavily marketed, creating some degree of controversy regarding their utility. However, as expressed in the recent revision of the American College of Cardiology (ACC)/ American Heart Association (AHA) guidelines, the role of BNP assays in the routine evaluation and management of HF patients remains to be defined (18). Furthermore, it is unclear what diagnostic value such assays may have in chronic stable HF patients. A heart-failure specific lab test might be particularly useful in older patients, for whom the diagnosis is often more challenging. However, it is known that atrial natriuretic peptide and possibly also BNP increases mildly as part of the aging process, so that the specificity of the assays for older vs younger patients needs to be defined *(43)*. Furthermore, because BNP appears to be increased in DHF as well as in systolic failure *(30)*, it may not be helpful in discriminating between these two disorders *(18)*. Atrial natriuretic peptide levels are indicative of CHF risk within groups of elderly *(31)*.

PROGNOSIS

Elderly patients with HF suffer substantial morbidity, manifested by chronic exercise intolerance *(20,44)*, and acute exacerbations leading to frequent hospitalization *(45–48)*. The severity of exercise intolerance and the frequency of hospitalization appear to be similar in elderly with systolic vs diastolic HF *(44,45,49–51)*. Within 3 to 6 mo, 30–50% of initially hospitalized older patients have been rehospitalized. This high rate of rehospitalization is associated with poor quality of life and high health care costs. Older HF patients also have a high rate of other morbid outcomes, including stroke and myocardial infarction *(52)*.

Heart failure mortality increases substantially with advancing age and is nearly threefold higher in the group aged 65–74 yr compared to those aged 25–54 yr *(53)*. In community-dwelling persons aged 65–74 yr, the 10 yr mortality was 50% in women and over 70% in men *(53)*. In the elderly who have been hospitalized, the prognosis is even worse, with 33% 1 yr mortality and >70% 5 yr mortality *(52)*. Mortality was similar in blacks and whites *(52)*. Dishearteningly, comparisons of population databases suggest that there has been no improvement in mortality over the last few decades *(52–54)*.

The annual mortality rate for *diastolic* HF in the Framingham Study was 8.9% per year, twice as high as nested case controls, although it was only half that reported for SHF (19.6%) *(12)*. Similar results were found in the Cardiovascular Health Study *(55)*. However, in elderly *hospitalized* patients, mortality is similar with diastolic and systolic HF *(see* Fig. 7) *(11,45, 49,56,57)*. An important observation in the Cardiovascular Health Study was that, given the higher prevalence among the elderly, the population attributable mortality risk in patients with DHF is higher than in those with SHF, highlighting the public health implications of DHF in the elderly *(55)*.

The predictors of mortality in older HF patients are similar to those in younger patients and include age, gender (worse in men), recent hospitalization, diabetes, LV dilation and systolic dysfunction, renal dysfunction, hyponatremia, reduced peak oxygen consumption, and increased minute ventilation/carbon dioxide production during exercise *(52,55,58,59)*.

MANAGEMENT

Management goals in elderly HF patients include relief of symptoms, improvement in functional capacity and quality-of-life, prevention of acute exacerbations, decreased hospital admissions, and prolongation of survival. In older patients, preservation of independence and maintenance of a satisfactory quality-of-life may be more important considerations than maximizing survival. Given the greater heterogeneity in older patients, individualized management plans are even more important. A systematic approach should combine several elements: diagnosis and staging of disease, search for reversible etiology,

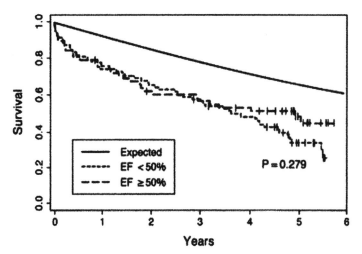

Fig. 7. Survival of patients admitted with congestive heart failure by ejection fraction. From ref. *11* with permission.

judicious use of medications, patient and caregiver education, enhancement of self-management skills, coordination of care across disciplines, and effective follow-up.

Disease Management

Hospital readmission rates for HF in elderly patients have remained unchanged over the past 15 yr. Furthermore, advances in pharmacological therapy have had minimal effects on mortality. This reflects underutilization of ACE inhibitors and β-blockers in the elderly *(60)*, insufficient patient support in overall disease management, including noncompliance with medications and diet, and inadequate discharge planning, patient education, and follow-up *(18,40)*. The patient and family must thoroughly understand the plans; individualization, repetition, and inclusion of spouse or other caregiver is particularly important in the education process. Every heart failure patient should have a scale, weigh themselves regularly, and know what steps to take if weight increases beyond prespecified ranges. Diuretic adjustments can be performed by nurses over the telephone, and in some cases by patients themselves, using individualized algorithms. There must be easy access to health care providers, so that problems can be addressed early to avoid decompensation. This can be facilitated with periodic telephone calls, frequent follow-up appointments, and monitoring programs utilizing the telephone and the Internet *(18)*.

There is undisputed evidence, specifically in older patients, of the efficacy of a multidisciplinary approach to care in reducing acute exacerbations leading to rehospitalization, improving quality-of-life, reducing total costs, and, in one study, increasing survival *(46,61–63)*. HF disease management teams are comprised of physicians, nurses, dietitians, social workers, home health specialists, pharmacists *(64)*, therapists, and aides *(46,64)*. Despite their specific efficacy and cost reductions in older patients *(65)*, HF management teams and programs are still underutilized *(18)*.

Heart failure disease management strategy should also include smoking and alcohol cessation, appropriate administration of pneumococcal and influenza vaccinations *(18)*, control of polypharmacy and over-the-counter medications, consideration of cardiac rehabilitation, and end-of-life care.

Older HF patients are often severely deconditioned, exhibiting skeletal muscle loss and severe exercise intolerance. Like younger patients, they should be encouraged to undertake moderate physical activity *(18)*. They may benefit from medically supervised exercise conditioning programs, which have been shown to improve exercise capacity in middle-aged SHF patients and cardiac transplant patients. Despite the obvious physiologic rationale and the demonstrated salutary effects on exercise capacity and quality of life, there is intense controversy and conflicting data regarding whether or not exercise training improves mortality in chronic HF of any type or in any age group. This critical, clinically important question is the subject of a proposed large multicenter randomized trial that has been approved but not yet funded by the National Heart, Lung, and Blood Institute.

End-of-life care is an element of HF disease management that is important to patients and their families but often inadequately addressed *(66)*. Given 1 yr mortality rates as high as 25–50% *(52)* and that the risk of sudden death is significant in HF, older patients with advanced HF can be considered to be terminally ill (i.e., New York Heart Association class III or IV). Patients should be offered assistance in developing a living will and assigning durable power of attorney. Detailed discussions of patient desires for intubation, resuscitation, invasive procedures, and feeding tubes while the patient is alert and competent are invaluable. (*See* Chapter 8 for a discussion of ethical and social issues in the elderly.) Pain, dyspnea, and anxiety are often inadequately treated in hospitalized elderly HF patients *(67)*. The judicious use of narcotics, sedatives, and other comfort measures are appropriate in terminal HF patients *(18)*.

Pharmacological Therapy

There is considerable controversy regarding drug therapy for HF in the elderly, given that data on drug therapy in very elderly patients (≥80 yr of age) are extremely sparse; no studies have evaluated treatment in residents of long-term-care facilities, and data on therapy for DHF, although comprises the majority of HF in the elderly, are minimal. Furthermore, although age, setting, and disease-specific data are sorely needed, several reports indicate that established therapies of proven efficacy are substantially underutilized in older patients who qualify for these therapies according to published guidelines *(60,68,69)*. For example, angiotensin-converting-enzyme (ACE) inhibitors and β-adrenergic antagonists are substantially underutilized in older patients with systolic dysfunction *(60,69)*. In addition, despite the fact that numerous randomized, controlled trials have shown a marked decrease in development of HF in elderly patients treated for systolic hypertension (*see* Table 4) *(70–73)*, community surveys consistently show undertreatment of hypertension, particularly among the elderly. Thus, while awaiting needed trials, outcomes in the older HF population could be improved by more appropriate and uniform application of existing, proven therapies.

SYSTOLIC HF

ACE Inhibitors

For the elderly as well as the young, the cornerstone of therapy of systolic HF is angiotensin-converting-enzyme inhibitors (ACEi) *(74)*. Subgroup analyses of individual studies and overviews of all randomized ACE inhibitor trials have concluded that they are as effective in reducing mortality and improving quality of life in older as in younger individuals *(75,76)*.

Table 4
Effect of Antihypertensive Therapy on Incident Heart Failure

Trial	N	Age range (yr)	Risk reduction (%)
European Working Party	840	>60	22
INDANA Group	884	60–79	32
Swedish Trial	1627	70–84	51
SHEP	4736	≥60	55
Syst-Eur	4695	≥60	36
STONE	1632	60–79	68

Source: Adapted from ref. 16.

There is controversy regarding the approach to patients who appear intolerant of ACEi. This occurs significantly more often in older than in younger patients. Several factors complicate the use of ACEi in older patients, including more frequent relative contraindications (absolute contraindications are uncommon) and increased susceptibility to side effects because of more frequent concomitant therapy with nonsteroidal anti-inflammatory agents and other antihypertensive agents. Despite these potential concerns, ACE inhibition should be attempted in nearly all elderly SHF patients.

There are a number of strategies that can be employed to optimize long-term tolerability to ACEi in older patients. ACEi, like most other medications, should be initiated in the older patient at low doses and titrated upward gradually, aiming toward doses used in conducted clinical trials with careful monitoring for adverse effects. Asymptomatic hypotension is common with ACEi therapy and, unless severe, should not be cause for discontinuation. Risk factors for severe first-dose hypotension include volume depletion from over-diuresis, severe LV dysfunction, baseline systolic blood pressure <100 mm Hg, hyponatremia, and advanced age. In these patients, volume depletion should be corrected beforehand, and ACEi therapy should begin at very low doses, with careful monitoring. Mild dry cough often decreases with time and, even when persistent, can often be tolerated when patients understand the significant survival benefit imparted by the drug (77). Among patients who are unable to tolerate standard doses of ACEi, data from the ATLAS study suggest (but do not prove) that doses of the long-acting ACE inhibitor lisinopril as low as 2.5–5 mg daily may be effective (78). Interestingly, this effect was observed particularly in older individuals (78).

Medication compliance studies demonstrate significant improvements in compliance with bid vs tid or qid regimens, and modest improvement in compliance with qd vs bid regimens. Cost is another important consideration for medication compliance, particularly for older patients on fixed incomes. There are currently at least seven ACEi approved for therapy of HF in the United States, and two of these (captopril and enalapril) are available in generic formulations in the United States. However, availability of generic formulations does not assure lower cost than active-patent proprietary medications do. It is important for health care providers to be aware of prevailing costs to the patient of the most common options among HF regimens. Because compliance with HF medications can be critical to both survival and symptom control, this information should be discussed frankly with patients at the time of initial prescription. (See Chapter 2 for a discussion of health care policy and costs.)

Angiotensin Receptor Blockers

An important and controversial question is whether or not angiotensin receptor blockers (ARBs) are acceptable alternatives to ACEi in the elderly SHF patient. Early data suggested the potential for superior tolerance and equal efficacy. ELITE-I (Evaluation of Losartan in the Elderly) was the first large, multicenter, randomized, controlled trial of any type of therapy ever performed specifically in older (≥65 yr) patients with systolic HF *(79)*. In this safety study, the ARB losartan was shown to have a lower rate of cough but not of renal dysfunction (the primary outcome) than the ACEi captopril. In the follow-up trial to determine the effect on mortality (ELITE II) 3152 patients older than 60 yr of age (mean: 71 yr) with systolic HF (left-ventricular ejection fraction ≤40%) were randomized to captopril 50 mg tid or losartan 50 mg qd *(80)*. Annual mortality was 11.7% in the losartan group and 10.4% in the captopril group. These data have been subjected to various interpretations, including assertions that ARBs are of equivalent efficacy for mortality reduction compared to ACEi. However, the statistical confidence intervals surrounding this outcome and post hoc power calculations from ELITE II do not support this, but rather support the statement that ARB therapy is neither superior to nor has been proven to be as effective as ACEi for mortality reduction in elderly patients with SHF. Furthermore, the trial data establishing the efficacy of ACEi are voluminous and compelling, in contrast to that available for ARBs. Thus, ACEi remains the initial therapy of choice *(18)*. However, an ARB is a suitable alternative in patients unable to tolerate ACEi.

Angiotensin receptor blocker therapy added to patients who continue to be severely symptomatic despite maximal ACEi therapy improves exercise tolerance and symptoms *(81)*. In the RESOLVD trial, the combination of an ARB with an ACEi appeared to be more favorable for LV remodeling than was either alone *(82)*. The recently reported VALHEFT trial added the ARB valsartan to existing therapy (which included ACE inhibitors and β-adrenergic antagonists in most patients) for moderate to severe SHF. Importantly, there was no upper age limit on enrollment. The mean age was 63 yr and out of 5010 patients, 53% were age 65 or older. There was no significant effect on the primary outcome of all-cause mortality. However, there was a 13% reduction in the secondary end-point of all-cause mortality and morbidity, a 28% reduction in hospitalizations, and improvement in quality-of-life. There was a small subgroup of patients (n = 366) who were on no ACEi therapy at baseline. These patients tended to be older (mean age: 67 yr) and had a significant, 45% reduction, in all-cause mortality. Several other ongoing trials will help further clarify the role of ARBs in the management of HF.

Hydralazine and Isosorbide Dinitrate

The combination of hydralazine 75 mg qid with isosorbide dinitrate 40 mg qid has adverse compliance and tolerability, is less effective than ACE inhibitor therapy on survival, and has minimal trial experience in older patients *(83)*. Nonetheless, this combination may be used as an adjunct to either ACE inhibitors or ARBs, or as an alternative to either ACE inhibitors or ARBs in older patients with contraindications or intolerance to these agents.

β-Adrenergic Receptor Antagonists

Multiple, large, randomized trials have conclusively proven that long-term β-blockade is beneficial in patients with systolic HF *(84–86)*. Patients up to the age of 80 have been included in these trials, and subgroup analyses indicate that β-blockers are as effective in older as in younger patients. Based on these findings, β-blockers should now be considered standard therapy in patients of all ages with stable, mild to moderate systolic HF in the absence of contraindications *(18)*. As with ACEi, however, the use of β-blockers may be problematic in the elderly. Relative contraindications to β-blockers, particularly bradyarrhythmias and chronic lung disease, are more prevalent in the elderly. To minimize the risk of adverse effects, β-blockers should only be initiated in patients who have been clinically stable without HF exacerbation for at least 4 wk, and appropriate doses of ACEi and diuretics. Starting doses should be low with very gradual upward titration.

Digoxin

The Digitalis Investigators Group (DIG) was one of the first large clinical HF intervention trials without an enrollment age limit. In patients with symptomatic systolic HF and sinus rhythm, the addition of digoxin to ACE inhibitor and diuretic therapy reduced HF symptoms and hospitalizations but had no effect on cardiovascular or all-cause mortality *(87)*. Importantly, the effects of digoxin were similar in younger and in older patients, including those over 80 yr of age *(88)*. Therefore, digoxin should be considered in patients who remain symptomatic despite treatment with ACE inhibitors and diuretics. Digoxin can improve symptoms in patients with higher NYHA class and more severe left-ventricular systolic dysfunction.

The volume of distribution and renal clearance of digoxin decline with age, and the therapeutic range for the serum digoxin level is lower in older than in younger patients specifically (0.5–1.5 ng/mL after age 70) *(89)*. In addition, serum digoxin levels over 1.5 ng/mL are associated with increased toxicity but no greater efficacy in older persons *(90)*. For these reasons, the dose of digoxin should be reduced in older persons, and 0.125 mg daily is an appropriate dose for most older patients with normal renal function. In patients with severe renal dysfunction, 0.125 mg one to three times weekly is often sufficient. With appropriate dosing, older patients may not be at increased risk for digoxin toxicity compared to younger patients *(88)*. The treatment of suspected or confirmed digoxin toxicity is similar in older and younger patients.

Diuretics

Diuretics are indispensable for the rapid relief of pulmonary congestion and peripheral edema and are necessary in most patients with moderate to severe HF to mitigate volume overload. However, with the exception of spironolactone, diuretics have not been shown to reduce mortality, and they may accelerate activation of the renin–angiotensin system. In addition, older patients are at increased risk for diuretic induced renal insufficiency and electrolyte disturbances. Therefore, the lowest dose capable of maintaining euvolemia (no jugular venous distension [JVD], edema, etc.) should be utilized. Although some patients with mild HF can be treated effectively with a thiazide diuretic, most will require a loop diuretic at a dose titrated to maintain euvolemia. When this is achieved, it is worthwhile to note the patient's weight at the time for use as a reference point. In patients with more severe HF or concomitant renal insufficiency, the addition of 2.5–10 mg metolazone daily may become necessary to achieve effective diuresis.

The addition of low-dose spironolactone (12.5–50 mg daily) to standard therapy (i.e., digoxin, diuretics, and ACE inhibitors) has been shown to reduce mortality by 25–30% in patients with severe symptoms (NYHA class III–IV). This benefit was felt to be independent of the modest or minimal diuresis obtained *(91)*. Importantly, benefits were similar in older and younger patients *(92)*. This agent is now recommended for treatment of SHF patients with recent or current NYHA class IV symptoms and no hyperkalemia *(18)*. Its role in patients with milder symptoms, particularly those already receiving β-adrenergic blocking agents, is unclear. Spironolactone is contraindicated in patients with advanced renal dysfunction or pre-existing hyperkalemia (serum potassium ≥5.0 meq/L); painful gynecomastia may occur in up to 10% of patients during long-term therapy. Caution should be exercised with this agent in patients with tenuous potassium homeostasis. The rate of hyperkalemia seems higher in clinical practice than that reported in the RALES clinical trial, perhaps resulting from selection bias. Furthermore, deaths have been reported in patients on this therapy who develop diarrhea *(93)*.

Most HF patients have an intrinsic "diuretic threshold," below which minimal diuresis occurs, even when repeated doses are administered. Thus, multiple daily doses are not usually necessary, are inconvenient for the patient, and can exacerbate urinary incontinence. Usually, a single morning oral dose somewhat above the diuretic threshold will provide effective control of salt and fluid retention. Need for escalating diuretic doses in a previously stable outpatient suggests disease progression, worsening renal function, poor absorption because of bowel edema, noncompliance, or other systemic complications. In selected patients, short-term use of low-dose dopamine or dobutamine is occasionally helpful in promoting diuresis by increasing renal flow. Nonsteroidal anti-inflammatory medications, frequently used in older patients, can cause relative diuretic resistance and should be discontinued if possible. During active diuresis, careful monitoring and replacement of electrolytes, particularly potassium and magnesium, are important; fluid restriction may be needed to avoid or alleviate hyponatremia *(94)*.

Approach to Therapy

Reversible causes of HF should be fully considered and pursued as appropriate. Careful education and follow-up should be provided to all patients, and those with moderate to severe disease should be referred to a disease management team if available. Patients with LV systolic dysfunction (ejection fraction ≤40%) should receive an ACEi. A β-blocker should be added as tolerated in patients who are stable, noncongested, and nonedematous and have mild to moderate symptoms. Diuretics are essential in order to relieve congestion and edema but should be adjusted precisely to the point of euvolumia. Spironolactone may be added in patients with severe (NYHA class III–IV) symptoms, despite the above measures. Digoxin should also be added in patients with persistent or severe symptoms, S_3 gallop, or severe LV systolic dysfunction. Patients with advanced or refractory symptoms should be referred to a HF specialist, particularly if they are suitable candidates for investigational treatments.

DIASTOLIC HF

The literature base regarding therapy for DHF is embarrassingly scant *(95)*, in contrast to SHF where numerous studies in thousands of patients have generated a rich evidence base to direct therapy; there is no single, large, multicenter trial for DHF *(18,95)*. This is remarkable given the high prevalence, substantial morbidity, and significant mortality of DHF *(96,97)*. This is particularly regrettable for the elderly who bear the brunt of DHF.

Given the lack of trial data, it is not surprising that most published HF management guidelines do not include DHF. A recent update to the joint ACC/AHA Guidelines for Evaluation and Management of Heart Failure noted the absence of published trial data to guide the management of this important disorder (18). Given this dearth of data, therapy must be empiric and both myths and controversies are plentiful (95). If one considers as a guide the almost breathtaking twists and turns experienced on the journey to definitive, evidence-based therapy for SHF during the past three decades (recall the biases in favor of inotropes and against β-blockers), then we are likely to see a number of surprising reversals during the journey we are beginning for DHF.

A survey of practitioners caring for elderly patients confirmed the confusion regarding the treatment of DHF, where, in contrast to SHF, no single pattern has emerged (98). Advances in DHF therapy have been hindered by lack of standard case definition, absence of a readily available, reliable test that characterizes and quantitates diastolic function, and a relatively poor understanding of the pathophysiology of DHF. Thankfully, as consensus emerges on case definition and preliminary data are reported, the pace of progress appears to be increasing (95).

General Approach

A majority of the general principles and strategies discussed for systolic HF, particularly in the disease management section, are applicable to DHF (18). Diuretics should be used for initial control of congestion and edema, as described for systolic HF. The approach to the patient with HF and a normal ejection fraction should begin with a search for a primary etiology. Most patients will be found to have hypertension as their main underlying condition (18). Screening for ischemic heart disease with a noninvasive stress test or coronary angiography should be considered in selected patients with chest pain and/or "flash pulmonary edema" to exclude severe coronary heart disease (18). When found, ischemia should be treated, invasively if indicated (18), because ischemia is a therapeutic target in its own right and also strongly impairs diastolic relaxation. A small but important number of patients will be found to have hypertrophic cardiomyopathy (99,100), with or without dynamic obstruction, undiagnosed valvular or coronary disease, and, rarely, amyloid heart disease (101).

Control of hypertension may be the most important treatment strategy for DHF. Chronic hypertension causes left-ventricular hypertrophy and fibrosis, which impair diastolic chamber compliance. Acute hypertension impairs diastolic relaxation. In addition, meta-analyses indicate that control of chronic, mild systolic hypertension in the elderly is a potent means of preventing the development of HF, and it is likely that the major portion of cases prevented are the result of DHF (see Table 4) (8,70–73). Although available data do not yet definitively address which antihypertensive agent is most beneficial for this purpose, the STOP-2 trial in the elderly (aged 70–84 yr) mildly favored ACE inhibitors (102). Furthermore, the early ALLHAT report showed that the diuretic chlorthalidone was superior to the α-adrenergic antagonist for prevention of CHF in older hypertensives (103).

Loss of atrial contraction is deleterious to LV filling, and atrial fibrillation with fast ventricular rate is a common precipitant of decompensated DHF. Therefore, sinus rhythm should be maintained (18). Achieving and maintaining sinus rhythm can be difficult in the elderly, where the incidence of atrial fibrillation is high. When sinus rhythm cannot be maintained, a more modest goal of rate control should be pursued.

Digoxin

Because most inotropes enhance early diastolic relaxation, digoxin might theoretically have a similar effect. Indeed, in the DIG study described earlier, which included a substantial number of elderly patients with preserved systolic function, results were similar regardless of ejection fraction, with symptomatic improvement and prevention of hospitalizations but no difference in overall mortality compared with placebo *(87)*. This suggests that digoxin could play a role in relieving symptoms, as suggested in the recently revised ACC/AHA guidelines *(18)*.

ACE Inhibitors

Angiotensin-converting-enzyme inhibitors (ACEi) and ARBs, which interfere with the renin–angiotensin system and its end-organ effects, are attractive as therapy for patients with DHF. As discussed earlier, these drugs are the cornerstone of systolic HF therapy, where they both reduce mortality and hospital admissions and improve exercise tolerance and symptoms. These effects in systolic HF are thought to be primarily the result of interference with the increased neurohormonal activation that is pivotal to the HF state. Patients with DHF also appear to have neuroendocrine activation, increased left-ventricular filling pressure, and decreased stroke volume similar to those with systolic failure *(20,30,51)*. Furthermore, ACEi and similar agents effectively control hypertension and reduce left-ventricular hypertrophy. In animal models of left-ventricular hypertrophy, renin–angiotensin activity is upregulated, and there is increased myocardial tissue angiotensin I conversion that impairs diastolic function *(104)*. In addition, increased renin–angiotensin activity appears to be a stimulus for myocardial fibrosis, which increases LV stiffness. In animals and in humans, ACE inhibition not only reduces even severe left-ventricular hypertrophy (LVH) but improves left-ventricular relaxation and also improves aortic distensibility *(104–108)*.

Preliminary clinical data in humans also appear favorable for ACEi. Aronow et al. showed that in a group of elderly (mean age: 80) patients with NYHA class III HF patients with presumptive diastolic dysfunction (EF >50%), enalapril significantly improved functional class, exercise duration, ejection fraction, diastolic filling, and left-ventricular mass *(109)*. In an observational study of 1402 patients admitted to 10 community hospitals, ACEi use in DHF patients was associated with substantially reduced all-cause mortality (odds ratio: 0.61) and CHF death (odds ratio: 0.55) *(110)*.

Despite these promising data, a provocative report by Dauterman et al. from a large database of hospitalized elderly patients with heart failure and relatively preserved ejection fractions recently introduced controversy, suggesting increased mortality in patients treated with ACEi *(95,111)*. The ultimate answer will, of course, come from appropriately powered randomized controlled trials. The European trial PEP–CHF is assessing the effect of the ACEi perindopril in elderly (age > 70 yr) HF patients with a LV ejection fraction ≥40% on death, HF admission, quality-of-life, and 6 min walk distance *(112)*.

Angiotensin Receptor Blockers

In a blinded randomized controlled crossover trial of 20 elderly patients with diastolic dysfunction and an exaggerated blood pressure response to exercise, the ARB losartan substantially improved exercise capacity (*see* Fig. 8) and quality-of-life, possibly by blocking the exercise induced elaboration of angiotensin-II and, subsequently, its adverse effect on LV relaxation via a reduction in exercise systolic blood pressure and pulse pressure

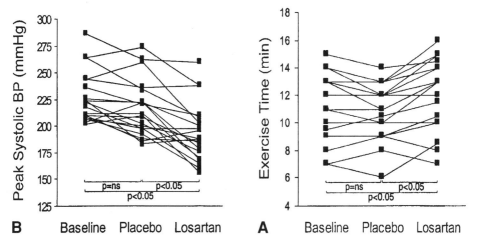

Fig. 8. Results of a blinded, randomized, crossover trial of the ARB losartan in 20 patients with diastolic dysfunction. Peak systolic blood pressure (left panel) was reduced and exercise time (right panel) was increased compared with placebo. From Warner et al., J Am Coll Cardiol 1999;33:1567–1572.

(113). The ongoing trial CHARM is assessing the effect of candesartan on death and hospital admission in HF patients with EF >40% and is due to report in year 2003 *(114)*.

Calcium Channel Antagonists

Calcium channel antagonists have often been suggested for DHF. In hypertrophic cardiomyopathy, a disorder in which diastolic dysfunction is common, verapamil appears to improve symptoms and objectively measured exercise capacity *(115–118)*. In laboratory animal models calcium antagonists, particularly dihydropyridines, prevent ischemia-induced increases in LV diastolic stiffness *(119)* and improve diastolic performance in pacing-induced HF *(120–122)*. However, negative inotropic calcium antagonists significantly impair early relaxation *(122–126)*. Negative inotropic calcium antagonists have, in general, demonstrated a tendency toward producing adverse outcomes in patients with systolic HF *(122)*. However, a trial conducted by Setaro, which examined 22 men (mean age: 65) with clinical HF despite ejection fraction >45% in a randomized double-blind placebo-controlled crossover trial of verapamil *(127)*, showed a 33% improvement in exercise time and significant improvements in clinico-radiographic HF scoring and peak filling rate. These improvements apparently occurred in the absence of a significant difference in blood pressure and ejection fraction.

β-Adrenergic Antagonists

β-Adrenergic antagonists have also been successful as therapy for hypertrophic obstructive cardiomyopathy *(128)* and they substantially improve mortality in SHF patients; they reduce blood pressure, assist in the regression of ventricular hypertrophy, and increase the ischemic threshold, all of hypothetical importance in DHF *(22,25,28,129,130)*. They may improve diastolic filling indirectly by increase in the time for diastolic filling because of negative chronotropism. However, this hypothesis has never been tested directly, and diastasis may not be compromised except at high heart rates. Furthermore, Cheng et al. and others have shown that early diastolic relaxation is enhanced by β-adrenergic drive and impaired by β-adrenergic blockade *(131,132)*. Therefore, controversies surrounding the use of β-blockers, like ACEi and calcium channel antagonists, will only be resolved with well-designed clinical trials. Notably, a significant percentage of elderly patients have relative contraindications to β-blockers.

CONCLUSION

Heart failure is common among the elderly; outcome is poor, and relevant data in this age group are minimal. The dearth of data in the presence of the large health care burden of heart failure on older persons in our society generates a wide range of important unanswered questions that need to be addressed with urgently needed research. Furthermore, the modest amount of currently available information is underutilized.

ACKNOWLEDGMENT

This work was supported by the National Institute of Aging grant no. RO1 AG18915.

REFERENCES

1. Kannel WB. Epidemiological aspects of heart failure. Cardiol Clin 1989;7(1):1–9.
2. Schocken DD. Epidemiology and Risk Factors for Heart Failure in the Elderly, 16(3): 2000, WB Saunders Co., Philadelphia, PA, pp. 407–418.
3. Kitzman DW, Gardin JM, Gottdiener JS, Arnold AM, Boineau R, Aurigemma GP, et al. Importance of heart failure with preserved systolic function in patients > or = 65 years of age. CHS Research Group. Cardiovascular Health Study. Am J Cardiol 2001;87:413–419.
4. Gottdiener JS, Arnold AM, Aurigemma GP, Polak JF, Tracy RP, Kitzman DW, et al. Predictors of congestive heart failure in the elderly: the Cardiovascular Health Study. J Am Coll Cardiol 2000;35: 1628–1637.
5. Chen YT, Vaccarino V, Williams CS, Butler J, Berkman LF, Krumholz HM. Risk factors for heart failure in the elderly: a prospective community-based study. Am J Med 1999;106:605–612.
6. Chae CU, Pfeffer MA, Glynn RJ, Mitchell GF, Taylor JO, Hennekens CH. Increased pulse pressure and risk of heart failure in the elderly. JAMA 1999;281:634–639.
7. Moser M, Hebert PR. Prevention of disease progression, left ventricular hypertrophy and congestive heart failure in hypertension treatment trials. J Am Coll Cardiol 1996;27:1214–1218.
8. Kramer K, Kirkman P, Kitzman DW, Little WC. Flash pulmonary edema: association with hypertension, reocurrence despite coronary revascularization. Am Heart J 2000;140:451–455.
9. Arnold JMO, Mrachiori GE, Imrie JR, Burton GL, Pflugfelder PW, Kostuk WJ. Large artery function in patients with chronic heart failure. Circulation 1991;84:2418–2425.
10. Luchi RJ, Snow E, Luche JM. Left ventricular function in hospitalized geriatric patients. J Am Geriatr Soc 1982;30:700–705.
11. Senni M, Tribouilloy CM, Rodeheffer RJ, Jacobsen SJ, Evans JM, Bailey KR, et al. Congestive heart failure in the community: a study of all incident cases in Olmsted County, Minnesota, in 1991. Circulation 1998;98:2282–2289.
12. Ramachandran S, Vasan RS, Larson MG, Benjamin EJ, Evans JC, Reiss CK, et al. Congestive heart failure in subjects with normal versus reduced left ventricular ejection fraction. J Am Coll Cardiol 1999; 33:1948–1955.
13. Gottdiener JS, Arnold AM, Marshall RJ, Aurigemma GP, Gardin JM, Rutledge JC, et al. LV function and congestive heart failure in the elderly—relevance of therapeutic trials. The Cardiovascular Health Study. Circulation 1998;98:S718 (abstract).
14. Devereux RB, Roman MJ, Liu JE, Welty TK, Lee ET, Rodeheffer R, et al. Congestive heart failure despite normal left ventricular systolic function in a population-based sample: the Strong Heart Study. Am J Cardiol 2000;86:1090–1096.
15. Kupari M, Lindroos M, Iivanainen AM, Heikkila J, Tilvis R. Congestive heart failure in old age: prevalence, mechanisms and 4-year prognosis in the Helsinki Ageing Study. J Intern Med 1997;241: 387–394.
16. Rich MW, Kitzman DW. Heart failure in octogenarians: a fundamentally different disease. Am J Geriatr Cardiol 2000;9:97–104.

17. Ogawa T, Spina RJ, Martin WH, Kohrt WM, Schechtman KB. Effect of aging, sex, and physical training on cardiovacular responses to exercise. Circulation 1992;86:494–503.

18. The ACC/AHA Task Force on Practice Guidelins (Committee to Revise the 1995 Guidelines for the Evaluation and Management of Heart Failure. ACC/AHA Guidelines for the Evaluation and Management of Chronic Heart Failure in the Adult: executive summary. Circulation 2001;38:2002–2113.

19. Cody R, Toree S, Clar M, Pnodolfina K. Age-related hemodynamic, renal, and hormonal differences among patients with congestive heart failure. Arch Intern Med 1989;149:1023–1028.

20. Kitzman DW, Higginbotham MB, Cobb FR, Sheikh KH, Sullivan M. Exercise intolerance in patients with heart failure and preserved left ventricular systolic function: failure of the Frank–Starling mechanism. J Am Coll Cardiol 1991;17:1065–1072.

21. Hundley WG, Kitzman DW, Morgan TM, Hamilton CA, Darty SN, Stewart KP, et al. Cardiac cycle dependent changes in aortic area and aortic distensibility are reduced in older patients with isolated diastolic heart failure and correlate with exercise intolerance. J Am Coll Cardiol 2001;38:796–802.

22. Little WC. Enhanced load dependence of relaxation in heart failure: clinical implications. Circulation 1992;85:2326–2328.

23. Hoit BD, Walsh RA. Diastolic dysfunction in hypertensive heart disease. In: Gaasch WH, LeWinter MM, eds. Left Ventricular Diastolic Dysfunction and Heart Failure. Lea & Febiger, Philadelphia, PA, 1994, pp. 354–372.

24. Gelpi RJ. Changes in diastolic cardiac function in developing and stable perinephritic hypertension in conscious dogs. Circ Res 1991;68:555–567.

25. Shannon RP, Komamura K, Gelpi RJ, Vatner SF. Altered load: an important component of impaired diastolic function in hypertension and heart failure. In: Lorell BH, Grossman W, eds. Diastolic Relaxation of the Heart, 2nd ed. Kluwer Academic, Norwell, MA, 1994, pp. 177–185.

26. Little WC, Ohno M, Kitzman DW, Thomas JD, Cheng CP. Determination of left ventricular chamber stiffness from the time for deceleration of early left ventricular filling. Circulation 1995;92:1933–1939.

27. Little WC, Braunwald E. Assessment of cardiac function. In: Braunwald E, ed. Heart Disease, 5th ed. WB Saunders, Philadelphia, PA, 1996, pp. 421–444.

28. Iriarte M, Murga N, Morillas M, Salcedo A, Etxebeste J. Congestive heart failure from left ventricular diastolic dysfunction in systemic hypertension. Am J Cardiol 1993;71:308–312.

29. Gandhi SK, Powers JE, Fowle KM, Rankin KM, Nomeir AM, Kitzman DW, et al. The pathogenesis of acute pulmonary edema associated with hypertension. N Engl J Med 2000;344:17–22.

30. Clarkson PBM, Wheeldon NM, MacFadyen RJ, Pringle SD, MacDonald TM. Effects of brain natriuretic peptide on exercise hemodynamics and neurohormones in isolated diatsolic heart failure. Circulation 1996;93:2037–2042.

31. Davis KM, Fish LC, Elahi D, Clark BA, Minaker KL. Atrial naturetic paptide levels in the prediction of congestive heart failure risk in frail elderly. JAMA 1992;267:2625–2629.

32. Bella JN, Palmieri V, Liu JE, Kitzman DW, Oberman A, Hunt SC, et al. Relationship between left ventricular diastolic relaxation and systolic function in hypertension: the hypertension genetic epidemiology network (hypergen) study. Hypertension 2001;38:424–428.

33. Arnett D, Devereux R, Rao DC, Kitzman DW, Oberman A, Hopkins P. A genome search in hypertensive African American and white siblings detects a locus mapping to chromosome 7 that influences variation in left ventricular mass: the HyperGEN Study. Circulation 1999;100:I–193.

34. Tang W, Arnett DK, Devereux RB, Atwood L, Kitzman DW, Rao DC. Linkage of left ventricular diastolic filling parameters to chromosome 5 in hypertensive African-Americans: the HyperGEN Study. Am J Cardiol 2002;15:621–627.

35. Vikstrom KL, Leinwand LA. The molecular genetic basis of familial hypertrophic cardiomyopathy. Heart Failure 1995;11:5–14.

36. Webster KA, Bishopric NH. Molecular aspects and gene therapy prospects for diastolic failure. Cardiol Clin 2000;18:621–635.

37. Vasan RS, Levy D. Defining diastolic heart failure: a call for standardized diagnostic criteria. Circulation 2000;101:2118–2121.

38. Yamamoto K, Burnett JC Jr, Bermudez EA, Jougasaki M, Bailey KR, Redfield MM. Clinical criteria and biochemical markers for the detection of systolic dysfunction (in process citation). J Card Failure 2000;6:194–200.

39. Ghali JK, Kadakia S, Cooper R, Liao Y. Bedside diagnosis of preserved versus impaired left ventricular systolic function in heart failure. Am J Cardiol 1991;67:1002–1006.

40. Nagueh SF, Middleton KJ, Kopelen HA, Zoghbi WA, Quinones MA. Doppler tissue imaging: a non-invasive technique for evaluation of left ventricular relaxation and estimation of filling pressures. J Am Coll Cardiol 1997;30:1527–1533.
41. European Study Group on Diastolic Heart Failure. How to diagnose diastolic heart failure. Eur Heart J 1998;19:990–1003.
42. Zile MR, Gaasch WH, Carroll JD, Feldman MD, Aurigemma GP, Schaer GL, et al. Heart failure with a normal ejection fraction: is measurement of diastolic function necessary to make the diagnosis of diastolic heart failure? Circulation 2001;104:779–782.
43. Davis KM, Fish LC, Minaker KL, Elahi D. Atrial natriuretic peptide levels in the elderly: differentiating normal aging changes from disease. J Gerontol 1996;51A:M95–M101.
44. Kitzman DW. Heart failure in the elderly: systolic and diastolic dysfunction. Am J Geriatr Cardiol 1995; 5:20–26.
45. Vinson JM, Rich MW, Sperry JC, Shah AS, McNamara T. Early readmission of elderly patients with congestive heart failure. J Am Geriatr Soc 1990;38:1290–1295.
46. Rich MW, Beckham V, Wittenberg C, Leven CL, Freedland KE, Carney R. A multidisciplinary intervention to prevent the readmission of elderly patients with congestive heart failure. N Engl J Med 1995; 333:1190–1195.
47. Krumholz HM, Parent EM, Tu N, Vaccarino V, Wang Y, Radford MJ, et al. Readmission after hospitalization for congestive heart failure among Medicare beneficiaries. Arch Intern Med 1997;157:99–104.
48. Philbin EF, Rocco TA Jr, Lindenmuth NW, Ulrich K, Jenkins PL. Clinical outcomes in heart failure: report from a community hospital-based registry. Am J Med 1999;107:549–555.
49. Pernenkil R, Vinson JM, Shah AS, Beckham V, Wittenberg C, Rich MW. Course and prognosis in patients ≥70 years of age with congestive heart failure and normal versus abnormal left ventricular ejection fraction. Am J Cardiol 1997;79:216–219.
50. Rich MW, Vinson JM, Sperry JC, Shah AS, Spinner LR, Chung MK, et al. Prevention of readmission in elderly patients with congestive heart failure: results of a prospective, randomized pilot study. J Gen Intern Med 1993;8:585–590.
51. Kitzman DW, Brubaker PH, Anderson RT, Brosnihan B, Stewart KP, Wesley DJ, et al. Isolated diastolic heart failure: does it exist? Characterization of an important syndrome among the elderly. J Am Coll Cardiol 2000;35:193A.
52. Croft JB, Giles WH, Pollard RA, Keenan NL, Casper ML, Anda RF. Heart failure survival among older adults in the United States: a poor prognosis for an emerging epidemic in the Medicare population (see comments). Arch Intern Med 1999;159:505–510.
53. Schocken DD, Arrieta MI, Leaverton PE, Ross EA. Prevalence and mortality rate of congestive heart failure in the United States. J Am Coll Cardiol 1992;20:301–306.
54. Senni M, Tribouilloy CM, Rodeheffer RJ, Jacobsen SJ, Evans JM, Bailey KR, et al. Congestive heart failure in the community: trends in incidence and survival in a 10-year period (see comments). Arch Intern Med 1999;159:29–34.
55. Marshall RJ, Gottdiener JS, Shemanski L, McClelland MS, Furberg C, Kitzman DW, et al. Outcome of congestive heart failure in the elderly: influence of left ventricular systolic function. The Cardiovascular Health Study. Circulation 1998;I–17:1064.
56. Taffet GE, Teasdale TA, Bleyer AJ, Kutka NJ, Luchi RJ. Survival of elderly men with congestive heart failure. Age Ageing 1992;21:49–55.
57. Aronow WS, Ahn C, Kronzon I. Prognosis of congestive heart failure in elderly patients with normal versus abnormal left ventricular systolic function associated with coronary artery disease. Am J Cardiol 1990;66:1257–1259.
58. Krumholz HM, Chen YT, Vaccarino V, Wang Y, Radford MJ, Bradford WD, et al. Correlates and impact on outcomes of worsening renal function in patients > or = 65 years of age with heart failure. Am J Cardiol 2000;85:1110–1113.
59. Davies LC, Francis DP, Piepoli M, Scott AC, Ponikowski P, Coats A. Chronic heart failure in the elderly: value of cardiopulmonary exercise testing in risk stratification. Heart 2000;83:147–151.
60. Krumholz HM, Wang Y, Parent EM, Modena MG, Petrillo M, Radford MJ. Quality of Care for elderly patients hospitalized with heart failure. Arch Intern Med 1997;157:2242–2247.
61. Stewart S, Marley JE, Horowitz JD. Effects of a multidisciplinary, home-based intervention on unplanned readmissions and survival among patients with chronic congestive heart failure: a randomised controlled study. Lancet 1999;354:1077–1083.

62. Stewart S, Vanderheyden M, Pearson S, Horowitz JD. Prolonged beneficial effects of a home-based intervention on unplanned readmissions and mortality among patients with congestive heart failure. Arch Intern Med 1999;159:257–261.

63. Tsuyuki RT, McKelvie RS, Arnold JM, Avezum A Jr, Barretto AC, Carvalho AC, et al. Acute precipitants of congestive heart failure exacerbations. Arch Intern Med 2001;161:2337–2342.

64. Gattis WA, Hasselblad V, Whellan DJ, O'Connor CM. Reduction in heart failure events by the addition of a clinical pharmacist to the heart failure management team: results of the Pharmacist in Heart Failure Assessment Recommendation and Monitoring (PHARM) Study. Arch Intern Med 1999;159: 1939–1945.

65. Whellan DJ, Gaulden L, Gattis WA, Granger B, Russell SD, Blazing MA, et al. The benefit of implementing a heart failure disease management program. Arch Intern Med 2001;161:2223–2228.

66. Levenson JW, McCarthy EP, Lynn J, Davis RB, Phillips RS. The last six months of life for patients with congestive heart failure. J Am Geriatr Soc 2000;48:S101–S109.

67. Baker R, Wu AW, Teno JM, Kreling B, Damiano AM, Rubin HR, et al. Family satisfaction with end-of-life care in seriously ill hospitalized adults. J Am Geriatr Soc 2000;48:S61–S69.

68. Aronow WS, Ahn C, Kronzon I. Comparison of incidences of congestive heart failure in older African-Americans, Hispanics, and whites. Am J Cardiol 1999;84:611–612.

69. Philbin EF. Current community practices in heart failure: understanding the underutilization of angiotensin-converting enzyme inhibitors. J Am Coll Cardiol 1997;29(2 (Suppl A):325.

70. Amery A, Birkenhager W, Brixko P, et al. Mortality and morbidity results from the European Working Party on High Blood Pressure in the Elderly Trial. Lancet 1985;I(8442):1349–1354.

71. Dahlof B, Lindholm L, Hannson L, Schersten B, Ekbom T, Wester PO. Morbidity and mortality in the Swedish Trial in Old Patients with Hypertension (STOP-Hypertension). Lancet 1991;338:1281–1285.

72. Stassen JA, Fagard R, Thijs L, et al. Randomised double-blind comparison of placebo and active treatment for older patients with isolated systolic hypertension. Lancet 1997;350:757–764.

73. Gong LS, Zhang W, Zhu Y. Shanghai Trial of Nifedipine in the Elderly (STONE). J Hypertens 2001; 14:1237–1245.

74. Braunwald E. Ace inhibitors—a cornerstone of the treatment of heart failure. N Engl J Med 1991;325: 351–353.

75. Garg R, Yusuf S. Overview of randomized trials of angiotensin-converting enzyme inhibitors on mortality and morbidity in patients with heart failure. JAMA 1995;273:1450–1456.

76. Flather M, Yusuf S, Kober L, Pfeffer M, Hall A, Murphy G, et al. Long-term ACE-inhibitor therapy in patients with heart failure or left-ventricular dysfunction: a systematic overview of data from individual patients. ACE-Inhibitor Myocardial Infarction Collaborative Group. Lancet 2000;355:1575–1581.

77. Kitzman DW. Heart failure and cardiomyopathy. In: Abrams WB, Beers MH, Berkow B, eds. The Merck Manual of Geriatrics, 3rd ed. Merck Research Laboratories, Whitehouse Station, NJ, 2000, pp. 900–914.

78. Packer M, Poole-Wilson PA, Armstrong PW, Cleland J, Horowitz JD, Massie BM, et al., and on behalf of the ATLAS study group. Comparative effects of low and high doses of the angiotensin-converting enzyme inhibitor, lisinopril on morbidity and mortality in chronic heart disease. Circulation 1999;100: 2312–2318.

79. Pitt B, Segal R, Martinez FA, Meurer G, Cowley A, Thomas I, et al. Randomized trial of losartan versus captopril in patients over 65 with heart failure (Evaluation of Losartan in the Elderly Study, ELITE). Lancet 1997;349:747–752.

80. Pitt B, Poole-Wilson PA, Segal R, Martinez FA, Dickstein K, Camm AJ, et al. Effect of losartan compared with captopril on mortality in patients with symptomatic heart failure: randomised trial—The Losartan Heart Failure Survival Study (ELITE II). Lancet 2000;355:1582–1587.

81. Hamroff G, Katz SD, Mancini D, Blaufarb I, Bijou R, Patel R, et al. Addition of angiotensin II receptor blockade to maximal angiotensin-converting enzyme inhibition improves exercise capacity in patients with severe congestive heart failure. Circulation 1999;99:990–992.

82. McKelvie RS, Yusuf S, Pericak D, Avezum A, Burns RJ, Probstfield J, et al. Comparison of candesartan, enalapril, and their combination in congestive heart failure: randomized evaluation of strategies for left ventricular dysfunction (RESOLVD) pilot study. The RESOLVD Pilot Study Investigators. Circulation 1999;100:1056–1064.

83. Cohn JN, Johnson GR, Ziesche S, et al. A comparison of enalapril with hydralazine-isosorbide dinitrate in the treatment of chronic congestive heart failure. N Engl J Med 1991;325:303–310.

84. Packer M, Bristow MR, Cohn JN, Colucci WS, Fowler MB, Gilbert EM, et al. The effect of carvedilol on morbidity and mortality in patients with chornic heart failure. N Engl J Med 1996;334:1349–1355.

85. Anon. Effect of metoprolol CR/XL in chronic heart failure: Metoprolol CR/XL Randomised Intervention Trial in Congestive Heart Failure (MERIT-HF). Lancet 1999;353:2001–2007.
86. CIBIS-II Investigators and Committees. The Cardiac Insufficiency Bisoprolol Study II (CIBIS-II): a randomised trial. Lancet 1999;353:9–13.
87. Digoxin Investigators Group. The effect of digoxin on mortality and morbidity in patients with heart failure. N Engl J Med 1997;336:525–533.
88. Rich MW, McSherry F, Williford WO, Yusuf S. Effect of age on mortality, hospitalizations, and response to digoxin in patients with heart failure: the DIG Study. J Am Coll Cardiol 2001;38:806–813.
89. Ware JA, Snow E, Luchi JM, Luchi RJ. Effect of digoxin on ejection fraction in elderly patients with congestive heart failure. J Am Geriatr Soc 1984;32:631–635.
90. Slatton ML, Irani WN, Hall SA, Marcoux LG, Page RL, Grayburn PA, et al. Does digoxin provide additional hemodynamic and autonomic benefit at higher doses in patients with mild to moderate heart failure and normal sinus rhythm? J Am Coll Cardiol 1997;29:1206–1213.
91. Cody R, Pitt B, Perez A, Betz P, for the RALES Investigators. The benefit of spironolactone in the RALES Trial is not primarily due to a diuretic effect. J Am Coll Cardiol 2000;35:212A.
92. Pitt B, Zannad F, Remme WJ, Cody R, Castaigne A, Perez A, et al. The effect of spironolactone on morbidity and mortality in patients with severe heart failure. N Engl J Med 1999;341:709–717.
93. Berry C, McMurray JJ. Serious adverse events experienced by patients with chronic heart failure taking spironolactone. Heart 2001;85:E8.
94. Leier CV, Dei Cas L, Metra M. Clinical relevance and management of the major electrolyte abnormalities in congestive heart failure: hyponatremia, hypokalemia, and hypomagnesemia. Am Heart J 1994; 128:564–574.
95. Kitzman DW. Therapy for diastolic heart failure: on the road from myths to multicenter trials. J Card Failure 2001;7:229–231.
96. Tresch DD, McGough MF. Heart failure with normal systolic function: a common disorder in older people. J Am Geriatr Soc 1995;43:1035–1042.
97. Committee on Evaluation and Management of Heart Failure. Guidelines for the evaluation and management of heart failure. J Am Coll Cardiol 1995;26:1376–1398.
98. Fleg J, Kitzman DW, Aronow WS, Rich MW, Gardin JM, Slone S. Physician management of patient with heart failure and normal versus decreased left ventricular systolic function. Am J Cardiol 1998;81: 506–509.
99. Lewis JF, Maron BJ. Clinical and morphologic expression of hypertrophic cardiomyopathy in patients ≥65 years of age. Am J Cardiol 1994;73:1105–1111.
100. Lewis JF, Maron BJ. Elderly patients with hypertrophic cardiomyopathy: a subset with distinctive left ventricular morphology and progressive clinical course late in life. J Am Coll Cardiol 1989;13:36–45.
101. Olson LJ, Gertz MA, Edwards WD, et al. Senile cardiac amyloidosis with myocardial dysfunction. Diagnosis by endomyocardial biopsy and immunohistochemistry. N Engl J Med 1987;317:738–742.
102. Hansson L, Lindholm L, Ekbom T, et al. Randomised trial of old and new antihypertensive drugs in elderly patients: cardiovascular mortality and morbidity in Swedish Trial in Old Patients with Hypertension–2 Study. Lancet 1999;354:1751–1756.
103. The Allhat Officers and Coordinators for the ALLHAT Collaborative Research Group. Major cardiovascular events in hypertensive patients randomized to doxazosin vs chlorthalidone: the antihypertensive and lipid-lowering treatment to prevent heart attack trial (ALLHAT). JAMA 2000;283:1967–1975.
104. Lorell BH, Grossman W. Cardiac hypertrophy: the consequences for diastole. J Am Coll Cardiol 1987; 9:1189–1193.
105. Lorell BH. Cardiac renin–angiotensin system in cardiac hypertophy and failure. In: Lorell BH, Grossman W, eds. Diastolic Relaxation of the Heart, 2nd ed. Kluwer Academic, Norwell, MA, 1996, pp. 91–99.
106. Oren S, Grossman E, Frohlich ED. Reduction in left ventricular mass in patients with systemic hypertension treated with enalapril, lisionopril, or fosenopril. Am J Cardiol 1996;77:93–96.
107. Friedrich SP, Lorell BH, Douglas PS, et al. Intracardiac ACE inhibition improves diastolic distensibility in patients with left ventricular hypertrophy due to aortic stenosis. Circulation 1992;86(Suppl I): I–119.
108. Lakatta E. Cardiovascular aging research: the next horizons. J Am Geriatr Soc 1999;47:613–625.
109. Aronow WS, Kronzon I. Effect of enalapril on congestive heart failure treated with diuretics in elderly patients with prior myocardial infarction and normal left ventricular ejection fraction. Am J Cardiol 1993;71:602–604.
110. Philbin EF, Rocco TA. The utility of angiotensin-converting enzyme inhibitors in heart failure with preserved left ventricular systolic function. J Am Coll Cardiol 1997;29(2 (Suppl A):321.

111. Dauterman KW, Go AS, Rowell R, Gebretsadik T, Gettner S, Massie BM. Congestive heart failure with preserved systolic function in a statewide sample of community hospitals. J Card Failure 2001;7: 221–228.

112. Cleland JG, Tendera M, Adamus J, Freemantle N, Gray CS, Lye M, et al. Perindopril for elderly people with chronic heart failure: the PEP–CHF study. The PEP investigators (see comments). Eur J Heart Failure 1999;1:211–217.

113. Abraham TP, Kon ND, Nomeir AM, Cordell AR, Kitzman DW. Accuracy of transesophageal echocardiography in preoperative determination of aortic anulus size during valve replacement. J Am Soc Echocardiogr 1997;10:149–154.

114. Swedberg K, Pfeffer M, Granger C, Held P, McMurray J, Ohlin G, et al. Candesartan in heart failure—assessment of reduction in mortality and morbidity (CHARM): rationale and design. Charm-Programme Investigators. J Card Failure 1999;5(3):276–282.

115. Vandenberg VF, Rath LS, Stuhlmuller P, Melton H, Skorton DJ. Estimation of left ventricular cavity area with on-line, semiautomated echocardiographic edge detection system. Circulation 1992;86:159–166.

116. Bonow RO, Leon MB, Rosing DR, Kent K, Lipson LC, Bacharach SL, et al. Effects of verapamil and propranolol on left ventricular systolic function and diatsolic filling in patients with coronary artery disease: radionuclide angiographic studies at rest and during exercise. Circulation 1981;65:1337–1350.

117. Bonow RO, Dilsizian V, Rosing DR, Maron BJ, Bacharach SL, Green MV. Verapamil-induced improvement in left ventricular diastolic filling and increased exercise tolerance in patients with hypertrophic cardiomyopathy: short- and long-term effects. Circulation 1985;72:853–864.

118. Udelson J, Bonow RO. Left ventricular diastolic function and calcium channel blockers in hypertrophic cardiomyopathy. In: Gaasch WH, ed. Left Ventricular Diastolic Dysfunction and Heart Failure. Lea & Febiger; Malvern, PA, 1996, pp. 465–489.

119. Serizawa T, Shin-Ichi M, Nagai Y, Ogawa T, Sato T, Nezu Y, et al. Diastolic abnormalities in low-flow and pacing tachycardia-induced ischemia in isolated rat hearts-modification by calcium antagonists. In: Lorell BH, Grossman W, eds. Diastolic Relaxation of the Heart, 2nd ed. Kluwer Academic, Norwell, MA, 1996, pp. 266–274.

120. Cheng CP, Pettersson K, Little WC. Effects of felodipine on left ventricular systolic and diastolic performance in congestive heart failure. J Pharmacol Exp Thera 1994;271:1409–1417.

121. Cheng CP, Noda T, Ohno M, Little WC. Differential effects of enalaprilat and felodipine on diastolic function during exercise in dogs with congestive heart failure. Circulation 1993;88(4):I–294.

122. Little WC, Cheng CP, Elvelin L, Nordlander M. Vascular selective calcium entry blockers in the treatment of cardiovascular disorders: focus on felodipine. Cardiovasc Drugs Ther 1995;9:657–663.

123. Ten Cate FJ, Serruys PW, Mey S, Roelandt JR. Effects of short-term administration of verapamil on left ventricular filling dynamics measured by a combined hemodynamic-ultrasonic technique in patients with hypertrophic cardiomyopathy. Circulation 1983;68:1274–1279.

124. Hess OM, Murakami T, Krayenbuehl HP. Does verapamil improve left ventricular relaxation in patients with myocardial hypertrophy? Circulation 1996;74:530–543.

125. Brutsaert DL, Rademakers F, Sys SU, Gillebert TC, Housmans PR. Analysis of relaxtion in the evaluation of ventricular function of the heart. Prog Cardiovasc Dis 1985;28:143–163.

126. Brutsaert DL, Sys SU, Gillebert TC. Diastolic failure: pathophysiology and therapeutic implications. J Am Coll Cardiol 1993;22:318–325.

127. Setaro JF, Zaret BL, Schulman DS, Black HR. Usefulness of verapamil for congestive heart failure associated with abnormal left ventricular diastolic filling and normal left ventricular systolic performance. Am J Cardiol 1990;66:981–986.

128. Sasayama S, Asanoi H, Ishizaka S, Kihara Y. Diastolic dysfunction in experiemental heart failure. In: Lorell BH, Grossman W, eds. Diastolic Relaxation of the Heart, 2nd ed. Kluwer Academic, Norwell, MA, 1994, pp. 195–202.

129. Colucci WS, Ribeiro JP, Rocco MB, Quigg RJ, Creager MA, Marsh JD, et al. Impaired chronotropic response to exercise in patients wtih congestive heart failure. Circulation 1989;80:314–323.

130. Udelson J, Bonow RO. Left ventricular diastolic function and calcium channel blockers in hypertrophic cardiomyopathy. In: Gaasch WH, LeWinter MM, eds. Left Ventricular Diastolic Dysfunction and Heart Failure. Lea & Febiger, Philadelphia, PA, 1994, pp. 462–489.

131. Cheng CP, Igarashi Y, Little WC. Mechanism of augmented rate of left ventricle filling during exercise. Circ Res 1992;70:9–19.

132. Cheng CP, Noda T, Nozawa T, Little WC. Effect of heart failure on the mechanism of exercise induced augmentation of mitral valve flow. Circ Res 1993;72:795–806.

IV CARDIAC SURGICAL CARE FOR THE ELDERLY

15

Surgical Treatment of Ischemic Heart Disease in the Elderly

Mauricio J. Garrido, MD,
Michael Argenziano, MD, and Eric A. Rose, MD

CONTENTS

BACKGROUND

The number of Americans over the age of 70 is steadily increasing. To meet the needs of this segment of the population, cardiac surgery centers have been broadening their inclusion criteria for coronary revascularization in the elderly. We have learned new lessons about both the successes and limitations of surgical treatment for coronary disease in this population. Patients who, just one decade ago, would not have been considered suitable surgical candidates are enjoying good outcomes today. Off-pump coronary artery bypass grafting is proving to be safer and less expensive than revascularization with cardiopulmonary bypass. Although risks of complications and hospital costs are higher in this population, the benefits of surgical intervention compared to medical treatment are clear in selected elderly patients. In this chapter, we will review the current literature on coronary revascularization in septuagenarians and octogenarians.

DEMOGRAPHICS

According to the 2000 US Census Bureau Report, people over the age of 80 comprise 3.4% of Americans today; this figure will increase to 4.4% (14.8 million) by 2025. It is estimated that 61% of this group will be women. The cohort of the population 70–74 yr of age will double in size over the next 25 yr *(1)*. The incidence of coronary artery disease

From: *Aging, Heart Disease, and Its Management: Facts and Controversies*
Edited by: N. Edwards, M. Maurer, and R. Wellner © Humana Press Inc., Totowa, NJ

increases with age. Up to 40% of Americans over the age of 80 experience serious cardio-vascular symptoms. In the year 2000, 1 in 58 people 65 and older died as a result of cardiac disease compared to 1 in 448 people between the ages of 45 to 64. Cardiac disease is the most common cause of all deaths in the United States and in the 65 yr and older group *(2)*. These statistics are bringing cardiac surgery into a new arena and are shaping the way we think about cardiac surgery in the elderly.

INDICATION FOR CORONARY REVASCULARIZATION IN THE ELDERLY

The American College of Cardiology/American Heart Association guidelines for coro-nary artery bypass grafting indicate that improvement in survival and quality-of-life are the primary indications for the procedure *(3)*.

Longevity

The current life expectancy in the United States is 77.1 yr and is estimated to increase to 80.6 yr by 2025. The US Census Bureau 1997 report on life expectancy by age group showed that at 65, 75, 80, and 85 yr of age, the life expectancy was 18, 11, 9, and 6 yr, respec-tively *(4)*. Realistic consideration of age-adjusted life expectancy plays an integral role in the decision to subject a patient over 80 with coronary artery disease to the perioperative risk of elective revascularization. Moreover, an elderly patient with limited predicted longevity may not benefit from the longer patency expected of an internal mammary artery conduit.

Three major historical studies that randomized patients to coronary artery bypass graft-ing versus medical therapy did not include the elderly. The effect of age on consideration for revascularization has not been widely studied. The University of Wisconsin retro-spectively reviewed the long-term outcome of 1689 US veterans after undergoing isolated primary coronary artery bypass grafting from 1972 to 1994. Patients were divided into three groups: I (<50 yr), II (51–70 yr) and III (>70 yr), all with comparable preoperative ejec-tion fraction. The 10 yr survival significantly diminished with increasing age at 74%, 68%, and 47% in groups I, II, and III, respectively. Survival comparison of the revascularized patients to age-matched population was done for each year after surgery. Interestingly, it was found that a significant difference in survival between revascularized and the age-matched population was realized at postoperative yr 4 and 8 in groups I and II, respec-tively. Group III showed no significant change in survival even at postoperative yr 10 *(5)*.

Unfortunately, the study did not identify the postoperative year at which a patient over 70 would have a benefit in survival over the general population *(5)*. We can only conclude that it is greater than 10 yr. Additionally, this retrospective study compared revascularized patients to the general population and not to patients with pre-existing coronary artery dis-ease who would have lower survival rates.

Quality-of-Life

Rumfeld evaluated changes in the health-related quality-of-life (HRQoL) for 1744 US veterans who underwent coronary artery bypass grafting. HRQoL was determined preop-eratively and at 6 mo follow-up. The mean age of study participants was 63 ± 9 yr and no age stratification was done in the analysis. Interestingly, this study found that the patients most likely to have an improvement in HRoQL were those who had the lowest preoperative HRQoL. Conversely, patients with high preoperative HRQoL experienced the greatest decline in HRQoL *(6)*. We can hypothesize that elderly patients with symptomatic coronary disease may have lower HRoQL preoperatively and, therefore, benefit from revascularization more than younger counterparts. Boucher studied 266 patients older than 70 yr of age who underwent revascularization and showed a significant decrease of NYHA functional class—from 3.2 to 1.6 at average follow-up of 30 mo *(6)*. Similar studies of 117 octogenarians showed a comparable decrease at 2 yr follow-up *(7,8)*.

CORONARY REVASCULARIZATION IN THE ELDERLY

Off-Pump vs On-Pump Coronary Artery Bypass Grafting

Multiple studies have demonstrated that off-pump coronary artery bypass grafting (OPCABG) is associated with a lower risk of perioperative morbidity than on-pump revascularization. Comparison of 104 OPCABG patients older than 75 yr to patients who underwent on-pump coronary artery bypass grafting demonstrated a significant benefit when cardiopulmonary bypass was not used. Although cardiac event-free and survival rates did not differ for elderly patients undergoing OPCABG, total intubation time (8 vs 18 h), intensive care unit stay (2.2 vs 3.5 d), and postoperative hospital stay (14 vs 20 d) were significantly shorter in the OPCABG group. Postoperative stroke and respiratory failure were significantly less frequent in the off-pump cohort *(9)*. A similar study of 53 patients 75 yr and older also demonstrated shorter hospital stays, in addition to lower transfusion requirements (0.4 vs 1.9 U of packed red blood cells), as well as a significantly lower perioperative mortality rate. There was no significant difference in postoperative myocardial infarction, atrial fibrillation, bleeding, neurologic complications, or renal failure *(10)*.

Retrospective series comparing off-pump to on-pump coronary artery bypass grafting for patients of all ages have demonstrated that OPCABG is a safe alternative with a lower incidence of major in-hospital adverse clinical events and a decreased requirement for medical resources *(11)*. In one of the largest studies conducted, the Northern New England Cardiovascular Disease Study Group, the perioperative patient outcome after 1741 OPCABG cases was compared to the outcome of 6126 conventional coronary artery bypass procedures. The investigators found no significant difference in perioperative mortality, intraoperative and postoperative stroke, mediastinitis, and return to the operating room for bleeding. Need for intra-aortic balloon pump support (2.3% vs 3.4%), the incidence of postoperative atrial fibrillation (21% vs 26%), and postoperative length of stay (5 vs 6 d) were significantly lower in the OPCABG group *(12)*.

In one of the few prospective randomized multicenter trials that compared OPCABG to conventional coronary artery bypass grafting, 142 patients were randomized to OPCABG. The mean age was 61 yr. Necessity to give blood products was significantly lower in the off-pump group (3% vs 13% of patients), and creatine kinase muscle–brain isoenzyme levels were 41% lower as well. No other significant differences in postoperative complications, quality-of-life, 1 mo mortality, and proportion of patients surviving free of cardiovascular events were found *(13)*.

Internal Mammary Artery Grafting

The patency of the left internal mammary artery (LIMA) to the left anterior descending artery is 95% at 10 yr. In comparison, the patency of saphenous vein grafts is approx 75%

at 5 yr. In younger patients, the relationship between the longer patency rates of arterial conduits and fewer future reoperations is clear. However, elderly patients requiring coronary revascularization may have limited longevity prior to surgery. In these cases, the primary indication for surgery may be solely quality-of-life. The excellent 10 yr patency of the internal mammary artery (IMA) is statistically not likely to be realized in select elderly patients because of their short age-adjusted life expectancy at the time of surgery.

Alexander et al. demonstrated that IMA use was a univariate predictor for lower short-term mortality for all age groups *(14)*. Additionally, Hahnemann University compared perioperative mortality of 188 octogenarians who underwent coronary artery bypass grafting with an IMA conduit to 286 with saphenous vein grafts only and found the difference not to be significant. Hospital mortality rates were 9% and 7%, respectively, and the deep sternal infection rate was similar in both groups, at 1.8% and 1.1%, respectively *(15)*. An analysis of 309 patients over 70 who underwent coronary revascularization included 227 utilizing the LIMA and 27 utilizing bilateral internal mammary arteries (BIMA). This analysis demonstrated a 30 d mortality rate of 3.5%, 3.7%, and 5.3% in the LIMA, BIMA, and solely saphenous vein graft conduit procedures, respectively, and it was concluded that there is no increased operative mortality with the use of the right internal mammary artery *(16)*. In contrast, a study by He retrospectively reviewed 512 patients older than 70 who underwent internal mammary artery grafting and found that BIMA and right internal mammary artery (RIMA) use was significantly associated with increased operative mortality when compared to LIMA use *(17)*. More data are necessary before drawing conclusions on operative risk associated with RIMA and BIMA coronary revascularization in the elderly.

Concomitant Disease

The Cardiac Surgery Reporting System of New York State determined the main risk factors for in-hospital death after adult open heart surgery. The major risk factors were recent myocardial infarction (odds ratio [OR] = 3.4), ejection fraction less than 20% (OR = 3.4), end-stage renal disease (OR = 3.2), reoperation (OR = 2.6), congestive heart failure (OR = 2.5), and diabetes (OR = 2.1). All of these comorbid conditions are more likely to be present in older patients and, therefore, can contribute to a higher perioperative mortality in the elderly *(18,19)*. Care should be taken to identify these risk factors during preoperative counseling.

RESULTS OF CORONARY REVASCULARIZATION IN THE ELDERLY

Mortality

Multiple studies have found in-hospital mortality rates after coronary artery bypass surgery of 3–8% in patients older than 70 (*see* Table 1) *(19)*. A large series of 964 patients 70 yr or older had a 95% in-hospital survival after coronary revascularization; a comparable series involving 67 octogenarians showed a 91% in-hospital survival rate. The University of Wisconsin study described earlier found a 10 yr mortality rate of 53% in patients over the age of 70 undergoing coronary revascularization. Another study of octogenarians who underwent coronary artery bypass grafting showed an actuarial survival of 87%, 80%, 77%, and 73% for the first 4 yr postoperatively *(24)*. In a group of 121 octogenarians, only 6% were discharged to a nursing home after coronary artery bypass grafting, with 92% discharged home. As discussed earlier, many studies have found similar or decreased perioperative morbidity and mortality with the off-pump approach.

Table 1
Short-Term Survival of Elderly Patients
Undergoing Coronary Artery Bypass Grafting

Author (ref.)	Age (yr)	n	In-hospital Mortality (%)
Peterson et al. (20)	>80	24,461	4.4
Salomon et al. (21)	>75	469	6.8
Canver et al. (5)	>70	218	3.2[a]
Edwards et al. (22)	>70	121	7.4
Deiwick et al. (23)	>80	61	8.2[a]

[a]Thirty day mortality.

Morbidity

POSTOPERATIVE MYOCARDIAL INFARCTION

The CADENCE Research Group (25) retrospectively compared the outcomes of coronary revascularization in 1034 patients divided into cohorts of 70–74, 75–79, and ≥80 yr of age. All three cohorts showed no significant difference in sex distribution, NYHA functional class, or number of grafts. The degree of urgency was lower in the youngest group in comparison to the older groups. They found no significant difference in the incidence of postoperative myocardial infarction, which were 4.5%, 3.4%, and 4.2% in the three groups, respectively. Additionally, a study of 463 patients over 70 undergoing coronary revascularization with or without valve repair demonstrated an impressively low perioperative myocardial infarction rate of 0.9%.

INTRA-AORTIC BALLOON PUMP (IABP) REQUIREMENT

Postoperative ventricular dysfunction is associated with increased mortality and prolonged intensive care unit stays. A meta-analysis of 1497 patients in two studies have shown that the rate of intra-aortic balloon pump (IABP) requirement after revascularization is 4.3% in patients over 70 yr of age (26). The rate of low output states was higher in patients who underwent revascularization with a combined valvular procedure (26,27). Deiwick demonstrated a higher rate of IABP requirement (10.9%) in 101 consecutive patients over 80 undergoing cardiac surgery compared with younger patients (23). Avery compared patients 65–75 yr of age ($n = 351$) to those older than 80 yr ($n = 104$) undergoing car-diac surgery, with the majority (72%) specifically undergoing coronary revascularization (28). They found a significant difference in rates of postoperative low output states (3% vs 11%, younger and older groups, respectively). Two studies showed that off-pump coronary revascularization had similar postoperative low output states in 2.2% (age > 75) and 2% (age > 70) of patients (28,29). In patients who underwent conventional revascularization with cardiopulmonary bypass, the rate of IABP requirement was higher than with OPCABG.

POSTOPERATIVE ARRHYTHMIA

Although arrhythmias after cardiac surgery occur in patients of all ages, it presents a greater problem for the elderly. Atrial fibrillation is the most frequent complication after coronary revascularization in the elderly and accounts for 95% of all postoperative tachyar-rhythmias *(30)*. The postoperative arrhythmia rate has been reported to be 49% in octoge-narians. Postoperative atrial fibrillation occurs significantly more often in octogenarians undergoing cardiac surgery than in patients 65–75 yr of age *(23)*. The potential complica-tions with advancing age from prophylactic anticoagulation cannot be dismissed.

NEUROCOGNITIVE COMPLICATIONS

The rate of major neurologic complications in patients undergoing coronary artery bypass grafting ranges from 1% to 6% for all ages. Causes of neurologic defects can result from embolic phenomena with air or atheromatous plaque, perioperative cerebral hypo-perfusion, or pre-existing carotid or cerebrovascular disease *(28)*. The pathophysiologic process that results in coronary disease can concomitantly cause extracranial and intracra-nial carotid disease. With aging, the risk of developing cerebrovascular disease increases and many of the older patients who undergo coronary revascularization today have pre-existing cerebrovascular disease. D'Agostino reports that among other risk factors, age and left main coronary stenosis greater than 60% are clinical predictors of significant carotid stenosis *(31)*.

During cardiopulmonary bypass, patients with advanced cerebrovascular disease are at risk of developing a watershed infarct at low-flow areas in the brain and thrombotic emboli from ulcerated carotid plaques. Interestingly, it appears that the majority of asymptomatic carotid artery lesions do not cause perioperative neurologic events. Studies of cerebral flow during cardiopulmonary bypass suggest that neurologic events can be avoided by maintenance of perfusion pressure of at least 50 mm Hg. In fact, adverse neurologic events associated with extracorporeal circulation result mainly from aortic atherosclerotic dis-ease, rather than from carotid disease *(32)*. This would explain the increased rate of stroke associated with aortic cross-clamping. Comparison of 104 OPCABG vs 74 traditional on-pump coronary revascularization procedures demonstrated a significantly increased rate of cerebral vascular accident perioperatively in patients undergoing cardiopulmo-nary bypass over 75 yr of age *(30)*. There are, however, several studies that do not show a significant difference in the rate of postoperative stroke with OPCABG as compared with cardiopulmonary bypass. Hernandez et al. conducted one of the largest studies comparing 6126 on-pump with 1741 off-pump coronary revascularizations in patients of all ages. The investigators demonstrated an adjusted rate of perioperative stroke of 1.81% and 1.34%, respectively, which were not significantly different.

SUMMARY

The age distribution of the US population will undergo a dramatic change in the next 25 yr. The aging population will be increasingly present in our medical offices and operat-ing rooms. We are beginning to find answers to the problems of managing coronary dis-ease in the elderly. Off-pump coronary artery bypass surgery provides a significant benefit when compared to conventional revascularization with cardiopulmonary bypass. With proper patient selection, outcomes from revascularization can be realized in the elderly that do not differ from those in younger patients. Patients in their seventh and eighth decade of life present complex and interesting problems with medical, financial, and ethical dimen-sions that will be clarified as we develop new approaches to their care.

REFERENCES

1. Hetzel L, Smith A. The 65 years and over population: 2000. Census 2000 Brief. US Census Bureau, October 2001.
2. Minino A, Smith B. Deaths: Preliminary Data for 2000. National Vital Statistics Report Oct 2001;49(12): 1–40.
3. Eagle KA, Guyton RA, Davidoff R, et al. ACC/AHA guidelines for coronary artery bypass graft surgery: a report of the American College of Cardiology/American Heart Association Task Force on Practice Guidelines. J Am Coll Cardiol 1999;34:1262–1364.
4. Life Expectancy by Age Group—1997 Data. US Census Bureau, 1997.
5. Canver CC, Nichols RD, Kroncke GM, et al. Influence of increasing age on long-term survival after coronary artery bypass grafting. Ann Thorac Surg 1996;62:1123–1127.
6. Rumsfeld JS, Magid DJ, O'Brien M, et al. Changes in health-related quality of life following coronary artery bypass graft surgery. Ann Thorac Surg 2001;72:2026–2032.
7. Boucher JM, Dupras A, Jutras N, et al. Long-term survival and functional status in the elderly after cardiac surgery. Can J Cardiol 1997;13:646–652.
8. Freeman WK, Schaff HV, O'Brien PC, et al. Cardiac surgery in the octogenarian: perioperative outcome and clinical follow-up. J Am Coll Cardiol 1991;18:29–35.
9. Ko W, Krieger KH, Lazenby WB, et al. Isolated coronary artery bypass grafting in one hundred consecutive octogenarian patients: a multivariate analysis. J Thorac Cardiovasc Surg 1991;102:532–538.
10. Hitoshi H, Amano A, Takahashi A. Off-pump coronary artery bypass grafting for elderly patients. Ann Thorac Surg 2001;72:2013–2019.
11. Koutlas TC, Elbeery JR, Chitwood WR, et al. Myocardial revascularization in the elderly using beating heart coronary artery bypass surgery. Ann Thorac Surg 2000;69:1042–1047.
12. McKay RG, Mennett RA, Boden WE, et al. A comparison of on-pump vs. off-pump coronary artery bypass surgery among low, intermediate, and high-risk patients: the Hartford Hospital experience. Connect Med 2001;65(9):515–521.
13. Hernandez F, Cohn WE, O'Connor GT, et al. In-hospital outcomes of off-pump versus on-pump coronary artery bypass procedures: a multicenter experience. Ann Thorac Surg 2001;72:1528–1534.
14. Dijk D, Nierich AP, Jaegere P, et al. Early outcome after off-pump versus on-pump coronary artery bypass surgery. Results from a randomized study. Circulation 2001;104:1761–1766.
15. Alexander KP, Anstrom KJ, Muhlbaier LH, et al. Outcomes of cardiac surgery in patients over 80 >= year: results from the National Cardiovascular Network. J Am Coll Cardiol 2000;35:731–738.
16. Morris RJ, Strong MD, Kresh JY, et al. Internal thoracic artery for coronary artery grafting in octogenarians. Ann Thorac Surg 1996;62(1):16–22.
17. Zaidi AM, Fitzpatrick AP, Grotte GJ, et al. Good outcomes from cardiac surgery in the over 70s. Heart 1999;82:134–137.
18. He GW, Acuff TE, Mack MJ, et al. Risk factors for operative mortality in elderly patients undergoing internal mammary artery grafting. Ann Thorac Surg 1994;57:1453–1460.
19. Hannan EL, Kilburn H, Shields E, et al. Adult open heart surgery in New York State. An analysis of risk factors and hospital mortality rates. JAMA 1990;264:2768–2774.
20. Peterson ED, Cowper PA, Pryor DB, et al. Outcomes of coronary artery bypass graft surgery in 24461 patients aged 80 years or older. Circulation 1995;92(Suppl II):II-85–II-91.
21. Salomon NW, Page US, Bigelow JC, et al. Coronary artery bypass grafting in elderly patients: comparative results in a consecutive series of 469 patients older than 75 years. J Thorac Cardiovasc Surg 1991; 101:209–217.
22. Edwards FH, Taylor AJ, Thompson L, et al. Current status of coronary artery operation in septuagenarians. Ann Thorac Surg 1991;52:265–269.
23. Deiwick M, Tandler R, Scheld HH, et al. Heart surgery in patients aged eighty years and above: determinants of morbidity and mortality. Thorac Cardiovasc Surg 1997;45:119–126.
24. Higgins TL, Estafanous FG, Paranandi L, et al. Stratification of morbidity and mortality outcome by preoperative risk factors in coronary artery bypass patients. JAMA 1992;267:2344–2348.
25. Slaughter MS, Ward HB. Surgical management of heart failure. Clin Geriatr Med 2000;16(3):567–592.
26. Talwalker NG, Damus PS, Durban LH, et al. Outcome of isolated coronary artery bypass surgery in octogenarians. J Cardiac Surg 1996;11:172–179.
27. Smith KM, Lamy A, Kent R, et al. Outcomes and costs of coronary artery bypass grafting: comparison between octogenarians and septuagenarians at a tertiary care center. CMAJ 2001;165(6):759–764.

28. Avery GJ, Ley SJ, Dick SE, et al. Cardiac surgery in the octogenarian: evaluation of risk, cost, and outcome. Ann Thorac Surg 2001;71:591–596.
29. Demers P, Cartier R. Multivessel off-pump coronary artery bypass surgery in the elderly. Eur J Cardiothorac Surg 2001;10:908–912.
30. Hirose H, Amano A, Takahashi A. Off-pump coronary artery bypass grafting for elderly patients. Ann Thorac Surg 2001;72:2013–2019.
31. Lazar HL, Menzoian JO. Coronary artery bypass grafting in patients with cerebrovascular disease. Ann Thorac Surg 1998;66:968–974.
32. D'Agostino RS, Svensson LG, Shahian DM, et al. Screening carotid ultrasonography and risk factors for stroke in coronary artery surgery patients. Ann Thorac Surg 1996;62:1714–1723.

16

Surgical Treatment of Heart Failure in the Elderly

Aftab R. Kherani, MD and Mehmet C. Oz, MD

INTRODUCTION

In the United States, there are an estimated 5 million people suffering from congestive heart failure (CHF), with 400,000 new cases being diagnosed annually *(1–3)*. The incidence of CHF increases exponentially with age and afflicts approx 10% of the population over the age of 85. Over 40% of CHF patients die within 2 yr of their diagnosis *(1,4,5)*. The economic impact of treating CHF patients is enormous, accounting annually for almost 1 million hospitalizations, 3 million office visits, and $35 billion dollars, representing 5% of total health care expenditures *(6–8)*. Many patients are treated medically with variable results. To provide value to society of the large investment that we are making in this patient population, we must explore all therapies that could result in improved patient survival and quality of life. Some of these options are surgical. Reparative options may include revascularization with or without valve repair or replacement. For severe cases of failure, mechanical circulatory support and transplantation may be indicated. Elderly patients are not exempt from the benefit that these procedures may provide and thus these options should be considered in this age group.

CARDIOVASCULAR TOLL OF AGING

Age is a significant independent risk factor for heart failure *(9)*. A series of changes that adversely affect the vasculature and the heart itself are responsible. These changes are interrelated and contribute to the higher incidence of failure seen in the elderly.

The arterial walls thicken *(10)* and stiffen with age. This leads to increased systolic arterial pressure and pulse-wave velocity, amplifying aortic impedance and afterload *(11)*.

From: *Aging, Heart Disease, and Its Management: Facts and Controversies*
Edited by: N. Edwards, M. Maurer, and R. Wellner © Humana Press Inc., Totowa, NJ

The result is an increase in left-ventricular wall thickness (this occurs even in normotensive individuals), the extent of which is directly related to the degree of hypertension (12).

The amount of fibrous tissue increases, and the sizes of individual myocytes increase, yet the number of cardiac myocytes decreases (13). Early diastolic filling declines with age, likely the result of fibrous myocardial changes and prolonged myocardial activation (calcium mediated) from the preceding systole. Meanwhile, late diastolic filling increases secondary to enhanced left atrial contraction (14), and left atrial size increases with age. The increased dependence upon the atrial kick and late diastolic filling on increasing left-ventricular preload results in older patients being more sensitive to atrial fibrillation (13).

With age, there is no conclusive data that demonstrate a decline in coronary blood flow (13). However, a variety of age-related neurohormonal changes have been demonstrated (15). They include increases in sympathetic activity (16), plasma catecholamine concentration (17), and, possibly, arterial α_1-adrenoreceptor density (18). Decreases have been established in parasympathetic activity, baroreceptor reflex activity, and response to β-adrenoreceptor stimulation (15).

Aging has a profound effect on the cardiovascular response to stress. After age 20, maximum work capacity and oxygen capacity decline by 10% every decade (19). In response to exercise, increases in peak heart rate and contractility are diminished in older patients. This, likely, is the result of the previously mentioned decrease in β-adrenoreceptor response that accompanies aging. The cardiovascular response to exercise in older patients mimics congestive failure in that the increased perfusion requirement peripherally is met mainly by preload reserve. This is in contrast to younger patients, who may rely upon sympathetic activation as well as β-adrenergic stimulation in response to exercise. Thus, older patients are increasingly prone to cardiovascular insufficiency when stressed (15).

TREATMENT OPTIONS

Intra-Aortic Balloon Counterpulsation

The intra-aortic balloon pump (IABP) can play an important role in the management of cardiogenic shock and is associated with a survival benefit when used in combination with thrombolytics in the setting of acute myocardial infarction (MI). Barron and colleagues (20) studied 23,180 patients who participated in the National Registry of Myocardial Infarction 2 and identified 7268 who received IABP support. Patients who received thrombolytic therapy alone had a mortality rate of 67%, whereas those receiving thrombolytics and IABP demonstrated a mortality rate of 49%. This observational study is being followed by the randomized, controlled TACTICS trial.

In elderly patients (≥70 yr of age), 35% of whom were in failure, Gutfinger and colleagues (21) found that preoperative utilization of IABP was helpful for patients set to undergo coronary artery bypass grafting. In this high-risk group, defined as having a greater incidence of failure or acute myocardial infarction, or lower ejection fraction, preoperative IABP use led to complication and mortality rates comparable to low-risk older patients.

Acorn Cardiac Support Device

The Acorn CSD (cardiac support device) (Acorn Cardiovascular, St. Paul, MN) is a polyester mesh knit that serves as a jacket around the ventricles. It has bidirectional compliance and assists the heart in minimizing the extent of dilatation and actually reducing the diameter of the ventricle slightly. Six sizes are available, and the surgeon does any minor trimming that may be necessary. Once fitted, the CSD is sewn posteriorly and laterally, just above or below the atrioventricular groove. A final set of anterior stay sutures is placed. CSD implantation can be performed at the time of another cardiac surgical procedure, such as valve repair/replacement or coronary artery bypass grafting (22).

Power and colleagues published the first large animal study examining the CSD (23). They paced 12 adult sheep into heart failure. They then implanted the CSD into each animal via a partial lower sternotomy and randomized the animals to device retention (wrap) or removal (sham). Pacing then continued for 28 d, after which time the Australian group observed significant differences in left-ventricular fractional shortening, degree of mitral valve regurgitation, and left-ventricular long axis area, all favoring the wrap group. A subsequent canine study out of the Henry Ford Hospital supported these findings (24). After 3 mo, dogs treated with the CSD demonstrated a significant decrease of almost 20% in left-ventricular end-diastolic volume ($p = 0.04$), compared with the just over 10% increase experienced by the control group ($p = 0.002$). The dogs with the device also demonstrated an increase in fractional area of shortening, compared to the decrease experienced by the control group. Additionally, CSD-treated animals demonstrated diminished myocyte hypertrophy and interstitial fibrosis compared to control dogs.

To date, the largest clinical trial was performed at Charité Universitätsklinikum, Humboldt-Universität zu Berlin, Germany, on 27 patients between April 1999 and March 2000 (25). In 11 cases, CSD placement was the only procedure performed. All patients were New York Heart Association (NYHA) class III or IV at the time of enrollment. All CSD-only patients survived the operation and were eventually discharged from the hospital, as there were no adverse events associated with the device at any time. Two patients died subsequent to discharge, one of decompensated heart failure (he had refused readmission for medical management), and the other of pneumonia several months after implantation. Three months following CSD placement, 56% of the patients were NYHA class I, 33% were class II, and 11% were class II/III. The left-ventricular ejection fraction (LVEF) increased significantly at 3 and 6 mo post-implantation, from 21.7 ± 1.5 to 27.6 ± 3.2 and 32.8 ± 4.9, respectively. Left-ventricular end-diastolic dimension (but not end-systolic dimension) decreased significantly at 3 and 6 mo, and the degree of mitral regurgitation decreased significantly at 3 mo (there was insufficient data to make a determination at 6 mo). Quality-of-life indices correlated with the objective improvement seen in these patients. This initial clinical safety trial supports CSD implantation as a means of improving cardiac function and symptoms in class III and IV heart failure patients in both the short and intermediate term.

Assist Devices

Left-ventricular assist devices (LVADs) have emerged as a potential therapeutic option for patients who are not transplant candidates (26). Advances in LVAD technology have also enabled select patients to be discharged to home with their device. This has proven to be both a safe and potentially cost-effective treatment for heart failure in certain patients (27). This option is a valid one for the population as a whole, including the elderly.

There are four types of assist devices: extracorporeal nonpulsatile pumps, total artificial hearts, extracorporeal pulsatile pumps, and implantable pulsatile devices.

Extracorporeal nonpulsatile pumps: These assist devices are simple, relatively inexpensive, and serve a limited role in postcardiotomy ventricular dysfunction. Although they have been used successfully in neonatal respiratory failure (extracorporeal membrane oxygenation), these devices have no significant role in the management of the elderly because of very poor long-term survival in patients over 75 (Abiomed database).

Total artificial hearts: This device provides an exciting alternative that has been highlighted in the press with the first human implantation of the AbioCor replacement heart in 2001. This device consists of two blood pumps coupled to an energy source. Data from a 30 d study in cows demonstrated no hemolysis and normal hemodynamics and end-organ function *(28)*. Early human results have also been encouraging, except for the recent occurrence of stroke in the first recipient of the device. Data from the Cardiowest device experience is also encouraging, although issues of portability and long-term reliability coupled with the lack of self-sufficient backup systems in the event of device failure limit the application of this device in elderly patients who are not transplant candidates.

Extracorporeal pulsatile devices: The third group, extracorporeal pulsatile devices, includes the Pierce–Donachy device (Thoratec Laboratories, Berkeley, CA) and the Abiomed device (Abiomed, Danvers, MA). These devices are used primarily for short-term support, as a bridge to transplantation and provide only limited potential for rehabilitation. Again, lack of "wearability," especially if transplant is not an option, limit the value of these technologies in older patients.

Implantable pulsatile devices: Finally, today's implantable pulsatile devices provide the greatest potential for outpatient rehabilitation with acceptable quality of life. They may serve not only as a bridge to transplantation but as a bridge to recovery in select patients. The Novacor (World Heart, Ottawa, Canada) and HeartMate (Thoratec, Pleasantville, CA) LVADs are examples of implantable pulsatile devices *(29)*. Both are implanted via a median sternotomy, with the pumping chamber placed within the abdominal wall. The inflow cannula is placed in the left-ventricular apex; the outflow tube is anastomosed to the ascending aorta (*see* Fig. 1) *(30)*. The use of these devices has led to promising results, allowing 91% of patients surviving implant to be discharged from the hospital; overall, 74% have survived to transplantation *(31)*.

Long-term LVAD support (exceeding 30 d) is indicated in patients whose 6 mo mortality is estimated at greater than 30% *(32–34)*. It can benefit several patient populations. The first consists of individuals with severe CHF who are awaiting transplantation and develop hemodynamic instability, making further delay to heart transplantation dangerous. LVAD support can minimize end-organ dysfunction and prevent death.

A second set of patients that may benefit from LVAD support are those who are not transplant candidates but require more than medical management to address their heart failure *(31)*. This is the newest patient population that has been targeted for device implantation. There is a growing body of literature that suggests that although supported, native myocardial function may improve to the point where transplantation is not necessary. This "bridge-to-recovery" hypothesis centers around LVAD-induced remodeling, also known as "reverse remodeling." Although the exact mechanisms involved in the various aspects of reverse remodeling are still being researched, there are data that supports LVAD-induced remodeling in the following areas *(35)*: (1) reversal of chamber enlargement and normalization of the end-diastolic pressure–volume relationship *(36)*, (2) decreased left-ventricular mass and regression of myocyte hypertrophy *(37,38)*, (3) increased contractility *(39)*, and (4) normalizing expression of genes-encoding proteins involved in calcium metabolism.

Reverse remodeling may allow recovery to such an extent that neither further LVAD support nor transplantation is needed as has been demonstrated in select patients with

Device	Duration	Type of support	Device Cost	Hospital Discharge
ABIOMED BVS 5000	Short	Uni, biventricular	$140,000 startup $12,400 per pump $64,500 console	No
Thoratec LVAD	Short/ Long	Uni, biventricular	$46,765 per pump* $1,500 per cannula $60,000 console $150,000 startup	No
Novacor LVAS	Long	Univentricular	Implant kit (pump/cannulae) $74,500 $55,000 console $ 196,000 startup (plus two implant kits)	Yes
Thoratec IP HeartMate	Long	Univentricular	$45,000 (pump)	No
Thoratec VE HeartMate	Long	Univentricular	$64,000 (pump) $278,450 startup	Yes

Fig. 1. Food and Drug Administration-approved ventricular assist devices. From DiGiorgi PL, Rao V, Oz MC. Which patient, which pump, in preparation.

nonischemic cardiomyopathy *(40)*. The final group of patients who may derive benefit from LVAD support consists of individuals who are not transplant candidates and will require lifelong LVAD support.

With the advent of wearable devices, outpatient LVAD support became a practical solution in 1998, when the Food and Drug Administration approved the Thermocardiosystems V-E Heartmate (*see* Fig. 2) and the Novacor LVAS for outpatient use. General criteria that should be met prior to discharge include *(41)*: (1) clinical stability, (2) training of patient and family in care and management of device, including how to deal with device malfunction, (3) patient and family are able to manage the device and driveline exit site, (4) patient has successfully completed an adequate number of day-trips away from the hospital, and (5) echocardiographic evidence that the native heart could temporarily provide adequate flow to sustain flow in the event of major device malfunction.

In Morales and colleagues' recent review of the outpatient LVAD experience, they studied 471 patients representing 61,237 support days. Only two died while at home, giving a mortality rate of 0.012 per outpatient year. Comparing this value with the 66% 1 yr mortality rate of status I, class IV heart failure patients and the 30% annual mortality rate of all patients on the transplant list *(42,43)* demonstrates that outpatient LVAD support can be an effective treatment option and is estimated to cost only $27 per day to maintain while at home. In fact, even LVAD support within the hospital setting is associated with a roughly 40% lower daily cost when compared with patients receiving conventional pretransplant therapy (i.e., IABP support in combination with inotropes) *(44)*.

We have recently completed the Randomized Evaluation of Mechanical Assistance for the Treatment of Congestive Heart Failure (REMATCH trial) *(45)*, which compares medical management and vented electric LVAD support in a randomized series of 129 heart failure patients who were not candidates for transplantation. This trial has demonstrated that LVAD placement is associated with a 48% reduction in mortality, by Kaplan–Meier

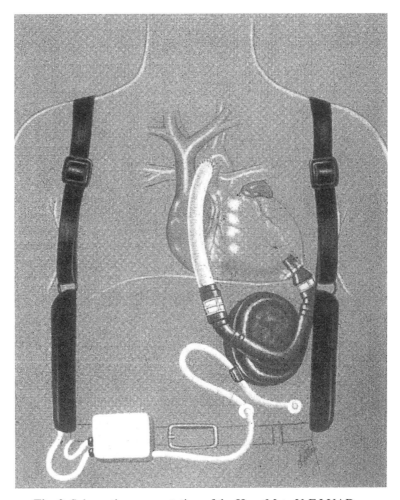

Fig. 2. Schematic representation of the HeartMate V-E LVAD.

survival analysis. Survival at 1 yr was 52% in the device group and 25% in the medical-therapy group ($p = 0.002$); at two years, survival rates were 23% and 8% ($p = 0.09$), respectively. Although the frequency of serious adverse events (e.g., device malfunction, infection, bleeding) in the device group was 2.35 times that in the medical-therapy group, the quality-of-life was significantly improved at 1 yr in the device group. The findings of the REMATCH trial will likely have a profound effect on how elderly patients suffering from end-stage heart failure are managed, with LVADs increasingly providing a valid surgical option.

The question of whether or not a LVAD should be implanted in the elderly, which may be adversely affected by cardiac pathology (the incidence of which increases in the elderly) remains. Valvular disease, most commonly aortic insufficiency, has been extensively investigated. Rao and colleagues demonstrated that pre-existing native or prosthetic valvular pathology does not increase the immediate perioperative risk of LVAD placement. Surgical intervention, especially oversewing of the aortic valve, expanded the population suitable for LVAD while not increasing either the short-term morbidity or mortality of LVAD implantation *(46)* (*see* Fig. 3).

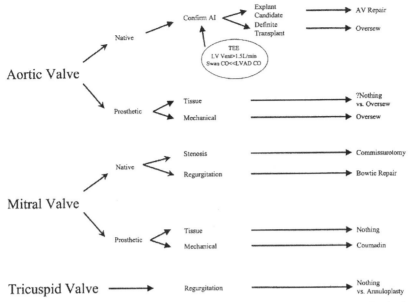

Fig. 3. Algorithm for the management of valvular disease during left-ventricular assist device support (AI = aortic insufficiency; AV = aortic valive; CO = cardiac output; LV = left ventricle; TEE = transesophageal echocardiohraphy).

In 1996, Smedira and colleagues examined the importance of age as a risk factor for outcome after placement of an implantable LVAD. In this study out of the Cleveland Clinic Foundation, all patients were the recipients of a HeartMate device. The majority of the patients over the age of 60 suffered from ischemic cardiomyopathy. In this subpopulation of the Cleveland Clinic's database (where the oldest patient was 69 yr of age), age was not a significant risk factor for outcome following implantable left-ventricular assist support. There was no significant difference in survival to transplantation or survival to discharge between the older and younger age groups *(47)*. These data are consistent with the conclusions drawn by Wareing and Kouchoukos, who found that older patients demonstrated comparable survival to younger recipients of postcardiotomy support *(48)*.

Transplantation

Although there is considerable promise surrounding outpatient implantable devices and despite a growing body of evidence supporting the use of LVADs as a potential bridge to recovery, assist devices continue to serve primarily as a bridge to transplantation. This raises the question of whether heart transplantation is a viable option in elderly patients. Between 1982 and 1999, less than 5% of all heart recipients (over 55,000 in the registry) were over the age of 65 *(49)*. So, how well do elderly patients tolerate transplantation? Several studies have reported no significant difference in survival following heart transplantation between older and younger patients *(50,51)*. Preoperatively, however, the latter set of patients was less stable hemodynamically. A subsequent study found that elderly patients (defined as at least 54 yr of age) demonstrated comparable survival to their younger counterparts. In fact, this study demonstrated the older population experiencing a lower rate of rejection (within 4 mo of transplantation) and a lower incidence of opportunistic infection. One hypothesis was that an age-associated weakening of immune function was responsible for these findings *(52)*. This point is still debatable, but what is established from these older studies is that survival after heart transplantation among select elderly patients is not statistically different from that of younger patients.

Blanche and colleagues recently published their findings from a study of heart transplantation in patients aged 70 and above. Their elderly recipients did have a higher preoperative left-ventricular ejection fraction and did receive a higher percentage of allografts from female donors. This being said, no statistically significant difference was observed between older and younger age groups with regard to the following *(53)*: (1) 30 d or to-discharge operative mortality, (2) actuarial survival at 1, 2, 3, and 4 yr, (3) duration of post-transplantation intensive care unit, (4) duration of total hospital stay, (5) total cost of hospitalization, (6) mean follow-up time, (7) incidence of cytomegalovirus (CMV) infection, and (8) incidence of rejection episodes.

With regard to various aspects of the perioperative period surrounding cardiac transplantation, certain older patients have comparable experiences to younger ones. Thus, bridging them to transplantation with the support of an LVAD may be a worthwhile endeavor.

CONTROVERSIES

Scarcity of Organs

Organs for transplantation are a scarce resource, and select older patients, even septagenarians, can do well following transplantation. However, most institutions can not justify allocating such a rare resource to the elderly, and many academic centers have age limits for potential heart recipients. One possible solution that would provide older patients with donor hearts, without affecting the number of hearts available to the existing recipient pool, is broadening the donor criteria in instances where the recipient is elderly. Some institutions are transplanting patients of advanced age, who would otherwise be too old to qualify as potential recipients, with hearts that otherwise would not be "suitable" for transplantation for various reasons. The ethical implications surrounding issue are significant.

Scarcity of Financial Resources

It is estimated that 30–40% of health-related costs are utilized in the care of patients in their last 18 mo of life *(54)*. Will major surgical intervention for elderly heart failure patients increase this already high percentage? Some studies have demonstrated that the hospital cost associated with cardiac surgery in very elderly patients exceeds that for younger patients. In the United Kingdom, numerous treatments provided by the National Health Service are not available to the elderly *(55)*.

Long-term LVAD support and transplantation are associated with a high fixed cost. Estimates of first-year costs (not including professional fees) associated with the two procedures are $192,154 and $176,605, respectively *(56)*. They become increasingly economical as postprocedure survival increases. From a monetary standpoint, this is the key question that must be answered when considering these surgical interventions in any patient, including the elderly. The longer that life expectancy can be extended in an outpatient setting, the more economic sense LVAD implantation and transplantation make.

Recent studies would suggest that older patients can benefit from cardiac surgery, including surgical intervention for heart failure. Elderly patients tolerate cardiac surgery well, with acceptable morbidity, mortality, and long-term outcome *(57,58)*. In elective operations these statistics are comparable for octogenarians and younger patients undergoing cardiac surgical procedures *(59)*. Surgical intervention for heart failure is being performed more frequently now as compared to the mid-1980s. There has been an accompanying decline in length of stay and mortality, and adjusted costs were not significantly different between 1990–1991 and 1994–1996 *(60)*. This suggests that surgical intervention for heart failure is effective both economically and therapeutically; the elderly may be among those who may benefit from such intervention.

REFERENCES

1. Slaughter MS, Ward HB. Surgical management of heart failure. Clin Geriatr Med 2000;16:567–592.
2. American Heart Association. Heart and Stroke Facts, Statistical Supplement. American Heart Association, Dallas, TX, 1998.
3. Smith WM. Epidemiology of congestive heart failure. Am J Cardiol 1985;55:3A.
4. Ho KKL, Anderson KM, Kannel WB, et al. Survival after the onset of congestive heart failure in Framingham Heart Study subjects. Circulation 1993;88:107.
5. Rodeheffer RJ, Jacobsen SJ, Gersch BJ, et al. The incidence and prevalence of congestive heart failure in Rochester, Minnesota. Mayo Clin Proc 1993;68:1143.
6. Frazier OH, Myers TJ. Surgical therapy for severe heart failure. Curr Probl Cardiol 1998;23:721–764.
7. National Heart, Lung, and Blood Institute: Congestive Heart Failure in the United States: a New Epidemic [data fact sheet]. National Heart, Lung, and Blood Institute, National Institutes of Health, Bethesda, MD, 1996.
8. O'Connell JB, Bristow MR. Economic impact of heart failure in the United States: time for a different approach. J Heart Lung Transplant 1994;13(Suppl):S107–S112.
9. Chen YT, Vaccarino V, Williams CS, et al. Risk factors for heart failure in the elderly: a prospective community-based study. Am J Med 1999;106:605–612.
10. Nagai J, Metter EJ, Earley EJ, et al. Increased carotid artery intimal-medial thickness in asymptomatic older subjects with exercise-induced myocardial ischemia. Circulation 1998;98:1504–1509.
11. Lakatta EG. Changes in cardiovascular function with aging. Eur Heart J 1990;11(Suppl):22–29.
12. Gerstenblith G, Fredricksen J, Yin FCP, et al. Echocardiographic assessment of normal adult aging population. Circulation 1977;56:273–278.
13. Lakatta EG. Cardiovascular aging in health. Clin Geriatr Med 2000;16:419–443.
14. Swinne CJ, Shapiro EP, Lima SD, et al. Age-associated changes in left ventricular diastolic performance during isometric exercise in normal subjects. Am J Cardiol 1992;69:823–826.
15. Priebe H-J. The aged cardiovascular risk patient. Br J Anaesth 2000;85:763–778.
16. Ebert TJ, Morgan BJ, Barney JA, Denahan T, Smith JJ. Effects of aging on baroreflex regulation of sympathetic activity in humans. Am J Physiol 1992;263:H798–H803.
17. Esler MD, Turner AG, Kaye DM, et al. Aging effects on human sympathetic neuronal function. Am J Physiol 1995;268:R278–R285.
18. Rudner XL, Berkowitz DE, Booth JV, et al. Subtype specific regulation of human vascular alpha1-adrenergic receptors by vessel bed and age. Circulation 1999;100:2336–2343.
19. Lakatta EG. Cardiovascular aging research: the next horizons. J Am Geriatr Soc 1999;47:613–625.
20. Barron HV, Every NR, Parson LS, Angeja B, Goldberg RJ, Gore JM, et al., for the Investigators in the National Registry of Myocardial Infarction 2. The use of intra-aortic balloon counterpulsation in patients with cardiogenic shock complicating acute myocardial infarction: data from the National Registry of Myocardial Infarction 2. Am Heart J 2001;141:933–939.
21. Gutfinger DE, Ott RA, Miller M, Selvan A, Codini MA, Alimadadian H, et al. Aggressive preoperative use of intraaortic balloon pump in elderly patients undergoing coronary artery bypass grafting. Ann Thorac Surg 1999;67:610–613.
22. Oz MC. Passive ventricular constraint for the treatment of congestive heart failure. Ann Thorac Surg 2001; 71:S185–S187.
23. Power JM, Raman J, Dornom A, Farish SJ, Burrell LM, Tonkin AM, et al. Passive ventricular constraint amends the course of heart failure: a study in an ovine model of dilated cardiomyopathy. Cardiovasc Res 1999;44:549–555.

24. Chaudhry PA, Mishima T, Sharov VG, Hawkins J, Alferness C, Paone G, et al. Passive epicardial containment prevents ventricular remodeling in heart failure. Ann Thorac Surg 2000;1275–1280.

25. Konertz WF, Shapland E, Hotz H, Dushe S, Braun JP, Stantke K, et al. Passive containment and reverse remodeling by a novel textile cardiac support device. Circulation 2001;104(Suppl I):I270–I275.

26. Gronda E, Mangiavacchi M, Frigerio M, et al. Determination of candidacy for mechanical circulatory support: importance of clinical indices. J Heart Lung Transplant 2000;19:S83–S88.

27. Morales DLS, Argenziano M, Oz MC. Outpatient left ventricular assist device support: a safe and economical therapeutic option for heart failure. Prog Cardiovasc Dis 2000;43:55–66.

28. Dowling RD, Etoch SW, Stevens KA, Johnson AC, Gray LA. Current status of the AbioCor implantable replacement heart. Ann Thorac Surg 2001;71:S147–S149.

29. Goldstein DJ, Oz MC, Rose EA. Implantable left ventricular assist devices. N Engl J Med 1998;339: 1522–1533.

30. Oz MC, Goldstein DJ, Rose EA. Preperitoneal placement of ventricular assist devices: an illustrated stepwise approach. J Cardiac Surg 1995;10:288–294.

31. Mehta SM, Aufiero TX, Pae WE Jr, Miller CA, Pierce WS. Combined registry for the clinical use of mechanical ventricular assist pumps and the total artificial heart in conjunction with heart transplantation: sixth official report—1994. J Heart Lung Transplant 1995;14:585–593.

32. Gronda E, Mangiavacchi M, Frigerio M, Oliva F, Andreuzzi B, Paolucci M, et al. Determination of candidacy for mechanical circulatory support: importance of clinical indices. J Heart Lung Transplant 2000;19:S83–S88.

33. Costanzo MR, Augustine S, Bourge R, et al. Selection and treatment of candidate for heart transplantation. A statement of health professionals from the Committee on Heart Failure and Cardiac Transplantation of the Council on Clinical Cardiology, American Heart Association. Circulation 1995;92:3593–3612.

34. Hunt SA, Frazier OH. Mechanical circulatory support and cardiac transplantation. Circulation 1998;97: 2079–2090.

35. Burkhoff D, Holmes JW, Madigan J, Barbone A, Oz MC. Left ventricular assist device-induced reverse ventricular remodeling. Prog Cardiovasc Dis 2000;43:19–26.

36. Levin HR, Oz MC, Chen JM, et al. Reversal of chronic ventricular dilation in patients with end-stage cardiomyopathy by prolonged mechanical unloading. Circulation 1995;91:2717–2720.

37. Altemose GT, Gritsus V, Jeevanandam V, et al. Altered myocardial phenotype after mechanical support in human with advanced cardiomyopathy. J Heart Lung Transplant 1997;16:765–773.

38. Zafeiridis A, Houser SR, Mattielo JA, et al. Gene expression of the cardiac Na+-Ca2+ exchanger in end-stage human heart failure. Circ Res 1994;75:443–453.

39. Dipla K, Mattiello JA, Jeevanandam V, et al. Myocyte recovery after mechanical circulatory support in humans with end-stage heart failure. Circulation 1998;97:2316–2322.

40. Jaski BE, Lingle RL, Reardon LC, Dembitsky WP. Left ventricular assist device as a bridge to patient a myocardial recovery. Prog Cardiovasc Dis 2000;43:5–18.

41. Morales DLS, Argenziano M, Oz MC. Outpatient left ventricular assist device support: a safe and economical therapeutic option for heart failure. Prog Cardiovasc Dis 2000;43:55–66.

42. Goldstein DJ, Rose EA. Cardiac allotransplantation. In: Rose EA, Stevenson LW, eds. Management of End-Stage Heart Disease. Lipincott–Raven, Philadelphia, PA, 1998, pp. 177–185.

43. Stevenson LW. When is heart failure a surgical disease? In: Rose EA, Stevenson LW, eds. Management of End-Stage Heart Disease. Lipincott–Raven, Philadelphia, PA, 1998, pp. 129–146.

44. Cloy MJ, Myers TJ, Stutts LA, Macris MP, Frazier OH. Hospital charges for conventional therapy versus left ventricular assist system therapy in heart transplant patients. ASAIO J 1995;41:M535–M539.

45. Rose EA, Gelijns AC, Moskowitz AJ, Heitjan DF, Stevenson LW, Dembitsky W, et al., for the Randomized Evaluation of Mechanical Assistance for the Treatment of Congestive Heart Failure (REMATCH) Study Group. Long-term use of a left ventricular assist device for end-stage heart failure. N Engl J Med 2001;345:1435–1443.

46. Rao V, Slater JP, Edwards NM, Naka Y, Oz MC. Surgical management of valvular disease in patients requiring left ventricular assist device support. Ann Thorac Surg 2001;71:1448–1453.

47. Smedira NG, Dasse KA, Patel AN, Vargo RL, Massad MG, McCarthy PM. Age-related outcome after implantable left ventricular assist system support. ASAIO J 1996;42:M570–M573.

48. Wareing TH, Kouchoukos NT. Postcardiotomy mechanical circulatory support in the elderly. Ann Thorac Surg 1991;51:443–447.

49. Hosenpud JD, Bennett LE, Keck BM, Boucek MM, Novick RJ. The registry of the International Society for Heart and Lung Transplantation: Seventeenth official report—2000. J Heart Lung Transplant 2000; 19:909.

50. Shaw BW Jr. Transplantation in the elderly patient. Surg Clin Am 1994;74:389–400.
51. Carrier M, Emery RW, Riley JE, et al. Cardiac transplantation in patients over 50 years of age. J Am Coll Cardiol 1986;8:285–288.
52. Renlund DG, Gilbert EM, O'Connell JB, et al. Clinical studies: age-associated decline in cardiac allograft rejection. Am J Med 1987;83:391–398.
53. Blanche C, Blanche DA, Kearney B, Sandhu M, Czer L, Kamlot A, et al. Heart transplantation in patients seventy years of age and older: a comparative analysis of outcome. J Thorac Cardiovasc Surg 2001; 121:532–541.
54. Van Weel C, Michels J. Dying, not old age, to blame for costs of health care. Lancet 1997;350:1159–1160.
55. Pathy J. Cardiac surgery in elderly patients: benefits and resource priorities. Heart 1999;82:121–122.
56. Moskowitz AJ, Rose EA, Gelijns AC. The cost of long-term LVAD implantation. Ann Thorac Surg 2001;71(3 Suppl):S203–S204.
57. Zaidi AM, Fitzpatrick AP, Keenan DJM, Odom NJ, Grotte GJ. Good outcomes from cardiac surgery in the over 70s. Heart 1999;82:134–137.
58. Deiwick M, Tandler R, Mollhoff T, Kerber S, Rotker J, Roeder N, et al. Heart surgery in patients aged eighty years and above: determinants of morbidity and mortality. Thorac Cardiovasc Surg 1997;45: 119–126.
59. Avery GJ, Ley SJ, Hill JD, Hershon JJ, Dick SE. Cardiac surgery in the octogenarian: evaluation of risk, cost, and outcome. Ann Thorac Surg 2001;71:591–596.
60. Polanczyk CA, Rohde LEP, Dec W, DiSalvo T. Ten-year trends in hospital care for congestive heart failure. Arch Intern Med 2000;160:325–332.

17

Cardiac Pacing and Defibrillators

Henry M. Spotnitz, MD

INTRODUCTION

General management of pacemakers and defibrillators has been well described previously *(1–3)*. A recent review of 2760 procedures at the Columbia–Presbyterian campus of New York Presbyterian Hospital revealed that 23% of pacemaker recipients and 5% of implantable cardioverter defibrillator (ICD) recipients were octogenarians. The 80 to 90 yr age group also accounted for 22% of pacemaker generator replacements and 5% of ICD generator replacements. The incidence of pacemaker insertion in patients older than 75 was 2.6% in a recent survey of noninstitutionalized adults. The efficacy and cost-effectiveness of pacemaker insertion in older patients are widely accepted *(1)*, but the appropriate role for ICD insertion in the elderly remains to be established. Problems with arrhythmia control devices in older patients include difficulty with venous access, device follow-up, effects of progressive deterioration of cardiac function, dementia/delerium during and after surgery, and complex issues encompassing patient motivation, quality-of-life, and cost. This chapter will discuss general management of pacemakers as well as issues specific to older patients.

From: *Aging, Heart Disease, and Its Management: Facts and Controversies*
Edited by: N. Edwards, M. Maurer, and R. Wellner © Humana Press Inc., Totowa, NJ

DISCUSSION OF PACEMAKERS

A "permanent pacemaker" consists of pacing leads *(2)* and a pacemaker generator. The generator contains a battery, a telemetry antenna, and integrated circuits. The power source is generally lithium iodide, but rechargeable and nuclear batteries have been used. The integrated circuits include programmable microprocessors providing memory functions, oscillators, amplifiers, and sensing circuits *(3)*. The integrated circuits employ CMOS (complimentary metal oxide semiconductor) technology, which can be damaged by ionizing radiation *(4)*. Current pacemakers can telemeter their internal status, the condition of their external connections, their programmed settings, and recent activity. Unfortunately, each device only responds to the programmer of its manufacturer.

A five-letter code describes pacemaker function *(5)*. The first three letters are in common usage. The first letter is the chamber paced; the second is the chamber sensed. The third letter describes the algorithm used to integrate pacing and sensing functions. Thus, fixed-rate ventricular and atrial pacemakers are VOO and AOO, respectively. Demand (rate inhibited) pacers for the same chambers would be VVI and AAI. VDD refers to a pacemaker that paces the ventricle only, but senses both the atrium and the ventricle *(6)*. DVI involves atrial and ventricular pacing, but only the ventricle is sensed. DDD is the most flexible of current designs.

Cellular membrane depolarization and repolarization allow automaticity of the cardiac chambers and the conduction system. In the resting state, the outer surface of the cell is positive and the interior of the cell is negative. Applying a negative current to the outside of the cell theoretically would produce a greater potential difference and more successfully depolarize the cell than a positive current. Empirically, such a relation is observed: Unipolar pacing thresholds are lowest when the negative terminal (cathode) of a pacing system is connected to the heart and the positive terminal (anode) is connected to ground *(7)*. Electrogram amplitude is not substantially dependent on polarity.

SPECIFIC DISORDERS POTENTIALLY REQUIRING PACING

Concern about indiscriminate recommendation for pacemaker insertion led to the development of Medicare guidelines (*see* Table 1). Supporting documentation may be required. Medicare divides indications into three categories: justified, never justified, and possibly justified. Symptomatic third-degree heart block and profound sinus bradycardia are not problematic if adequately documented. Evaluation of sinus bradycardia with rates in the 50s can be quite complex. Symptoms must be shown to be causally related to the underlying bradyarrhythmia. Documentation of this is likely to require Holter monitoring. Medicare allows pacemakers in support of long-term necessary drug therapy for medical conditions such as supraventricular arrhythmias, ventricular tachycardia, hypertension, and angina. Although new indications for pacemaker therapy may be well supported by clinical research, recognition of such advances by Medicare is often slow. An electrophysiology (EP) study is often helpful in defining proper treatment *(8)*.

Pacing is indicated in sinus node dysfunction either when symptomatic bradycardia is present or when symptomatic bradycardia is caused by administration of drugs required for treatment of ancillary conditions. Causes of sinus node dysfunction include coronary artery disease, cardiomyopathy, and reflex influences.

First degree heart block represents prolongation of the PR interval. Second-degree block involves incomplete dissociation of the atria and ventricles, which results in either

Table 1
Medicare Guidelines for Cardiac Pacemaker Implantation

Accepted in symptomatic patients with chronic conditions
  Atrioventricular (AV) block
    Complete (third degree)
    Incomplete (second degree)
      Mobitz I
      Mobitz II
    Incomplete with 2:1 or 3:1 block
  Sinus node dysfunction (symptomatic)
    Sinus bradycardia, sinoatrial block, sinus arrest
    Bradycardia–tachycardia syndrome
Controversial
  In symptomatic patients
    Bifascicular/trifascicular intraventricular block
    Hypersensitive carotid sinus syndrome
  In asymptomatic patients
    Third-degree block
    Mobitz II
    Mobitz II AV block following myocardial infarction
    Congenital AV block
    Sinus bradycardia <45 bpm with long-term necessary drug therapy
    Overdrive pacing for ventricular tachycardia
Not warranted
  Syncope of undetermined cause
  In asymptomatic patients
    Sinus bradycardia, sinoatrial block, sinus arrest
    Bundle branch blocks
    Mobitz I

Source: Modified from AMA Council on Scientific Affairs. The use of cardiac pacemakers in medical practice. JAMA 1985.

progressive PR prolongation and dropped beats (Wenckebach, Mobitz I, usually AV nodal block) or frequently dropped beats without prior progression of the PR interval [Mobitz II, usually in the His–Purkinje system *(9)*]. Third-degree block is diagnosed when complete atrioventricular (AV) dissociation is present and the atrial rate exceeds the ventricular rate. Left and right bundle branch blocks and left anterior and posterior hemiblocks complete the spectrum of conduction system blocks recognizable by electrocardiogram. The etiology of AV block includes ischemic heart disease, idiopathic fibrosis, cardiomyopathy, iatrogenic damage, AV node ablation, Lyme disease, bacterial endocarditis, lupus erythematosis, and congenital heart disease. In general, pacing is always indicated for symptomatic second- and third-degree AV block.

Neurally mediated reflex disorders include carotid sinus hypersensitivity, vasovagal syncope, and rare entities such as micturation-induced and deglutition syncope *(10)*. Both cardioinhibitory (asystole >3 s) and vasodepressor (marked fall in blood pressure despite adequate heart rate) components of reflex-mediated syncope are recognized. The indication for pacemaker insertion is determined by symptoms and clinical judgment based on the duration of asystole. Tilt-table testing provides objective data. Current trends favor pacemaker insertion for asystolic intervals >3 s; medical therapy is favored for vasodepressor syncope, even with substantial sinus bradycardia *(11)*. Dual-chamber (DDD or VDD) pacing is strongly favored for this population because of beneficial effects of AV synchrony on both stroke volume and symptoms.

FEATURES OF PERMANENT PACING

Atrioventricular synchrony is important for maintenance of ventricular filling and stroke volume. In the normal heart, stroke volume is increased 5–15% by AV synchrony (vs the asynchronous state) *(12,13)*. In the presence of left-ventricular hypertrophy, older age, and heart failure, atrial contraction is of even greater quantitative significance *(14)*. Apical pacing of the right-ventricle disrupts the normal sequence of activation, because depolarization spreads slowly and progressively over the ventricular walls rather than spreading rapidly and symmetrically through the conduction system.

The hypothesis that abnormalities of the sequence of activation can impair mechanical performance of the left ventricle has been established experimentally, but recent developments have increased the clinical relevance of this finding. Thus, disruption of the activation sequence is believed to explain the ventricular–aortic gradient reduction in hypertrophic obstructive cardiomyopathy (HOCM) with DDD pacing *(15–17)*. Conversely, some clinical studies suggest that right-ventricular (RV) outflow tract pacing may improve stroke volume compared to apical pacing because of favorable effects on activation sequence *(18)*. Biventricular pacing with leads in the RV apex and coronary sinus in patients with advanced cardiomyopathy and an intraventricular conduction defect is believed to improve LV function by "ventricular resynchronization"—restoring simultaneous contraction of the septum and free wall *(19)*.

The functional algorithm of DDD pacemakers includes the lower rate, the upper rate, and the AV delay *(20)*. If the atrial rate falls between the upper and lower rate limits, the pacemaker will maintain a 1:1 response between the right atrium (RA) and RV. If the atrial rate falls to the lower rate limit, the pacemaker initiates atrial pacing. If the atrial rate exceeds the upper rate limit, the pacemaker lowers the ventricular rate to the upper rate limit. Loss of AV synchrony results when pacing at the upper rate limit, resembling a Wenckebach effect.

The algorithm for ventricular pacing includes a programmable AV delay. Timing starts when an atrial electrogram or pacing stimulus is detected. If no ventricular depolarization is detected within the allowed interval, the ventricle is paced. With atrial pacing, the actual P-wave may occur as much as 100 ms after the pacing artifact. This is accounted for by using a longer AV delay during atrial pacing than during atrial tracking.

At times of high metabolic demand, cardiac output is physiologically potentiated by increased myocardial contractility, increased venous return, and increased heart rate. In patients with a normal sinus node rate response to exercise and complete AV block, dual-chamber pacemakers restore both AV synchrony and, by tracking the atrium, a normal rate response. With dual-chamber pacing and sinus node incompetence (no atrial rate increase with exercise) or with single-chamber ventricular pacing, alternative methods of assessing and compensating for metabolic demand are needed. Pacemakers with this capability are identified by the letter "R" (for "rate responsive") added to the three-letter pacemaker code. Either body vibration *(21)* or respiratory rate *(22)* is commonly employed to estimate demand in commercial products. Other indicators under evaluation include body temperature *(23)*, venous oxygen saturation *(24)*, QT interval *(25)*, RV systolic pressure *(26)*, and RV stroke volume *(27)*. All proposed and implemented indicators can produce aberrant increases in heart rate *(28)*. For example, a pacemaker that senses body vibration may cause tachycardia during a bumpy car ride. Elderly patients with sedentary lifestyles are unlikely to benefit substantially from rate-responsive pacing, and adverse effects can result from elevated heart rates in patients with evolving coronary disease.

Enthusiasm for dual-chamber pacing continues to increase. Because of the development of mode switching and the observation that sinus rhythm may be better maintained by atrial than ventricular pacing, paroxysmal atrial fibrillation is no longer considered a contraindication to this type of pacing *(29)*. Similarly, dual-chamber pacing is now recommended for reflex-mediated syncope with cardioinhibitory features *(11)*. Whether or not the additional complexity of dual-chamber pacing is warranted in elderly patients who do not suffer from pacemaker syndrome is debatable. Either VVI or VVIR pacing is most appropriate for chronic atrial fibrillation patients with bradycardia. AAIR is appropriate for cardiac allograft recipients who experience either sinus arrest or sinus bradycardia *(30)*.

In unipolar systems, the patient's body serves as a ground for anodal conduction; leads containing only a single conductor carry the negative current to the heart. Bipolar lead designs involve two conductors electrically isolated by insulation. Bipolar pacing systems are resistant to electrical "noise" (oversensing) and adventitious pacing of the diaphragm or chest wall. These advantages are offset by the increased engineering complexity of containing two conductors in a single structure. Bipolar leads are more prone to structural breakdown of its insulation or conductors, which can lead to important forms of pacemaker malfunction *(2,31)*. Bipolar leads tend to be thicker, stiffer, and less easily maneuvered than unipolar leads. Flexibility facilitates J-bends and reduces the risk of perforating the right ventricular apex. Recent bipolar leads are similar in diameter to unipolar leads, but long-term durability remains to be proven.

Positive lead fixation techniques are preferable, particularly in locations with minimal trabeculation. Positive fixation involves a small wire spiral or "screw" at the tip of the lead. A fixed screw may be covered with soluble material to promote venous passage. Alternatively, a retractable screw may be used, which is either extended or retracted by rotation of the pin at the lead tip. Axial clockwise rotation of these leads during fixation provides tactile feedback about the firmness and reproducibility of the fixation site.

Tined leads use miniature anchors in a variety of shapes and sizes that secure the lead tip by wedging between myocardial trabeculae. Tined leads require a larger introducer than screw-in leads do and are not as secure in ventricles which are either smooth walled (as in corrected transposition of the great vessels) or massively dilated. Tined leads are also less secure in atrial insertion. However, many have achieved excellent results with these leads *(32,33)*.

TEMPORARY PACING

Acute bradycardia can be treated with transthoracic pacing, temporary endocardial pacing, or chronotropic drugs like atropine or isoproterenol. Right ventricle perforation has become less likely with current endocardial lead designs, but this complication must be considered if hypotension develops following temporary wire removal.

Bradycardia after cardiac surgery is usually treated with pacing using temporary atrial and ventricular epicardial wires. Potential problems include loss of right atrium or right ventricle capture and loss of right atrium sensing. Competition between an atrial pacemaker and the patient's intrinsic rhythm can precipitate either atrial fibrillation or atrial flutter. If atrial sensing is inadequate, pacing the atrium at a rate that is considerably faster than the intrinsic rate can reduce competition. Reversing polarity or inserting an independent ground wire in the skin under local anesthesia may alleviate problems with temporary epicardial pacing. The output of the external generator should be set at least twice as high as the threshold and measured daily.

Pacing rate and AV delay may affect hemodynamics in patients following cardiac surgery. If systemic vascular resistance is constant, mean arterial pressure is directly correlated to cardiac output. Following the mean pressure as the rate is varied can optimize cardiac output. Rate adjustments should be examined over intervals of less than 20 s to minimize reflex effects. The rate yielding the highest sustained mean arterial pressure should also produce the highest cardiac output.

PACEMAKER INSERTION

Recent trends favor pacemaker and ICD surgery in EP laboratories as well as operating rooms *(34)*. Infection control is critical *(35)*; operating room standards for air quality should be enforced. Pacemakers can be inserted in an EP laboratory by one skilled surgeon and one skilled circulating nurse. This is satisfactory unless complications such as angina, transient ischemic attack, patient disorientation, or lidocaine toxicity arise. Also, the presence of an anesthesiologist during pacemaker insertion may be warranted in patients who are likely to experience adverse intraoperative effects or are simply unstable as a result of dementia, delirium, myocardial ischemia, heart failure, anxiety, or ventricular tachycardia. Vancomycin reactions (Red Man syndrome), pacing-induced ventricular fibrillation, air embolism, and Stokes–Adams attacks may occur, albeit rarely, requiring assistance of a skilled specialist. Intraoperative mortality can result from hemorrhage or myocardial infarction. Good clinical judgment about when an anesthesiologist is essential is an important issue, particularly in the elderly. If English is not the patient's first language, a translator can be immensely helpful.

The type of monitoring employed during pacemaker implantation can be crucial. Pacing artifacts that fail to capture may not be distinguishable from those that do solely on the basis of electrocardiogram (ECG) R-wave detection systems. Regular signaling from the monitor can be elicited in an asystolic patient despite subthreshold pacing. Oxygen-saturation monitors, on the other hand, signal only during blood flow. Additionally, palpation of temporal, facial, or radial artery pulses can be valuable for confirming the presence of an adequate pulse.

Venous access choices include the following: which side will be employed and whether or not a cutdown or percutaneous venipuncture will be used. Cutdown approaches to the cephalic, external jugular, and internal jugular system have been described *(34,36)*. Subclavian venipuncture has recently been modified *(31,37)* in an effort to reduce the frequency of subclavian crush. Subclavian puncture is associated with a low incidence of pneumo/hemothorax and major venous injury *(38)*. Venous access is effectively impossible in a patient with superior vena cava syndrome or subclavian/innominate vein thrombosis (e.g., with chronic dialysis, mediastinal tracheostomy, or multiple pacemaker leads). Access from below is possible *(35,39)*, but the potential for venous thrombosis and pulmonary embolism is a concern. One useful approach described is a right parasternal mediastinotomy. The right atrium is exposed for a Seldinger approach with small introducers through an atrial pursestring suture *(40)*. Technical details of pacemaker insertion and generator replacement have been described *(38)*.

Although cosmetic appearance may seem a secondary concern for the octogenarian, good technique is critical in order to minimize the risk of developing pressure necrosis in patients with poor nutrition. In addition, patients with prior injuries or history of surgery/radiotherapy from breast cancer can present formidable technical problems.

Standard recommendations for wound care include keeping wounds dry until the follow-up office visit 7–10 d postoperatively. Any wound drainage should be cultured, and prophylactic antibiotics should be started while awaiting culture results. We have abandoned aspiration of the rare postoperative hematoma in favor of close observation, unless infection is an issue or spontaneous drainage appears imminent.

Early hospital discharge after pacemaker insertion is feasible in patients who have an adequate escape rhythm. After monitoring and recovery from sedation, patients are ambulated and instructed in range of motion exercises for the shoulder. A chest radiograph is obtained to document lead position and rule out hemo/pneumothorax or pericardial enlargement. Lead displacement can be the result of technical error, physical resistance from uncooperative patients, and other factors. Because a small percentage of lead displacement is probably unavoidable *(32,33)*, patients who might suffer death or injury in the event of abrupt pacemaker failure should be observed in the hospital overnight on telemetry. Lead displacement in ambulatory patients has not occurred more frequently than in hospitalized patients.

COMPLICATIONS OF PACEMAKER INSERTION

The incidence of early complications of pacemaker implantation in one recent large series was 6.7%, of which 4.9% required reoperation *(39)*, figures that were comparable in patients over 65 to those under 65 (6.1% and 4.4%, respectively) *(41)*. Lead displacement, pneumothorax, and cardiac perforation were the most common complications. The reported incidence of late complications was 7.2% *(39)*. Death is a rare complication of pacemaker insertion *(34,39,41)*. Lethal technical complications include lead displacement, venous or cardiac perforation *(2,34,39)*, air embolism, and ventricular tachycardia or fibrillation.

The incidence of endocardial lead displacement with early lead designs was greater than 10% *(42)*. With tined and positive fixation leads, this figure has fallen to the range of 2% *(2,32,33,39,41–44)*. The overall incidence of this complication was 1.5% for both atrial and ventricular leads in all locations in a recent review of experience at the Columbia–Presbyterian Medical Center *(34)*. If the lead length is too short, a deep breath in the upright position can result in lead displacement. If the lead length is too long, an unintended loop may form in the atrium or ventricle, causing arrhythmias or lead displacement.

Bradycardia is a common indication for pacemaker insertion in patients with inoperable coronary artery disease, but an increase in heart rate can be detrimental. Angina, myocardial infarction or death can result from pacemaker-induced increases in heart rate. Hemopneumothorax and pericardial tamponade can result from injury to the heart, arterial, or venous system. The Seldinger technique can lead to such injuries when not applied correctly. In patients over 65, pneumothorax has been related to subclavian puncture *(41)*.

Loss of AV synchrony produces symptoms related to contraction of the atria against closed AV valves and reflex effects. The resulting constellation of symptoms is known as pacemaker syndrome *(45)*. These symptoms are quite variable, but severely affected patients are reluctant to allow pacemaker magnet testing. Symptoms are relieved immediately by conversion from VVI to dual-chamber pacing.

Our experience with lead entrapment is 3 firmly entangled leads in 1000 lead implants. Entrapment of a pacemaker lead in the chordae tendineae can be treated by application of lead extraction techniques *(46,47)* and an open procedure. To avoid the increased risk associated with lead extraction, all three of the leads were capped and abandoned. There were no untoward consequences of abandoning these leads. This experience taught us to avoid the anatomic center of the right ventricle when implanting positive fixation leads. This problem has not recurred in more than 750 subsequent pacemaker implants.

Pacemaker infection appears as frank sepsis, intermittent fever with vegetations, or inflammation, purulence, and drainage at the pacemaker pocket. Established infection in implanted prosthetic devices can be suppressed but rarely eliminated by antibiotics. Antibiotic suppression may result in temporary resolution of drainage from a pacemaker or ICD pocket, but a relapse usually occurs several months later *(48,49)*. Negative cultures from pacemaker erosion may encourage the clinician to move the generator to a fresh, adjacent site. However, recurrent erosion usually results. Clinical resolution of recurrent device erosion in such individuals almost always requires removal of all hardware and insertion of a new device from a fresh site *(48,49)*. Operator inexperience was recently shown to increase the incidence of erosions, infections, hematoma, and lead displacement early after pacemaker insertion *(44)*.

The pulse width delivered to the ventricular lead should be at least twice the threshold value. Adjusting generator output to a safe minimum can prolong pacemaker generator longevity and prevent premature battery depletion. Because of early instability of pacing thresholds, we make this adjustment 1 yr following insertion of new pacemaker leads. Electrical component failures are rare. Over the past 10 yr, we have seen three pacemaker and ICD generator failures, requiring urgent device replacement. New pacemakers and leads may contain design flaws that will not become apparent for many years *(2,50)*.

Pacemaker dysfunction can be caused by mechanical defects in leads, lead displacement, or errors in connecting the lead to the generator. Most commonly, dysfunction represents scarring at the lead–myocardial interface, changes in myocardial properties as a result of tissue necrosis or drug effects, or a poor initial choice of lead position. Undersensing is a failure to sense atrial or ventricular electrograms, manifested as an atrial or ventricular pacing artifact that should have been inhibited by a preceding (unsensed) beat. In a dual-chamber pacemaker, undersensing may also appear as failure to pace the ventricle after an atrial P-wave. Such complications may be resolved by programming increased generator sensitivity, but this can increase the risk of oversensing. The latitude for reprogramming can be estimated by examining telemetered electrograms *(39)*.

Oversensing is inappropriate pacemaker inhibition or triggering in unipolar systems that can result from detection of myopotentials (muscular activity). This can occur without compromise of lead integrity and may be correctable by reprogramming to reduce pacemaker sensitivity. Such problems in bipolar systems may indicate breakdown of lead insulation.

A deflection on the ventricular lead immediately after the atrial-pacing artifact could signal either a premature ventricular contraction or far-field sensing of an atrial depolarization. Many pacemakers deal with this ambiguity by pacing the ventricle at a very short (100 ms) AV delay. Observation of this phenomenon, known as "safety pacing," indicates that the pacemaker is detecting a signal during the AV delay (20). Complexities of dual-chamber pacemaker programming involve blanking and refractory periods used to compensate either for crosstalk or for the onset of atrial fibrillation, or to prevent retrograde AV conduction from producing pacemaker-mediated tachycardia (see below). Crosstalk is ameliorated by bipolar lead systems.

Pacing threshold is expected to increase over 7–14 d after lead insertion and then stabilize after about 6 wk. Exit block refers to a rising pacing threshold resulting from edema or scarring at the lead tip–myocardial interface. This phenomenon, which is believed to be related to inflammatory changes at the lead tip, is ameliorated by steroid eluting leads (2, 51). Exit block may be corrected by programming increased amplitude or pulse width, but this shortens battery life. In unipolar systems, pacing of chest wall and/or diaphragm may result from high generator output.

Suspected lead fracture, whether resulting from insulation or conductor breaks, is often demonstrable by chest X-ray. Lead impedance of less than 300 Ω suggests an insulation break, whereas high lead impedance (more than 1000 Ω) may suggest conductor problems. Telemetered electrograms, if available, should be monitored for noise while the patient hyperventilates, coughs, bends, and swings his arms. Pacemaker malfunction related to body movement is an indication for lead replacement or repair. Dysfunctional leads should be capped. Lead removal is potentially traumatic and probably should be deferred unless infection or mechanical problems are an issue. The probability of lead fracture has, in the past, been increased by design errors, bipolar construction, certain forms of polyurethane insulation, and epicardial insertion (50). Technical factors may include tight ligatures applied to the lead without an anchoring sleeve, kinking, lead angulation, and "subclavian crush" (2,31,37). An unusual form of lead fracture affects the Telectronics Accufix atrial screw-in lead. A J-bend near the lead tip is maintained by a retention wire bonded to the lead body with polyurethane. The retention wire proved susceptible to fracture, followed by extrusion and cardiovascular injury. More than 45,000 of these leads were implanted. The manufacturer recommended fluoroscopic lead surveillance and lead removal if retention wire fracture is detected (52–54). We have discussed technical aspects of this elsewhere (38).

Subclavian crush refers to entrapment of a pacemaker lead between the clavicle and first rib in the costoclavicular ligament. The lead is believed to be subjected to high levels of stress during body movement, with early lead failure as a result. This problem pertains to leads implanted by percutaneous puncture of the subclavian vein and may be avoided with cephalic cutdown. Techniques employed to minimize this problem have been described (2,31,37).

Pneumothorax/hemothorax are also almost exclusively the result of technical problems related to percutaneous subclavian venipuncture. In our experience with pacemaker insertion in more than 1000 patients by cephalic cutdown, hemopneumothorax has not occurred. In a recent review of 1088 consecutive implants by subclavian puncture, the overall incidence of pneumothorax was 1.8% (44). However, deaths have occurred because of complications of subclavian puncture during pacemaker implantation.

Fifteen percent of pacemaker implants were replacements (55). Complications of pacemaker generator replacement include infection, lead damage, connector problems, and asystole during the transition from the old generator to the new. Relatively minor conduction problems at the time of initial pacemaker implant may progress to severe pacemaker dependence by the time of generator replacement. Ambulatory surgery is usually appropriate.

As a practical matter, we no longer reverse coumadin for pacemaker generator replacement, unless lead replacement is anticipated *(56)*. Patients with leads more than 10 yr old should be carefully evaluated for pacemaker dysfunction prior to generator replacement. A Holter monitor should be obtained if lead dysfunction is suspected. Rising pacing threshold may indicate impending lead failure.

POSTOPERATIVE TESTING/FOLLOW-UP

Whether patients with implanted pacemakers or ICDs should receive antibiotic prophylaxis prior to dental work and other procedures that may cause transient bacteremia is controversial, but it is not recommended by the AHA/ACC guidelines. We recommend prophylaxis for 3 mo after device insertion, allowing time for the pacing leads to become endothelialized.

Pacemakers require periodic testing both to confirm sensing and pacing function and to detect battery depletion. Current standards involve testing these functions at 1 to 3 mo intervals. Whether follow-up should be done by trans-telephonic monitoring, clinic, or office visits is under dispute *(57–59)*. Trans-telephonic monitoring alleviates transportation issues for elderly patients, but some are either too anxious or unable to manage the process. In addition to reduced travel for patients, reduced office volume, and time saved for the physician, many commercial services provide emergency monitoring on a 24 h basis, which can be very helpful for managing apprehensive patients.

Pacemaker programming should be done by trained, experienced personnel. In urgent situations in which programmers are not available, a manufacturer's representative may be able to help with programming. Trans-telephonic programming is not currently available. Basic programming for current DDD pacing includes electrogram sensitivity and pacing stimulus amplitude/pulse width for both the atrium and ventricle. Lower rate, upper rate, atrioventricular delay, and refractory periods for atrial and ventricular sensing are programmable. Programmable rate responsiveness, unipolar/bipolar configuration, and many other options are available.

We initially program newly inserted pacemakers to stimulation amplitude and pulse width higher than nominal. When the patient comes in for an initial office visit, pacing thresholds are retested, and amplitude and pulse width are adjusted to nominal levels if pacing thresholds are appropriate. Details of pacemaker programming have been described elsewhere *(34,50)*. Some current pacemakers are capable of automated threshold adjustment.

Office programming allows most problems detected by transtelephonic or Holter monitoring to be corrected. The etiology of specific patient symptoms can often be elicited by examining real-time electrograms or stored data. Adjustments may include not only sensitivity or pacing output but also pacing mode for new onset atrial fibrillation *(60)* or sinus node incompetence related to medication changes. Problems requiring reoperation include lead displacement, lead fracture, insulation degradation, and exit block *(39,41)*.

INNOVATIONS AND SPECIAL PROBLEMS

Many DDD pacemaker recipients suffer from both sinus bradycardia and intermittent, paroxysmal atrial fibrillation (sick sinus syndrome). A standard DDD pacemaker responds to atrial fibrillation by pacing at the upper rate limit. Although DDD pacing was initially felt to be contraindicated in atrial fibrillation, the current view is that atrial pacing may decrease the frequency of paroxysmal atrial fibrillation. Mode switching achieves a useful compromise *(61)*. Mode switching can be triggered by a programmed upper rate limit or by comparing the observed atrial rate to predictions based on the patient's activity level. If an atrial tachyarrhythmia is detected, the pacemaker switches to VVIR pacing until the atrial rate decreases to the normal range.

A DDD pacemaker can participate in a re-entrant arrhythmia, pacemaker-mediated tachycardia (PMT) *(62)*. This involves retrograde conduction through the AV node, as might occur following a premature ventricular depolarization. If the pacemaker senses the resulting atrial depolarization and the ventricle is paced, a recurring cycle is set up that could continue indefinitely at the upper rate limit of the pacemaker. This problem can be minimized by avoiding high upper rate limits in patients with retrograde conduction and by adjusting the post ventricular atrial refractory period (PVARP) so that the pacemaker will ignore atrial depolarizations for 300–350 ms after the QRS complex. Current pacemaker circuits also have built-in safeguards that attempt to break re-entrant arrhythmias by periodic interruption of continuous pacing at the upper rate limit. In addition, pacemaker telemetry provides notification when upper rate limit pacing suspicious of PMT has been observed.

An increasing problem especially in elderly patients is the need for general surgery in the presence of pacemaker dependence *(63)*. Certain procedures, like hip replacement, require unipolar cautery, making electromagnetic interference with pacemaker function more likely. A multi-step evaluation should be carried out before surgery is begun. The manufacturer and model of the pacemaker must be identified. If the patient's pacemaker card is not available, the service or physician performing pacemaker follow-up may be helpful. A radiograph of the pacemaker may reveal radio-opaque markers, which identify the manufacturer and model, or the X-ray appearance may uniquely identify the pacemaker, if an appropriate reference source is available *(64,65)*. After the pacemaker has been identified, its operating modes, programmability, polarity, end-of-life indicators, and other critical information should be determined. A programmer for the pacemaker should be obtained. Pacemakers with telemetry should be interrogated with the programmer before surgery to determine the pacemaker's operating parameters and to confirm proper function. The next issue is whether or not the patient is pacemaker dependent. If the electrocardiogram reveals ventricular pacing of every beat, the consequences of abrupt pacemaker failure during surgery must be determined, as electrocautery can result in pacemaker failure *(63)*. This is best determined by judicious testing with the programmer. Pacemaker dependence may increase during anesthesia, because of withdrawal of sympathetic stimulation. If the patient is pacemaker dependent, backup pacing or chronotropic agents should be available during surgery. In addition, the pacemaker should be programmed to the VOO, DOO, or VVT mode to counteract possible inhibition by electromagnetic interference *(63)*.

Manufacturers recommend that electrocautery should not be employed in pacemaker patients, but this is impractical. If electrocautery must be used, unipolar cautery is far inferior to bipolar cautery. Unipolar pacemakers are also more susceptible to interference from electrocautery than bipolar pacemakers are. At a minimum, electrical interference from the electrocautery may be misinterpreted by pacemaker sensing circuits as a rapid heart rate, resulting in pacemaker inhibition. This inhibition is reversible when the interference stops. Cautery can also cause pacemaker reprogramming or reversion of the pacemaker to a backup mode. Backup modes differ for different units. A common backup mode is VOO. Finally, electrocautery can cause complete and permanent loss of pacing, although this is rare *(63)*.

One approach to avoiding pacemaker inhibition is to program sensing off and to increase the rate to minimize competition with the intrinsic heart rate. However, competition with spontaneous beats can occur, including a risk of induction of atrial fibrillation or ventricular tachycardia in susceptible patients. In view of this, the pacemaker should be returned to a sensing mode as soon as possible after the completion of surgery.

A permanent magnet placed over a pacemaker closes a magnetic reed switch and converts the pacemaker to "magnet mode." Magnet mode behavior is not the same for all pacemakers. In some, a magnet initiates the VOO mode, making the pacemaker insensitive to electrocautery. Other pacemakers will convert to VOO for a few beats and then revert to the underlying program. Most current generators perform a "threshold margin" test under the influence of a magnet; this investigates the adequacy of the pacing margin by decreasing the output in a predictable pattern.

A promising approach to the problem of fibrosis at the lead–myocardial interface involves incorporation of a pellet of dexamethasone at the lead tip. This has resulted in a reproducible improvement in early lead thresholds, which is superior statistically to performance of conventional leads *(51)*. The clinical performance of these leads makes them the lead of choice for patients who require lead replacement for early exit block. The long-term (>1 yr) performance of steroid eluting leads has not yet been defined.

Cognitive impairment, which may be induced by sedation, can either create serious problems in patients requiring surgery under local anesthesia or exaggerate underlying bradycardia. Patients with dementia or disorientation may manually explore their surgical wound, forcing emergent induction of general anesthesia. Confusion and thrashing can result in pacemaker lead displacement postoperatively. A vigil conducted by family members at the bedside may palliate this problem. Every effort should be made to anticipate and avoid such problems.

Atrioventricular node ablation is used to control ventricular rate response in patients with atrial fibrillation refractory to medical management. One approach is to ablate the AV node, place a temporary wire, and then send the patient to the operating room for permanent pacemaker insertion. Ventricular escape rhythm is often poor in these patients, favoring positive fixation leads and high pacemaker output in the early postoperative period. Alternatively, the pacemaker can be placed and allowed to heal prior to ablation, theoretically reducing the risk of lead displacement and avoiding the need for overnight hospitalization.

Transvenous pacing in ICD recipients has stringent requirements for lead performance. The possibility of cross-talk between devices can result in inappropriate ICD shocks or failure of the ICD to detect and correct a potentially lethal ventricular arrhythmia. Although techniques have been described for simultaneous implantation of an independent pacemaker and an ICD in the same patient *(66)*, currently the preferred solution is the use of ICDs with integrated DDD pacing capability.

HOCM or hypertrophic obstructive cardiomyopathy can cause LV outflow obstruction with angina and/or syncope. Permanent RV pacing at AV intervals sufficient to pre-excite the right ventricle decreases outflow gradients in some patients with HOCM *(15–17)*. A reduction in the incidence of sudden death has also been reported with this approach in patients with a history of syncope, but an ICD may be indicated in selected patients *(67)*.

End-stage cardiomyopathy and heart failure tend to progress with advancing age. Advanced therapies like cardiac transplantation or current left-ventricular assist devices are inappropriate for most octogenarians, but biventricular pacing may be widely applicable. Although clinical improvement has been modest in early trials and requires a QRS duration of greater than 120 ms, this therapy is very helpful in selected patients *(19,68)*.

Overdrive pacing techniques have been described for ventricular tachycardia (VT), Wolff–Parkinson–White syndrome, and atrial flutter *(69,70)*. Implantable pacemaker–defibrillators are under development for atrial fibrillation. Anti-tachycardia ventricular pacing for VT has been integrated into ICD therapy.

ENVIRONMENTAL ISSUES

Electromagnetic interference can result from electrocautery, cellular telephones, magnetic resonance imagers *(71)*, microwaves, diathermy, arc welders, powerful radar and radio transmitters, and theft detectors in department stores. Any defective electrical appliance or motor, including electric razors, lawn mowers, or even an electric light can be problematic. The importance of electrical noise to a pacemaker recipient is related to his or her degree of pacemaker dependence. Most pacemaker recipients are not pacemaker dependent; therefore, a brief period of pacemaker dysfunction will not result in loss of consciousness. Pacemaker-dependent patients who work in electrically noisy environments are likely to benefit from the added protection of bipolar pacing systems. Patients with cellular telephones should maintain several inches of separation between the telephone and the pacemaker generator *(72)*.

Mechanical problems can be caused by lithotripsy, trauma, dental equipment, and even bumpy roads. Trauma associated with motor vehicle accidents has resulted in pacemaker damage and disruption of pacemaker wounds *(73)*. Vibration in subways or automobiles can produce symptoms annoying to patients with vibration sensors in rate-responsive units. Patients with poor escape rhythms, who could suffer death or injury in the event of abrupt pacemaker failure, should be discouraged from exposure to deceleration injury, as can occur during traditional contact sports as well as basketball, handball, downhill skiing, surfing, diving, mountain climbing, and gymnastics. Participants in these activities should realize that abrupt pacemaker failure could occur in the event of lead displacement related to trauma.

The integrated circuits of current pacemakers can be damaged by radiotherapy. If the pacemaker cannot be adequately shielded from the radiation field, it may be necessary to remove and replace it or move the pacing system to a remote site.

Indications for lead extraction include chronic infection and life-threatening mechanical defects *(52–54)*. Some have suggested that any dysfunctional pacemaker lead should be removed. Until recently, the techniques for extraction of a transvenous lead included either external traction or thoracotomy/cardiotomy, employing inflow occlusion or cardiopulmonary bypass. Chronically implanted leads may be densely fibrosed to the RV myocardium, vena cava, innominate, and subclavian veins. Lead extraction has been advanced by techniques described by Byrd *(46,47)*. A carefully sized stylet is passed inside the central channel to the tip of the lead, where it locks by uncoiling, allowing traction to be applied to the lead tip. A long plastic sheath slightly larger than the pacing lead is passed over the lead to the tip. Countertraction is applied to the myocardium with the sheath while traction is applied to the lead tip with the locking stylet. Success with this technique has been greater than 90%, with a 3% chance of serious morbidity or death. Laser-based systems have also been used *(74)*. Technical details have been described *(34,46,47)*. Extraction of leads implanted for more than 10 yr is both difficult and tedious.

In contrast to ICD recipients, quality-of-life is not a major concern for most pacemaker recipients. Although many clinics require periodic visits, the model of trans-telephonic monitoring with office visits only for problems is quite viable. This latter system involves a preop visit, a 10 d postop visit, and a 1 yr visit to adjust output; unless functional problems or impending battery depletion are detected, no additional visits are necessary. Some recipients are never happy with their pacemaker because of issues related to body image, vague symptoms with no clear etiology, or concerns that life will be artificially prolonged. With regard to the latter issue, the value of continuation of pacemaker therapy or generator replacement in patients with advanced debilitation has been discussed *(75)*.

AUTOMATIC IMPLANTABLE CARDIAC DEFIBRILLATORS

More than 400,000 deaths occurring annually in the United States are classified as sudden and likely to be caused by arrhythmias *(76)*. Mirowski conceptualized the implantable defibrillator in the late 1960s. He overcame numerous conceptual, engineering, and financial obstacles and participated in a successful clinical trial of his device in the early 1980s *(77)*. Today's ICD reflects dramatic and resource-intensive growth in technology. The therapeutic efficacy of the ICD in survivors of sudden death is well established. Increasingly sophisticated clinical trials, clinical experience, and the passage of time have only emphasized the survival advantages of the ICD over other modalities, including anti-arrhythmic drugs and subendocardial resection. The ICD is associated with the lowest sudden death mortality (1–2%/yr) of any known form of therapy *(78–81)*. The ICD is expensive ($12,000–$20,000 generator, $2000–$8000 lead system), with discomfort and lifestyle issues. The role of prophylactic ICD insertion is under study.

Clinical trials, including CASH, AVID, MUSST, CIDS, and MADIT, have demonstrated advantages for ICD therapy *(82–89)*. Only The CABG Patch Trial, which compared CABG to CABG+ICD, failed to demonstrate ICD benefits compared to CABG *(90)*. Trials focus now on prophylactic ICD insertion, its cost-effectiveness, and the formidable expense of widespread use of such therapy.

The clinical success of the ICD spurred an intense engineering effort that has increased battery life beyond 5 yr and added broad programmability while reducing size and weight to that of a large pacemaker. Lead systems have evolved from epicardial patches requiring thoracotomy to effective endocardial systems *(78–81)*, potentiated by biphasic shocks *(91)* and "hot can" technology *(92)*. These advances make pectoral implant feasible and preferable for most patients. Implantation is performed by electrophysiologists with increased frequency. Abdominal implantation is now reserved for special cases. Diagnostic advances include downloadable real-time and stored electrograms *(93)*. VVI, DDD, and insensible anti-tachycardia pacing have been successfully integrated into ICDs *(94)*. Accelerated development has put pressure on the Food and Drug Administration to rapidly approve new technology. In 1995, when the US Health Care Finance Administration refused to allow Medicare reimbursement to support device development, ICD development moved overseas.

A straightforward ICD candidate has suffered a documented cardiac arrest in the absence of acute myocardial infarction and is proven unsuitable for anti-arrhythmic drug or surgical therapy based on programmed electrical stimulation studies in the EP laboratory. However, many patients who suffer cardiac arrest do not have inducible VT on EP study, and many patients with a history of syncope and presyncope have inducible VT but no history of a clinical arrhythmia. Many antiarrhythmics have negative inotropic and pro-arrhythmic effects *(95,96)*. Serial EP studies of drug efficacy have been discredited in clinical trials *(91)*. In mid-1996, the Food and Drug Administration (FDA) approved an indication for prophylactic ICD insertion based on early termination of the MADIT Trial *(87)*. If EP studies demonstrate inducible VT in patients with nonsustained VT and history of myocardial infarction, an ICD is indicated.

Implantable cardioverter–defibrillators employ two basic lead systems: one for ventricular pacing/rate sensing and the other to deliver the defibrillation current. These systems are usually bipolar leads, but a unipolar ventricular lead paired with an "active can" delivers the defibrillation current in some designs. Algorithms intended to distinguish supraventricular arrhythmias from VT based on QRS morphology have fallen into disfavor, and rate alone is currently used to determine when a patient requires treatment, resulting in a substantial incidence of inappropriate therapy *(78,97)*. Addition of a bipolar atrial lead allows atrial pacing or differentiation of supraventricular arrhythmias from VT. Subcutaneous patch leads and arrays are available for patients with high defibrillation thresholds (DFTs). Leads come in standard lengths for pectoral implants and long lengths for abdominal implants. Positive fixation leads are available and desirable. The ICD contains a high-energy battery and a capacitor to step up the output voltage to 600–800 V at 35–40 J. Biphasic (positive and negative phases) shocks can reduce DFTs. The device includes integrated circuits and a telemetry antenna. A broad range of programmable diagnostic and therapeutic functions are supported.

Most potential ICD recipients would be at high mortality/morbidity risk for any surgical procedure. Accordingly, therapy of ischemia, heart failure, and systemic illnesses should be optimized before ICD implantation. Ischemia has been more lethal in our experience than an ejection fraction of below 15% has been. When ischemia is severe, the patient may be operable only with ancillary coronary artery bypass grafting (CABG), percutaneous transluminal coronary angioplasty (PTCA), IABP, or deferral of DFT measurement.

The epicardial approach *(98,99)* is now rarely useful (e.g., in patients who require ICD implantation during cardiac surgery). Even this has been discouraged since the CABG Patch Trial demonstrated increased infectious complications *(92)*. Extrapericardial ICD patches cause less fibrotic reaction, less impairment of diastolic properties *(100,101)*, and less potential for graft impingement than intrapericardial leads. Biphasic waveforms, improved leads, high output "hot can" generators, and ancillary subcutaneous patches and arrays contribute to a high rate of success for the endocardial approach. A surgical technique has been described *(34)*.

The DFT is critical to ICD insertion. Its measurement requires induction of ventricular fibrillation (VF). The DFT should be at least 10 J less than the maximum output of the ICD. If DFTs are not adequate with optimized endocardial leads, an axillary subcutaneous patch or array may help by distributing the defibrillation current over the lateral LV. Collaboration with an electrophysiologist is advisable during DFT measurement and ICD programming. DFT measurement can depress LV function *(102,103,103a)* and result in a low-output state. Fortunately, this is rare. The mortality of ICD insertion with present techniques is on the order of 1% *(93)*. Complications include myocardial infarction, heart failure, lead displacement, infection, and venous occlusion.

We keep ICD recipients on telemetry until a postoperative EP evaluation that includes confirmation of pacing thresholds and sensing. DFT measurement is usually not repeated.

Personnel should be trained to use an ICD magnet to inhibit inappropriate shocks triggered by lead displacement or supraventricular arrhythmias. We prefer 24 h of vancomycin and gentamycin followed by 5 d of ciprofloxacin for antibiotic prophylaxis. A postoperative office visit is scheduled 7–14 d after discharge.

At the postoperative office visit, lead position, patient symptoms, and the surgical wound are assessed. If drainage is present, the wound is cultured and treated appropriately. For persistent sterile drainage, ciprofloxacin or bactrim is administered for 10 d, and the patient is asked to keep the wound dry until it heals.

Implantable cardioverter–defibrillators require outpatient EP evaluation at 1 to 3 mo intervals to cycle the capacitors, confirm battery life, test pacing thresholds, and download electrograms. The electrograms define aborted charging cycles and arrhythmias. Programming is adjusted accordingly. For patients reporting an ICD shock, telemetry downloads confirm proper ICD function, detect inappropriate shocks, and can detect electrical noise and oversensing that may indicate a need for lead revisions.

The ICD battery life is now typically more than 60 mo. Generator replacement can be complicated by infection, myocardial infarction, or death. One reason for this is the progression of heart failure and/or coronary artery disease. Replacement is now commonly done under local anesthesia, with sedation during DFT measurement. DFT measurement may be deferred if the risk of the test appears greater than the risk of sudden death. Patients are usually discharged on the same day, unless the high-voltage lead is replaced.

The incidence of lead failure progresses with implant duration. Approximately 50% of ICD recipients require lead revision at 10 yr of follow-up (104–107). Problems include lead fracture, high DFTs, oversensing, undersensing, and exit block. The incidence of transvenous lead displacement is 7% and fracture is 6% at 2-yr follow-up (107). Oversensing can be caused by insulation damage in the ICD pocket. Oversensing is usually corrected with a new transvenous rate-sensing lead, preferably of the positive fixation type. Outer insulation damage inside the defibrillator pocket may be reparable with silicone sleeves, silicone glue, and ligatures (108). Patch leads can fail because of either conductor fracture or distortion by fibrosis. DFTs may increase with cardiac enlargement, which shifts the left ventricle leftward, away from the original lead system. High DFTs can be corrected by insertion of a new transvenous defibrillator lead, a subcutaneous patch, and/or a high-output generator.

The benefits and liabilities of the ICD for treatment of VT/VF in patients who are candidates for cardiac allografting is under investigation (109,110). Transvenous ICDs are likely to be advantageous in this group if the cost of treatment can be reduced.

Quality-of-life issues include the discomfort and distress of repeated shocks and mandatory outpatient visits. These are particularly trying for elderly patients and are an important part of the decision to implement ICD therapy. Dramatic progress has been made in reduction of ICD size, but ICDs remain bulky compared to current pacemakers. Although many patients are elated to be rescued from a malignant arrhythmia by their ICD, others find their plights distressing (111–113). Many ICD patients do not comply with recommended restrictions concerning automobile driving. Fortunately, the reported rate of accidents in ICD recipients is low (114).

Implantable cardioverter–defibrillator therapy is expensive, but the cost of VT/VF management in the absence of an ICD is also substantial. The incremental cost per year-of-life added has been estimated at $10,000–$200,000 (115–117). Substantial reduction in the cost of ICD generators and leads is necessary before potential benefits of widespread implementation of ICD prophylaxis can be widely realized.

REFERENCES

1. Rosenheck S, Geist M, Weiss A, Hasin Y, Weiss TA, Gotsman MS. permanent cardiac pacing in octogenarians. Am J Geriatr Cardiol 1995;4(6):42–47.
2. Mond HG, Helland JR. Engineering and clinical aspects of pacing leads. In: Ellenbogen KA, Kay GN, Wilkoff BL, eds. Clinical Cardiac Pacing. WB Saunders, Philadelphia, PA, 1995, p. 69.
3. Ireland JR, Kay GN. Pulse generator circuitry. In: Ellenbogen KA, Kay GN, Wilkoff BL, eds. Clinical Cardiac Pacing. WB Saunders, Philadelphia, PA, 1995, p. 419.
4. Rodriguez F, Filimonov A, Henning A, et al. Radiation-induced effects in multiprogrammable pacemakers and implantable defibrillators. PACE 1991;14:2143.
5. Bernstein AD, Camm AJ, Fletcher R, et al. The NASPE/BPEG generic pacemaker code for antibrady-arrhythmia and adaptive-rate pacing and antitachy-arrhythmia devices. PACE 1987;10:794.
6. Wiegand UK, Potratz J, Bode F, Schreiber R, Bonnemeier H, Peters W, et al. Cost-effectiveness of dual-chamber pacemaker therapy: does single lead VDD pacing reduce treatment costs of atrioventricular block? Eur Heart J 2001;22(2):174–180.
7. Sokes KB, Kay GN. Artificial electric cardiac stimulation. In: Ellenbogen KA, Kay GN, Wilkoff BL, eds. Clinical Cardiac Pacing. WB Saunders, Philadelphia, PA, 1995, p. 3.
8. Nelson SD, Kou WH, EdBuitleir M, et al. Value of programmed ventricular stimulation in presumed carotid sinus syndrome. Am J Cardiol 1987;60:1073.
9. Wharton JM, Ellenbogen KA. Atrioventricular conduction system disease. In: Ellenbogen KA, Kay GN, Wilkoff BL, eds. Clinical Cardiac Pacing. WB Saunders, Philadelphia, PA, 1995, p. 304.
10. Jaeger FJ, Fouad-Tarazi FM, Casle LW. Carotid sinus hypersensitivity and neurally mediated syncope. In: Ellenbogen KA, Kay GN, Wilkoff BL, eds. Clinical Cardiac Pacing. WB Saunders, Philadelphia, PA, 1995, p. 333.
11. Sra JS, Jazayeri MR, Avitall B, et al. Comparison of cardiac pacing with drug therapy in the treatment of neurocardiogenic (vasovagal) syncope with bradycardia or asystole. N Engl J Med 1993;328:1085.
12. Mitchell JH, Gilmore JP, Sarnoff SJ. The transport function of the atrium: factors influencing the relation between mean left atrial pressures and left ventricular end-diastolic pressure. Am J Cardiol 1962; 9:237.
13. Leclercq C, Gras D, Le Hellco A, et al. Hemodynamic importance of preserving the normal sequence of ventricular activation in permanent cardiac pacing. Am Heart J 1995;129:1133.
14. Prech M, Grygier M, Mitkowski P, Stanek K, Skorupski W, Moszynska B, et al. Effect of restoration of AV synchrony on stroke volume, exercise capacity, and quality-of-life: can we predict the beneficial effect of a pacemaker upgrade? Pacing Clin Electrophysiol 2001;24(3):302–307.
15. Fananapazir L, Cannon RO III, Tripodi D, et al. Impact of dual-chamber permanent pacings in patients with obstructive hypertrophic cardiomyopathy with symptoms refractory to veapamil and b-adrenergic blocker therapy. Circulation 1992;85:2149.
16. Erwin JP III, Nishimura RA, Lloyd MA, Tajik AJ. Dual chamber pacing for patients with hypertrophic obstructive cardiomyopathy: a clinical perspective in 2000. Mayo Clin Proc 2000;75(2):173–180.
17. Gadler F, Linde C, Daubert C, McKenna W, Meisel E, Aliot E, et al. Significant improvement of quality of life following atrioventricular synchronous pacing in patients with hypertrophic obstructive cardiomyopathy. Data from 1 year of follow-up. PIC study group. Pacing In Cardiomyopathy. Eur Heart J 1999;20(14):1044–1050.
18. Karpawich PP, Mital S. Comparative left ventricular function following atrial, septal, and apical single chamber heart pacing in the young. Pacing Clin Electrophysiol 1997;20(8 Pt 1):1983–1988.
19. Leclercq C, Cazeau S, Ritter P, Alonso C, Gras D, Mabo P, et al. A pilot experience with permanent biventricular pacing to treat advanced heart failure. Am Heart J 2000;140(6):862–870.
20. Barold SS. Timing cycles and operational characteristics of pacemakers. In: Ellenbogen KA, Kay GN, Wilkoff BL, eds. Clinical Cardiac Pacing. WB Saunders, Philadelphia, PA, 1995, p. 567.
21. Lau CP, Butrous GS, Ward DE, et al. Comparison of exercise performance of six rate-adaptive right ventricular cardiac pacemakers. Am J Cardiol 1989;63:833.
22. Kay GN, Bubien RS, Epstein AE, et al. Rate-modulated cardiac pacing based on transthoracic impedance meaurements of minute ventilation: correlation with exercise gas exchange. J Am Coll Cardiol 1989; 14:1283.
23. Sellers TD, Fearnot NE, Smith HJ. Temperature controlled rate-adaptive pacing. In: Ellenbogen KA, Kay GN, Wilkoff BL, eds. Clinical Cardiac Pacing. WB Saunders, Philadelphia, PA, 1995, p. 201.

24. Kay GN, Bornzin GA. Rate-modulated pacing controlled by mixed venous oxygen saturation. In: Ellenbogen KA, Kay GN, Wilkoff BL, eds. Clinical Cardiac Pacing. WB Saunders, Philadelphia, PA, 1995, p. 212.

25. Connelly DT, Rickards AF. The evoked QT potential. In: Ellenbogen KA, Kay GN, Wilkoff BL, eds. Clinical Cardiac Pacing. WB Saunders, Philadelphia, PA, 1995, p. 250.

26. Yee R, Bennett TD. Rate-adaptive pacing controlled by dynamic right ventricular pressure (dp/dtmax). In: Ellenbogen KA, Kay GN, Wilkoff BL, eds. Clinical Cardiac Pacing. WB Saunders, Philadelphia, PA, 1995, p. 187.

27. Salo R, O'Donoghue S, Platia EV. The use of intracardiac impedance-based indicators to optimize pacing rate. In: Ellenbogen KA, Kay GN, Wilkoff BL, eds. Clinical Cardiac Pacing. WB Saunders, Philadelphia, PA, 1995, p. 234.

28. Furman S. Rate-modulated pacing. Circulation 1990;82:1081.

29. Hesselson AB, Parsonnet B, Bernstein AD, et al. Deleterious effects of long-term single-chamber ventricular pacing in patients with sick sinus syndrome: the hidden benefits of dual chamber pacing. J Am Coll Cardiol 1992;15:1542.

30. Cooper MW, Smith CR, Rose EA, Schneller SJ, Spotnitz HM. Permanent transvenous pacing following orthotopic heart transplantation. J Thorac Cardiovasc Surg 1992;104:812–816.

31. Magney JE, Flynn DM, Parsons JA, et al. Anatomical mechanisms explaining damage to pacemaker leads, defibrillator leads, and failure of central venous catheters adjacent to the sternoclavicular joint. PACE 1993;16:445.

32. Mond H, Sloman G. The small tined pacemaker lead—absence of dislodgement. PACE 1980;3:171.

33. Mond HG, Hua W, Wang CC. Atrial pacing leads: the clinical contribution of steroid elution. PACE 1995;18:1601.

34. Spotnitz HM. Practical considerations in pacemaker-defibrillator surgery. In: Edmunds LH Jr, ed. Cardiac Surgery in the Adult. McGraw-Hill, New York, 1997, pp. 793–831.

35. Da Costa A, Kirkorian G, Cucherat M, Delahaye F, Chevalier P, Cerisier A, et al. Antibiotic prophylaxis for permanent pacemaker implantation: a meta-analysis. Circulation 1998;97(18):1796–1801.

36. Belott PH, Reynolds DW. Permanent pacemaker implantation. In: Ellenbogen KA, Kay GN, Wilkoff BL, eds. Clinical Cardiac Pacing. WB Saunders, Philadelphia, PA, 1995. p. 447.

37. Mathur G, Stables RH, Heaven D, Ingram A, Sutton R. Permanent pacemaker implantation via the femoral vein: an alternative in cases with contraindications to the pectoral approach. Europace 2001;3(1): 56–59.

38. Byrd CL. Recent developments in pacemaker implantation and lead retrieval. PACE 1993;16:1781.

39. Kiviniemi MS, Pirnes MA, Eranen HJ, Kettunen RV, Hartikainen JE. Complications related to permanent pacemaker therapy. Pacing Clin Electrophysiol 1999;22(5):711–720.

40. Hoyer MH, Beerman LB, Ettedgui JA, Park SC, del Nido PJ, Siewers RD. Transatrial lead placement for endocardial pacing in children. Ann Thorac Surg 1994;58(1):97–101; discussion 101–102.

41. Link MS, Estes NA III, Griffin JJ, Wang PJ, Maloney JD, Kirchhoffer JB, et al. Complications of dual chamber pacemaker implantation in the elderly. Pacemaker Selection in the Elderly (PASE) Investigators. J Interv Cardiac Electrophysiol 1998;2(2):175–179.

42. Brewster GM, Evans AL. Displacement of pacemaker leads-a 10-year survey. Br Heart J 1979;42:266.

43. Perrins EJ, Sutton R, Kalebic B, et al. Modern atrial and ventricular leads for permanent cadiac pacing. Br Heart J 1981;46:196.

44. Aggarwal RK, Connelly DT, Ray SG, et al. Early complications of permanent pacemaker implantation: no difference between dual and single chamber systems. Br Heart J 1995;73:571.

45. Ellenbogen KA, Stambler BS. Pacemaker syndrome. In: Ellenbogen KA, Kay GN, Wilkoff BL, eds. Clinical Cardiac Pacing. WB Saunders, Philadelphia, PA, 1995, p. 419.

46. Smith HJ, Fearnot NE, Byrd CL, et al. Five-years experience with intravascular lead extraction. U.S. Lead Extraction Database. PACE 1994;17:2016.

47. Byrd CL. Management of implant complications. In: Ellenbogen KA, Kay GN, Wilkoff BL, eds. Clinical Cardiac Pacing. WB Saunders, Philadelphia, PA, 1995, p. 491.

48. Chua JD, Wilkoff BL, Lee I, Juratli N, Longworth DL, Gordon SM. Diagnosis and management of infections involving implantable electrophysiologic cardiac devices. Ann Intern Med 2000;133(8):604–608.

49. Molina JE. Undertreatment and overtreatment of patients with infected antiarrhythmic implantable devices.Ann Thorac Surg 1997;63(2):504–509.

50. Furman S, Benedek ZM, Andrews CA, et al. Long-term follow-up of pacemaker lead systems: establishment of standards of quality. PACE 1995;18:271.

51. Mond H, Stokes KB. The electrode-tissue interface: the revolutionary role of steroid elution. PACE 1992;15:95.
52. Parsonnet V. The retention wire fix. (editorial). PACE 1995;18:955.
53. Brinker JA. Endocardial pacing leads: the good, the bad, and the ugly. (editorial; comment). PACE 1995; 18:953.
54. Daoud EG, Kou W, Davidson T, et al. Evaluation and extraction of the Accufix atrial J lead. Am Heart J 1996;131:266.
55. Silverman BG, Gross TP, Kaczmarek RG, et al. The epidemiology of pacemaker implantation in the United States. Public Health Rep 1995;110:42.
56. Goldstein DJ, Losquadro W, Spotnitz HM. Outpatient pacemaker procedures in orally anticoagulated patients. Pacing Clin Electrophysiol 1998;21(9):1730–1734.
57. Sweesy MW, Erickson SL, Crago JA, et al. Analysis of the effectiveness of in-office and transtelephonic follow-up in terms of pacemaker system complications. PACE 1994;17:2001.
58. Gessman LJ, Vielbig RE, Waspe LE, et al. Accuracy and clinical utility of transtelephonic pacemaker follow-up. PACE 1995;18:1032.
59. Goldschlager N, Ludmer P, Creamer C. Follow-up of the paced outpatient. In: Ellenbogen KA, Kay GN, Wilkoff BL, eds. Clinical Cardiac Pacing. WB Saunders, Philadelphia, PA, 1995, p. 780.
60. Aronow WS. Management of the older person with atrial fibrillation. J Am Geriatr Soc 1999;47(6): 740–748.
61. Ovsyshcher IE, Katz A, Bondy C. Initial experience with a new algorithm for automatic mode switching from DDDR to DDIR mode. PACE 1994;17:1908.
62. Love CJ, Hayes DL. Evaluation of pacemaker malfunction. In: Ellenbogen KA, Kay GN, Wilkoff BL, eds. Clinical Cardiac Pacing. WB Saunders, Philadelphia, PA, 1995, p. 656.
63. Madigan JD, Choudhri AF, Chen J, Spotnitz HM, Oz MC, Edwards N. Surgical management of the patient with an implanted cardiac device: implications of electromagnetic interference. Ann Surg 1999; 230(5):639–647.
64. Castle LW, Cook S. Pacemaker radiography. In: Ellenbogen KA, Kay GN, Wilkoff BL, eds. Clinical Cardiac Pacing. WB Saunders, Philadelphia, PA, 1995, p. 539.
65. Morse D, Parsonnet V, Gessman L, Droege T, Shimmel JB, Bernstein AD, et al. A Guide to Cardiac Pacemakers, Defibrillators, & Related Products. Droege Computing Services, Durham, NC, 1996.
66. Spotnitz HM, Ott GY, Bigger JT Jr, Steinberg JS, Livelli F Jr. Methods of implantable cardioverter–defibrillator–pacemaker insertion to avoid interactions. Ann Thorac Surg 1992;53(2):253–257.
67. Maron BJ, Shen WK, Link MS, Epstein AE, Almquist AK, Daubert JP, et al. Efficacy of implantable cardioverter–defibrillators for the prevention of sudden death in patients with hypertrophic cardiomyopathy. N Engl J Med 2000;342(6):365–373.
68. Reuter S, Garrigue S, Bordachar P, Hocini M, Jais P, Haissaguerre M, et al. Intermediate-term results of biventricular pacing in heart failure: correlation between clinical and hemodynamic data. Pacing Clin Electrophysiol 2000;23(11 Pt 2):1713–1717.
69. den Dulk K, Wellens HJJ. Antitachycardia pacing: clinical considerations. In: Ellenbogen KA, Kay GN, Wilkoff BL, eds. Clinical Cardiac Pacing. WB Saunders, Philadelphia, PA, 1995, p. 735.
70. Bonnet CA, Fogoros RN. Clinical experience with antitachycardia pacing. In: Ellenbogen KA, Kay GN, Wilkoff BL, eds. Clinical Cardiac Pacing. WB Saunders, Philadelphia, PA, 1995, p. 744.
71. Lauck G, von Smekal A, Wolke S, et al. Effects of nuclear magnetic resonance imaging on cardiac pacemakers. PACE 1995;18:1549.
72. Barbaro V, Bartolini P, Donato A, et al. Do European GSM mobile cellular phones pose a potential risk to pacemaker patients? PACE 1995;18:1218.
73. Brown KR, Carter W Jr, Lombardi GE. Blunt trauma-induced pacemaker failure. Ann Emerg Med 1991;20:905.
74. Epstein LM, Byrd CL, Wilkoff BL, Love CJ, Sellers TD, Hayes DL, et al. Initial experience with larger laser sheaths for the removal of transvenous pacemaker and implantable defibrillator leads. Circulation 1999;100(5):516–525.
75. Manganello TD. Disabling the pacemaker: the heart-rending decision every competent patient has a right to make. Health Care Law Mon 2000;3–15.
76. Weaver WE, Cobb LA, Hallstrom AP, et al. Factors influencing survival after out-of-hospital cardiac arrest. J Am Coll Cardiol 1986;7:752.
77. Mirowski R, Reid PR, Mower MM, et al. Termination of malignant ventricular arrhythmia with an implantable automatic defibrillator in human beings. N Engl J Med 1980;303:322.

78. Zipes DP, Roberts D. Results of the international study of the implantable pacemaker cardioverter–defibrillator. A comparison of epicardial and endocardial lead systems. Circulation 1995;92:59.

79. Shahian DM, Williamson WA, Svensson LG, et al. Transvenous versus transthoracic cardioverter–defibrillator implantation. J Thorac Cardiovasc Surg 1995;109:1066.

80. Fitzpatrick AP, Lesh MD, Epstein LM, et al. Electrophysiological laboratory, electrophysiologist-implanted, nonthoracotomy-implantable cardioverter/defibrillators. Circulation 1994;89:2503.

81. Kim SG, Roth JA, Fisher JD, et al. Long-term outcomes and modes of death of patients treated with nonthoracotomy implantable defibrillators. Am J Cardiol 1995, 75:1229.

82. Moss AJ, Hall WJ, Cannom DS, Daubert JP, Higgins SL, Klein H, et al. Improved survival with an implanted defibrillator in patients with coronary disease at high risk for ventricular arrhythmia. Multicenter Automatic Defibrillator Implantation Trial Investigators. N Engl J Med 1996;335(26):1933–1940.

83. The Antiarrhythmics Versus Implantable Defibrillators (AVID) Investigators. A comparison of anti-arrhythmic drug therapy with implantable defibrillators in patients resuscitated from near-fatal ventricular arrhythmias. N Engl J Med 1997;337:1576–1583.

84. Anon. Causes of death in the Antiarrhythmics Versus Implantable Defibrillators (AVID) Trial. J Am Coll Cardiol 1999;34(5):1552–1559.

85. Hohnloser SH. Implantable devices versus antiarrhythmic drug therapy in recurrent ventricular tachycardia and ventricular fibrillation. Am J Cardiol 1999;84(9A):56R–62R.

86. Klein H, Auricchio A, Reek S, Geller C. New primary prevention trials of sudden cardiac death in patients with left ventricular dysfunction: SCD–HEFT and MADIT-II. (Review) Am J Cardiol 1999;83(5B): 91D–97D.

87. Prystowsky EN, Nisam S. Prophylactic implantable cardioverter defibrillator trials: MUSTT, MADIT, and beyond. Multicenter Unsustained Tachycardia Trial. Multicenter Automatic Defibrillator Implantation Trial. Am J Cardiol 2000;86(11):1214–1215.

88. Klein HU, Reek S. The MUSTT study: evaluating testing and treatment. J Interv Cardiac Electrophysiol 2000;4(Suppl 1):45–50.

89. Capucci A, Aschieri D, Villani GQ. The role of EP-guided therapy in ventricular arrhythmias: beta-blockers, sotalol, and ICD's. J Interv Cardiac Electrophysiol 2000;4(Suppl 1):57–63.

90. Bigger JT Jr. Prophylactic use of implanted cardiac defibrillators in patients at high risk for ventricular arrhythmias after coronary-artery bypass graft surgery. Coronary Artery Bypass Graft (CABG) Patch Trial Investigators. N Engl J Med 1997;337(22):1569–1575.

91. Block M, Breithardt G. Optimizing defibrillation through improved waveforms. PACE 1995;18:526.

92. Libero L, Lozano IF, Bocchiardo M, Marcolongo M, Sallusti L, Madrid A, et al. Comparison of defibrillation thresholds using monodirectional electrical vector versus bidirectional electrical vector. Ital Heart J 2001;2(6):449–455.

93. Horton RP, Canby RC, Roman CA, et al. Diagnosis of ICD lead failure using continuous event marker recording. PACE 1995;18:1331.

94. Luceri RM. Initial clinical experience with a dual chamber rate responsive implantable cardioverter defibrillator. Pacing Clin Electrophysiol 2000;23(11 Pt 2):1986–1988.

95. Boineau JP, Cox JL. Slow ventricular activation in acute myocardial infarction. A source of reentrant premature ventricular contractions. Circulation 1973;49:702.

96. The Cardiac Arrhythmia Suppression Trial (CAST) Investigators. Preliminary report: effect of encainide and flecainide on mortality in a randomized trial of arrhythmia suppression after myocardial infarction. N Engl J Med 1989;321:406–412.

97. Winkle RA, Mead RH, Ruder MA, et al. Long-term outcome with the automatic cardioverter–defibrillator. J Am Coll Cardiol 1989;13:1353.

98. Spotnitz, HM. Surgical approaches to ICD insertion. In: Spotnitz HM, ed. Research Frontiers in Implantable Defibrillator Surgery. RG Landes, Austin, TX, 1992, p. 23.

99. Watkins L Jr, Taylor E Jr. Surgical aspects of automatic implantable cardioverter–defibrillator implantation. PACE 1991;14:953.

100. Auteri JS, Jeevanandam V, Bielefeld MR, et al. Effects of location of AICD patch electrodes on the left ventricular diastolic pressure–volume curve in pigs. Ann Thorac Surg 1991;52:1052.

101. Barrington WW, Deligonul U, Easley AR, Windle JR. Defibrillator patch electrode constriction: an underrecognized entity. Ann Thorac Surg 1995;60:1112.

102. Spotnitz HM. Effects of ICD insertion on cardiac function. In: Spotnitz HM, ed. Research Frontiers in Implantable Defibrillator Surgery. RG Landes, Austin, TX, 1992, p. 98.

103. Park WM, Amirhamzeh MMR, Bielefeld MR, et al. Systolic arterial pressure recovery after ventricular fibrillation/flutter in humans. PACE 1994;17:1100.

103a. Hauser RG, Kurschinski DT, McVeigh K, et al. Clinical results with nonthoracotomy ICD systems. PACE 1993;16:141.

104. Mattke S, Muller D, Markewitz A, et al. Failures of epicardial and transvenous leads for implantable cardioverter defibrillators. Am Heart J 1995;130:1040.

105. Roelke M, O'Nunain, Osswald S, et al. Subclavian crush syndrome complicating transvenous cardio-verter defibrillator systems. PACE 1995;18:973.

106. Argenziano M, Spotnitz HM, Goldstein DJ, Weinberg AD, Dizon JM, Bigger JT Jr. Longevity of lead systems in patients with implantable cardioverter–defibrillators. Circulation 2000;102:II–397.

107. Jones GK, Bardy GH, Kudenchuk PJ, et al. Mechanical complications after implantation of multiple-lead nonthoracotomy defibrillator systems: implications for management and future systems design. Am Heart J 1995;130–327.

108. Dean DA, Livelli FL Jr, Bigger JT Jr, Spotnitz HM. Safe repair of insulation defects in ICD leads. PACE 1996;19:678 (abstract).

109. Jeevanandam V, Bielefeld MR, Auteri JS, et al. The implantable defibrillator: an electronic bridge to cardiac transplantation. Circulation 1992;86:II–276.

110. Bolling SF. Implantable cardioverter-defibrillators as a bridge to cardiac transplantation. In: Spotnitz HM, ed. Research Frontiers in Implantable Defibrillator Surgery. RG Landes, Austin, TX, 1992, p. 57.

111. May CD, Smith PR, Murdock CL, Davis MJE. The impact of implantable cardioverter defibrillator on quality-of-life. PACE 1995;18:1411.

112. Ahmad M, Bloomstein L, Roelke M, Bernstein AD, Parsonnet V. Patients' attitudes toward implanted defibrillator shocks. Pacing Clin Electrophysiol 2000;23(6):934–938.

113. Kohn CS, Petrucci RJ, Baessler C, Soto DM, Movsowitz C. The effect of psychological intervention on patients' long-term adjustment to the ICD: a prospective study. Pacing Clin Electrophysiol 2000;23 (4 Pt 1):450–456.

114. Akiyama T, Powell JL, Mitchell LB, Ehlert FA, Baessler C. Resumption of driving after life-threatening ventricular tachyarrhythmia. N Engl J Med 2001;345(6):391–397.

115. Hoffmaster B. The ethics of setting limits on ICD therapy. Can J Cardiol 2000;16(10):1313–1318.

116. Stanton MS, Bell GK. Economic outcomes of implantable cardioverter–defibrillators. Circulation 2000; 101(9):1067–1074.

117. O'Brien BJ, Connolly SJ, Goeree R, Blackhouse G, Willan A, Yee R, et al. Cost-effectiveness of the implantable cardioverter-defibrillator: results from the Canadian Implantable Defibrillator Study (CIDS). Circulation 2001;103(10):1416–1421.

18 Postoperative Management of the Geriatric Patient

Hugh R. Playford, MB, BS, FANZCA, FFICANZCA

INTRODUCTION

Aging is seemingly a simple process. However, the biological process of aging (senescence) is extremely complex and not purely time related. In fact, its rate is not only individual, but it may fluctuate at different stages of an individual's life *(1)*. Aging demonstrates its greatest biological impact in the fourth decade and slows toward the eighth and ninth decades.

Health care in most developed nations has improved dramatically over the past century *(2)*. The reductions in the death rates in early life have led to significant improvements in life expectancy. Further gains are undoubtedly more difficult to achieve and often more costly *(3)*. Although there have been significant achievements in modifying the processes *associated* with aging, there is nothing currently available that can modify or reverse senescence directly.

The interaction of improving life expectancy with falling fertility rates will lead to an explosion in numbers, both absolute and relative, of the very old. This group will experience disability and debilitation (up to one-third will be demented by age 85), utilize polypharmacy, and maintain very low incomes *(4,5)*. Caring for these patients will lead to massive clinical, administrative, financial, and social challenges in the decades to come (*see* Chapter 1).

From: *Aging, Heart Disease, and Its Management: Facts and Controversies*
Edited by: N. Edwards, M. Maurer, and R. Wellner © Humana Press Inc., Totowa, NJ

DIFFERENCES

Physiological Changes

CARDIOVASCULAR FUNCTION

The causes of the heterogeneous changes in cardiovascular function in the elderly are difficult to distinguish from those related to senescence and those attributed to atherosclerotic cardiovascular disease (*see* Chapter 9 on age-related changes in cardiovascular function). Nevertheless, changes within the vascular wall (thickening and decreased compliance) contribute to arterial hypertension and increased afterload. The heart increases in size, largely through an increase in left-ventricular wall mass as cardiac myocytes hypertrophy in response to systolic hypertension. Contractility in the elderly may remain close to normal at rest but lacks the ability to increase sufficiently for exercise.

Functionally, ejection fraction and stroke volume change little with normal aging, but considerable change may result from superimposed cardiovascular disease. Left-ventricular relaxation is impaired, prolonging early diastolic filling, and there is an increased reliance upon atrial contraction to contribute to late diastolic filling. The crucial role of atrial contraction in the elderly partially explains the critical cardiovascular collapse that occurs when the atrium's contribution is lost, such as during atrial fibrillation.

Myocardial fibrosis can impair cardiac conduction increasing the propensity for cardiac dysrhythmias and conduction block *(6)*. At a receptor level, a decrease in adrenergic affinity impairs the cardiovascular response to β-adrenergic stimulation. Thus, in response to hemodynamic stress, the heart rate response, mediated by β-adrenergic stimulation, is blunted with age.

RESPIRATORY

Deciding whether to ascribe changes in respiratory function that occur with age to "normal aging" or to pathophysiologic processes can be challenging. Nevertheless, it is well documented that there is significant deterioration in pulmonary function with age *(7–9)*.

Anatomical pulmonary changes associated with aging include bronchiolar narrowing resulting from alterations in the supporting connective tissues. Decreased elasticity and increased collagen deposition cause alveolar duct size to increase and the alveolar sacs to flatten. These physiologic changes largely account for the decrease in elastic recoil, increase in pulmonary compliance, decrease in oxygen-diffusion capacity, earlier airway closure contributing to increased ventilation–perfusion mismatching, small airway closure resulting in air trapping, and decreased expiratory flow rates *(7)*.

Within the chest wall, compliance decreases with changes to the thoracic spine and the costovertebral and costochondral joints. This rigidity impairs thoracic muscular expansion of the chest, and, as a result, chest expansion is more dependent on diaphragmatic and abdominal muscular excursion. Although diaphragmatic mass is preserved, it is functionally impaired *(10,11)*, contributing to the minimal respiratory reserve in the elderly during situations requiring a high minute ventilation *(7)*. Additionally, protective reflexes of the upper airway are impaired in the elderly, significantly increasing the risk of aspiration.

These anatomical differences cause predictable changes in respiratory function. Residual volume and functional residual capacity increase with preservation of total lung capacity. The increases in closing volume contribute to airway closure in the dependent areas of the lung during normal tidal breathing and, thus, lower arterial oxygen tension in the aged.

There are decreases in forced vital capacity and expiratory flow. Small-airway closure increases dead-space ventilation. Mismatching of ventilation–perfusion is increased.

Gas exchange is significantly altered. Ventilation–perfusion mismatch increases the alveolar–arterial oxygen gradient. Diffusion capacity also declines in the elderly—males at a rate greater than females. The hypoxic response is variably impaired, but the ventilatory response to hypercapnia tends to be blunted, presumably as a result of changes to neural inputs and lung mechanics.

In summary, aging can diminish upper airway protective reflexes and markedly reduced pulmonary reserve in the face of even mild forms of respiratory failure.

NEUROLOGICAL FUNCTION

Hearing, vision, memory, motor efficiency, and strength decrease with advancing age (*see* Chapter 6 for more details). Although performance on timed tasks declines after the second decade, intelligence does not. Anatomically, brain size declines with variable studies of cerebral blood flow and oxygen consumption.

Of greater clinical concern is dementia, which increases in prevalence by 400% between the ages of 65 and 85; approximately one-third of those individuals over 85 are demented to some degree *(12,13)*. The exact incidence of delirium in the ICU is unknown but regarded as high *(14)*, given the elderly patient is at a higher risk for its development *(15)*.

The incidence of epilepsy increases with age *(16)*, probably because of a vascular mechanism, but it also should be noted that critically ill elderly patients are at greater risk of developing nonconvulsive status epilepticus *(17)*.

RENAL FUNCTION

The kidney undergoes structural and functional changes after the third or fourth decade. By the eighth decade, renal size has declined by 20–30% and renal volume by 40%. The loss of renal mass is predominantly cortical with primarily vascular changes. By the eighth decade, the number of glomeruli has declined by 40% and there is some loss of medullary parenchyma and an increase in medullary fibrosis.

Renal plasma flow (RPF) decreases by about 10% per decade after the fourth decade. The RPF decrease is not paralleled by a decline in blood pressure, suggesting that the decline is probably the result of intravascular pathology (atheroma, sclerosis) or increased renal vascular resistance *(18)*.

The decline in glomerular filtration rate (GFR) with age has been well studied. In a longitudinal study *(19)*, mean true creatinine clearances fell from 140 mL/min/1.73 m^2 between the ages of 25 and 34 to 97 mL/min/1.73 m^2 between ages 75 and 84. During that same time period, mean serum creatinine rose insignificantly because skeletal muscle mass decrease. This reinforces the inadequacy of serum creatinine to assess renal function. Estimates of creatinine clearance (mL/min) may be calculated using the Cockcroft–Gault formula *(20)*:

$$\text{CrCl (mL/min)} = \frac{(140 - \text{age [yr]}) \times \text{Weight (kg)}}{72 \times \text{Creatinine (mg/dL)}}$$

Creatinine clearance is lower in females, and thus, the above formula requires adjustment (i.e., multiply the result by a factor of 0.85). Of interest, there appears to be a minimal decline in GFR in healthy subjects and a pronounced decrease in GFR in those with coexisting cardiovascular disease *(21)*. This suggests that ischemia is the principle reason for the decline in renal function; it is not the result of age-related effects.

Along with the age-associated decline in GFR, there is a decline in tubular function. The net effects of aging on the kidney include a decreased ability to conserve sodium and a diminished concentrating ability. Sodium wasting is increased because of elevations in atrial natriuretic peptide (ANP), decreased aldosterone response, and a decreased response to β-adrenergic stimulation. The implications of these changes are that during instances when the body requires maximum sodium conservation (e.g., hypovolemia), the elderly kidneys excrete sodium inappropriately. Conversely, as excretion of sodium is partly dependent on GFR, the time taken to excrete a large sodium load is often prolonged, resulting in intravascular volume overload.

Aging alters potassium excretion by a number of mechanisms. First, the loss of tubules reduces active transport into the tubular lumen; second, renin release is blunted with lower angiotensin and aldosterone generation; and third, tubular responsiveness to aldosterone appears limited in the elderly. Additionally, concurrent medications such as β-blockers, angiotensin-converting-enzyme inhibitors, and potassium-sparing diuretics also contribute to the hyperkalemia.

Generally, acid–base homeostasis is maintained in the elderly. However, there is an impaired excretion of acute acid loads, largely explained by the decreased production of ammonia (to buffer the acid). Thus, the elderly are much more prone to severe metabolic acidosis.

Total-body water decreases with age from 60% for men and women in the fourth decade to about 50% in the eighth decade. As a consequence, water gains and losses in older patients have a more pronounced effect on body-fluid osmolality. Compounding the situation is a decrease in maximal urinary concentrating ability that becomes more prominent with age, probably as a result of decreased medullary hypertonicity *(22)*. At age 80, the maximal urinary concentration is often 400–500 mOsmol/kg, compared with a maximal concentrating capacity of 1100-1200 mOsmol/kg at age 30. Additionally, the diluting capacity of the kidney and water excretion are impaired in the elderly.

Despite the significant alteration in the elderly population in dealing with sodium and water, the management of hyponatremia, hypernatremia, and water overload and dehydration differs little from the management utilized in younger population.

GASTROINTESTINAL SYSTEM, AND NUTRITION

Intestinal motility may be significantly reduced in the elderly but with only limited clinical importance *(23)*. Gastric emptying for liquids and solids may be impaired by up to 50% in one-quarter of people over age 70. The absorptive surface of the small intestine is reduced by up to 20% and mesenteric blood flow is reduced by as much as one-third. However, there is sufficient intestinal reserve such that these changes translate into only small differences in speed and total amount of absorption *(24)*.

The size of the liver declines with age and may become very small in the elderly *(25)*. In infants, the liver makes up 4% of the total body weight; however, by 80 yr, this percentage has declined to one-half of that. The reduction in liver mass is largely a result of declines in both total hepatic blood flow and portal venous flow.

Despite these changes, overall liver function tests change little in the elderly. The reduction in hepatic blood flow causes a reduction in first-pass clearance of drugs, but the enzymatic function appears to be only marginally affected. Synthetic function of the liver also appears to be well preserved in the elderly. As a result, the elderly liver would be expected to have little functional impairment, but, nonetheless, diminished reserve when stressed. Care should also be exercised in managing drugs that are metabolized hepatically.

Aging is associated with a reduction in lean body mass, the net result of a decline in muscle mass and in total-body water. Energy expenditure also decreases. Furthermore, malnutrition is common (up to 30–40% of the elderly hospitalized population), largely secondary to diminished intake.

Pancreatic function is essentially maintained. In fact, pancreatic insufficiency is almost always related to disease and not to age. Nonetheless, glucose intolerance is common, secondary to peripheral resistance to insulin.

ENDOCRINE FUNCTION

Over the last decade, there has been a realization that hormonal function plays a significant role in senescence. However, the debate continues regarding exactly how endocrine function contributes to aging.

Advancing age is strongly associated with a diminished capacity to metabolize a glucose load (26). Healthy older adults have higher plasma glucose levels when fasting, which decline at a slower rate after a glucose load. The higher prevalence of diabetes and impaired glucose tolerance among older individuals has been demonstrated. The hyperglycemia is related to both peripheral tissue insulin resistance and, to a variable extent, declining pancreatic insulin secretion as a result of disease. Not all of the hyperglycemia can be attributed to senescence; significant behavioral and pathological processes also interplay.

Plasma renin levels decrease by 30–50% in the elderly; as a result, plasma concentrations of aldosterone are also diminished. This carries with it the potentially life-threatening complication of hyperkalemia, particularly in the critical care setting of significant fluid and electrolyte fluctuations.

Thyroid abnormalities increase with age and are common in the elderly population. Hypothyroidism, in particular, may go unrecognized in the elderly.

THERMOREGULATION

Temperature regulation has significant consequences postoperatively in the elderly. They are more susceptible to the development of hypothermia and, subsequently, resistant to rewarming. They have a reduced sense of external temperature changes and require greater external thermal stimuli to respond to temperature extremes (e.g., adding clothes). Despite this, the elderly seem to prefer lower-temperature environments (27). Many medications acting via the hypothalamus (opioids, barbituates, benzodiazepines, antipsychotics, tricyclic antidepressants) may also interfere with thermoregulation (28). These drugs modify centrally mediated vasoconstriction and the shivering response.

The elderly have a decreased ability to produce heat. The basal metabolic rate (BMR) diminishes with the normal aging process. Poor nutrition resulting in reduced subcutaneous fat can cause reduced heat-generating substrate and decreased insulation when cold. Superimposed endocrine disorders (i.e., hypothyroidism) further increase the risk of hypothermia in the elderly (29).

There is also increased heat loss in the elderly. Insulation is not only impaired by decreased subcutaneous fat but also by decreased total-body water, lowering the thermal buffering capacity. Once hypothermic, the normal autonomic vasoconstrictor response is markedly impaired. Immobilization, as a result of disease states, reduces the behavioral options available to the elderly when faced with cold. Shivering is often impaired by both diminished muscle mass and the effects of medications.

Pharmacological Changes

Pharmacotherapy in the elderly is affected by an age-related decline in most organ function, reduction in receptor response, and a loss of water content and an increase in the fat content of the body *(30)*. Alterations in both pharmacodynamics and pharmacokinetics play a crucial role in the management of the postoperative elderly patient (*see* Chapter 5). Some of the adverse effects in the elderly can be ascribed to pharmacodynamic effects in the setting of alterations in organ function; however, pharmacokinetics also change with aging.

As demonstrated, chronological age does not necessarily predict the biological condition of a patient. Thus, predictive pharmacokinetic models based solely on age are, at best, a guide only. Elderly patients are more likely to be taking multiple medications chronically, increasing the chance of drug interactions.

Absorption is impaired as a result of changes in the intestinal epithelium, splanchnic blood flow, and gut motor function. Drugs absorbed passively are altered the least. Compounds absorbed by active mechanisms (calcium, iron, vitamins) may be absorbed at lower rates in the elderly *(30)*. The reduction in hepatic blood flow and first-pass clearance may cause higher oral bioavailablity of compounds undergoing significant first-pass elimination.

Bioavailability for drugs administered by the subcutaneous or intramuscular route is dependent on tissue perfusion. An elderly individual with marginal tissue perfusion will have unpredictable absorption of drugs delivered via these routes. Additionally, the decreased subcutaneous tissue of the elderly may inadvertently cause subcutaneously administered drugs to be delivered via the intramuscular route.

The most important pharmacokinetic change in the elderly is a decrease in renal drug excretion. Drugs that are predominantly excreted by the kidney will have significant reductions in total clearance and their doses should be adjusted in the elderly. Drugs dependent on the kidney for delivery to their site of action (e.g., loop diuretics) are also less effective in the setting of renal dysfunction.

Age has a variable impact upon the liver's drug-metabolizing capability. Overall, however, it is thought that the inter-individual variation in metabolic drug clearance exceeds the age-related decline *(30,31)*. Anatomical mechanisms reducing hepatic blood flow and first-pass metabolism have been previously noted. Pathological changes, particularly those related to poor nutrition, consistently impair hepatic metabolism. Reports of the effects of age on hepatic enzyme induction have been conflicting, possibly reflecting high variability among elderly individuals.

The alteration in body compartments of the elderly (greater fat content and lower water proportion) decreases the volume of distribution for hydrophilic drugs and increases it for lipophilic drugs. The elderly have higher plasma levels of hydrophilic drugs and lower plasma levels of lipophilic drugs. Plasma albumin changes little with age, creating only subtle changes in plasma protein binding.

Unfortunately there is a relative paucity of data regarding pharmacodynamic changes in the elderly *(30)*. The β-adrenergic receptor has reduced sensitivity to both agonists and antagonists in the elderly *(32)*. As a result, there is reduced chronotropy and inotropy to isoprenaline and a reduced hypotensive effect to β-adrenergic blockade *(33)*. Atropine has a reduced chronotropic effect, likely to be secondary to changes in the muscarinic nervous system. Conversely, the sensitivity (but not actual number) of $Na^+ K^+$-ATPase is increased with age. Particularly in the setting of hypokalemia, elderly patients are at higher risk of digitalis toxicity.

Opioids are frequently used in the postoperative management of the elderly. Even with weight-appropriate doses, greater sensitivity has been demonstrated with increased sedation and respiratory depression (33,34). Similarly, benzodiazepines require judicious use with a greater risk of exaggerated effect.

In particular, drug therapy involving hemodynamics, neurological function, and coagulation must be monitored extremely closely in the elderly postoperative patient.

STANDARDS OF CARE

In this era of evidence-based medicine, for postoperative patients there is a glaring deficiency of information specifically pertaining to the elderly. Usually excluded from randomized controlled trials, information relating to the elderly has generally been based upon uncontrolled cohort trials with only a limited number of outcome measures (usually mortality). The diverse nature of the studies to a large degree precludes rigorous scientific overview.

There are also relatively few "Standards of Care" for the general population that translate seamlessly to the elderly patient. Nevertheless, in extrapolating routine care from younger to older patients, we do so without firm evidence-based foundations.

Transfusion

In any critically ill patient, but particularly in the elderly, one of the most challenging aspects of care revolves around fluid administration and hemodynamic support. Even in the general population, there exists limited data to guide decisions for blood product transfusion. Although consensus panels provide an algorithmic approach (35), much transfusion practice has varied widely and is, in fact, considered inappropriate (36,37). A limited supply of blood products, as well as evidence associating over-transfusion with unfavorable outcomes (38), has led to increased scrutiny of transfusion practice.

Among patients admitted to an intensive care unit, one well-conducted trial concluded that maintaining hemoglobin levels between 7.0 and 9.0 g/dL resulted in significantly lower in-hospital mortality than those subjects managed with more liberal hemoglobin strategy (10.0–12.0 g/dL) (39). It should be noted that 30 d mortality between the groups was not significantly different. Of significance, the mortality difference was greater in parameters that were younger (<55 yr) and less severely ill. These differences were not noted in subjects older than 55 yr. No further analysis of the elderly was reported. A subgroup of patients with cardiac disease had no 30 d mortality difference between the two transfusion strategies. Importantly, a 54% reduction in red cell units transfused was noted in patients with lower hemoglobin goals.

A separate study of elderly patients undergoing hip repair concluded that hemoglobin levels as low as 8 g/dL did not influence 30 or 90 d mortality (40,41). If the hematocrit falls below 28, the incidence of intraoperative and postoperative myocardial events in elderly patients undergoing noncardiac surgery was greater (42).

Specifically in patients undergoing cardiac surgery, widely variable outcomes of allogenic transfusions have been demonstrated, making conclusions difficult to draw (43–46).

Of elderly patients experiencing or suffering an acute myocardial infarct, a large retrospective study has suggested a significant survival benefit if transfused when the hematocrit drops below 33 (47).

Overall, the evidence, although lacking in completeness, suggests that the hematocrit be kept above 28–33 in elderly patients at risk for myocardial ischemia; for those not at risk for myocardial ischemia, a lower, less well-defined transfusion threshold may be appropriate.

Delirium and Agitation

The elderly postoperative patient is at high risk for developing agitation and delirium. The incidence of these adverse events has been estimated to range between 15 % and 50% among the hospitalized elderly (15,48,49). Up to 83% of elderly patients admitted to the ICU develop delirium (14,50). It would be expected that the incidence of delirium will continue to increase as the population ages. Major risk factors for agitation and delirium (such as older age, drug interactions, postoperative state, metabolic abnormalities, infection, and history of dementia) are frequently present in the elderly. Delirium and agitation have major ramifications associated with increased in-hospital and postdischarge mortality and prolonged hospital length of stay (15,51). Unfortunately, most postoperative wards, and indeed ICUs, foster a state of sensory deprivation and overload, with excessive noise, hearing and visual impairment, pain, and sleep deprivation.

Recently, the Confusion Assessment Method (CAM) has been developed and validated as a method allowing nonpsychiatrists to assess delirium both in the general hospital wards and in the ICU (14,50,52).

Despite our improvements in assessing delirium, there has been little success with interventional studies. Most have focused on the management of delirium, using either pharmacological or physical methods. One preventive trial tackled six risk factors for development of delirium in general medical patients over 70 yr of age (49). Patients enrolled in the intervention group had a lower incidence of delirium with fewer total episodes and shorter duration. Nevertheless, recurrence rates and severity of delirium were not different in the control group.

Hyperglycemia

Management of hyperglycemia using intensive insulin therapy has developed into an important tool in the postsurgical population. In patients admitted to a single intensive care unit in Belgium (of whom 62% had undergone cardiac surgery), intensive insulin therapy (to maintain the blood glucose between 80 and 100 mg/dL) reduced intensive care mortality from 8.0% to 4.6% (a median unbiased estimate of the reduction in mortality of 32%) (53). These results were translated to similarly impressive figures regarding in-hospital mortality. Sepsis as a cause of death was affected most significantly. Reductions were noted in bloodstream infections by 46%, acute renal failure requiring dialytic therapy by 41%, and critical illness polyneuropathy by 44%. Other significant reductions were noted in a median number of red cell transfusions, prolonged ventilation, and prolonged intensive care length of stay (53). No subgroup analysis was performed according to age, although it is expected that the results would translate to the aged. With such impressive results, there has been attention redirected at glycemic control in the critically ill postsurgical patient. Caution must be advised until these results have been replicated in a wider, multi-center trial.

CONTROVERSIES

The significant changes in an individual both in senescence and pathology, not unexpectedly, have led to wide ranges in outcome. Rates of return to independent living vary tenfold in apparently similar studies involving the elderly post-trauma *(54)*. Age alone is a poor predictor of mortality and quality-of-life among the critically ill *(40)*. In fact, illness severity has a greater impact upon hospital mortality than age *(55,56)*.

That variation in outcome is also noted in studies of mortality and chronic morbidity in the elderly after prolonged mechanical ventilation. After a prolonged ICU stay, patients over age 70 had an in-hospital mortality rate of 53% and high levels of neuropsychiatric disability in the survivors *(57)*. Additionally, these outcomes were derived at high cost (up to US $60,000/survivor). Other studies have failed to differentiate age as the major determinant of resource utilization in the ICU *(58,59)*. However, an attempt to pool several studies has suggested that the 1 yr survival of the critically ill over 85 yr of age is a sobering 30%, with much of the mortality soon after ICU discharge *(1,60,61)*.

After critical illness, a significant number of the elderly return home with adequate, but not necessarily premorbid, functional ability *(62)*. It appears that, as with mortality, pre-hospital functional status, comorbidities, and severity of illness are the greatest predictors of long-term morbidity *(55,56)*.

Specifically relating to coronary artery bypass grafting, patients presenting for cardiac surgery usually have significant comorbidities and more advanced cardiovascular disease, leading to presentation later in their disease course. Studies have yielded conflicting outcome results with continuing controversy in some institutions regarding the role of such operations in those patients age 80 and older *(63)*. Nevertheless, there appears to be an increasing body of evidence supporting the reasonable safety of the procedure. The trend has been one of decreasing mortality over the last two decades *(63–68)*.

Among those patients admitted to the ICU after their coronary artery bypass grafts, the risk of perioperative morbidity increases with age. Several series, not unexpectedly, demonstrate that the elderly ≥80 yr of age are susceptible to atrial arrhythmias (20–60%) *(69, 70)*, respiratory failure (4–20%) *(70)*, renal insufficiency (2.5–19%) *(71,72)*, and cerebrovascular events (2–20%) *(71,73)*. With increasing numbers of elderly patients undergoing cardiac surgery, the postoperative challenge revolves around preventing and managing these complications.

Given that outcome studies better correlate mortality in the elderly with severity of illness than with age, there have been attempts to develop predictive models to discriminate between those patients who would be expected to do well and those who would not. Despite the promise of severity scoring systems (such as APACHE II and III, SAPS) over the last two decades, the ability of these instruments to accurately and meaningfully predict outcome in the individual patient remains poor irrespective of age. This presents a greater problem for the elderly, who were either excluded or underrepresented in the datasets used to develop and validate the scores. Furthermore, specific scoring systems developed to address those deficiencies in the elderly perform poorly *(74)*.

As much as objective evidence regarding treatment of the elderly with critical illness is sought, the ability and applicability to make decisions in the individual patient currently remains highly questionable.

REFERENCES

1. Saul P. Saving lives almost over. How should we treat the very elderly? In: Keneally J, ed. Australasian Anaesthesia. Australian and New Zealand College of Anaesthetists, Melbourne, 2001, pp. 143–148.
2. Campion EW. The oldest old. N Engl J Med 1994;330(25):1819–1820.
3. Olshansky SJ, Carnes BA, Desesquelles A. Demography. Prospects for human longevity. Science 2001; 291(5508):1491–1492.

4. Anon. Canadian study of health and aging: study methods and prevalence of dementia. Canadian Medical Association Journal 1994;150(6):899–913.
5. Anderson G, Kerluke K. Distribution of prescription drug exposures in the elderly: description and implications. J Clin Epidemiol 1996;49(8):929–935.
6. Fleg JL, Kennedy HL. Cardiac arrhythmias in a healthy elderly population: detection by 24-hour ambulatory electrocardiography. Chest 1982;81(3):302–307.
7. Chan ED, Welsh CH. Geriatric respiratory medicine. Chest 1998;114(6):1704–1733.
8. Enright PL, Kronmal RA, Higgins M, Schenker M, Haponik EF. Spirometry reference values for women and men 65 to 85 years of age. Cardiovascular health study. Am Rev Respir Dis 1993;147(1):125–133.
9. Pack AI, Millman RP. The lungs in later life. In: Fishman AP, ed. Pulmonary Diseases and Disorders. McGraw-Hill, New York, 1988, pp. 79–90.
10. Polkey MI, Harris ML, Hughes PD, et al. The contractile properties of the elderly human diaphragm. Am J Respir Crit Care Med 1997;155(5):1560–1564.
11. Tolep K, Higgins N, Muza S, Criner G, Kelsen SG. Comparison of diaphragm strength between healthy adult elderly and young men. Am J Respir Crit Care Med 1995;152(2):677–682.
12. Morrison JH, Hof PR. Life and death of neurons in the aging brain. Science 1997;278(5337):412–419.
13. Katzman R. Human nervous system. In: Masoro EJ, ed. Handbook of Physiology; Section 11: Aging. Oxford University Press, New York, 1995, pp. 325–344.
14. Ely EW, Margolin R, Francis J, et al. Evaluation of delirium in critically ill patients: validation of the Confusion Assessment Method for the Intensive Care Unit (CAM-ICU). Crit Care Med 2001;29(7): 1370–1379.
15. Francis J, Martin D, Kapoor WN. A prospective study of delirium in hospitalized elderly. JAMA 1990; 263(8):1097–1101.
16. Tallis R, Hall G, Craig I, Dean A. How common are epileptic seizures in old age? Age Ageing 1991;20(6): 442–448.
17. Litt B, Wityk RJ, Hertz SH, et al. Nonconvulsive status epilepticus in the critically ill elderly. Epilepsia 1998;39(11):1194–1202.
18. Lindeman RD. Renal and urinary tract function. In: Masoro EJ, ed. Handbook of Physiology; Section 11: Aging. Oxford University Press, New York, 1995, pp. 485–503.
19. Rowe JW, Andres R, Tobin JD, Norris AH, Shock NW. The effect of age on creatinine clearance in men: a cross sectional and longitudinal study. J. Gerontol. 1976;31:155–163.
20. Cockcroft DW, Gault MH. Prediction of creatinine clearance from serum creatinine. Nephron 1976; 16(1):31–41.
21. Lindeman RD, Tobin JD, Shock NW. Association between blood pressure and the rate of decline of renal function with age. Kidney Int 1984;26:861–864.
22. Rowe JW, Shock NW, DeFronzo RA. The influence of age on the renal response to water deprivation in man. Nephron 1976;17(4):270–278.
23. Holt PR. The gastrointestinal tract. In: Masoro EJ, ed. Handbook of Physiology; Section 11, Aging. Oxford University Press, New York, 1995, pp. 505–554.
24. Iber FL, Murphy PA, Connor ES. Age-related changes in the gastrointestinal system. Effects on drug therapy. Drugs Aging 1994;5(1):34–48.
25. Howell TH. Organ weights in nonagenarians. J Am Geriatr Soc 1978;26(9):385–390.
26. Halter JB, Beard JC, Porte D Jr. Islet function and stress hyperglycemia: plasma glucose and epinephrine interaction. Am J Physiol 1984;247(1 Pt 1):E47–E52.
27. Taylor NA, Allsopp NK, Parkes DG. Preferred room temperature of young vs aged males: the influence of thermal sensation, thermal comfort, and affect. J Gerontol A Biol Sci Med Sci 1995;50(4):M216–M221.
28. Ballester JM, Harchelroad FP. Hyperthermia: how to recognize and prevent heat-related illnesses. Geriatrics 1999;54(7):20–24.
29. Manning B, Stollerman GH. Hypothermia in the elderly. Hosp Pract (Off Ed) 1993;28(5):53–60, 64–70.
30. Turnheim K. Drug dosage in the elderly. Is it rational? Drugs Aging 1998;13(5):357–379.
31. Schmucker DL. Aging and drug disposition: an update. Pharmacol Rev 1985;37(2):133–148.
32. O'Malley K, Kelly JG, Swift CG. Responsiveness to drugs. In: Swift CG, ed. Clinical Pharmacology in the Elderly. Marcel Dekker, New York, 1987, pp. 83–101.
33. Lamy PP. Physiological changes due to age. Pharmacodynamic changes of drug action and implications for therapy. Drugs Aging 1991;1(5):385–404.
34. Feely J, Coakley D. Altered pharmacodynamics in the elderly. Clin Geriatr Med 1990;6(2):269–283.

35. Anon. Practice strategies for elective red blood cell transfusion. American College of Physicians. Ann Intern Med 1992;116(5):403–406.
36. Hebert PC, Wells G, Martin C, et al. A Canadian survey of transfusion practices in critically ill patients. Transfusion Requirements in Critical Care Investigators and the Canadian Critical Care Trials Group. Crit Care Med 1998;26(3):482–487.
37. Surgenor DM, Wallace EL, Churchill WH, Hao SH, Chapman RH, Poss R. Red cell transfusions in total knee and total hip replacement surgery. Transfusion 1991;31(6):531–537.
38. Spiess BD, Ley C, Body SC, et al. Hematocrit value on intensive care unit entry influences the frequency of Q-wave myocardial infarction after coronary artery bypass grafting. The Institutions of the Multicenter Study of Perioperative Ischemia (McSPI) Research Group. J Thorac Cardiovasc Surg 1998;116(3): 460–467.
39. Hebert PC, Wells G, Blajchman MA, et al. A multicenter, randomized, controlled clinical trial of transfusion requirements in critical care. Transfusion Requirements in Critical Care Investigators, Canadian Critical Care Trials Group. N Engl J Med 1999;340(6):409–417.
40. Chelluri L, Grenvik A, Silverman M. Intensive care for critically ill elderly: mortality, costs, and quality of life. Review of the literature. Arch Intern Med 1995;155(10):1013–1022.
41. Chelluri L. Critical illness in the elderly: review of pathophysiology of aging and outcome of intensive care. J Intensive Care Med 2001;16:114–127.
42. Hogue CW Jr, Goodnough LT, Monk TG. Perioperative myocardial ischemic episodes are related to hematocrit level in patients undergoing radical prostatectomy. Transfusion 1998;38(10):924–931.
43. Goodnough LT, Johnston MF, Toy PT. The variability of transfusion practice in coronary artery bypass surgery. Transfusion Medicine Academic Award Group. JAMA 1991;265(1):86–90.
44. Goodnough LT, Soegiarso RW, Birkmeyer JD, Welch HG. Economic impact of inappropriate blood transfusions in coronary artery bypass graft surgery. Am J Med 1993;94(5):509–514.
45. Surgenor DM, Wallace EL, Churchill WH, Hao SH, Chapman RH, Collins JJ Jr. Red cell transfusions in coronary artery bypass surgery (DRGs 106 and 107). Transfusion 1992;32(5):458–464.
46. Stover EP, Siegel LC, Parks R, et al. Variability in transfusion practice for coronary artery bypass surgery persists despite national consensus guidelines: a 24-institution study. Institutions of the Multicenter Study of Perioperative Ischemia Research Group. Anesthesiology 1998;88(2):327–333.
47. Wu WC, Rathore SS, Wang Y, Radford MJ, Krumholz HM. Blood transfusion in elderly patients with acute myocardial infarction. N Engl J Med 2001;345(17):1230–1236.
48. Levkoff SE, Evans DA, Liptzin B, et al. Delirium. The occurrence and persistence of symptoms among elderly hospitalized patients. Arch Intern Med 1992;152(2):334–340.
49. Inouye SK, Bogardus ST Jr, Charpentier PA, et al. A multicomponent intervention to prevent delirium in hospitalized older patients. N Engl J Med 1999;340(9):669–676.
50. Ely EW, Inouye SK, Bernard GR, et al. Delirium in mechanically ventilated patients: validity and reliability of the confusion assessment method for the intensive care unit (CAM-ICU). JAMA 2001;286(21): 2703–2710.
51. McCusker J, Cole M, Abrahamowicz M, Primeau F, Belzile E. Delirium predicts 12-month mortality. Arch Intern Med 2002;162(4):457–463.
52. Inouye SK, van Dyck CH, Alessi CA, Balkin S, Siegal AP, Horwitz RI. Clarifying confusion: the confusion assessment method. A new method for detection of delirium. Ann Intern Med 1990;113(12):941–948.
53. van den Berghe G, Wouters P, Weekers F, et al. Intensive insulin therapy in the surgical intensive care unit. N Engl J Med 2001;345(19):1359–1367.
54. Young L, Ahmad H. Trauma in the elderly: a new epidemic? Aust N Z J Surg 1999;69(8):584–586.
55. Pompei P, Charlson ME, Ales K, MacKenzie CR, Norton M. Relating patient characteristics at the time of admission to outcomes of hospitalization. J Clin Epidemiol 1991;44(10):1063–1069.
56. Narain P, Rubenstein LZ, Wieland GD, et al. Predictors of immediate and 6-month outcomes in hospitalized elderly patients. The importance of functional status. J Am Geriatr Soc 1988;36(9):775–783.
57. Montuclard L, Garrouste-Orgeas M, Timsit JF, Misset B, De Jonghe B, Carlet J. Outcome, functional autonomy, and quality of life of elderly patients with a long-term intensive care unit stay. Crit Care Med 2000;28(10):3389–3395.
58. Chelluri L, Pinsky MR, Donahoe MP, Grenvik A. Long-term outcome of critically ill elderly patients requiring intensive care. JAMA 1993;269(24):3119–3123.
59. Wu AW, Rubin HR, Rosen MJ. Are elderly people less responsive to intensive care? J Am Geriatr Soc 1990;38(6):621–627.

60. Swinburne AJ, Fedullo AJ, Bixby K, Lee DK, Wahl GW. Respiratory failure in the elderly. Analysis of outcome after treatment with mechanical ventilation. Arch Intern Med 1993;153(14):1657–1662.

61. Kollef MH. Do age and gender influence outcome from mechanical ventilation? Heart Lung 1993;22(5): 442–449.

62. Power M, Chelluri L. Critical illness in the elderly: survival, quality of life, and costs. Crit Care Med 1999;27(12):2829–2830.

63. Smith KM, Lamy A, Arthur HM, Gafni A, Kent R. Outcomes and costs of coronary artery bypass grafting: comparison between octogenarians and septuagenarians at a tertiary care centre. Canadian Medical Association Journal 2001;165(6):759–764.

64. Glower DD, Christopher TD, Milano CA, et al. Performance status and outcome after coronary artery bypass grafting in persons aged 80 to 93 years. Am J Cardiol 1992;70(6):567–571.

65. Tsai TP, Chaux A, Matloff JM, et al. Ten-year experience of cardiac surgery in patients aged 80 years and over. Ann Thorac Surg 1994;58(2):445–450; discussion 450–451.

66. Akins CW, Daggett WM, Vlahakes GJ, et al. Cardiac operations in patients 80 years old and older. Ann Thorac Surg 1997;64(3):606–614; discussion 614–615.

67. Hannan EL, Burke J. Effect of age on mortality in coronary artery bypass surgery in New York, 1991–1992. Am Heart J 1994;128(6 Pt 1):1184–1191.

68. Peterson ED, Cowper PA, Jollis JG, et al. Outcomes of coronary artery bypass graft surgery in 24,461 patients aged 80 years or older. Circulation 1995;92(9 Suppl):II85–II91.

69. Cane ME, Chen C, Bailey BM, et al. CABG in octogenarians: early and late events and actuarial survival in comparison with a matched population. Ann Thorac Surg 1995;60(4):1033–1037.

70. Curtis JJ, Walls JT, Boley TM, Schmaltz RA, Demmy TL, Salam N. Coronary revascularization in the elderly: determinants of operative mortality. Ann Thorac Surg 1994;58(4):1069–1072.

71. Ko W, Gold JP, Lazzaro R, et al. Survival analysis of octogenarian patients with coronary artery disease managed by elective coronary artery bypass surgery versus conventional medical treatment. Circulation 1992;86(5 Suppl):II191–II197.

72. Edwards FH, Clark RE, Schwartz M. Coronary artery bypass grafting: the Society of Thoracic Surgeons National Database experience. Ann Thorac Surg 1994;57(1):12–19.

73. Peigh PS, Swartz MT, Vaca KJ, Lohmann DP, Naunheim KS. Effect of advancing age on cost and outcome of coronary artery bypass grafting. Ann Thorac Surg 1994;58(5):1362–1366; discussion 1366–1367.

74. Jandziol AK, Ridley SA. Validation of outcome prediction in elderly patients. Anaesthesia 2000;55(2): 107–112.

19

Incidence and Management of Complications of Surgical Treatment in the Elderly

Eugene Kukuy, MD *and Niloo M. Edwards,* MD

CONTENTS

INTRODUCTION

It is axiomatic that as our population ages, we face increasing numbers of older patients undergoing cardiac surgical procedures. Most studies on postcardiac surgical outcomes in older patients suggest that the frequency of complications is higher than in younger subjects but that the incidence of these complications is steadily decreasing. Additionally, it would appear that the increased incidence of complications may be more related to the increased incidence of comorbidities rather than to age itself and that delayed referral for intervention may increase the probability of adverse outcomes. Mortality and morbidity rates for the elderly undergoing elective cardiac surgical procedures are low and comparable to the risks in younger patients; however, emergent operative intervention carries a significantly higher risk of adverse outcome in the older patient, and the elderly are more likely to undergo emergency cardiac surgery than younger patients.

A study of perioperative determinants of morbidity and mortality found that patients older than age 75 had an overall morbidity of 54%, but when subdivided by urgency of operation, the morbidity for elective operations dropped to 3% and was comparable to 1.5% morbidity for patients younger than 75 *(1)*. Avery compared patients older than 80

From: *Aging, Heart Disease, and Its Management: Facts and Controversies*
Edited by: N. Edwards, M. Maurer, and R. Wellner © Humana Press Inc., Totowa, NJ

Table 1
In-House Mortality for All Patients Undergoing Coronary Artery
Bypass Surgery at Columbia–Presbyterian Medical Center from 1991–1999

Operative priority	Mortality for age ≥75	Mortality for age 18–74
Elective	0.9%	1.3%
Urgent	5.1%	2.7%
Emergent	12.1%	7.5%
Overall	3.7%	2.2%

Table 2
Morbidity Defined by a Series of In-House Complications
Including Cerebrovascular Accident, Pulmonary Embolus,
Wound Infection, and So Forth

Operative priority	Morbidity for age ≥75	Morbidity for age 18–74
Elective	14.3%	11.7%
Urgent	18.2%	16.3%
Emergent	32.9%	26.2%
Overall	17.6%	14.3%

to patients between the ages of 65 and 75. They found that the older cohort had increased hospital mortality (13.5% vs 3.4%, $p = 0.0004$), but when divided by urgency of operation the mortality difference was no longer significant (7.3% vs 2.8%, $p = NS$) (2). An analysis of all coronary artery bypass patients done between 1991 and 1999 at Columbia–Presbyterian, which compared 1072 patients older than 75 to 4022 patients younger than 75, demonstrated that the overall mortality for the older group was 3.7% in comparison to 2.2%. However, when analyzed by operative urgency, the operative mortality for emergency operations in the older cohort was 12.1% compared to 7.5% in the younger cohort, and this fell to 0.9% mortality for older patients compared to 1.3% in the younger patient who underwent elective bypass surgery (see Table 1). The same trend was noted in an analysis of postoperative morbidity for the same patient populations. Although overall morbidity was 17.6% in older subjects versus 14.3% in younger subjects, the morbidity for emergency operations was 32.9%, a figure that fell to 14.3% for elective operations in the elderly group (see Table 2). Similarly, an Emory study comparing outcomes of octogenarians to patients in their sixties and seventies found that although older patients had more preoperative risk factors, including lower ejection fraction and a higher frequency of emergency surgery, the overall mortality for the older patient group was 9.1% but was only 8.2% when bypass surgery was performed electively compared to 24.1% when done emergently (3).

Whereas patient selection may account for most of the differences in outcomes for elective operations, these data also suggest that the reluctance to operate on the elderly may contribute to the increased morbidity and mortality in the older patient because these patients may represent higher-risk emergency operative candidates. The decision not to operate should be made based on comorbidities rather than age alone. In fact, if the patient would be a candidate under emergency circumstances, then surgery should be seriously considered while it is still elective.

The following sections will examine the more common complications encountered following cardiac operations in the elderly.

STROKE

Cerebral complications represent one of the more devastating adverse outcomes following cardiac surgery. Unfortunately the incidence of neurologic complications increases with age *(4,5)*. Age older than 70 is the leading risk factor for fatal strokes, nonfatal strokes, transient ischemic attacks, coma, confusion, and decreased intellectual function after bypass surgery *(6)*. The incidence of perioperative neurologic events increases exponentially with age *(7)*, but, fortunately, many of the cognitive changes are transient and will resolve within 6 mo for over half of the patients *(8)*. A large prospective study involving 4941 patients in the Veterans Administration (VA) system found increasing age to be a predictor of stroke by both univariate and multivariate analysis *(9)*; however, similar large studies have isolated history of stroke, female gender, and ascending aortic arteriosclerosis as risk factors for stroke with no independent association with age. This suggests that the incidence of stroke may be more a function of comorbid risk factors than of age alone. Certainly, increasing age is associated with aortic calcification, with one-third of octogenarians who undergo cardiac surgery having significant aortic disease *(10)*. The impact of aortic disease on stroke is exacerbated by the manipulation and application of an aortic cross-clamp *(11)*. Early off-pump bypass surgery data suggest that this operation may be optimally suited for the older patient population, perhaps because of decreased aortic manipulation, clamping, and cannulation. Additionally, new cannulation technologies that allows isolation of the head vessels from the remainder of the systemic circulation, a single aortic cross-clamp technique, increased cardiopulmonary bypass perfusion pressure, and use of epicardial ultrasound to identify "low-risk" aortic cannulation sites carry the promise of reducing stroke rates in high-risk populations such as the elderly.

Intrinsic carotid disease carries a similarly high risk of perioperative stroke for all patients. In our experience, the probability of carotid disease increases from 6.9% (in patients under 75) to 13.2% in patients over 75. The presence of a carotid bruit has indicated an increased risk of stroke of 2.9% from 0.7% *(12)*; however, it is less clear whether simultaneous or staged operations provide the greater advantage for carotid and cardiac disease.

POSTOPERATIVE ISCHEMIA

Although a low output state postoperatively is more common in the over-80 patient population, when compared to patients aged 65–75 (10.7% vs 3.1%) *(2)*, the need for intra-aortic balloon pump placement is more frequent (3.7%) when compared to patients in their sixties (1.5%) or seventies (2.1%) *(3)*, and numerous clinical studies demonstrate that the older patients are more likely to have multivessel coronary artery disease *(13)*. The incidence of Q-wave myocardial infarction is similar in all age groups *(2)*. The treatment of postoperative ischemia should focus on evaluation of graft patency and the realization that the elderly patient has less reserve in all organ systems. In addition, one must keep in mind that heart replacement options may be limited in this patient population, although there is data to support transplantation with reasonable outcomes in the patient over age 70 (*see* Chapter 16) *(14)*.

GASTROINTESTINAL COMPLICATIONS

Gastrointestinal hemorrhage followed by acute pancreatitis and acute acalculous chole-cystitis are the most common abdominal complications following cardiac surgery *(15)*. Perioperative hypotension, prolonged cardiopulmonary bypass, use of vasoconstrictive agents, arrhythmias, hemorrhage, pre-existing vascular disease, and aortic atherosclerosis increase the likelihood of gastrointestinal complications *(16,17)*. The reported incidence of these complications varies from 0.12% to 2%, and most major centers may expect to see a major abdominal complication at least once a month. Older age plays a role because many of the risk factors for developing these complications occur more frequently in the elderly. Age is a particularly strong predictor of postoperative gastrointestinal bleeding *(16,17)*; we have seen a statistically significant increase in gastrointestinal bleeding in patients over 75 when compared to younger patients (2.3% vs 1.5%, $p < 0.05$).

Postoperative confusional states, lower pain thresholds, and reluctance to subject the older patient to a second procedure often delay diagnosis and intervention. The time from the onset of abdominal symptoms to the start of definitive treatment is about 3 d *(16)*. Unfortunately, invasive monitoring with a pulmonary artery catheter is inadequate to detect or prevent splanchnic ischemia; therefore, a low threshold of suspicion and early involve-ment of a general surgeon is the key to optimizing outcome. Physicians are often reluctant to consider either invasive diagnostic measures or aggressive general surgical interven-tions because of the recent cardiac operation, but the results of such expectant management are universally poor.

Complicated peptic ulcer disease, with either bleeding or perforation, is the most com-mon abdominal complication following cardiac surgery and usually presents at the end of the first postoperative week. Initial treatment should include endoscopy for both diag-nosis and treatment. Continued bleeding or free air should warrant expeditious surgical intervention. The abdominal incision should be placed as low as possible to protect the sternal incision from abdominal contamination.

After cardiac surgery, 25–35% of patients develop asymptomatic hyperamylasemia and 1–2% develop acute pancreatitis. However, the incidence of mild pancreatitis in this patient population may be underreported *(15)*. Routine postoperative lab tests should include a serum amylase level. If this is significantly elevated, enteral feeding should be postponed. The indications to operate do not differ from those in the general population; again, delay in diagnosis can lead to considerable morbidity and mortality.

The incidence of acute cholecystitis is approx 0.2–0.5% and also appears to be increased in the older (>70) postcardiac surgery patient. Symptoms usually develop 5–15 d post-operatively, and the etiology is acalculous in about 35% of patients *(15)*. The causes for acalculous cholecystitis in this population are the same as for other groups, with patients developing progressive gallbladder distention and subsequent impaired bladder wall blood flow with the risk of wall necrosis. The initial test of choice is an abdominal ultrasound, reserving HIDA scanning for those in whom the diagnosis is unclear. Medical manage-ment includes antibiotics and hydration. The definitive surgical treatment is cholecystec-tomy; however, in the unstable patient, who cannot tolerate an operation, percutaneous cholecystostomy is an excellent option. Mortality rates for this complication can range as high as 65–100%.

Bowel ischemia is less common than other gastrointestinal complications (0.02–0.3%) and is also associated with advanced age. Risk factors include the need for emergency sur-gery and perioperative hypotension. It usually presents 1 wk after surgery, with the gradual onset of severe abdominal pain. The diagnosis can be difficult to make because many signs like acidosis, leukocytosis, and melena are not specific. Sigmoidoscopy may play a role if the patient has colonic ischemia and angiography may be helpful for patients with small-bowel ischemia. A mini-laparotomy at the bedside or formal abdominal exploration may be necessary to make the diagnosis. Aggressive surgical management with resection of necrotic bowel is necessary because the prognosis for patients with transmural bowel ischemia is uniformly fatal with medical management.

ARRHYTHMIAS

Atrial fibrillation is the most common postoperative complication following cardiac surgery and increases in frequency with patient age (2). This complication is discussed in more detail in Chapter 11.

PULMONARY COMPLICATIONS

Prolonged intubation resulting from respiratory failure and pneumonia is the most frequent postoperative complications seen in the elderly patient. Reintubation rates are higher in patients over 80 when compared to patients 65–75 yr of age (7.9% vs 1.1%) (2), and the frequency of pneumonia and prolonged intubation (>5 d) are also increased. In our experience respiratory failure was higher in patients over age 75 when compared to younger patients (8.6% vs 6.8%), and it appears to be related to sedation, pulmonary toilet, and less functional reserve. Many elderly are easily sedated by even the mildest analgesics and have decreased respiratory drive and cough. Aggressive pulmonary toilet as well as judicious use of pain medication can greatly reduce the frequency of this complication.

Late-occurring pleural effusions after cardiac surgery are also common, most of which are small, left-sided, asymptomatic, and require no treatment. Bloody effusions tend to occur within the first 2 wk of surgery, whereas serous effusions are more likely to occur more than 4 wk postoperatively. Symptomatic effusions requiring treatment are infrequent (0–4%) (18), and most can be drained by thoracentesis, or tube thoracostomy if the effusion persists. Earlier thoracentesis of pleural effusions may be beneficial in the elderly, who have decreased pulmonary reserve and in whom treatment with diuretics may have deleterious renal and hemodynamic consequences.

RENAL FAILURE

Preoperative renal dysfunction is an important risk factor for increased morbidity—particularly in the elderly. The need for postoperative dialysis may be more frequent in the elderly. Although most studies demonstrate a higher percentage of the elderly requiring postoperative dialysis, these numbers do not reach statistical significance. In general, avoidance of nephrotoxic drugs and minimizing the use of vasocontrictors is recommended. Careful attention to hydration status is important because many of these patients are admitted as outpatients for catheterization followed by surgery. The double insult of contrast dye and cardiopulmonary bypass in the underhydrated elderly will result in acute renal dysfunction. Some have advocated the use of renal dopamine, the use of pulsatile cardiopulmonary bypass, and the maintenance of higher bypass pressures as protective adjuncts. The balance between use of moderate doses of vasopressors to maintain higher systemic pressures and the negative vasoconstrictive must be made on an individual basis.

COST

The elderly cardiac surgery patient does, however, utilize a greater proportion of resources. Rady et al. found that although the older patient constituted 14% of ICU admissions, they accounted for 22% of ICU length of stay, and postoperative morbidity doubled the median length of stay in the ICU *(1)*. Katz and Chase noted that the postoperative length of stay is 2 d longer and hospital charges were 13% more in the elderly *(19)*. Furthermore, Avery's study demonstrated a 3-d increase in length of stay for patients older than age 80 with an associated 26.8% ($4818) higher direct cost.

Shorter hospitalizations and appropriate post-hospital disposition is aided by a more proactive approach to the elderly. A higher percentage of older patients will require discharge to skilled nursing or rehabilitation facilities, which can be aided by identifying and initiating discharge planning early in the patients' hospital course.

CONCLUSION

The morbidity and mortality for elderly patients undergoing cardiac surgery are higher than for younger patient cohorts. However, it appears that this is more related to a higher incidence of comorbidities and urgency of operation than to age alone. There is a three-fold increase in mortality for emergency operations in the elderly, when compared to younger patients. We need to focus more on comorbidities in selecting older patients for surgery rather than on patient age. Unfortunately, current practice often delays surgical involvement based solely on age, until operative intervention is precipitated by an acute decompensation, fulfilling the prediction that older patient have poorer outcomes.

Despite this, acceptable morbidity and mortality in the older patient population has been achieved by optimizing their care. We must recognize that this population has a smaller reserve in all organs and that low flow appears to play a major role in the development of many complications perioperatively. As a result, hemodynamic status must be optimized not only intraoperatively and postoperatively, but also preoperatively. We also need to modify the way in which we practice; options including off-pump bypass surgery, single cross-clamp technique, and higher cardiopulmonary bypass pressures should all be incorporated into planning operative intervention in the elderly. In addition we need to focus on the further research and prospective randomized trials that specifically study older patients so that we can provide evidence-based care for the older patient, not just extrapolate management based on data from younger patients.

REFERENCES

1. Rady MY, Ryan T, Starr N. Perioperative determinants of morbidity and mortality in elderly patients undergoing cardiac surgery. Crit Care Med 1998;26(2):225–235.
2. Avery GJ, Ley SJ, Hill JD, Hershon JJ, Dick SE. Cardiac surgery in the octogenarian: evaluation of risk, cost and outcome. Ann Thorac Surg 2001;71:591–596.
3. Craver JM, Puskas JD, Weintraub WW, Shen Y, Guyton RA, Gott JP, et al. 601 octogenarians undergoing cardiac surgery: outcome and comparison with younger age groups. Ann Thorac Surg 1999;67: 1104–1110.
4. Aziz S, Grover F. Cardiovascular surgery in the elderly. Cardiol Clin 1999;17(1):213–231.
5. Alexander KP, Anstrom KJ, Muhlbaier LH, Grosswald RD, Smith PK, Jones RH, et al. Outcomes of cardiac surgery in patients >80 years: results from the national cardiovascular network. J Am Coll Cardiol 2000;35:731–738.
6. Edwards FH, Clark RE, Schwartz M. Coronary artery bypass grafting: the society of thoracic surgeons national database experience. Ann Thorac Surg 1994;57:12–19.

7. Truman KJ, McCarthy RJ, Najafi H, et al. Differential effects of advances age on neurologic and cardiac risk factors of coronary artery operations. J Thorac Cardiovasc Surg 1992;104:1510–1517.

8. Newman MF, Schell RM, Croughwell N, et al. Pattern and time course of cognitive dysfunction following cardiopulmonary bypass. Anesth Anal 1993;76:S294.

9. Almassi GH, Sommers T, Moritz TE, et al. Stroke in cardiac surgical patients: determinants and outcome. Ann Thorac Surg 1999;68:391–398.

10. Davila-Roman VG, Kouchoukos NT, Schechtman KB, Barilai B. Atherosclerosis of the ascending aorta is a predictor of renal dysfunction after cardiac operations. J Thorac Cardiovasc Surg 1999;117:111–116.

11. Stump DA, Jones TJJ, Rorie KD. Neuropsychological monitoring and outcomes in cardiovascular surgery. J Cardiol Vasc Anesth 1999;13:600–613.

12. Reed GL, Singer DE, Picard EH, et al. Stroke following coronary artery bypass surgery. A case-control estimate of the risk from carotid bruits. N Engl J Med 1988;319:1246–1250.

13. Tsai TP, Chaux A, Matloff JM, et al. Ten year experience of cardiac surgery in patients aged 80 years and over. Ann Thorac Surg 1994;58:445–451.

14. Blanche C, Blanche DA, Kearney B, et al. Heart transplantation in patients seventy years of age and older: a comparative analysis of outcome. J Thorac Cardiovasc Surg 2001;121:532–541.

15. Sakorafas GH, Tsiotos GG. Intra-abdominal complications after cardiac surgery. Eur J Surg 1999;165: 820–827.

16. Ott MJ, Buchman TG, Baumgartner WA. Postoperative abdominal complications int cardiopulmonary bypass patients:a case controlled study. Ann Thorac Surg 1995;59:1210–1213.

17. Ohri SK, Desai JB, Gaer JAR, et al. Intra-abdominal complications after cardiopulmonary bypass. Ann Thorac Surg 1991;52:826–831.

18. Light RW, Rogers JT, Cheng D, et al. Large pleural effusions occurring after coronary artery bypass grafting. Ann Intern Med 1999;130:891–896.

19. Katz NM, Chase GA. Risks of cardiac operations for elderly patients: reduction of the age factor. Ann Thorac Surg 1997;63:1309–1314.

20 Valvular Heart Disease in the Elderly Population

Windsor Ting, MD and Craig R. Smith, MD

INTRODUCTION

Since the first successful valve operations were reported in the 1950s and 1960s *(1–4)*, valvular surgery has gradually increased in frequency and currently comprises close to 15% of all adult cardiac operations *(5,6)*. However, the precise percentage of valve operations compared to other cardiac procedures at each institution varies, as a reflection of different geographic locations and referral patterns. According to the American Heart Association and the Society of Thoracic Surgeons, more than 95,000 heart valve operations were performed in American adults in 1999 *(5,6)*. Commensurate with the quantitative increase in valve procedures are the dramatic advances achieved in cardiac surgery, improvement in the results of valvular surgery, and the overall quality of prosthetic valves during the past 50 yr. Not surprisingly, the mean age of patients undergoing valve surgery has gradually increased during the same period. In 1999, nearly 60% of the 95,000 valve operations were performed among individuals 65 yr and older *(5)*.

From: *Aging, Heart Disease, and Its Management: Facts and Controversies*
Edited by: N. Edwards, M. Maurer, and R. Wellner © Humana Press Inc., Totowa, NJ

The increasing number of older patients undergoing valve surgery also reflects the changing demographic profile of the overall population. At the present time, 12.5% of the US population is over the age of 65 *(7)*. In 1990, almost 7 million Americans were 80 yr and older and is currently the fastest growing age group; their numbers are predicted to double in less than 30 yr *(7–10)*.

There have been many reports of valve surgery in septuagenarians, octogenarians, and even nonagenarians *(11–17)*. While the operative mortality is higher in these patient cohorts, it is still within an acceptable range. After successful valve surgery in elderly patients, the mid-term and long-term outcomes have been salutary; the actuarial survival rates of these patients have achieved levels close to their age-matched population norms. From the ensuing discussion in this chapter, it is clear that advanced age is not a contraindication to valve surgery. However, valve surgery in this cohort of elderly patients has special challenges and considerations, and decision-making regarding management issues can be difficult.

EPIDEMIOLOGY

Cardiovascular disease is the leading cause of death in the United States *(5,7)*. It is a disease that becomes even more prominent in the elderly population and more prevalent with an aging population *(7)*. The Cardiovascular Health Study, a prospective longitudinal study of more than 5000 men and women 65 yr or older, has provided valuable data on cardiovascular disease in the elderly *(18)*. Based on clinical and echocardiographic evaluation, this population-based study reported the overall incidence of aortic valve sclerosis (leaflet thickening or calcification, or both) at 26%, aortic stenosis (AS) at 2%, and prior aortic valve replacement (AVR) at 0.5%. The incidence of these pathological findings was further increased among patients 75 yr or older, suggesting a significant influence of age on the progression of AS. An echocardiographic evaluation of 58 subjects who were 90 and older showed 30% had some evidence of AS, suggesting the prevalence of aortic valvular disease in the elderly *(19)*.

Another population-based study, the Helsinki Aging Study, randomly selected 577 men and women within the age groups 55–71, 75–76, 80–81, and 85–86 yr to undergo echocardiographic evaluation. Aortic insufficiency (AI), mostly mild, and calcific aortic valve, also mostly mild, was documented in 29% and 53% of the subjects respectively. Critical AS (calculated valve area ≤0.8 cm^2) was present in 2%. All cases of AS were in the three older age groups, and 50% of these subjects with critical AS were symptomatic which rendered them potential candidates for valve surgery *(20)*.

These studies suggest aortic valve disease, especially aortic stenosis, is prevalent among the elderly and increases with advancing age. Other valvular diseases including mitral valve disease, multiple valve disease, and prosthetic valve degeneration, have been investigated to lesser extent in the elderly population. They appear to be less common but are nevertheless an important aspect of valve surgery in this group of patients.

ETIOLOGY AND ASSOCIATED CARDIAC PATHOLOGY

The decrease in rheumatic heart disease in conjunction with an increase in the elderly population has altered the profile of valvular heart disease in developed countries *(21)*. While geographic location and referral pattern can also influence the composition of valvular pathology from one institution to another, some general patterns are apparent.

Among all elderly patients requiring aortic valve surgery, AS is the most common. In one report, the underlying pathology was AS in approx 70% of the cases, AI 15% and mixed AS/AI 15% *(22)*.

Degenerative AS, also known as senile idiopathic calcific AS, is characterized by increased leaflet thickness, stiffening, calcification, and the absence of commissural fusion *(18)*. It is the most common cause of AS in elderly patients and has a frequency that increases with the increasing age of patients requiring AVR *(18,20,23,24)*. The similarities of early degenerative AS to atherosclerosis, and the association of degenerative AS to advanced age, male gender, smoking, hyperlipidemia, hypertension, and diabetes suggests the condition is more than a "wear-and-tear" or aging phenomenon *(18,25–27,29)*.

Congenital bicuspid aortic valve with progressive calcification, whereas a more common cause of AS among patients in their 50's and 60's requiring AVR, remains a significant cause of AS among patients in their 70's and 80's *(30)*.

Rheumatic heart disease also contributes to AS in elderly patients, although to a lesser degree than in the past. These older individuals lived during an earlier era when rheumatic fever was common or had come from geographic locations where rheumatic fever was common until recently *(31)*.

With a large number of patients having undergone cardiac surgery during the past several decades, some of these individuals, now in their 70's and older, need valve surgery. In one series of 113 consecutive cardiac reoperations among patients 80 yr and older, 30% were valvular procedures and 25% were combined coronary artery bypass grafting (CABG) and valve operations *(9)*. These valvular reoperations, either as a sole procedure or in combination with CABG, comprise a small but likely an increasing proportion of elderly patients presenting for valve surgery.

Geographic location has a significant influence on the etiology of valve disease in the elderly. Angelini and associates examined 500 valve specimens from patients (mean age 70.4 yr, 0.9 male to 1.0 female ratio, 55% female) undergoing valve surgery at one medical center in Italy from 1991 to 1993 *(32)*. They reported that rheumatic disease was responsible for 50% of the underlying aortic valve pathology and 60% of mitral valve pathology. These percentages are higher than other reports and most likely a result of the geographic location of the institution and its referral base.

The presence of concomitant cardiac disease, either other diseased valve or CAD, is seen in many elderly patients. In Lie's study of 237 autopsy specimens from elderly patients, multiple cardiac disorders were common and the extent of coronary atherosclerosis was similar to findings reported in younger patients who died from CAD *(33)*. In Burr's series of more than 2000 valve operations in the elderly, approx 7% of the cases were multiple valve procedures and 46% needed concurrent CABG *(34)*. In Pupello's report of more than 2000 valve operations in the elderly, 48% underwent concurrent CABG *(35)*. In a smaller report of 46 elderly patients (mean age 78.5 yr) who underwent AVR for AS, 57% needed combined AVR/CABG *(36)*.

Among the elderly with AS, the primary pathology is confined to the valve and left-ventricular function is usually preserved albeit the presence of significant left-ventricular hypertrophy. In contrast, mitral valve disease in elderly patients, either ischemic in nature or as some other anatomical pathology, frequently occurs with concurrent myocardial dysfunction *(37)*. This difference between aortic and mitral valve diseases can have clinical implications in terms of the early postoperative management and surgical outcomes.

SPECIAL FEATURES OF PREOPERATIVE EVALUATION

After the diagnosis of valvular disease has been established, and prior to surgery, patients are evaluated with several questions in mind. At what stage is the patient's disease relative to the natural history of the disease process? Are there any co-morbidities? What are the risks of surgery? What is the probable duration of survival with and without surgery? What will be the quality-of-life after surgery? These issues are no different in an elderly patient who is being evaluated for valve surgery. The chronological age should be recognized as but one of many factors affecting the physiological condition of the patient, and a critical item in estimating the probable longevity of the patient with and without the valve operation *(38)*.

Since advanced age is more likely to be associated with co-morbidities, it underscores the importance of a thorough evaluation. Elderly patients undergoing aortic or mitral valvular surgery frequently undergo CABG concurrently, although the percentage varies from one series to another. In one series reported by Davis et al., 51% of the AVR and 55% of the mitral valve procedures among patients 70 or older had concomitant CABG *(37)*. Information regarding CAD and the severity of CAD is helpful in decision making with regards to a concurrent procedure that may contribute to additional operative mortality and morbidity.

That the more common postoperative complications after cardiac surgery in the elderly are known also helps to direct special attention in several areas. Organ systems that are associated with significant complications include the cerebral circulation, pulmonary function, renal function and cardiac arrhythmia. The presence of any abnormality should be known before surgery, and, optimally managed prior to surgery.

INDICATIONS FOR SURGERY

There is no report in the medical literature that advocates advanced age alone is a contraindication to surgery. However, most would recommend a more cautious approach in reserving surgery for symptomatic patients or for those in whom ventricular dysfunction will soon develop based on the natural history of the disease *(7,38,39)*. This approach is generally applicable for all types of valvular disease.

The benefits of AVR for symptomatic AS are well established *(40,41)*. For example, it is known that once heart failure complicates critical aortic stenosis, the patient is significantly disabled and the mean-life expectancy without surgery is less than 2 yr *(7,42)*. Even though AVR is associated with a higher-operative mortality and morbidity in the elderly, this management strategy appears equally sound for older patients with symptomatic AS *(36,39,43)*. Symptomatic AS should be operated on regardless of age.

A more controversial area is the issue of surgery among the less symptomatic or asymptomatic elderly patients with AS. Most reports, including several prospective studies, presented data that questioned the benefit of early surgery in asymptomatic AS *(44,45)*. However, some reported that asymptomatic AS could progress rapidly and lead to adverse outcomes, suggesting a role for early surgery in these patients *(46,47)*. In a study to select patients with asymptomatic AS who may benefit from early surgery, Rosenhek and associates followed 128 subjects with asymptomatic AS and concluded that delayed surgery until the appearance of symptoms is appropriate for most patients. However, they also found that patients with moderate to severe valvular calcification and a rapid increase in aortic-jet velocity were associated with a very poor prognosis, and these patients would benefit from early surgery, even in the absence of any symptoms *(48)*.

For elderly patients with symptomatic valvular disease and severe comorbidity that precludes surgery, there is a paucity of nonsurgical, palliative procedures that are currently associated with a satisfactory outcome. Mitral stenosis may be the only exception. Sutaria examined 20 octogenarians (mean age 83 yr) with severe, symptomatic mitral stenosis, most of whom were not surgical candidates. These individuals were treated instead with percutaneous mitral balloon valvotomy *(49)*. There was no procedure-related mortality and improvements in objective cardiac parameters were observed in mean mitral valve area (0.8 to 1.8 cm^2), valvular gradient (12 to 6 mm Hg), and cardiac output (3 to 4 l/min). Among the 20 patients, all reported immediate symptomatic improvement, 80% were improved by at least one New York Heart Association functional class, and 35% had sustained symptomatic improvement at one year. These findings were confirmed in another study in which balloon mitral valvotomy was compared between younger and older patients (mean 71 yr). Although procedural success was higher in the younger groups, complications, improvement in functional class, and restenosis rate were similar *(50)*. Findings of these studies suggested that balloon valvotomy might provide acceptable palliation in selected patients who are not surgical candidates.

SPECIAL SITUATIONS AND CONTROVERSIES

Infective Endocarditis

Infective endocarditis has been observed with increasing frequency in the elderly as a result of the aging population and the prevalence of underlying valvular pathology among these individuals *(51)*. At present, 50% of endocarditis cases are in patients aged 60 and older *(51)*. Some reports suggest endocarditis has different clinical features in the elderly when compared to a younger population *(52,53)*.

Terpening and colleagues compared endocarditis in three age groups: 60 yr and older, 40–60, and less than 40 *(53)*. Staphylococcal and streptococcal species were responsible for approx 80% of endocarditis in all age groups, as noted by Centrell as well as others *(51, 52,54)*. Although far less frequent causes of endocarditis, enterococci, Streptococcus bovis, and coagulase-negative staphylococci were more commonly observed in the elderly patients.

These reports also observed more frequent errors and delays in diagnosis because symptoms in elderly patients were less severe or attributed to another condition *(53–55)*. The absence of a murmur did not eliminate the diagnosis of endocarditis *(54)*. While vascular procedures and a nosocomial source were reported as common sources of infection in elderly patients, the presence of underlying valve pathology had been reported in 60% of patients *(54,55)*. A satisfactory evaluation of the heart valves for vegetations might be impeded by the coexistence of valvular abnormalities *(55)*. Finally, overall mortality was close to 45% in the elderly patients, 35% in the 40–60 yr age group and 9% in the less than 40 yr age group *(56)*. According to another report, the overall 1 yr survival in elderly patients with endocarditis was approx 25% *(55)*.

However, in a more recent report, Gagliardi and colleagues disputed these findings. They showed that the clinical presentation, characteristics, and outcomes of endocarditis were similar between the two age groups if prosthetic valve endocarditis and intravenous drug-related endocarditis were excluded *(56)*. While coronary artery disease and malignancy were more common in the elderly, there were no other differences relative to comorbidities, valve involvement, and complications. Gagliardi also confirmed that streptococcal and staphylococcal species were the most common causative organisms in both age groups, and enterococcal species was a distant third but similar in prevalence between age groups. Based on their findings, Gagliardi concluded that age was not a predictor of mortality in either age group. Accordingly, endocarditis in the elderly population should be treated early and aggressively, including surgery if indicated.

Using the same exclusion criteria, Netzer's findings were similar to Gagliardi except in several areas (57). While Gagliardi reported both valves were equally involved regardless of age, Netzer reported that the mitral valve was more frequently involved in the elderly, and the aortic valve in the younger patients. After valve surgery, Netzer noted that older patients were more likely to develop postoperative complications including prosthetic valve dysfunction, tamponade, renal failure, arrhythmias, and the need for a second surgical intervention.

SELECTION OF PROSTHETIC VALVE

There are several general principles concerning valve selection that are applicable regardless of the patient's age. While mechanical and tissue prosthetic valves have improved in quality, the performance of these valves does not match that of a native valve in terms of hemodynamics, thrombo-embolic complications, and durability. Accordingly, diseased valve should be repaired whenever feasible. While the aortic valve is normally not repairable, this is not the case with the mitral valve. In mitral valve surgery, for both mitral regurgitation and mitral stenosis, reconstruction of the mitral valve and/or annuloplasty is frequently feasible and should be given preference.

Jabara and associates examined the efficacy of mitral valve repair in 79 patients aged 70 yr and older. Close to 90% of the patients in the study had either prolapse of the posterior leaflet (56%) or both leaflets (32%). Resection of the posterior leaflet was undertaken in 76%, and ring annuloplasty in 96%. Among the surviving patients (96%), only one patient required reoperation for mitral regurgitation, and excellent short-term and long-term results were reported (58).

If valve replacement is necessary, there are few agreements on valve selection whether the patient is young or old. Generally, a bioprosthetic valve is the valve of choice for an elderly patient, but as in any patient, the decision must be tailored to each patient and should include consideration of such factors as: the presence of any contraindications to anticoagulation therapy, the need for long-term anticoagulation for other reasons, prior valve surgery or other cardiac procedures, and patient preference (59–64). The potential benefits of bioprosthetic valves in the elderly are well established and include the avoidance of anticoagulation that may be associated with more bleeding complications with advancing age, the longer durability of tissue valves in elderly patients, and a reduced incidence of thromboembolism. While bioprosthetic valves are less durable than mechanical valves, this feature is of lesser importance in a group of patients whose life expectancy is unlikely to exceed the life span of a bioprosthesis.

Pupello and colleagues evaluated the failure rates of the Carpentier-Edwards bioprosthetic valve implanted in 500 patients by age. They observed that the valve failure rate was significantly reduced after the age of 70 yr compared to younger patients who received

Table 1
Freedom from Structural Deterioration
in Bioprostheses: Effects of Valve Position and Age

Valve site vs age	10 yr	15 yr
Aortic bioprostheses	98%	77%
65–69 yr	95%	
70–74 yr	99%	
Mitral bioprostheses	79%	56%
65–69 yr	70%	
70–74 yr	90%	

Adapted from Burr LH. Porcine bioprostheses in the elderly: clinical performance by age groups and valve positions. Ann Thorac Surg 1995;60:S264–S269.

the same bioprosthetic valve *(65)*. In a later study including an even larger cohort of elderly patients from the same investigators, they confirmed their earlier observations, and, in addition, estimated the overall structural failure rate at 0.6% per patient year, and a slightly higher failure rate of bioprosthesis in the mitral position *(65)*.

Burr and associates reviewed the results of more than 2000 bioprosthetic valve operations in patients 65 yr and older, examining parameters such as valve position and age of patient. They observed a significant difference in the durability of a bioprosthetic valve in the aortic and mitral positions. In their study, they showed freedom from structural deterioration for tissue AVR was 98% at 10 yr, and 77% at 15 yr. By comparison in tissue MVR, it was 79% at 10 yr, and 56% at 15 yr. When structural deterioration was evaluated in terms of patient age, they found freedom from structural deterioration for tissue AVR was 95% in patients aged 65–69, and 99% in patients 70–74. In contrast, for tissue MVR, it was 70% in patients 65–69, and 90+% for 70 and older *(34)*. Table 1 summarizes these findings. Based on these findings, they recommend a tissue prosthetic valve in the aortic position for patients 65 yr and older, and in the mitral position for patients 70 yr and older.

The Veterans Affairs Cooperative Study on Valvular Disease was one of very few randomized, multi-center study comparing mechanical and tissue prosthetic valve. The study randomized 575 men, either AVR or MVR but not both, to either a mechanical or tissue valve *(66)*. While the patients in this study were younger (mean age 59 yr ± 8 yr), it nevertheless provided valuable information. The study found no differences in mortality from all causes or valve-related complications between tissue and mechanical valves at eleven years. The authors concluded that a bioprosthetic valve should be recommended for patients 60 yr and older.

Kobayashi and associates also confirmed a higher rate of structural deterioration among patients with bioprosthetic valves in comparison to mechanical valves when patients of all age categories were being considered, however, no such difference was observed in patients 70 yr or older *(67)*. Equally important, bioprosthetic valves were associated with a lower rate of major bleeding complications and this benefit was maintained beyond the age of 70 yr. However, there were no differences in thromboembolic complications and infective endocarditis between the two types of valves.

Some surgeons prefer the mechanical valve for older patients. This preference is based on the improving life expectancy of the elderly and the increasing likelihood of an older person to outlive his or her bioprosthetic valve. Valve reoperation in an elderly patient is associated with significant mortality and morbidity. Finally, with lower dosage of warfarin, the risk of bleeding has been reduced (68).

Several studies have supported this line of thinking. One such study by Ninet and colleagues retrospectively compared 93 patients with a mechanical valve with 113 patients with a bioprosthesis, all were 70 and older, who underwent aortic valve replacement between 1982 and 1996. They reported that bleeding complications are equivalent in mechanical and tissue valves (68). Of note, the actuarial overall survival and freedom from valve-related death were not significantly different the two groups.

While most surgeons prefer a stented bioprosthetic valve or a mechanical valve in an elderly patient, some have reported excellent results with the stentless aortic heterograft (69). An excellent outcome with the Ross procedure has also been reported in patients between the age of 60 and 70 yr (70). However, the use of the stentless prosthetic valve or the Ross procedure in an older patient should be tempered by the greater complexity of these operations, the longer aortic cross-clamp times, experience of the surgeon, and whether the benefits of these special valves would be realized in the elderly patients.

RESULTS

The goals of valve surgery generally include replacement or repair of the diseased valve with an acceptable operative mortality and morbidity, life prolongation, and improvement in the quality of life after surgery. According to the STS Cardiac Surgery National Database, the risk-adjusted operative mortality for all patients was 4% for aortic valve replacement and 6% for mitral valve replacement (6). How do elderly patients after valvular surgery fare in terms of these goals?

Operative Mortality and Survival

In Burr's report of 2000 valve replacements with bioprosthesis, the overall operative mortality of all patients was 9.5%. Operative mortality rates according to different age groups were as follows: 7% for age 65–69, 10% for age 70–74, 11% for age 75–79, 15% for age 80–84, and 18% for age 85 yr or older (34). The operative mortality was higher for MVR compared to AVR, 13.5% and 6.5% respectively. Table 2 summarizes the operative mortality reported by Burr and associates.

Logeais and associates reported the outcomes of 200 consecutive patients aged between 80 and 90 yr who underwent AVR, AVR/MVR, or AVR/CABG from 1978 to 1992. The overall operative mortality in this series was 11.5%, and the actuarial survival at 1, 3 and 5 yr for the surviving patients was 82%, 75% and 57%. These survival rates were similar to the life expectancy for individuals of the same age but without AS (11). In Khan's series of 61 patients (mean age 83.5 years, range 80–89) who underwent cardiac valve procedures, the operative mortality was also 11.5%. Actuarial survival at 1 and 5 yr was 85% and 66%, respectively (15). In Bessou's series of 140 patients 80 and over (mean 82.5 yr), the overall operative mortality was 9%. Actuarial survival for these patients at 1, 5, and 8 yr was 86%, 57%, and 54% (14).

In Tseng's series of 247 patients 70 and older (mean age 76 yr) who underwent isolated AVR at Johns Hopkins Medical Center from 1980 to 1995, the operative mortality was

Table 2
Operative Mortality After Valvular Surgery

Operative parameters	Mortality (%)
Overall	9.5
Effect of age	
65–69 yr	7
70–74 yr	10
75–79 yr	11
80–84 yr	15
>85 yr	18
Aortic valve replacement	6.5
Mitral valve replacement	13.5
Single valve replacement	7.5
Concurrent procedure	12

Adapted from Burr LH. Porcine bioprosthesis in the elderly: clinical performance by age groups and valve positions. Ann Thorac Surg 1995;60:S264–S269.

6%. For the survivors in this series, actuarial survival at 1, 5, and 10 yr was 90%, 69%, and 41% *(71)*. In Aranki's series of patients 70 and older (mean age 77 yr) who underwent isolated AVR or combined AVR/CABG between 1980 and 1992, the operative mortality was close to 7% *(13)*. In Bessone's report of 219 patients 70 and older undergoing either isolated AVR or AVR/CABG, the long-term survival at 7 yr was 77% for the isolated AVR and 57% for the AVR/CABG *(72)*.

Overall, the operative mortality rates of elderly patients who underwent valvular surgery were higher than those reported for all patients in the STS Cardiac Surgery National Database, the mortality rates ranging from 6% to 16% and generally increasing with advanced age. The differences in operative mortality among different reports may be explained by different study designs, differences in the mean age of study subjects, different time periods when the study was undertaken, and other unspecified reasons.

Impact of Gender, CABG, and Previous Cardiac Surgery

The addition of concomitant procedures in the elderly increased the operative mortality an additional 5% to 12%, depending on the nature of the concurrent procedure.

In one series of 71 patients (mean age 82 yr), the overall operative mortality was 13%; it was 6% among those patients who underwent AVR alone, and 19% for those patients who underwent AVR/CABG *(17)*.

Coronary artery bypass grafting appears to negatively influence the operative mortality to a greater extent in female compared to male patients. In one series of 717 patients at least 70 yr of age (mean age 77 yr) reported by Aranki, the overall operative mortality was 7%, whereas for AVR alone it was 4%, and for AVR/CABG it was 9% *(13)*. In this report, the operative morality of combined AVR and CABG among women was 10% but the operative mortality of the same operation among men was 7%. Multivariate logistic regression analysis showed CABG was a predictor of operative mortality in women but not in men.

Predictors of Mortality

The higher mortality associated with valvular surgery in the elderly patient is well established by the aforementioned discussion. Identification of the risk factors that are connected with the high mortality is important because the information will assist in better patient selection, improve patient counseling prior to surgery, enable risk stratification, and possibly lead to a better outcome among these patients.

In Tseng's series, poor left-ventricular function, preoperative pacemaker insertion, and postoperative infection were predictors of early mortality *(71)*. In addition, they found chronic obstructive pulmonary disease, urgency of operation, and postoperative renal failure were independent predictors of poor long-term survival.

In Bessou's report, age over 83 and the presence of comorbidities at the time of surgery were the major parameters that influenced long-term survival *(14)*.

In Fremes's series of 469 patients greater than 70 yr old (mean age 74 yr) undergoing valvular procedures with or without CABG, the predictors of operative mortality were urgent operation, mitral or double valve surgery, coronary artery disease especially if CABG was not performed, female gender, and left-ventricular dysfunction *(73)*. While no risk analysis was undertaken, Pupello's report of more than 2000 patients (mean age 74 yr) undergoing valve surgery underscored the higher risk of urgent valvular surgery. In this study, the operative mortality of elective valve surgery was 8.5%, urgent surgery was 15%, and emergent surgery was 34% *(65)*.

In Milano's report of 355 elderly patients (mean age 74 yr), the predictors of operative mortality were duration of cardiopulmonary bypass, urgency of operation, and left ventricular ejection fraction of 45% or less *(22)*.

In Kahn's series, preoperative intensive care unit stay and New York Heart Association function class IV predicted operative mortality whereas perioperative complications affected intermediate and long-term survival *(15)*.

The predictors of mortality in valvular surgery among patients 70 yr and older do not include several risk factors of CABG in a similar cohort of elderly patients. While it is unclear whether the predictors of CABG mortality among elderly patients can be extrapolated to valve surgery, these additional risk factors summarized by Blanche and associates are worthy of mention. They include previous myocardial infarction, triple-coronary artery disease, postoperative stroke, congestive heart failure, preoperative intra-aortic balloon pump, chronic renal disease, peripheral and cerebrovascular disease, and female gender *(9)*.

Postoperative Complications

Two types of complications characterize valvular procedures, those that are valve-related and those that are procedure-related. The timing of these complications is different with procedure-related complications occurring early, whereas valve-related complications mostly taking place months to years after the initial surgery.

Valve-related complications include bleeding from the anticoagulation therapy, thromboembolism, hemolysis, endocarditis, paravalvular leak, and prosthetic dysfunction, some of which may result in the need for another valve procedure. There are reports that suggest bleeding from anticoagulation is increased in the elderly *(74)*, but others do not *(75)*. Aside from bleeding related to anticoagulation, there is no evidence to suggest other prosthetic valve complications occur at a different frequency in the elderly.

In contrast, some procedure-related complications, although seen in all age groups, appear to be more common in the elderly after valvular operations. In Ruygrok's series of patients in their 70's who underwent aortic valve surgery between 1980 to 1989, the post-operative complications were similar to patients in their 60's undergoing the same operation except for a higher stroke rate (4.5% vs 1.5%) *(12)*. In Pupello's study of 2000 patients, approx 50% experienced some post-operative complications. The most common morbidities were low cardiac output (12%), respiratory failure (12%), atrial fibrillation (19%), renal failure (7%), and stroke (3%) *(65)*. In Morell's report of AVR in the elderly (mean age 78.5 yr), the most important complications were pneumonia (9%), stroke (6.5%), and complete heart block requiring a pacemaker (6.5%) *(36)*. Many reports listed low cardiac output, respiratory failure, and stroke as the major causes of postoperative complications *(14)*.

Quality-of-Life

There have been comparatively few reports on the quality-of-life after valvular surgery in the elderly. Because the quality-of-life is dependent in part on disease symptoms, the fact that most studies have reported significant symptom improvement after valve surgery is an important observation. Pupello and associates investigated the quality-of-life among their elderly valve patients and found that they scored significantly better on SF-36 than age-adjusted norms *(65)* while another groups found their elderly patients had scores on SF-36 almost equal to age-matched population norms *(71)*.

Conclusions

Overall, studies have shown a pattern in which the operative mortality begins to increase, by one to two percent after the age of 60. But by age 80 and older, the operative mortality is three to five times higher when compared to patients 60 and younger. The immediate postoperative course of these older patients is notable for more frequent complications of low cardiac output, respiratory failure, and stroke. After valve surgery, symptomatic improvement in the elderly patient is generally excellent, and the actuarial survival rates approximate those of age-matched controls. The quality of life after surgery has not been reported extensively but a few studies suggested that it is equal to or better than age-matched population norms.

ANTICOAGULATION THERAPY

The risk of anticoagulation plays a pivotal role in valve selection, especially in the elderly. The high incidence of postoperative atrial fibrillation after valve surgery in the elderly also makes anticoagulation therapy an essential management issue. This topic is covered in greater detail elsewhere in this book (*see* Chapter 11). The benefit of long-term warfarin therapy is limited by bleeding complications, a risk that may be more pronounced in the elderly population. A higher incidence of adverse reactions, the greater likelihood of associated medical problems, use of multiple medications, and increased vascular fragility are reported to be contributory *(74)*. However, whether bleeding complications from anticoagulation are increased among the elderly patients is an issue that remains controversial and the data conflicting.

Beyth and Landefeld analyzed seven studies comprising more than 14,000 patients showed that warfarin therapy among patients 60 yr and older were twice as likely to have a bleeding complication. In contrast, seven other studies with nearly 3000 patients did not show an increase in bleeding complications (74).

Gurwitz and colleagues also analyzed the bleeding complications of 321 patients on warfarin therapy during an 8 yr period at an outpatient anticoagulation clinic. They reported the overall incidence of minor bleeding was 19% with the greatest risk during the first 3 mo of therapy. Major bleeding complications were observed in 4% of the patients and they occurred mostly during the first 2 yr after initiation of warfarin therapy. However, they found that age is not an independent risk factor for minor or major bleeding complications (75).

FUTURE DEVELOPMENTS

Incremental improvements that have moved valvular surgery forward are expected to continue in the future. However, two recent developments have generated a great deal of excitement and hold the potential of becoming important milestones in cardiac surgery. One is robotically assisted port-access mitral valve surgery and the other is a modified maze procedure using a surgical radiofrequency ablation probe. Both of these developments will also have special efficacy in valvular surgery among elderly patients.

Longer stay in the intensive care unit, prolonged ventilatory support, extended hospitalization, slow convalescence, and other complications characterize the postoperative course of elderly patients who undergo valvular surgery. These are the very same problems that port-access surgery with or without robotic assistance promises to alleviate (76–80).

Recent advances in computer technology, robotic engineering, and instrumentation have made possible the performance of cardiac surgery through small port access incisions. Mohr and associates reported the use of robotically assisted approach in 131 CABG, most of which were mammary artery harvest but there were 15 CABG via a median sternotomy, and 3 total endocscopic CABG on a beating heart (78). In addition, there were 17 endoscopic mitral valve repairs in the series.

Realizing the potential benefits of robotically assisted mitral valve surgery, we at Columbia-Presbyterian Medical Center have recently initiated a clinical trial to evaluate the efficacy of robotically assisted mitral valve repair. In addition, we are utilizing the robot in repairs of atrioseptal defect and CABG. While the robotically assisted mitral valve repair trial is currently in the early stage of implementation, several patients have already undergone this innovative operation at our institution. Results of the clinical trial await completion of the study.

Up to 10% of patients aged 60 yr and older have atrial fibrillation, a percentage that is even higher among elderly patients with valvular disease (81–84,90). Chronic atrial fibrillation will frequently persist after correction of the underlying valve disease and impact on valve selection (82,85). Finally, restoration of a sinus rhythm lowers thromboembolic risk and improves the quality-of-life (85). The maze procedure described by Cox is highly effective in the treatment of atrial fibrillation but the procedure can be complex and time consuming (86–90). More recently, we and others are studying the efficacy of a simplified left-atrial maze procedure performed using a surgical radiofrequency ablation probe (85,86,89,91). According to our experience, which is an ongoing clinical study, this procedure prolongs the aortic cross-clamp time by 10–15 min. Most of these simplified maze procedures have been performed during mitral valve surgery. In Pasic's experience with this same procedure, freedom from atrial fibrillation was 100% intraoperatively, 25% at 1 wk, 60% at 1 mo, and 90% at 6 mo postoperatively (91). If this simplified maze procedure can significantly reduce the incidence of chronic atrial fibrillation as suggested by several studies, it will have an important role in valvular surgery in the elderly patients.

CONCLUSIONS

In this chapter, we have discussed the prominence of valvular disease, especially aortic stenosis, in the elderly population. Many of these patients also have concurrent CAD and required CABG during their valvular surgery. While surgery should be approached judiciously in the presence of other comorbid diseases, the indications for surgery are no different from younger patients. Valvular surgery should never be denied on the basis of chronological age alone. Infective endocarditis is observed with increasing frequency in the older patients. Therapeutic approaches including surgery should be pursued aggressively as in younger patients. Valve selection for an elderly patient remains controversial. Generally a bioprosthesis is selected in order to avoid anticoagulation therapy. However, a strong case could be made for a mechanical valve as well. The operative mortality for valvular surgery is higher in the elderly, ranging from 6% to 12%. A concurrent cardiac procedure, such as CABG, increases the mortality. The most important predictors of mortality in the elderly are left-ventricular dysfunction, urgency of operation, advancing age, and severe comorbidities. Hospitalization is longer in the elderly, with higher complication rates of respiratory failure, stroke, and arrhythmias. For survivors, symptomatic improvement is excellent and long-term survival approximates that of age-matched norms. Robotic assisted port access mitral valve repair and a simplified maze procedure using a surgical radiofrequency ablation probe are two recent developments that hold promises in valvular surgery among elderly patients

REFERENCES

1. Bailey CP, Jamison WL, Nichols HT. Commissurotomy for rheumatic aortic stenosis. Circulation 1951; 9:22–31.
2. Lillehei CW, Gott VL, De Wall RA, et al. The surgical treatment of stenotic or regurgitant lesions of the mitral and aortic valves by direct vision utilizing a pump-oxygenator. J Thorac Cardiovasc Surg 1958;35: 154–191.
3. Harken DE, Soroff HS, Taylor WJ, et al. Partial and complete prostheses in aortic insufficiency. J Thorac Cardiovasc Surg 1960;40:744–762.
4. Starr A, Edwards ML. Mitral replacement: clinical experience with a ball-valve prosthesis. Ann Surg 1961;154:726–740.
5. 2002 Heart and Stroke Statistical Update. www.americanheart.org
6. STS national database: STS U.S. cardiac surgery database 2000 executive summary www.ctsnet.org
7. Thibault GE. Too old for what? N Engl J Med 1993;328:946–950.
8. Barringer F. Prospects for the elderly differ widely by sex. New York Times. November 10, 1922:A1.
9. Blanche C, Khan S, Chaux A, et al. Cardiac reoperations in octogenarians: Analysis of outcomes. Ann Thorac Surg 1999;67:93–98.
10. Specer G. US Bureau of the Census: Projections of the population of the United States by age, sex, and race; 1988 to 2080. Washington, DC:US Government Printing Office, 1989. Current Population Reports; Series P-25; no. 1018.
11. Logeais Y, Roussin R, Langanay T, et al. Aortic valve replacement for aortic stenosis in 200 consecutive octogenarians. J Heart Valve Dis 195;4(Suppl 1):S64–S71.
12. Ruygrok PN, Barratt-Boyes BG, Agnew TM, et al. Aortic valve replacement in the elderly. J Heart Valve Dis 1993;2:550–557.
13. Aranki SF, Rizzo RJ, Couper GS, et al. Aortic valve replacement in the elderly. Effect of gender and coronary artery disease on operative mortality. Circulation 1993;88:II17–II23.

14. Bessou JP, Bouchart F, Angha S, et al. Aortic valve replacement in 140 octogenarians. Operative risk, mid term and long term results. Cardiovasc Surg 1997;5:117.
15. Khan JH, McElhinney DB, Hall TS, Merrick SH. Cardiac valve surgery in octogenarians: improving qual-ity of life and functional status. Arch Surg 1998;133:887–893.
16. Tsai TP, Denton TA, Chaux A, et al. Results of coronary artery bypass grafting and/or aortic or mitral valve operation in patients > or = 90 years of age. Am J Cardiol 1994;74:960–962.
17. Culliford AT, Galloway AC, Colvin SB, et al. Aortic valve replacement for aortic stenosis inpersons aged 80 years and over. Am J Cardiol 1991;67:1256–1260.
18. Stewart BF, Siscovick D, Lind BK, et al. Clinical factors associated with calcific aortic valve disease. J Am Coll Cardiol 1997;29:630–634.
19. Tunick PA, Freedberg RS, Kronzon I. Cardiac findings in the very elderly: analysis of echocardiography in fifty-eight nonagenarians. Gerontology 1990;36:206–211.
20. Lindroos M, Kupari M, Heikkilä J, Tilvis R. Prevalence of aortic valve abnormalities in the elderly: an echographic study of a random population sample. J Am Coll Cardiol 1993;21:1220–1225.
21. Rose AG. Etiology of valvular heart disease. Curr Opinion Cardiol 1996;11:98–113.
22. Milano A, Guglielmi C, De Carlo M, et al. Valve-related complications in elderly patients with biologi-cal and mechanical aortic valves. Ann Thorac Surg 1998;66:S82–S87.
23. Roberts WC, Perloff JD, Constantino T. Severe valvular aortic stenosis in patients over 65 years of age. Am J Cardiol 1971;27:497–506.
24. Sells S, Scully RE. Aging changes in the aortic and mitral valves. Am J Pathol 1965;46:345.
25. Gotoh T, Kuroda T, Yamasawa M, et al. Correlation between lipoprotein(a) and aortic valve sclero-sis assessed by echocardiography (the JMS Cardiac Echo and Cohort Study). Am J Cardiol 1995;76: 928–932.
26. Mohler ER, Sheridan MJ, Nichols R, et al. Development and progression of aortic valve stenosis:athero-sclerosis risk factors-a causal relationship? A clinical morphologic study. Clin Cardiol 1991;14:995–999.
27. Aronow WS, Schwartz KS, Koenigsberg M. Correlation of serum lipids, calcium, and phosphorus, diabetes mellitus and history of systemic hypertension with presence or absence of calcified or thickened aortic cusps or root in elderly patients. Am J Cardiol 1987;59:998–999.
28. Deutscher S, Rockette HE, Krishnaswami V, et al. Diabetes and Hypercholesterolemia among patients with calcific aortic stenosis. J Chronic Ds 1984;37:407–415.
29. Lindroos M, Kupari M, Valvanne J, et al. Factors associated with calcific aortic valve degeneration in the elderly. Eur Heart J 1994;15:865–870.
30. Roberts WC. The congenitally bicuspid aortic valve. A study of 85 autopsy patients. Am J Cardiol 1970; 26:72–83.
31. Waller BF. Rheumatic and non-rheumatic conditions producing valvular heart disease. Cardiovasc Clin 1986;16:3–104.
32. Angelini A, Basso C, Grassi G, et al. Surgical pathology of valve disease in the elderly. Aging 1994;6: 225–237.
33. Lie JT, Hammond PI. Pathology of the senescent heart: anatomic observations on 237 autopsy studies of patients 90 and 105 yeas old. Mayo Clin Proc 1988;63:552–564.
34. Burr LH, Jamieson E, Munro I, et al. Porcine bioprosthesis in the elderly: clinical performance by age groups and valve operations. Ann Thorac Surg 1995;60:S264–S269.
35. Pupello DF, Bessone LN, Lopez E, et al. Long-term results of the bioprosthesis in elderly patients: impact on quality of life. Ann Thorac Surg 2001;71:S244–S248.
36. Morell VO, Daggett WM, Pezzella AT, et al. Aortic stenosis in the elderly: result of aortic valve replace-ment. J Cardiovasc Surg 1996;37:33–35.
37. Davis EA, Gardner TJ, Gillinov AM. Valvular disease in the elderly: influence on surgical results 1993; 55:333–337.
38. Marzo KP, Herling IM. Valvular disease in the elderly. Cardiovasc Clin 1993;23:175–207.
39. Sprigings DC, Forfar JC. How should we manage symptomatic aortic stenosis in the patient who is 80 or older? Br Heart J 1995;74:481–484.
40. Schwarz F, Baumann P, Manthey J, et al. The effect of aortic valve replacement on survival. Circulation 1982;66:1105–1110.
41. Horstkotte D, Loogen F. The natural history of aortic valve stenosis. Eur Heart J 1988;9:(Suppl E):57–64.
42. Smith N, McAnulty JH, Rahimtoola SH. Severe aortic stenosis with impaired left ventricular function and clinical heart failure: results of valve replacement Circulation 1978;58:255–264.

43. Livanainen AM, Lindroos M, Tilvis R, et al. Natural history of aortic valve stenosis of varying severity in the elderly, Am J Cardiol 1996;78:97–101.
44. Pellikka PA, Nishimura RA, Bailey KR, Tajik AJ. The natural history of adults with asymptomatic, hemodynamically significant aortic stenosis. J Am Coll Cardiol 1990;15:1012–1017.
45. Faggiano P, Ghizzoni G, Sorgato A, et al. Rate of progression of valvular aortic stenosis in adults. Am J Cardiol 1992;70:229–233.
46. Otto CM, Burwash IG, Legget ME, et al. Prospecttive study of asymptomatic valvular aortic stenosis: clinical, echocardiographic, and exercise predictors of outcome. Circulation 1997;95:2262–2270.
47. Carabello BA. Timing of valve replacement in aortic stenosis: moving closer to perfection. Circulation 1997:95:2242–2243.
48. Rosenhek R, Binder T, Porenta G, et al. Predictors of outcome in severe, asymptomatic aortic stenosis, N Engl J Med 2000;343:611–617.
49. Sutaria N, Elder AT, Shaw TR. Mitral balloon valvotomy for the treatment of mitral stenosis in octogenarians. J Am Geriat Soc. 2000;48:971–974.
50. Krasuski RA, Warner JJ, Peterson G, et al. Comparison of results of percutaneous balloon mitral commissurotomy in patients aged > or = 65 years with those in patients aged <65 tears. Am J Cardiol 2001; 88:994–1000.
51. Dhawan VK. Infective endocarditis in elderly patients. Clin Infect Dis 2002;34:806–812.
52. Cantrell M, Yoshikawa TT. Infective endocarditis in the aging patient. Gerontology 1984;30:316–326.
53. Terpening MS. Infective endocarditis: clinical features in young and elderly patients. Am J Med 1987;84: 626–634.
54. Thell R, Martin FH, Edwards JE. Bacterial endocarditis in subjects 60 years of age and older. Circulation 1975;51:174–182.
55. Werner GS, Schulz R, Fuchs JB, et al. Infective endocarditis in the elderly in the era of transesophageal echocardiography: clinical features and prognosis compared with younger patients. Am J Med 1996;100: 90–97.
56. Gagliardi JP, Nettles RE, McCarty DE, et al. Native valve infective endocarditis in elderly and younger adult patients: comparison of clinical features and outcomes with use of the Duke criteria and the Duke Endocarditis Database. Clin Infect Dis 1998;26:1165–1168.
57. Netzer ROM, Zollinger E, Seiler C, Cerny A. Native valve infective endocarditis in elderly and younger adult patients: comparison of clinical features and outcomes with use of the Duke Criteria. Clin Infect Dis 1999;28:933–934.
58. Jebara VA, Dervanian P, Acar C, et al. Mitral valve repair using Carpentier techniques in patients more than 70 years old. Early and late results. Circulation 1992;86(Suppl):II53–II59.
59. Akins CW, Carroll DR, Buckley MJ. Late results with Carpentier-Edwards porcine bioprosthesis. Circulation 1990;82(Suppl 4):65–74.
60. Holper K, Wottke M, Lewe T. Bioprosthetic and mechanical valves in the elderly: benefits and risks. Ann Thorac Surg 1995;60:S443–S446.
61. Myken PS, Caidahl K, Larsson P, et al. Mechanical versus biological valve prosthesis: a 10-year comparison regarding function and quality of life. Ann Thorac Surg 1995;60:447–452.
62. Gehlot A, Mullany CJ, Ilstrup D, et al. Aortic valve replacement in patients aged 80 years and older: early and long-term results. J Thorac Cardiovasc Surg 1996;111:1026–1036.
63. Borkon AM, Soule LM, Baugham KL. Aortic valve selection in the elderly patient. Ann Thorac Surg 1988;46:270–277.
64. Jamieson WRE, Burr LH, Munro AI, et al. Cardiac valve replacement in the elderly: clinical performances of biological prostheses. Ann Thorac Surg 1989;48:173–185.
65. Pupello DF, Bessone LN, Hiro SP, et al. The Carpentier-Edwards bioprosthesis: a comparative study analyzing failure rates by age. J Card Surg 1988;3:369–374.
66. Hammermeister KE, Sethi GK, Henderson WG, et al. A comparison of outcomes in men 11 years after heart-valve replacement with a mechanical valve or bioprosthesis. N Engl J Med 1993;328:1289–1296.
67. Kobayashi Y, Eishi K, Nagata S, et al. Choice of replacement valve in the elderly. J Heart Valve Dis 1997;6:404–409.
68. Ninet J, Tronc F, Robin A, et al. Mechanical versus biological isolated aortic valvular replacement after the age of 70: equivalent long-term results. Eur J Cardiothorac Surg 1998;13:84–89.
69. van Nooten GJ, Caes F, Francois K, et al. Toronto stentless aortic valve replacement in elderly patients. S Afri Med J 1996;86:C69–C73.

70. Schmidtke C, Bechtel M, Noetzold A, et al. Up to seven years of experience with the Ross procedure in patients >60 years of age. J Am Coll Cardiol 2000;36:1173–1177.
71. Tseng EE, Lee CA, Cameron DE, et al. Aortic valve replacement in the elderly. Risk factors and long-term results. Ann Surg 1997;225:793–802.
72. Bessone LN, Pupello DF, Hiro SP, et al. surgical management of aortic valve disease in the elderly: a longitudinal analysis. Ann Thorac Surg 1988;46:264–269.
73. Fremes SE, Goldman BS, Ivanov J, et al. Valvular surgery in the elderly. Circulation 1989;80:177–190.
74. Beyth RJ, Landefeld CS. Anticoagulants in older patients: a safety perspective. Drug Aging 1995;6: 45–54.
75. Gurwitz JH, Goldberg RJ, Holden A, et al. Age-related risks of long-term oral anticoagulant therapy. Arch Intern Med 1988;148:1733–1736.
76. Glower DD, Landolfo KP, Clements F, et al. Mitral valve operation via port access versus median sternotomy. Eur J Cardiothorac Surg 1998;14(Suppl 1):S143–S147.
77. Zenati MA. Robotic heart surgery. Cardiol Rev 2001;9:287–294.
78. Mohr FW, Falk V, Diegeler A, et al. Computer-ehanced robotic cardiac surgery: experience in 148 paitents. J Thorac Cardiovasc Surg 2001;121:842–853.
79. Falk V, Diegler A, Walther T, et al. Developments in robotic cardiac surgery. Curr Opin Cardiol 2000; 15:378–387.
80. Kappert U, Schneider J, Cichon R, et al. Closed chest totally endoscopic coronary artery bypass surgery: fantasy or reality? Curr Cardiol Rep 2000;2:558–563.
81. Cox JL, Schuessler RB, Lappas DG, Boineau JP. An 8½-year clinical experience with surgery for atrial fibrillation. Ann Surg 1996;224:267–275.
82. Alfieri O, Benussi S. Mitral valve surgery with concomitant treatment of atrial fibrillation. Cardio Rev 2000;8:317–321.
83. Takami Y, Yasuura K, Takagi Y, et al. Partial maze procedure is effective treatment for chronic atrial fibrillation associated with valve disease. J Card Surg 1999;14:103–108.
84. Kosaki Y, Kawaguchi AT, Isobe F, et al. Modified maze procedure for patients with atrial fibrillation undergoing simultaneous open heart surgery. Circulation 1995;92:II359–II364.
85. Sie HT, Beukema WP, Misier AR, et al. Radiofrequency modified maze in patients with atrial fibrillation undergoing concomitant cardiac surgery. J Thorac Cardiovasc Surg 2001;122:212–215.
86. Chen MC, Guo BF, Chang JP, et al. Radiofrequency and cryoablation of atrial fibrillation in patients undergoing valvular operations. Ann Thorac Surg 1998;65:1666–1672.
87. Cox JL, Boineau JP, Schuessler RB, et al. Modification of the maze procedure for atrial flutter and atrial fibrillation: I. Rationale and surgical results. J Thorac Cardiovasc Surg 1995;110:473–484.
88. Cox JL, Jaquiss RDB, Schuessler RB, et al. Modification of the maze procedure for atrial flutter and atrial fibrillation: II Surgical techniques of the maze II procedure. J Thorac Cardiovasc Surg 1995;110: 485–495.
89. Sandoval N, Velasco VM, Orjuela H, et al. Concomitant mitral valve or atrial septal defect surgery and the modified Cox-mze procedure. Am J Cardiol 1996;77:591–596.
90. Kawaguchi AT, Kosakai Y, Sasako Y, et al. Risks and benefits of concomitant maze procedure for atrial fibrillation associated with organic heart disease. J Am Coll Cardiol 1996;28:985–990.
91. Pasic M, Bergs P, Muller P, et al. Intraoperative radiofrequency maze ablation for atrial fibrillation: the Berlin modification. Ann Thorac Surg 2001;72:1484–1490.

INDEX